Progress in Epileptic Disorders
Volume 10
International Epilepsy Colloquium –
Cleveland

**Extratemporal Lobe
Epilepsy Surgery**

Progress in Epileptic Disorders
Volume 10
International Epilepsy Colloquium –
Cleveland

Extratemporal Lobe
Epilepsy Surgery

Mohamad Z. Koubeissi
Robert J. Maciunas

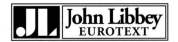

ISBN: 978-2-7420-0772-1
ISSN: 1777-4284
Vol. 10

Dedication:
To the memory of my father,
Zakaria Koubeissi (1930-2010).
MZK

Published by
Éditions John Libbey Eurotext
127, avenue de la République, 92120 Montrouge, France
Tel.: +33 (0)1 46 73 06 60
Website: www.jle.com

John Libbey Eurotext
42-46 High Street, Esther, Surrey, KT10 9KY
United Kingdom

Contents

Section V:
Surgery and outcome of extratemporal lobe epilepsies

Foreword

Epilepsy is a common neurologic disease, and medications achieve adequate seizure control in only 60% to 70% of cases. Medically-intractable epilepsy results in enormous economic burdens and increased mortality. A number of studies have shown that resective surgery in patients with pharmacoresistant epilepsy is significantly superior to medical management in terms of increasing survival and quality of life. However, epilepsy surgery continues to be underutilized. This book aims to familiarize physicians with recent advances in the diagnostic work up, surgical procedures, and outcome of extratemporal lobe epilepsy surgery.

Patients with medically refractory extratemporal lobe epilepsy, especially those with normal brain imaging studies, make up a disproportionate number of suboptimal outcomes after epilepsy surgery compared with patients with temporal lobe epilepsy. Seizure semiology, functional neuroimaging techniques, neuropsychological assessment, and intracranial electroencephalography are among the methods used for identification of surgical candidates. In addition, a number of centers have been investigating novel methods, such as assessing the significance of intracranially-recorded high-frequency oscillations, to help identify the epileptogenic zone in such patients. Moreover, precise localization of eloquent cortex is essential in the neurosurgical treatment of medically intractable extratemporal lobe epilepsy and brain tumors. While electrocortical stimulation mapping continues to be the gold standard for cortical mapping, a number of less invasive investigational method have been used, including spectral analysis of the electrocorticogram and functional magnetic resonance imaging. Such recent techniques have furthered our ability to identify epileptic and normal cortical tissue, without reducing the importance of the seizure semiology and EEG in the surgical evaluation.

Extratemporal lobe epilepsy surgery was the topic of the International Epilepsy Colloquium held in Cleveland in May 2010. This book is divided into five major sections, similar to the design of the Colloquium, and features contributions from many of the leaders in the field, including epileptologists, neurophysiologists, neurosurgeons, and neuropsychologists, as well as experts in neuroradiology and electrical engineering. A section is devoted to the semiology of extratemporal seizures and another to non-invasive neurophysiological evaluation of extratemporal lobe epilepsy. These are followed by sections on neuroimaging, invasive evaluation, and outcome of extratemporal lobe epilepsy surgery. Standard clinical methods, such as neuropsychology and depth electrode evaluation, are intermixed with rather investigational methods, such as thermocoagulation, deep brain stimulation, and electrical source imaging. We hope that this book will increase the familiarity of physicians with extratemporal lobe epilepsy surgery and contribute to increasing the utility of surgery in medically-refractory patients.

Editors

List of Authors

Bassel Abou-Khalil, Vanderbilt University Medical Center, Department of Neurology, Nashville, USA

Sebastian Bauer, Interdisciplinary Epilepsy Center, Department of Neurology, UKGM Marburg & Philipps-University of Marburg, Marburg, Germany

Mustapha Benmekhbi, University Hospitals, Strasbourg, France

Gregory K. Bergey, Johns Hopkins Epilepsy Center, Department of Neurology, Johns Hopkins University School of Medicine, Baltimore, USA

Warren T. Blume, London Health Sciences Centre, University Campus, Epilepsy Unit; University of Western Ontario, London, Canada

Alain Bouthillier, Neurosurgery Service, Notre-Dame Hospital, University of Montreal, Quebec, Canada

Richard C. Burgess, Cleveland Clinic Epilepsy Center, Cleveland, USA

Mar Carreño, Epilepsy Unit, Hospital Clínic, Barcelona, Spain

Francesco Cardinale, "C. Munari" Epilepsy Surgery Centre, Ospedale Niguarda Ca' Granda, Milano, Italy

Laura Castana, "C. Munari" Epilepsy Surgery Centre, Ospedale Niguarda Ca' Granda, Milano, Italy

Hélène Catenoix, Department of Functional Neurology and Epileptology, Pierre-Wertheimer Hospital, Hospices Civils de Lyon, Bron, France; University of Lyon, Lyon, France; Institut Fédératif des Neurosciences de Lyon, Lyon, France; Inserm, U879, Bron, France

Mackenzie C. Cervenka, Department of Neurology, The Johns Hopkins University School of Medicine, Baltimore, USA

Dominique Chaussemy, University Hospitals, Strasbourg, France

Massimo Cossu, "C. Munari" Epilepsy Surgery Centre, Ospedale Niguarda Ca' Granda, Milano, Italy

Nathan E. Crone, Department of Neurology, The Johns Hopkins University School of Medicine, Baltimore, USA

Beate Diehl, Institute of Neurology, University College London and National Hospital for Neurology and Neurosurgery, Queen Square, London, United Kingdom

John S. Duncan, Department of Clinical and Experimental Epilepsy, Institute of Neurology, University College London, National Hospital for Neurology and Neurosurgery and National Society for Epilepsy, UCLH NHS Foundation Trust, Queen Square, London, United Kingdom

Suela Dylgjeri, University Hospitals, Strasbourg, France

Philip S. Fastenau, Department of Neurology, Case Western Reserve University School of Medicine, University Hospitals Case Medical Center, Cleveland, USA

Stefano Francione, "C. Munari" Epilepsy Surgery Centre, Ospedale Niguarda Ca' Granda, Milano, Italy

Eliana Garzon, Electroencephalography Section, Division of Neurology, University Hospital, São Paulo School of Medicine, University of São Paulo, Brazil

Karolien Goffin, Division of Nuclear Medicine, University Hospital Leuven, Leuven, Belgium

Jean Gotman, Montreal Neurological Institute, Montreal, Quebec, Canada

Francesca Gozzo, "C. Munari" Epilepsy Surgery Centre, Ospedale Niguarda Ca' Granda, Milano, Italy

Marc Guénot, Department of Functional Neurosurgery, Pierre-Wertheimer Hospital, Hospices Civils de Lyon, Bron, France; University of Lyon, Lyon, France; Institut Fédératif des Neurosciences de Lyon, Lyon, France; Inserm, U879, Bron, France

Walter J. Hader, Calgary Epilepsy Programme, Department of Clinical Neurosciences, University of Calgary, Alberta, Canada

Hajo M. Hamer, Interdisciplinary Epilepsy Center, Department of Neurology, Philipps-University of Marburg, Marburg, Germany

Giannina M. Holloway, London Health Sciences Centre, University Campus, Epilepsy Unit; Professor, University of Western Ontario, London, ON, Canada

Jean Isnard, Department of Functional Neurology and Epileptology, Pierre-Wertheimer Hospital, Hospices Civils de Lyon, Bron, France; University of Lyon, Lyon, France ; Institut Fédératif des Neurosciences de Lyon, Lyon, France; Inserm, U879, Bron, France

Julia Jacobs, Department of Neuropediatrics, University of Freiburg, Germany

George I. Jallo, Division of Pediatric Neurosurgery, Johns Hopkins University School of Medicine, Baltimore, Maryland, USA

Christophe C. Jouny, Johns Hopkins Epilepsy Center, Department of Neurology, Johns Hopkins University School of Medicine, Baltimore, USA

Pierre Kehrli, University Hospitals, Strasbourg, France

Mohamad Z. Koubeissi, Department of Neurology, University Hospitals Case Medical Center, Case Western Reserve University, Cleveland, USA

Isabella Krotofil, Epilepsy Center, Department of Neurology, University of Munich, Munich, Germany

Samden D. Lhatoo, Epilepsy Center, University Hospitals – Case Medical Center, Cleveland, USA

Tobias Loddenkemper, Division of Epilepsy and Clinical Neurophysiology, Department of Neurology, Harvard Medical School, Children's Hospital Boston, USA

Giorgio Lo Russo, "C. Munari" Epilepsy Surgery Centre, Ospedale Niguarda Ca' Granda, Milano, Italy

Hans O. Lüders, The Neurological Institute, Department of Neurology, University Hospitals Case Medical Center, Cleveland, USA

Robert J. Maciunas, The Neurological Institute, University Hospitals Case Medical Center Western Reserve University Cleveland, USA

Joseph Madsen, Department of Pediatric Neurosurgery, Harvard Medical School, Children's Hospital Boston, USA

Roberto Mai, "C. Munari" Epilepsy Surgery Centre, Ospedale Niguarda Ca' Granda, Milano, Italy

Ramez Malak, Calgary Epilepsy Programme, Department of Clinical Neurosciences, University of Calgary, Alberta, Canada

François Mauguière, Department of Functional Neurology and Epileptology, Pierre-Werthei-mer Hospital, Hospices Civils de Lyon, Bron, France; University of Lyon, Lyon, France; Institut Fédératif des Neurosciences de Lyon, Lyon, France; Inserm, U879, Bron, France

Dang Khoa Nguyen, Neurology Service, Notre-Dame Hospital, University of Montreal, Quebec, Canada

Soheyl Noachtar, Epilepsy Center, Department of Neurology, University of Munich, Munich, Germany

Lino Nobili, "C. Munari" Epilepsy Surgery Centre, Ospedale Niguarda Ca' Granda, Milano, Italy

Andre Palmini, Neurology Service & Epilepsy Surgery Program, Hospital São Lucas Faculty of Medicine and the Brain Institute (InsCer), Pontificia Universidade Católica do Rio Grande do Sul (PUCRS), Porto Alegre, Brazil

Pablo F. Recinos, Division of Pediatric Neurosurgery, Johns Hopkins University School of Medicine, Baltimore, USA

Violette Renard Recinos, Division of Pediatric Neurosurgery, Johns Hopkins University School of Medicine, Baltimore, USA

Felix Rosenow, Epilepsy Center Hessen, Department of Neurology, UKGM Marburg & Philipps-University of Marburg, Marburg, Germany

Fergus J. Rugg-Gunn, Department of Clinical and Experimental Epilepsy, Institute of Neurology, University College London, National Hospital for Neurology and Neurosurgery and National Society for Epilepsy, UCLH NHS Foundation Trust, Queen Square, London, United Kingdom

Dragos Sabau, Departments of Neurology, Comprehensive Epilepsy Program, University Hospital, Indianapolis, USA

Americo C. Sakamoto, Epilepsy Surgery Center, Department of Neurosciences and Behavioral Sciences, Ribeirão Preto School of Medicine, University of São Paulo, Brazil

Vicenta Salanova, Departments of Neurology, Comprehensive Epilepsy Program, University Hospital, Indianapolis, USA

David R. Sandeman, Department of Neurosurgery, Frenchay Hospital, Bristol, United Kingdom

Maysa Sarhan, University Hospitals, Strasbourg, France

Ivana Sartori, "C. Munari" Epilepsy Surgery Centre, Ospedale Niguarda Ca' Granda, Milano, Italy

Marco Schiariti, "C. Munari" Epilepsy Surgery Centre, Ospedale Niguarda Ca' Granda, Milano, Italy

Elisabeth M.S. Sherman, Calgary Epilepsy Programme, Department of Clinical Neurosciences, University of Calgary, Alberta, Canada

Marc Sindou, Department of Functional Neurosurgery, Pierre-Wertheimer Hospital, Hospices Civils de Lyon, Bron, France; University of Lyon, Lyon, France; Institut Fédératif des Neurosciences de Lyon, Lyon, France

Caspar Stephani, Department of Clinical Neurophysiology, University of Göttingen, Göttingen, Germany

Werner Surbeck, Neurosurgery Service, Notre-Dame Hospital, University of Montreal, Quebec, Canada

Laura Tassi, "C. Munari" Epilepsy Surgery Centre, Ospedale Niguarda Ca' Granda, Milano, Italy

John P. Turnbull, University Hospitals of Cleveland, Case Medical Center, Institute of Neurology, Epilepsy Center, Cleveland, USA

Jamie Van Gompel, Department of Neurosurgery, Mayo Clinic, Rochester, USA

Wim Van Paesschen, Department of Neurology, University Hospital Leuven, Leuven, Belgium

Tonicarlo R. Velasco, Epilepsy Surgery Center, Department of Neurosciences and Behavioral Sciences, Ribeirão Preto School of Medicine, University of São Paulo, Brazil

Christian Vollmar, National Hospital for Neurology and Neurosurgery, Queen Square, London, United Kingdom; Department of Neurology, Epilepsy Center, University of Munich, Munich, Germany

James W. Wheless, Le Bonheur Comprehensive Epilepsy Program, Le Bonheur Children's Hospital and The University of Tennessee Health Science Center, Memphis, USA

Thomas Witt, Department of Neurosurgery, Comprehensive Epilepsy Program, University Hospital, Indianapolis, USA

Greg A. Worrell, Department of Neurology, Mayo Clinic, Rochester, USA

Robert Worth, Department of Neurosurgery, Comprehensive Epilepsy Program, University Hospital, Indianapolis, USA

Marcin Zarowski, Division of Epilepsy and Clinical Neurophysiology, Department of Neurology, Harvard Medical School, Children's Hospital Boston, USA; Polysomnography and Sleep Research Unit, Department of Developmental Neurology, Poznan University of Medical Sciences, Poznan, Poland

Section I:
Semiology of extratemporal lobe epilepsy

Overview

Jamie VanGompel[1], Greg A. Worrell[2]

Departments of [1]Neurosurgery and [2]Neurology, Mayo Clinic, Rochester, MN, USA

■ Introduction

The World Health Organization estimates that epilepsy is the cause of 1% of the global burden of disease based on productive years lost to disability or premature death (Murray 1994; Engel Jr, 2008). Partial, or localization related epilepsy, is the most common seizure disorder, and approximately 30% of patients will experience physically and socially disabling seizures despite anti-epileptic drugs (AEDs) (Kwan & Brodie, 2000; Kwan *et al.*, 2010). The majority of studies show that patients who fail to respond to initial first-line AED trial, have a low probability of being seizure-free with additional drug trials (Kwan & Brodie, 2000). A widely quoted study showed that 47% of patients respond to the first AED, 13% respond to the second AED, and only 3% respond to a third drug or multiple drugs (Kwan & Brodie, 2000). Generally, after failing 2 AED due lack of efficacy individuals are considered to have drug-resistant epilepsy (DRE) (Kwan *et al.*, 2010).

Partial epilepsy is classified according to the lobar region generating a patients habitual seizures, *e.g.* temporal lobe epilepsy (TLE), frontal lobe epilepsy, parietal lobe epilepsy, and occipital lobe epilepsy. Epilepsy surgery can be considered in each of these epilepsy types, but the efficacy and relative risk of functionally significant morbidity varies. Anterior temporal lobectomy is the most common and successful epilepsy surgery, and represents a major success in treatment of partial epilepsy (Engel Jr, 2008). The current chapter is directed at extratemporal lobe epilepsy (ETLE), but it is instructive to consider why temporal lobe epilepsy surgery is so often successful. Drug-resistant TLE most commonly arises from the highly epileptogenic anterior medial temporal lobe (amygdala, hippocampus, parahippocampus, and anterior temporal neocortex). This network is anatomically well defined, and the surgical approach is not so much a precise surgical strike but rather complete destruction. Outside the anterior-medial temporal lobe locating the entire epileptic network generating seizures is often difficult unless there is an MRI lesion.

■ Extratemporal lobe epilepsy

Neocortical epilepsy is commonly used to distinguish medial temporal lobe epilepsy (amygdala, hippocampus, entorhinal cortex, parahippocampus) from lateral (neocortical) temporal lobe epilepsy and ETLE (Luders and Comair, 2001). Partial epilepsy outside the temporal lobe is neocortical, and includes frontal lobe epilepsy, parietal lobe epilepsy, and occipital lobe epilepsy. In addition, seizures from insular cortex (a region of cerebral cortex folded deep within the lateral sulcus between the temporal and frontal lobes) can be differentiated from mesial temporal (Penfield & Faulk, 1955). In the following we provide a brief overview of anatomy and function of extratemporal lobes, followed by discussion of parital epilepsy in that region. There are some broad guidelines, that can help localize seizures to a particular lobar region. These must be applied cautiously, however, because seizures can begin in clinically silent areas of brain without signs or symptoms. Similarly, focal seizures are not always associated with clear scalp EEG correlates at onset given that a sizable region, ~7 cm^2 for interictal spikes (Tao et al., 2005), of cortex must be synchronously involved to generate a detectable scalp correlate. Given that neocortical seizures can begin in clinically silent areas without definitive scalp EEG correlates, and may rapidly propagate, localizing ETLE seizure onset is a challenge. The difficulty is most evident in the absence of an MRI lesion, when distinguishing between ETLE and temporal lobe seizures based on scalp EEG and semiology can be a real challenge. In these cases seizure onset localization has to be done with cautiously, and rely on concordance of clinical, EEG, structural and functional imaging clues. These steps may lead, but certainly not always (Bien et al., 2009), to a hypothesis for the lobar localization of seizure onset and phase II invasive monitoring with intracranial EEG.

■ Frontal lobe epilepsy

A detailed, and widely referenced, volume describing the electro-clinico-anatomical features of frontal lobe epilepsy is available has been published (Chauvel et al., 1992). The frontal lobe is separated from the parietal lobe by the central sulcus that separates primary motor cortex from parietal lobe sensory cortex, and inferiorly it is separated from the temporal lobe by the slyvian fissure (Figure 1). The frontal lobes make up approximately 30% of the neocortex. The frontal lobes are not a single functional entity, and are divided in to motor, pre-motor, and prefrontal regions (Miller & Cummings, 2007). While motor and pre-motor areas can be considered independent functional units, the pre-motor cortex is more complex and is further divided in sub regions (Miller & Cummings, 2007). Using functional arguments, the prefrontal cortex can be subdivided into orbital, dorsolateral, and cingulate cortex (Miller & Cummings, 2007).

Frontal lobe epilepsy is a common disorder, and represents a significant medical challenge. Traumatic brain injury is a common cause of FLE, in particular convexity and orbital frontal lobe injury. FLE seizures have wide range of etiologies including genetic, traumatic, and cryptogenic. Similar to all partial epilepsy infectious and inflamatory etiologies are also seen. Because of the proximity to the sinuses, direct infectious injury is not uncommon.

Frontal lobe seizure semiology includes simple partial, complex partial, and secondarily generalized (Chauvel et al., 1992). Because of the connection between lateral orbital frontal lobe to anterior temporal lobe the semiology of frontal lobe seizures can mimic temporal lobe epilepsy. Features suggestive of frontal lobe seizures include, i) brief seizures,

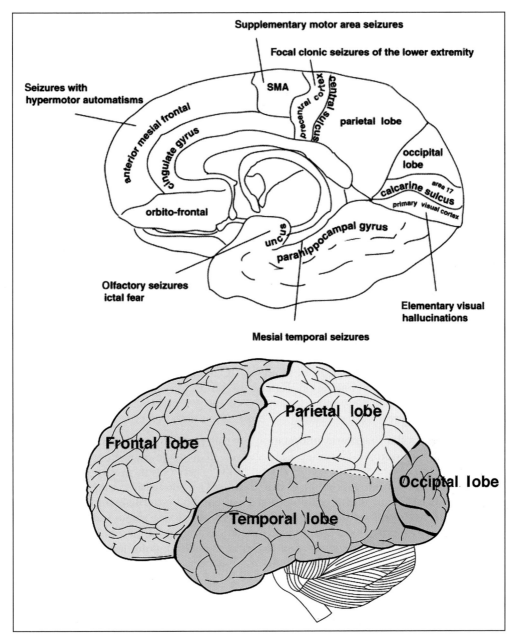

Figure 1. Anatomy of the human brain. Top: mesial view of the brain. Bottom: lateral view of brain and lobar structures.

ii) complex partial with minimal post-ictal confusion, iii) rapid 2nd generalization. In absence of an MRI lesion, distinguishing between orbital frontal and temporal lobe seizures based on EEG and semiology is ill advised.

Supplementary motor: The onset of seizure is often associated with posturing of the upper extremity, and may be contralateral or bilateral. The fencing posture, bicycling automatism are commonly seen. Also there may be vocalization or speech arrest.

Cingulate: autonomic signs and symptoms, fear, vocalization.

Frontopolar: forced thoughts, adversive eye movements.

Orbital frontal: olfactory hallucinations, oral automatisms, autonomic signs. Difficult to clearly distinguish from medial TLE.

Dorsal lateral frontal convexity: seizures begining over the dorsal lateral convexity include a large area of potentially clinical silent cortex. Clinically the seizures often are associated with versive head and eye movements and speech arrest.

Opercular: often associated with mastication, salivation, swallowing, laryngeal constriction, speech arrest.

Precentral gyrus (motor cortex): simple partial seizures in motor cortex produce rhythmic focal twitching of topographical defined muscle groups. The focal marching of clonic activity as a seizure spreads over motor cortex, *i.e.* Jacksonian march, is one of the signature semiologies in epilepsy.

Case of frontal lobe epilepsy: a 32 year old female presented with history of recurrent febrile seizures at age 1. From age 3 to 25 she was seizure free without AED. Otherwise her perinatal, birth, and developmental history were normal. At age 25 she experienced the onset of recurrent stereotypical seizures characterized by an epigastric rising sensation, deja vu, fear, and followed by loss of awareness. Clinically she exhibited bilateral upper extremity automatisms, and agitation. Rarely, the seizures 2nd generalized. They clustered around her menses, and were more frequent with sleep deprivation, and missed medications. The seizures were both nocturnal and diurnal, but most common during wakefulness.

Figure 2 provides the diagnostic information for this pateints case. Her 1.5 tesla seizure protocol MRI was normal. Her scalp EEG showed frequent midline frontal epileptiform discharges (*Figure 2A*). An interictal and ictal SPECT were obtained, and the subtraction ictal-interical SPECT co-registered to MRI (SISCOM) is shown in (*Figure 2B*). Based on the interictal EEG and seizure semiology the patient had extensive implantation with subdural electrodes and medial temporal lobe depth electrodes (*Figures 2C and D*). The patients habitual seizures were capture with chronic intracranial EEG monitoring (*Figure 2E*) and demonstrated to originate from the right medial temporal lobe. She underwent a focal mesial frontal neocortical resection, and has been seizure free for the past 5 years (she remains on AEDs).

▪ Parietal lobe epilepsy

In series of ETLE parietal lobe epilepsy is relatively infrequent, and typically of order of 5% (Engel et al., 2007). The parietal lobe is anatomically defined (*Figure 1*) by the central sulcus (separating parietal and frontal lobes), the parieto-occipital sulcus (separating parietal and occipital lobes), sylvian fissure (separating parietal from temporal lobe), and the inter-hemispheric fissure (separating the two cerebral hemispheres). The parietal lobe contains primary somatosensory cortex within the postcentral gyrus (Broadman area 3). The posterior parietal area (posterior to the postcentral gyrus) is subdivided into superior (Broadman areas 5 and 7) and inferior parietal (Broadman areas 39 and 40) lobules.

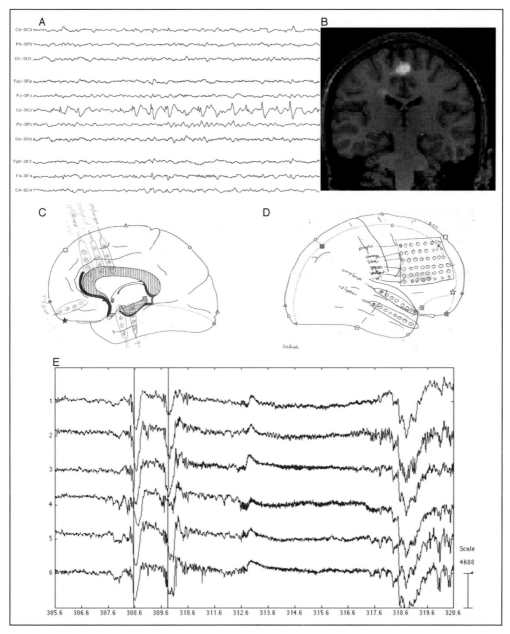

Figure 2. Clinical data from evaluation of case. **A.** Scalp EEG showing midline frontal epileptiform sharp waves. **B.** SISCOM study showing mesial frontal ictal hyper-perfusion. **C-D.** Schematic of implantation of intracranial electrodes. **E.** Seizure recorded from mesial frontal electrodes (bipolar montage).

The posterior parietal areas integrate sensory information and are involved in guidance of limb, eye movement, and visuospatial processing. The two hemispheres have functional different roles, with the dominant hemisphere involved in language and math. The non-dominant hemisphere is involved in visual spatial relationships.

Seizures originating from the parietal lobe can be partial, progress to complex partial or secondarily generalized tonic-clonic seizures (Williamson *et al.*, 1992). The interesting phenomena of reflex epilepsy can occur, whereby a particular movement or other somatosensory stimulus can provoke a seizure (So & Schaüble, 2004).

Post-central gyrus (primary sensory cortex): simple partial seizures most commonly produce positive sensations of tingling and electrical like sensation. Less common is sensation of numbness or pain. Similar to primary motor cortex, patients may describe a "Jacksonian march", were the sensation marches according to the sensorimotor homonculus face (Penfield and Jasper, 1954).

Posterior parietal cortex: somatic illusions associated with distortion of position of arms and legs or posture occur. Patients may experience vertigo, visual illusions or complex hallucinations. Commonly visual illusions with images spatially distorted (metamorphopsia) or persist (palinopsia). Linguistic disturbances (alexia with agraphia) and miscalculations are seen in dominant parietal lobe, and spatial disorientation is associated with non-dominant parietal lobe. Rarely ictal or post-ictal Gertsmann's syndrome occur (writing disability (agraphia or dysgraphia), arithmetic difficulties (acalculia or dyscalculia), left-right confusion, and finger agnosia.

■ Occipital lobe epilepsy

The occipital lobe is located at the back of cerebral hemispheres, behind the parietal and temporal lobes, and is the anatomical region of primary and associated visual cortex. The primary visual cortex, called striate cortex or V1 (Broadman area 17), is in the medial occipital lobe along the calcarine sulcus. The extrastriate regions functionally connected to striate cortex perform a range of downstream visual processing including, color discrimination, motion perception, and visuospatial processing.

The occipital lobes account for a relatively small fraction of partial epilepsy, estimated to be ~ 5-10% of epilepsy cases. Occipital epilepsy can be symptomatic, and associated with an underlying structural abnormality. Because of the location at the posterior head, the occipital lobes are susceptible to traumatic injury. Other common etiologies include vascular injuries and neoplasm. Idiopathic (presumed genetic) occipital lobe epilepsy are not uncommon, and begin in childhood and are often benign. In the authors experience, partial seizures arising directly from visual cortex often spread slowly and are more likely to remain partial without generalization. They may, however, progress to complex partial seizures, or more widely and 2nd generalized.

Seizures originating from the occipital lobes often are associated with primary visual phenomena such as white or colored flashing, flickering lights. The visual hallucination can be bilateral, or lateralized and indicating contra-lateral primary visual cortex. Less common is negative phenomena with loss of vision, or blind spots. Complex visual hallucinations are often described such as an image or movie. There can be eyelid blinking and eye movements. Post-ictal visual deficits include blind spots and distorted vision are the occipital lobe correlate to a Todd's paresis. If these findings are lateralized they are useful for cerebral lateralization of epileptgenic zone.

▪ Insular epilepsy

Insular cortex is a region of neocortex folded underneath the operculum within the lateral sulcus, between the temporal lobe and the frontal lobe.

The insula plays a fundamental role in emotion, autonomic function, and regulation of the body's homeostasis. Functions also include perception, self-awareness, and interpersonal experience. The insula is divided into anterior and posterior regions, The anterior region has primarily limbic connections and is involved in sensory and autonomic function. The posterior insular region has a more complex integrative function, and has mainly neocortical connections.

The possibility of insular cortex seizures were first suggested by Penfield and Jasper (Penfield & Jasper, 1954; Penfield & Faulk, 1955), and they recognized that that the seizures could mimic temporal lobe seizures. Insular cortex has extensive connections to the limbic system (amygdala, hippocampus, entorhinal cortex, and cingulate).

Stereotactic depth electrode implantation has made recording and stimulation studies in the insula possible. In a brain region not accessible to subdural strips and grids, depth electrodes can be safely passed thorough the overlying operculum using structural MRI and angiography image-guided stereotactic techniques to avoid critical vasculature.

In a recent study (Isnard et al., 2004), stimulation of 144 sites in the insular cortex of 50 patients was reported. The 139 reported evoked clinical responses in these patients were divided into somatosensory responses, viscerosensitve response, and other types.

Stimulation induced somatosensory responses included neutral or unpleasant non-painful paresthesiae (pins & needles or electric like current), warm sensation, and also painful electrical discharge. In 49 of the 58 evoked somatosensory responses the symptoms were contralateral to stimulation, 6 were ipsilateral, and 3 bilateral. The evoked responses affected focal regions, such as lips, cheeks, face, tongue, pharynx, or larger areas including hand, limb, neck and face.

Unpleasant visceral sensations located in the pharyngolaryngeal region that included constriction and strangulation and pain were recorded. Also recorded were symptoms suggestive mesial temporal lobe seizures and included abdominal heaviness, unpleasant ascending epigastric sensation, nausea and sudden flush. Less common were complex auditory illusions (muffling of sounds), hallucinations (buzzing and whistling), dysarthria, sensation of unreality, sensations of whole-body displacement in space, olfactogustatory response, and facial sweating.

▪ Electroencephalography

Scalp and intracranial EEG are cornerstones of seizure localization and epilepsy surgery evaluation. Interictal (between seizures) epileptiform spikes and sharp waves, and seizures is often useful in localizing epileptogenic brian. Scalp video-EEG emerged in the 1970's as a way to obtain rigourous electro-clinical correlation of seizures, and has become an indespensible tool for characterizing seizure type and region of seizure onset. The practice of EEG, v-EEG and intracranial EEG has undergone very little change over the past 3 decades. However, there is emerging data to support that the clinical bandwidth of current clinical EEG may be too restricted, and that activity outside the clinical bandwidth is important (Curio, 2000; Vanhatalo et al., 2005).

Scalp Interictal EEG: the distribution of IEDs in patients with focal extratemporal epilepsy can be highly variable. One study showed that 55% of frontal lobe epilepsy patients had either generalized IED or focal IED in regions other than the epileptogenic zone (Vadlamudi et al., 2004). It has been established that an epileptic focus in the deep frontal lobe can produce secondarily generalized IEDs with rapid interhemispheric spread (Loiseau, 1992). Despite the presence of generalized IEDs, these cases can still benefit from frontal lobe resections (Vadlamudi et al., 2004). It is not uncommon that the scalp EEG is unremarkable in ETLE. The absence of IEDs is likely related to the volume of focal epileptogenic brain that does not generate detectable IEDs on scalp EEG. Previous studies have shown that approximately 7 cm^2 of neocortex must be activated to produce IEDs on scalp EEG (Tao et al., 2005).

From these studies, it is reasonable to conclude the presence of widespread IEDs or the absence of IEDS should not preclude patients from consideration of potentially curative epilepsy surgery. Multiple studies do, however, report that the presence of generalized IEDs and/or generalized slowing of the background activity are related to poor outcome in neocortical extratemporal epilepsy surgery (Janszky et al., 2000), and that the presence of focal IEDs is associated with excellent outcome (Holmes et al., 2000). In contrast, several other studies did not find any association between the spatial distribution of IEDs and surgery outcome (Quesney et al., 1992; Quesney et al., 1992; Quesney, 2000).

Scalp Ictal EEG onset pattern: The localization value of ictal scalp EEG in frontal lobe epilepsy was investigated by Talairrach et al. (Talairach et al., 1992) concluded that a fast frequency ictal discharge was associated with successful epilepsy surgery in a group of patients with predominantly lesional frontal lobe epilepsy. Similarly, a focal beta frequency (> 13-25 Hz) discharge at ictal onset, called focal ictal beta, has been associated with excellent surgical outcome in lesional and nonlesional frontal lobe epilepsy (Worrell et al. 2002).

Intracranial EEG: A focal fast frequency ictal onset pattern on iEEG (Figure 2E) has also been associated with favorable outcome in ETLE epilepsy surgery. Previous studies investigating iEEG ictal onset patterns and surgery outcome in patients with normal MRI and ETLE (Park et al., 2002) (Wetjen et al., 2009) reported that focal low voltage fast or beta frequency spiking was associated with favorable surgical outcome. Rhythmic slow sinusoidal activity or rhythmic spike/sharp waves were associated with poor outcome.

■ Epilepsy surgery

Epilepsy surgery is an effective and safe therapy for carefully selected patients with drug-resistant partial epilepsy (Cascino et al., 1993; Engel, 1996; Luders & Comair, 2001). There is now widespread consensus (Neurology consensus practice parameter [Engel et al., 2003]) that epilepsy surgery should be considered for patients with drug-resistant localization related partial epilepsy. In particular, patients with lesional epilepsy have surgically remediable epilepsy syndromes. The majority of these patients will experience a significant reduction in seizure frequency following surgical resection of the region of epileptic brain (Cascino et al., 1992; 1993; Engel Jr, 2008; Engel et al., 2007; Luders & Comair, 2001; Radhakrishnan et al., 1998).

Patients with MRI lesional epilepsy are the most favorable candidates for surgical resection. The underlying structural pathology and association with functionally critical brain regions are important variables when evaluating a patient's candidacy for surgical treatment. The goal of epilepsy surgery is to eliminate, or dramtically reduce seizures to improve their quality of life. In the era of MRI the most common operation currently is a focal resection of epileptic brain tissue, e.g., a focal corticectomy. The rationale for surgical treatment is that removing the epileptogenic zone, i.e., site of seizure onset and initial seizure propagation will eliminate seizures. The high diagnostic yield of MRI to identify the common pathological substrates, e.g., post-traumatic encephalomalcia, vascular malformation, tumor, malformations of cortical development is well established in patients with DRE (Table I). Selected patients will require functional neuroimaging, i.e., PET, SPECT, functional MRI, and possibly chronic intracranial EEG monitoring to localize the region of seizure onset. The cornerstones of the presurgical evaluation are i) clinical history and neurological exam; ii) scalp video-EEG to record the patients habitual seizures; iii) seizure protocol MRI; and for some patients iv) functional neuroimaging (SPECT, PET, MRS, fMRI), MEG, WADA testing, and chronic intracranial EEG monitoring (iEEG).

Table I. Surgical outcomes for ETLE partial epilepsy

Localization	Outcomes
Related partial	Excellent*
Extratemporal lobe epilepsies	
MRI lesional (pathological substrate)	(66-72%) 72% (Mosewitch et al., 2000) 66% (Smith et al., 1997) 67% (Cascino et al., 1992)
MRI non lesional (cryptogenic)	(25-41%) 41% (Mosewich et al., 2000) 37% (Chapman et al., 2005) 29% (Smith et al., 1997) 25% (Cascino et al., 1992)

References

- Bien CG, Szinay M, Wagner J, Clusmann H, Becker AJ, Urbach H. Characteristics and surgical outcomes of patients with refractory magnetic resonance imaging-negative epilepsies. *Arch Neurol* 2009; 66: 1491-99.
- Cascino GD, Boon P, Fish DR. Surgically remedial lesional syndromes. In: J.J. Engel, ed. *Surgical Treatment of the Epilepsies*. New York: Raven Press, 1993.
- Cascino GD, Jack CR, Parisi JE, Marsh WR, Kelly PJ, Sharbrough FW, et al. MRI in the presurgical evaluation of patients with frontal lobe epilepsy and children with temporal lobe epilepsy: pathologic correlation and prognostic importance. *Epilepsy Res* 1992; 11: 51-9.
- Cascino GD, Kelly PJ, Sharbrough FW, Hulihan JF, Hirschorn KA, Trenerry MR. Long-term follow-up of stereotactic lesionectomy in partial epilepsy: predictive factors and electroencephalographic results. *Epilepsia* 1992; 33: 639-44.
- Chapman K, Wyllie E, Najm I, Ruggieri P, Bingaman W, Luders J, et al. Seizure outcome after epilepsy surgery in patients with normal preoperative MRI. *J Neurol Neurosurg Psychiatry* 2005; 76: 710-13.

- Chauvel P, Delgado-Escueta AV, Halgren E, Bancaud J. *Frontal Lobe Seizures and Epilepsies*. New York: Raven Press, 1992.
- Curio G. Ain't no rhythm fast enough: EEG bands beyond beta. *J Clin Neurophysiol* 2000; 17: 339-40.
- Engel Jr, J. Surgical treatment for epilepsy: too little, too late? *JAMA* 2008; 300: 2548.
- Engel J, Pedley TA, Aicardi J, Dichter MA, Moshé S. *Epilepsy: a Comprehensive Textbook*. Philadelphia: Lippincott Williams & Wilkins, 2007.
- Engel J, Wiebe S, French J, Sperling M, Williamson P, Spencer D, et al. Practice parameter: temporal lobe and localized neocortical resections for epilepsy: report of the Quality Standards Subcommittee of the American Academy of Neurology, in association with the American Epilepsy Society and the American Association of Neurological Surgeons. *Neurology* 2003; 60: 538-47.
- Engel JJ. Principles of epilepsy surgery. In: Shorvon S, Dreifuss F, Fish DR, eds. *The Treatment of Epilepsy*. Oxford: Blackwell, 1996.
- Murray CJL, Lopez AD. *Global Comparative Assessments in the Health Sector: Disease Burden, Expenditure, Intervention Packages*. Geneva: World Health Organization, 1994.
- Holmes MD, Born DE, Kutsy RL, Wilensky AJ, Ojemann GA, Ojemann LM. Outcome after surgery in patients with refractory temporal lobe epilepsy and normal MRI. *Seizure* 2000; 9: 407-11.
- Isnard J, Guénot M, Sindou M, Mauguière F. Clinical manifestations of insular lobe seizures: a stereo-electroencephalographic study. *Epilepsia* 2004; 45: 1079-90.
- Janszky J, Jokeit H, Schulz R, Hoppe M, Ebner A. EEG predicts surgical outcome in lesional frontal lobe epilepsy. *Neurology* 2000; 54: 1470-76.
- Kwan P, Brodie MJ. Early identification of refractory epilepsy. *N Engl J Med* 2000; 342: 314-9.
- Kwan P, Arzimanoglou A, Berg AT, Brodie MJ, Allen Hauser W, Mathern G, et al. Definition of drug-resistant epilepsy: consensus proposal by the ad hoc Task Force of the ILAE Commission on Therapeutic Strategies. *Epilepsia* 2010; 51: 1069-77.
- Loiseau P. Childhood absence epilepsy. In: Bureau M, Roger J, eds. *Epileptic Syndromes in Infancy, Childhood and Adolescence*. London: John Libbey, 1992.
- Luders JJ, Comair Y. *Epilepsy Surgery*. Philadelphia: Lippincott Williams & Wilkins, 2001.
- Miller BL, Cummings JL. *The Human Frontal Lobes: Functions and Disorders*. New York: The Guilford Press, 2007.
- Mosewich RK, So EL, O'Brien TJ, Cascino GD, Sharbrough FW, Marsh WR, et al. Factors predictive of the outcome of frontal lobe epilepsy surgery. *Epilepsia* 2000; 41: 843-49.
- Park SA, Lim SR, Kim GS, Heo K, Park SC, Chang JW, et al. Ictal electrocorticographic findings related with surgical outcomes in nonlesional neocortical epilepsy. *Epilepsy Res* 2002; 48: 199-206.
- Penfield W, Jasper H. *Epilepsy and the Functional Anatomy of the Human Brain*. Boston: Little Brown, 1954.
- Penfield W, Fauk ME. The insula; further observations on its function. *Brain* 1955; 78: 445-70.
- Quesney LF. Intracranial EEG investigation in neocortical epilepsy. *Adv Neurol* 2000; 84: 253-74.
- Quesney LF, Constain M, Rasmussen T, Olivier A, Palmini A. Presurgical EEG investigation in frontal lobe epilepsy. *Epilepsy Res* 1992; 5 (Suppl): 55-69.
- Quesney LF, Constain M, Rasmussen T, Stefan H, Olivier A. How large are frontal lobe epileptogenic zones? EEG, ECoG, and SEEG evidence. *Adv Neurol* 1992; 57: 311-23.
- Radhakrishnan K, So EL, Silbert PL, Jack CRJ, Cascino GD, Sharbrough FW, O'Brien PC. Predictors of outcome of anterior temporal lobectomy for intractable epilepsy: a multivariate study. *Neurology* 1998; 51: 465-71.
- Smith JR, Lee MR, King DW, Murro AM, Park YD, Lee GP, et al. Results of lesional *vs.* nonlesional frontal lobe epilepsy surgery. *Stereotact Funct Neurosurg* 1997; 69: 202-9.

- So EL, Schäuble BS. Ictal asomatognosia as a cause of epileptic falls: simultaneous video, EMG, and invasive EEG. *Neurology* 2004; 63: 2153-4.
- Talairach J, Bancaud J, Bonis A, Szikla G, Trottier S, Vignal JP, *et al*. Surgical therapy for frontal epilepsies. *Adv Neurol* 1992; 57: 707-32.
- Tao JX, Ray A, Hawes-Ebersole S, Ebersole JS. Intracranial EEG substrates of scalp EEG interictal spikes. *Epilepsia* 2005; 46: 669-76.
- Vadlamudi L, So EL, Worrell GA, Mosewich RK, Cascino GD, Meyer FB, Lesnick TG. Factors underlying scalp-EEG interictal epileptiform discharges in intractable frontal lobe epilepsy. *Epileptic Disord* 2004; 6: 89-95.
- Vanhatalo S, Voipio J, Kaila K. Full-band EEG (FbEEG): an emerging standard in electroencephalography. *Clin Neurophysiol* 2005: 116: 1-8.
- Wetjen NM, Marsh WR, Meyer FB, Cascino GD, So E, Britton JW, *et al*. Intracranial electroencephalography seizure onset patterns and surgical outcomes in nonlesional extratemporal epilepsy. *J Neurosurg* 2009; 110: 1147-52.
- Williamson PD, Boon PA, Thadani VM, Darcey TM, Spencer DD, Spencer SS, *et al*. Parietal lobe epilepsy: diagnostic considerations and results of surgery. *Ann Neurol* 1992; 31: 193-201.
- Worrell G, So EL, Kazemi J, O'Brien TJ, Mosewich RK, Cascino GD, *et al*. Focal ictal beta discharge on scalp EEG predicts excellent outcome of frontal. *Epilepsia* 2002; 43: 277-82.

Introduction to extratemporal lobe epilepsy

Soheyl Noachtar, Isabella Krotofil

Epilepsy Center, Department of Neurology, University of Munich, Munich, Germany

■ Introduction

Before the introduction of electroencephalography, a detailed analysis of seizure semiology was the only way to classify epileptic seizures. Careful clinical observations and detailed reports of seizure semiology by the patient or other observers are still essential for the proper management of epileptic patients. Modern video techniques combined with simultaneous EEG recordings have dramatically improved our knowledge of epileptic seizure semiology and provided information on localization and lateralization of the epileptogenic zone. Seizure semiology plays an important role in the pre-surgical work-up, particularly when analyzed independently of other pre-surgical tests (EEG monitoring, neuroradiology, etc.) (Noachtar & Borggraefe, 2009). Visual analysis of seizure semiology is prone to interobserver bias (Bleasel et al., 1997). Quantitative analysis of movements during video-recorded seizures introduced objective criteria for the analysis of seizure semiology (Li et al., 2002; Mirzadjanova et al., 2010; O'Dwyer et al., 2007; Silva Cunha et al., 2003).

Electrical stimulation of the cortex in a wake patients provided us with a wealth of information on the function of the cortex which allowed conclusions on the localization of the epileptogenic zone based on the analysis of seizure semiology (Penfield & Jasper, 1954). It was assumed that if electrical stimulation of a given cortical area produced a symptom that habitually occurred during an epileptic seizure, then the patient's seizures activate the same region that is stimulated. Therefore, these cortical regions producing the clinical symptoms of the seizure semiology are defined as the symptomatogenic zone (Lüders & Awad, 1992). However, if seizures originate in silent areas of the cortex they remain asymptomatic unless the epileptic activation reaches the eloquent cortex which leads to the clinical seizure semiology.

■ How to classify epileptic seizures?

Diagnostic schemes for seizures and epilepsy are published by the ILAE (International League against Epilepsy) regularly to adjust clinical guidelines according to recent research. In 2001 a diagnostic scheme for people with epileptic seizure and epilepsy was proposed by the ILAE in order to aid clinicians in daily routine (Engel, 2001). A strictly semiological approach is essential in order to achieve clearness in seizure classification. Only then seizure semiology can serve as a independent piece of information to be used for localization and lateralization of the epileptogenic zone (Noachtar *et al.*, 1998; Luders *et al.*, 1998).

Epileptic seizures are characterized by a variety of signs and symptoms. Conventional seizure analysis is based on visual expert opinion and mainly focuses on the predominant ictal features. The following four categories are involved in the ictal phenomena of epileptic seizures (Noachtar & Peters, 2009):
– sensorial sphere;
– autonomic sphere;
– consciousness;
– motor sphere.

While symptoms corresponding to several of the above-listed spheres occur simultaneously during most epileptic seizures, ictal phenomena of one or the other sphere almost always predominate *(Table I)*. Only few seizure types involve only one category *(Table II)*. For example an aura exclusively affects the sensorial sphere. Due to the absence of objective signs, the examiner has to rely on the patient's depiction of the aura. Since they occur at the onset of seizures they provide an extremely useful information about the localization and lateralization of the seizure onset zone. For example, visual auras usually occur at the beginning of the seizures in patients with occipital lobe epilepsy. Somatosensory auras arise contralaterally to the hemisphere of seizure onset in paracentral epilepsy and have a high lateralization value.

Many seizures are associated with a disturbance of consciousness. However, only for some seizures the disturbance is the predominant feature of the seizure. For example, generalized tonic-clonic seizures are always associated with impairment of consciousness. As generalized tonic-clonic motor phenomena here constitute the predominant seizure symptomatology, the seizure is classified as a motor seizure.

Table I. Spheres and seizure type

Sphere	Seizure type
Perception	Aura
Autonomic phenomena	Autonomic seizure
Consciousness	Dialeptic seizure
Motor phenomena	Motor seizure

Table II. Seizure type with regard to motor activity and level of consciousness

Seizure type			Motor activity	Consciousness
Aura			Unchanged	Normal
Dialeptic seizure ("absence")			Absent (or minimal)	Disturbed
Motor seizure	Simple motor seizure	Clonic seizure	Clonic	Normal or disturbed
		Tonic seizure	Tonic	
		Tonic-clonic seizure	Tonic-clonic	
		Myoclonic seizure	Myoclonic	
		Versive seizure	Versive	
		Epileptic spasm	Spasm	
	Complex motor seizure	Automotor seizure	Distal (hand, oral) automatisms	Normal or disturbed
		Hypermotor seizure	Pronounced, poximal musculature	
		Gelastic seizure	Laughing	
Special seizures		Atonic seizure	Reduction of tone	Normal or disturbed
		Astatic seizure	Drop; unknown of tonic and/or atonic	Normal or disturbed
		Akinetic seizure	Inability to initiate or maintain movements	Normal
		Aphasic seizure	Unchanged	Normal
		Negative myoclonic seizure	Brief muscle atonia	Normal
		Hypomotor seizure	Absent (or minimal)	No interpretation possible (newborns, severely retarded patients)

So far several terms are presently used for seizures with disturbed consciousness according to the EEG results and the underlying epilepsy syndrome. For example, the alteration of consciousness is labeled *absence seizure* if the patient has generalized 3 Hz spike wave complexes in the EEG, whereas the same clinical seizure would be called *complex partial seizure* if the patient had focal epilepsy or the EEG showed focal epileptiform discharges. Terms like "pseudo absence" have been proposed for these seizures in patients with focal epilepsy (Bancaud & Talairach, 1992), because the term absence is exclusively used for patients with generalized epilepsy in the seizure classification of the International League Against Epilepsy (ILAE, published in (Commission on Classification and Terminology of the International League Against Epilepsy, 1981). Thus, different terms ("absence" or "complex-partial seizure") were used, although the seizure semiology may be clinically indistinguishable. To avoid this confusion the term "dialeptic seizure" was introduced for ictal episodes with an alteration of consciousness as main manifestation, disregarding the underlying type of epilepsy (Lüders et al., 1998; Noachtar et al., 1998). The term dialeptic derives from the Greek verb "dialepein", which means "to stand still", "to interrupt" or "to pass out".

Seizures with motor phenomena as main manifestations are called motor seizures.

Autonomic seizures are extremely rare. The predominant symptomatology for this type of seizure is an objectively documented alteration of the autonomic system (i.e., tachycardia documented by ECG recording) regardless of whether the patient is aware of the seizure.

Seizures that cannot be assigned to any of the four groups outlined above are included in the group labeled "special seizures". This category includes primarily seizures characterized as "negative" ictal phenomena (atonic seizure, negative myoclonic seizure, etc.).

The semiological seizure classification (Lüders et al., 1998; Noachtar et al., 1998) (Table III) enables clinicians to classify seizures as precise as possible according to the available information. For example, an epileptic seizure of a patient can be classified as an "epileptic seizure" if no further information were available. If the seizure was primarily characterized by motor phenomena, it can be classified as a "motor seizure". If the motor seizure affected the right arm, but further specification was not possible, it can be classified as a "right arm motor seizure". If clonic jerking of the right arm is present during the seizure, the seizure classification would be "right arm clonic seizure". Thus, the more information we get on the seizure semiology, the more precise we can classify the seizure. This is a typical setting encountered in clinical practice; we frequently initially have little information on the seizure semiology if a patient is seen first in the emergency room or the outpatient clinic but we gradually achieve more information as more seizures were observed by others who can provide more detailed descriptions of the seizure semiology.

■ Status epilepticus

Essentially any seizure types discussed above can manifest as status epilepticus, although this clinical experience has not been evaluated in detail (Rona et al., 2005). Typical examples in extratemporal epilepsy are unilateral clonic status ("epilepsia partialis continua"), generalized tonic-clonic status ("grand mal status"), and so called non-convulsive status epilepticus which is characterized by disturbance of awareness and consciousness with minor motor manifestations. The term non-convulsive status is broad and includes a variety of status forms such as dialeptic status, automotor status, and also rare examples such as aphasic status (Rona et al., 2005). In daily practice, the term "non-convulsive status" is usually used as a synonym for dialeptic or automotor status. Dialeptic or automotor status can be localized only by EEG and imaging studies.

Table III. Semiological seizure classification

Epileptic seizure	Aura		Somatosensory aura* Visual aura* Auditory aura* Olfactory aura Gustatory aura Autonomic aura Abdominal aura Psychic aura
	Autonomic seizure*		
	Dialeptic seizure?	Typical dialeptic seizure?	
	Motor seizure*	Simple-motor seizure*	Myoclonic seizure* Epileptic spasm* Tonic-clonic seizure Tonic seizure* Clonic seizure* Versive seizure*
		Complex-motor seizure?	Hypermotor seizure? Automotor seizure? Gelastic seizure
	Special seizure		Aphasic seizure? Akinetic seizure * Atonic seizure * Astatic seizure Negative myoclonic seizure * Hypomotor seizure?
Paroxysmal event			

Modifier * = left/right/axial/generalized/bilateral asymmetric.
Modifier ° = lateralizing signs occurring during this seizure types are listed separately.

■ The localizing significance of different seizure types

Auras

Auras usually occur at the beginning of a seizure ("warning symptoms") for seconds up to minutes. Usually, they evolve into other seizure types due to the spread of the epileptiform discharge, although they may be seen in isolation as well. Several different forms of auras have been described (*Table III*). Since auras are the first clinical expression of a seizure, they frequently provide extremely useful localizing information about the seizure onset zone (Palmini & Gloor, 1992). However, frequently the aura is used to determine the localization of the epileptogenic zone. This approach constitutes the inverse problem of seizure semiology. Spread of epileptic activity may lead to false localization of the epileptogenic zone by aura type if the seizures start in a so called silent area of the cortex and the first clinical symptoms such as the aura are due to spread of the epileptic activity (Noachtar & Peters, 2009; Rossetti & Kaplan, 2010). Thus, one should be aware that there is not a 1:1 relationship between aura and localization of the epileptogenic zone but a probability that the epileptogenic zone is in the vicinity of the symptomatogenic zone. Although, for instance abdominal auras are typical for temporal lobe epilepsy, they are reported less frequently in extratemporal epilepsy such as frontal lobe epilepsy (Henkel *et al.*, 2002) seizures. An abdominal aura is associated with TLE with a probability of 73.6%.

The evolution of an abdominal aura into an automotor seizure, however, increases the probability of TLE to 98.3% (Henkel et al., 2002). Whereas in frontal lobe epilepsy, abdominal auras are followed by tonic seizures in 66%, this was not the case in any temporal lobe epilepsy patient (Henkel et al., 2002).

The propagation of aura symptoms during a seizure point to the functional cortical representation

The typical march of a somatosensory aura reflects the spreading activation of the epileptiform discharge on the contralateral somatosensory cortex which is organized somatotopically. Ipsilateral or bilateral, poorly described sensations of the trunk or distal extremities have rarely been observed in patients with seizures arising from the supplementary sensormotor area or the secondary sensory area (Penfield & Jasper, 1954; Morris et al., 1988).

Simple visual auras such as "bright spots" or "dark spots" as well as field defects result from epileptic activation of the visual field, especially of the striate and most likely also parts of the parastriate cortex (Noachtar, 2001). In occipital lobe epilepsy unilateral visual auras can lateralize the seizure onset to the contralateral hemisphere (Williamson et al., 1992; Salanova et al., 1992). Auras usually consist of "positive" phenomena such as an rising abdominal sensation, a tingling sensation of a limb or visual hallucinations (bright spots etc.) but they can also show "negative" phenomena such as ictal blindness as a reflection of for example occipital lobe epileptic activation. Due to rapid contralateral spread this ictal blindness usually occupies the entire visual field.

■ Disturbance of the autonomic sphere

Epileptic activation of the so called autonomic cortical centers including the basal frontal region and the anterior cingulate gyrus can evoke autonomic symptoms affecting only the autonomic system such as tachycardia, altered breathing or sweating without the occurrence of other auras or motor phenomena (Penfield & Jasper, 1954; Luders et al., 1998). Most of these symptoms are purely subjective and should be classified as an autonomic aura. But similar reactions occur as a response to the first seizure symptoms, especially in patients with other auras or focal motor seizures as the result of fear that the seizure will evolve further. Such responses to seizure symptoms should not be classified as autonomic auras. Otherwise, autonomic alterations which were observed (mydriasis, sweating, flushing) or documented by polygraphic recordings (EEG, ECG, blood pressure) should be classified as autonomic seizures. An increase in heart rate is frequently observed at seizure onset but could be secondary to the fear that a seizure is coming up or as a result of increased ictal motor activity. However, pure ictal tachycardia without any other clinical symptoms is highly correlated with a temporal rather than extratemporal epileptogenic zone (Weil et al., 2005).

■ Consciousness

Some seizure types consist mainly of an alteration of consciousness. Patients do not respond at all or only to a limited to extent to external stimuli during this seizure type. Patients are usually not aware of these episodes and cannot recall them later. It

Consciousness is difficult to define both, theoretically and even more practically (Gloor, 1986). We proposed the term dialeptic seizures if disturbance of consciousness is the predominant feature of the seizure and there is no or only minimal motor activity (Lüders et al., 1998; Noachtar et al., 1998). This seizure type is called absence if the patient has a generalized epilepsy and complex partial seizure if the patient has focal epilepsy by the International League Against Epilepsy Classification (Commission on Classification and Terminology of the International League Against Epilepsy, 1981).

Dialeptic seizures may occur in focal epilepsies as well (Bancaud & Talairach, 1992; Noachtar et al., 2000). However, there is little information about the frequency and the differences in the semiology of dialeptic seizures occurring in extratemporal and temporal epilepsy. Dialeptic seizures in frontal lobe epilepsy are termed as "frontal absence" or "pseudo-absence" because of their similar appearance to absence seizures in generalized epilepsies (Bancaud & Talairach, 1992; Swartz, 1992). Dialeptic seizures in focal epilepsies usually last longer than 20 seconds in comparison to generalized absence which typically last less than 20 seconds (Noachtar, 2000). Isolated examples of dialeptic seizures in patients with extratemporal lesions have been documented (Noachtar et al., 2000). The pathogenesis of dialeptic seizures in patients with focal epilepsies is poorly understood (Noachtar et al., 2000). An ictal SPECT study demonstrated that the thalamus and upper brain stem are involved in disturbance of consciousness in different types of focal epileptic seizures: impairment of consciousness showed a strong association with secondary hyper-perfusion in the thalamic/upper brainstem region (Lee et al., 2002).

Consciousness is usually not impaired at that time t tonic or clonic activity begins in simple motor seizures such as unilateral tonic or clonic seizures (Manford et al., 1996; Noachtar & Arnold, 2000; Werhahn et al., 2000). However, if tonic or clonic activity is the result of spread of epileptiform activity from the parietal, occipital or temporal lobe into the frontal lobe, consciousness is usually altered at the onset of unilateral clonic or tonic seizures. Generalized clonic seizures only very rarely occur with preserved consciousness (Bell et al., 1997) as well as generalized tonic seizures, which are common in patients with Lennox-Gastaut- syndrome.

■ Seizures characterized by motor phenomena

Ictal motor manifestations are divided into two major groups (simple and complex motor seizures) based on the type of motor symptoms (Table III).

■ Simple motor seizures

These seizures are characterized by unnatural, relatively simple movements which resemble movements which can be reproduced by electrical stimulation of the primary and supplementary sensormotor areas. Simple motor seizures can be divided into the following subtypes depending on the duration of the muscle contraction, the rhythmicity of movement repetition, and the muscles involved: myoclonic seizures, clonic seizures, tonic seizures, epileptic spasms, versive seizures, and tonic-clonic seizures. These motor symptoms can occur as the only manifestation of epileptic activity and rest focal or they can evolve to each other during an epileptic seizure by spreading of epileptic discharges. Tonic seizures evolved into clonic seizures occurred more frequently in patients with frontal lobe than with parieto-occipital lobe epilepsy (Werhahn et al., 2000). Myoclonic seizures which predominantly affect the shoulders and proximal arms are typical for patients with juvenile myoclonic epilepsy (Janz & Christian, 1957). In extratemporal lobe epilepsy the primary motor cortex or premotor areas are most likely involved in the generation of this seizure type.

Unilateral clonic activity occurs frequently in patients with frontal lobe epilepsy as the inital seizure symptom (Loddenkemper & Kotagal, 2005) and arise from epileptic activation of the contralateral primary motor cortex. Focal clonic seizures mostly affect the distal segments of the extremities, *e.g.* the hand or the face. Clonic activity may show a march, the so called Jacksonian progression from the distal to the proximal parts of the extremities, reflecting the spreading activation of the primary motor cortex (Penfield & Jasper, 1954; Manford *et al.*, 1996). Clonic activity could be reproduced by electrical stimulation of the primary motor cortex and prefrontal areas (Penfield & Jasper, 1954). Electrical stimulation of the supplementary sensormotor area can elicit distal clonic movements, but only very rarely (Lim *et al.*, 1996). In patients with frontal lobe epilepsy, clonic seizures tend to occur early in the seizure evolution. Clonic seizures which preceed a tonic seizure appeared only in frontal lobe epilepsy whereas clonic seizures followed a tonic seizure may also occur in patients with parieto-occipital and temporal lobe epilepsy (Werhahn *et al.*, 2000).

Tonic seizures in patients with focal epilepsy preferentially affect proximal muscle groups on both sides of the body (Bleasel & Lüders, 2000). Tonic seizures are common in patients with frontal lobe epilepsy (62%) and rare in temporal lobe epilepsy (1.7%) (Werhahn *et al.*, 2000). Strictly unilateral tonic seizures have a high lateralizing significance, pointing to a contralateral seizure onset (Werhahn *et al.*, 2000). Tonic seizures may also occur in parieto-occipital lobe epilepsy due to spread of the ictal epileptic activity into the frontal lobes and reflects the close relationship between the parieto-occipital and frontal regions.

Versive seizures consist of a sustained, unnatural turning of the eyes and head, forced and involuntary to one side are frequently seen in patients with different focal epilepsies (O'Dwyer *et al.*, 2007; Wyllie *et al.*, 1986). These seizures are the expression of epileptic activation of the frontal eye field and the motor areas anterior to the precentral gyrus that is contralateral to the side to which the eyes turn (Penfield & Jasper, 1954).

Tonic-clonic seizures have a typical evolution with bilateral tonic posturing which is followed by bilateral clonic activity. Focal seizure types may precede the generalized tonic-clonic seizure depending on the cortical region where the seizures originated.

■ Complex motor seizures

Complex motor seizures consist of motor seizures during which the patient performs movements that imitate natural movements (automatisms), except that they are inappropriate for the situation and which are relatively complex and tend to involve different body segments moving in different planes. Complex motor seizures are subdivided into three types depending on the characteristics of the automatisms.

Hypermotor seizures are characterized by complex sequences of movement which primarily affect the proximal body segments and result in large stereotypically repeated movements with violent appearance *(Figure 1)*. This seizure type is frequently seen in patients with frontal lobe epilepsy arising from mesial frontal or supplementary sensormotor area cortex (Morris *et al.*, 1988, Williamson *et al.*, 1985). However, spread of epileptic activity, into

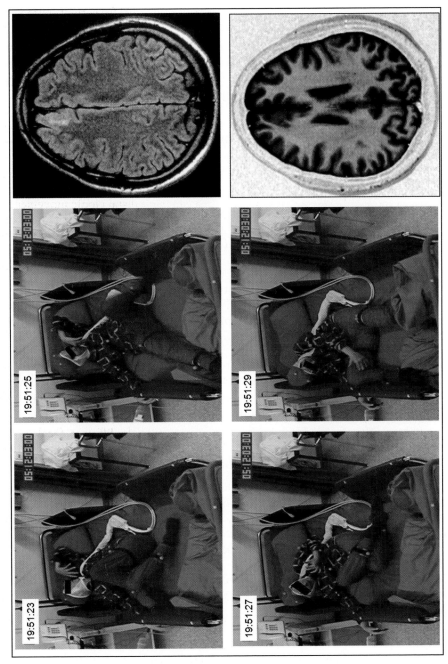

Figure 1. Several images of the course of a hypermotor seizure characterized by prominent trunk and proximal limb movements in a 33-year-old-woman with right mesial frontal lobe epilepsy since age 10. MRI of the brain (FLAIR and T1 weighted images) revealed a cortical dysplasia in the mesial aspect of the right superior frontal gyrus.

the frontal lobe or the supplementary sensormotor area cortex from a remote seizure onset zone is also a frequent cause of hypermotor seizures (Lüders & Noachtar, 2001) e.g. ictal spreading from the temporal lobe to the dorso-lateral and mesial frontal regions can also cause complex movements of the limbs and trunk (Kotagal et al., 2003). Consciousness may be preserved during this seizure type. The bizarre appearance of the seizure and the preserved consciousness frequently lead to the erroneous diagnosis of non-epileptic (psychogenic) pseudo seizures (Kanner et al., 1990).

Automotor seizures are characterized by manual and oral automatisms and are typical for temporal lobe epilepsy but may also occur in patients with extratemporal epilepsy (Manford et al., 1996). In frontal lobe epilepsy, automotor seizures are reported to arise from orbitofrontal regions (Bancaud & Talairach, 1992).

The symptomatogenic zone of automotor seizure onset is not clearly defined, but there is some evidence that epileptic activation of the anterior cingulate gyrus leads to distal automatisms with preserved responsiveness (Loddenkemper & Kotagal, 2005; Talairach et al., 1973).

Ictal "laughing" is the main feature in gelastic seizures and frequently is associated with hypothalamic hamartomas (Berkovic et al., 1988). Gelastic features may also occur rarely during seizures of patients with frontal lobe epilepsy (Kotagal et al., 2003). Gelastic seizures may be preceded or followed by other seizure types.

There is a group of seizures that cannot be classified in one of the four types described earlier (auras, autonomic, dialeptic, or motor seizures). Most of these seizures characteristically have a negative influence on motor (atonic, akinetic) or cognitive (aphasic) activity and may result from epileptic inhibition of the symptomatogenic zone.

Atonic seizures are characterized by a sudden reduction of postural tone that results in a loss of posture (head drop, falls, etc.). These seizures are often preceded by a brief myoclonic seizure with propulsion or retropulsion. They are frequently seen in patients Lennox-Gastaut-syndrome and are most probably the result of epileptic activation of the inhibitory centers in the brain stem (e.g., nucleus reticularis gigantocellularis) via fast cortico-reticulo-spinal systems (Lai & Siegel, 1988; Magoun & Rhines, 1946) or by spreading into negative motor areas (Lüders et al., 1995; Ikeda et al., 2000). However, focal atonia involving only distal parts of the body has been reported and was labeled ictal paresis or inhibitory seizure (So, 1995). It is sometimes difficult to distinguish these patients, in whom focal atonia occurs and consciousness is disturbed, from those with postictal (Todd) paralysis and non-epileptic mechanisms, such as migraine and transient ischemic attacks. It is possible that some of these seizures reflect ictal activation of the negative motor areas (Noachtar & Luders, 1999). Electrical stimulation of these areas causes an inability to perform voluntary movements and, in addition, very frequently various degrees of atonia are seen in distal muscle groups (fingers, hands, face, tongue) (Lüders et al., 1995).

Astatic seizures are characterized by epileptic falls, which can be due to atonic, myoclonic, or tonic seizures. Frequently, a myoclonic seizure leads to a loss of balance and the fall is produced by an atonia, which occurs immediately after the initial myoclonic jerk. The pathogenesis is unclear.

Negative myoclonic seizures, which are also called epileptic negative myoclonus, consist of short (ca. 30-400 ms) phases of muscle atonia and cause a brief interruption of muscle activity. The seizure is expressed clinically only during muscle innervation, *i.e.*, it does not occur when the patient is at rest (Tassinari & Gastaut, 1969). Generalized as well as focal negative myoclonic seizures have been described (Guerrini *et al.*, 1993). Polygraphic recordings showed that these seizures are frequently preceded by epileptiform discharges in the central region (20-30 msec before the atonia). There is much evidence for a causal sudden inhibition of tonic innervation of the motor neurons, which is reflected in the silent period of the EMG. The cortex regions giving rise to negative myoclonic seizure by epileptic activation could be the primary somatosensory motor cortex (Ikeda *et al.*, 2000) and the premotor cortex (Baumgartner *et al.*, 1996). A postcentral generator, which inhibits tonic motor activity, was identified in a patient with postcentral focal cortical dysplasia and hyperexcitability of the postcentral cortex (Noachtar *et al.*, 1997).

Akinetic seizures are characterized by an inability to perform voluntary movements. By definition consciousness is not disturbed during this seizure type so that the patient can be tested about the akinetic symptoms (Noachtar & Lüders, 1999; 2000). The inability to initiate and maintain voluntary movements may involve the entire body or only parts of it. Such seizures probably arise from epileptic activation of the so-called negative motor areas in the mesial frontal and inferior frontal gyri, which are identified by electrical cortical stimulation of the frontal lobe (Lüders *et al.*, 1995; Noachtar & Luders, 1999).

Aphasic seizures are characterized by an inability to speak or to comprehend language. However, consciousness is preserved by definition. Aphasic seizures most probably reflect epileptic activation of cortical language areas in the speech dominant hemisphere (Fakhoury *et al.*, 1994).and occur frequently in patients with mesial temporal lobe epilepsy (Kotagal *et al.*, 2003) rather than in frontal lobe epilepsy.

If the extent of motor activity is reduced or totally absent this seizure should be classified as a hypomotor seizure when the state of consciousness cannot be assessed during or after the seizure, *i.e.* newborns, infants, and severely mentally retarded patients. Most likely consciousness is affected in a considerable number of patients, although this cannot be tested in these patients (Acharya *et al.*, 1997). However, the pathogenetic mechanisms involved in the arrest of motor activity may be different in some hypomotor seizures.

■ Seizure evolution

Epileptic seizures frequently evolve from one seizure type into another. It is a well-established fact that the initial seizure symptoms provide information on the location of the seizure onset zone. The initial symptoms such as auras reflect activation of the symptomatogenic cortex, which is likely to be close to the seizure onset zone (Palmini & Gloor, 1992). However, seizures may arise in silent cortical regions that do not express any clinical symptoms and in such cases the epileptic activation remains unnoticed. Abdominal aura followed by an automotor seizure is frequently seen in patients with temporal lobe epilepsy and less common in epileptogenic activation of extratemporal regions (Henkel *et al.*, 2002). Responsiveness can be preserved during automatisms if the seizure origin is in the non-dominant hemisphere (Ebner *et al.*, 1995; Noachtar *et al.*, 1992). Other clinical phenomena such as somatosensory aura followed by unilateral tonic posturing and head version are the characteristics of frontal or paracentral epilepsy and appear contralateral to the side of the seizure onset (Janszky et al., 2001).

The termination of seizures also provides lateralizing information. The end of generalized tonic-clonic seizures was asymmetric in 65% of the patients and the unilateral clonic jerks at the end of the seizures were ipsilateral to the hemisphere of seizure onset in 80% of the patients (Leutmezer et al., 2002; Trinka et al., 2002).

■ Ictal lateralizing phenomena

Most patients with medically intractable extratemporal epilepsy who are considered for epilepsy surgery show ictal lateralizing phenomena such as dystonic hand posturing, version, ictal speech, postictal aphasia, ictal vomiting, unilateral clonic seizures, postictal paresis, postictal aphasia, and preserved responsiveness during automatisms. Most reports included patients with temporal lobe and less frequently patients with extratemporal epilepsy (Bleasel et al., 1997; O'Dwyer et al., 2007; Chee et al., 1993; Leutmezer & Baumgartner, 2002).

The positive predictive value of most lateralizing seizure phenomena is correct in 80-100%. This important lateralizing information should be considered in the classification of epileptic seizures (Lüders et al., 1998; Noachtar et al., 1998; Noachtar & Lüders, 1997).

References

- Acharya JN, Wyllie E, Lüders HO, Kotagal P, Lancman M, Coelho M. Seizure symptomatology in infants with localization-related epilepsy. Neurology 1997; 48: 189-96.

- Bancaud J, Talairach J. Clinical semiology of frontal lobe seizures. In: Chauvel P, Delgado-Escueta AV, Halgren E, Bancaud J, eds. Frontal Lobe Seizures and Epilepsies. New York: Raven Press, 1992, 3-58.

- Baumgartner C, Podreka I, Olbrich A, Novak K, Serles W, Aull S, et al. Epileptic negative myoclonus: An EEG-single-photon emission CT study indicating involvement of premotor cortex. Neurology 1996; 46: 753-8.

- Bell WL, Walczak TS, Shin C, Radtke RA. Painful generalised clonic and tonic-clonic seizures with retained consciousness. J Neurol Neurosurg Psychiatry 1997; 63: 792-5.

- Berkovic SF, Andermann F, Melanson D, Ethier RE, Feindel W, Gloor P. Hypothalamic hamartomas and ictal laughter: evolution of a characteristic epileptic syndrome and diagnostic value of magnetic resonance imaging. Ann Neurol 1988; 23: 429-39.

- Bleasel A, Kotagal P, Kankirawatana P, Rybicki L. Lateralizing value and semiology of ictal limb posturing and version in temporal lobe and extratemporal epilepsy. Epilepsia 1997; 38: 168-74.

- Bleasel A, Lüders HO. Tonic seizures. In: Lüders HO, Noachtar S, eds. Epileptic Seizures: Pathophysiology and Clinical Semiology. New York: Churchill Livingstone, 2000, 389-411.

- Chee MW, Kotagal P, Van Ness PC, Gragg L, Murphy D, Luders HO. Lateralizing signs in intractable partial epilepsy: blinded multiple-observer analysis. Neurology 1993; 43: 2519-25.

- Commission on Classification and Terminology of the International League Against Epilepsy. Proposal for a revised clinical and electroencephalographic classification of epileptic seizures. Epilepsia 1981; 22: 489-501.

- Ebner A, Dinner DS, Noachtar S, Luders H. Automatisms with preserved responsiveness: a lateralizing sign in psychomotor seizures. *Neurology* 1995; 45: 61-4.

- Engel J, Jr. A proposed diagnostic scheme for people with epileptic seizures and with epilepsy: report of the ILAE Task Force on Classification and Terminology. *Epilepsia* 2001; 42: 796-803.

- Fakhoury T, Abou-Khalil B, Peguero E. Differentiating clinical features of right and left temporal lobe seizures. *Epilepsia* 1994; 35: 1038-44.

- Gloor P. Consciousness as a neurological concept. *Epilepsia* 1986; 27: S14-S26.

- Guerrini R, Dravet C, Genton P, Bureau M, Roger J, Rubbioli G, Tassinari CA. Epileptic negative myoclonus. *Neurology* 1993; 43: 1078-83.

- Henkel A, Noachtar S, Pfander M, Luders HO. The localizing value of the abdominal aura and its evolution: a study in focal epilepsies. *Neurology* 2002; 58: 271-6.

- Ikeda A, Ohara S, Matsumoto R, Kunieda T, Nagamine T, Miyamoto S, *et al.* Role of primary sensorimotor cortices in generating inhibitory motor response in humans. *Brain* 2000; 123 (Pt 8): 1710-21.

- Janszky J, Fogarasi A, Jokeit H, Ebner A. Lateralizing value of unilateral motor and somatosensory manifestations in frontal lobe seizures. *Epilepsy Res* 2001; 43: 125-33.

- Janz D, Christian W. Impulsiv-Petit mal. *Dtsch Z Nervenheilk* 1957; 176: 346-86.

- Kanner AM, Morris HH, Luders H, Dinner DS, Wyllie E, Medendorp SV, Rowan AJ. Supplementary motor seizures mimicking pseudoseizures: some clinical differences. *Neurology* 1990; 40: 1404-7.

- Kotagal P, Arunkumar G, Hammel J, Mascha E. Complex partial seizures of frontal lobe onset statistical analysis of ictal semiology. *Seizure* 2003; 12: 268-81.

- Lai YY, Siegel JM. Medullary regions mediating atonia. *J Neurosci* 1988; 8: 4790-6.

- Lee KH, Meador KJ, Park YD, King DW, Murro AM, Pillai JJ, Kaminski RJ. Pathophysiology of altered consciousness during seizures: Subtraction SPECT study. *Neurology* 2002; 59: 841-6.

- Leutmezer F, Baumgartner C. Postictal signs of lateralizing and localizing significance. *Epileptic Disord* 2002; 4: 43-8.

- Leutmezer F, Lurger S, Baumgartner C. Focal features in patients with idiopathic generalized epilepsy. *Epilepsy Res* 2002; 50: 293-300.

- Li Z, Martins da Silva A, Cunha JP. Movement quantification in epileptic seizures: a new approach to video-EEG analysis. *IEEE Trans Biomed Eng* 2002; 49: 565-73.

- Lim SH, Dinner DS, Luders HO. Cortical stimulation of the supplementary sensorimotor area. *Adv Neurol* 1996; 70: 187-97.

- Loddenkemper T, Kotagal P. Lateralizing signs during seizures in focal epilepsy. *Epilepsy Behav* 2005; 7: 1-17.

- Luders H, Acharya J, Baumgartner C, Benbadis S, Bleasel A, Burgess R, *et al.* Semiological seizure classification. *Epilepsia* 1998; 39: 1006-13.

- Lüders HO, Awad IA. Conceptual considerations. In: Lüders HO, ed. *Epilepsy Surgery*. New York: Raven Press, 1992, 51-62.

- Lüders HO, Dinner DS, Morris HH, Wyllie E, Comair YG. Cortical electrical stimulation in humans. The negative motor areas. *Adv Neurol* 1995; 67: 115-29.

- Lüders HO, Noachtar S. *Atlas of Epileptic Seizures and Syndromes*. Philadelphia: Saunders; 2001.

- Magoun HW, Rhines R. An inhibitory mechanism in the bulbar reticular formation. *J Neurophysiol* 1946; 9: 165-71.

- Manford M, Fish DR, Shorvon SD. An analysis of clinical seizure patterns and their localizing value in frontal and temporal lobe epilepsies. *Brain* 1996; 119: 17-40.

- Mirzadjanova Z, Peters AS, Remi J, Bilgin C, Silva Cunha JP, Noachtar S. Significance of lateralization of upper limb automatisms in temporal lobe epilepsy: A quantitative movement analysis. *Epilepsia* 2010; 51: 2140-6.
- Morris HH, Dinner DS, Luders H, Wyllie E, Kramer R. Supplementary motor seizures: clinical and electroencephalographic findings. *Neurology* 1988; 38: 1075-82.
- Noachtar S, Arnold S. Clonic seizures. In: Lüders HO, Noachtar S, eds. *Epileptic Seizures: Pathophysiology and Clincal Semiology.* New York: Churchill Livingstone, 2000, 412-24.
- Noachtar S, Borggraefe I. Epilepsy surgery: a critical review. *Epilepsy Behav* 2009; 15: 66-72.
- Noachtar S, Desudchit T, Lüders HO. Dialeptic seizures. In: Lüders HO, Noachtar S, eds. *Epileptic Seizures: Pathophysiology and Clinical Semiology.* New York: Churchill Livingstone, 2000, 361-76.
- Noachtar S, Ebner A, Dinner DS. Das Auftreten von Automatismen bei erhaltenem Bewusstsein. Zur Frage der Bewusstseinsstörung bei komplex-fokalen Anfällen. In: Scheffner D, ed. *Epilepsie 91.* Reinbek: Einhorn-Presse Verlag, 1992, 82-7.
- Noachtar S, Holthausen H, Lüders HO. Epileptic negative myoclonus. Subdural EEG recordings indicate a postcentral generator. *Neurology* 1997; 49: 1534-7.
- Noachtar S, Lüders HO. Akinetic seizures. In: Lüders HO, Noachtar S, eds. *Epileptic Seizures Pathophysiology and Clinical Semiology.* New York: Churchill Livingstone; 2000, 500.
- Noachtar S, Lüders HO. Classification of epileptic seizures and epileptic syndromes. *Textbook of Stereotactic and Functional Neurosurgery* 1997: 1763-74.
- Noachtar S, Luders HO. Focal akinetic seizures as documented by electroencephalography and video recordings. *Neurology* 1999; 53: 427-9.
- Noachtar S, Peters AS. Semiology of epileptic seizures: a critical review. *Epilepsy Behav* 2009; 15: 2-9.
- Noachtar S, Rosenow F, Arnold S, Baumgartner C, Ebner A, Hamer H, *et al.* Semiologic classification of epileptic seizures. *Nervenarzt* 1998; 69: 117-26.
- Noachtar S. Seizure semiology. In: Lüders HO, ed. *Epilepsy: Comprehensive Review and Case Discussions.* London: Martin Dunitz Publishers, 2001, 127-40.
- O'Dwyer R, Silva Cunha JP, Vollmar C, Mauerer C, Feddersen B, Burgess RC, *et al.* Lateralizing significance of quantitative analysis of head movements before secondary generalization of seizures of patients with temporal lobe epilepsy. *Epilepsia* 2007; 48: 524-30.
- Palmini A, Gloor P. The localizing value of auras in partial epilepsies. *Neurology* 1992; 42: 801-8.
- Penfield W, Jasper H. *Epilepsy and the Functional Anatomy of the Human Brain.* Boston: Brown Little & Co; 1954.
- Rona S, Rosenow F, Arnold S, Carreno M, Diehl B, Ebner A, *et al.* A semiological classification of status epilepticus. *Epileptic Disord* 2005; 7: 5-12.
- Rossetti AO, Kaplan PW. Seizure semiology: an overview of the "inverse problem". *Eur Neurol* 2010; 63: 3-10.
- Salanova V, Andermann F, Olivier A, Rasmussen T, Quesney LF. Occipital lobe epilepsy: electroclinical manifestations, electrocorticography, cortical stimulation and outcome in 42 patients treated between 1930 and 1991. Surgery of occipital lobe epilepsy. *Brain* 1992; 115: 1655-80.
- Silva Cunha JP, Vollmar C, Li Z, Fernandes J, Feddersen B, Noachtar S. Movement quantification during epileptic seizures: a new technical contribution to the evaluation of seizure semiology. *Proceedings of the 25th Annual International Conference of the IEEE EMBS, Cancun, Mexico, September 17-21.* 2003.
- So NK. Atonic phenomena and partial seizures. A reappraisal. *Adv Neurol* 1995; 67: 29-39.
- Swartz BE. Pseudo-absence seizures: A frontal lobe phenomenon. *J Epilepsy* 1992; 5: 80-93.
- Talairach J, Bancaud J, Geier S, Bordas-Ferrer M, Bonis A, Szikla G, Rusu M. The cingulate gyrus and human behaviour. *Electroencephalogr Clin Neurophysiol* 1973; 34: 45-52.

- Tassinari CA, Gastaut H. A particular form of muscular inhibition in epilepsy: the related epileptic silent period. *Topical Probl Psychiatr Neurol* 1969; 10: 178-86.
- Trinka E, Walser G, Unterberger I, Luef G, Benke T, Bartha L, *et al*. Asymmetric termination of secondarily generalized tonic-clonic seizures in temporal lobe epilepsy. *Neurology*. 2002; 59: 1254-6.
- Weil S, Arnold S, Eisensehr I, Noachtar S. Heart rate increase in otherwise subclinical seizures is different in temporal versus extratemporal seizure onset: support for temporal lobe autonomic influence. *Epileptic Disord* 2005; 7: 199-204.
- Werhahn KJ, Noachtar S, Arnold S, Pfander M, Henkel A, Winkler PA, Luders HO. Tonic seizures: their significance for lateralization and frequency in different focal epileptic syndromes. *Epilepsia* 2000; 41: 1153-61.
- Williamson PD, Spencer DD, Spencer SS, Novelly RA, Mattson RH. Complex partial seizures of frontal lobe origin. *Ann Neurol* 1985; 18: 497-504.
- Williamson PD, Thadani VM, Darcey TM, Spencer DD, Spencer SS, Mattson RH. Occipital lobe epilepsy: clinical characteristics, seizure spread patterns, and results of surgery. *Ann Neurol* 1992; 31: 3-13.
- Wyllie E, Lüders H, Morris HH, Lesser RP, Dinner DS. The lateralizing significance of versive head and eye movements during epileptic seizures. *Neurology* 1986; 36: 606-11.

The ictal semiology
of prefrontal epilepsies

Samden D. Lhatoo[1], David R. Sandeman[2]

[1] *Epilepsy Center, University Hospitals – Case Medical Center, Cleveland, USA*
[2] *Department of Neurosurgery, Frenchay Hospital, Bristol, United Kingdom*

■ Introduction

Using a classification based broadly on cytoarchitectural characteristics, the frontal lobe can be subdivided into the motor, premotor and prefrontal areas. Many authors further subdivide these areas on a functional and anatomical basis although variable interpretations of subdivision unfortunately complicate matters. The supplementary sensorimotor areas (SSMA), the pre-SSMA, the anterior mesial frontal cortex, the orbitofrontal cortex, the frontopolar regions and the anterior cingulate regions for example, are often treated as distinct from the prefrontal region which is often considered only in its lateral aspect. For the purpose of this chapter and review, we consider the prefrontal cortex as encompassing the anterior, dorsolateral cortex and frontal pole, comprising Brodmann areas 8, 9, 10, 11, 45, 46 and 47. Whilst crucial to many aspects of higher cognitive functioning, these areas are largely silent to electrical discharges and seizures arising in these areas become symptomatic only on spread to nearby eloquent cortex. These symptomatogenic areas include the frontal eye fields, supplementary eye fields, negative motor and motor language areas in the premotor cortex, SSMA in the mesial mid-frontal lobe and the primary motor cortex in the posterior mesial frontal and posterior lateral frontal lobe. They are also within or closer to the premotor/motor areas than the prefrontal cortex. However, are there specific semiological patterns and identifiable seizure networks in the spread of seizures of prefrontal lobe epilepsy that point to and facilitate clinical diagnosis? We review the available literature and discuss our own experience of the various seizure types seen in these epilepsies.

■ Methodological problems in literature

The ictal semiology of any focal epilepsy is a result of the ictal involvement of one or more symptomatogenic zones (Rosenow, 2004). However, several factors confound the clinical application of this simple relationship. The dialeptic and automotor manifestations of a focal seizure for example, usually cannot be pinned to a specific brain region with reproducible certainty. Where clinical manifestations can be confidently attributed to "eloquent" cortex, the area of symptomatogenicity is often neither within, nor in close proximity to the epileptogenic zone (Rosenow, 2004). In certain well studied focal epilepsy syndromes, mesial temporal lobe epilepsy due to hippocampal sclerosis for example, clinical diagnosis based on careful semiological analysis is plausible enough. However, with many of the frontal epilepsies, a confident clinical diagnosis of subtype (premotor, prefrontal, frontopolar, orbitofrontal, anterior cingulate or mesial frontal) is much more difficult. A good example of this difficulty is the bilateral asymmetric tonic seizure arising from the SSMA. This can constitute the dominant manifestation of epilepsies of disparate origins within the frontal lobe, having been reported in mesial frontal, orbitofrontal, dorsolateral, frontopolar, anterior cingulate epilepsies and even epilepsies arising from brain regions posterior to the central sulcus (Green et al., 1980; Morris et al., 1988; So, 1994; Salanova et al., 1995; Bleasel, 1996; Ohara et al., 2004). Conversely and confusingly, there are reports of SSMA epilepsies that do not include the bilateral asymmetric tonic seizure in their manifestation although these situations are more likely exceptional (Blume et al., 1991; Chauvel, 1992; Williamson et al., 1992a; Williamson et al., 1992b; Chauvel, 1995; Salanova et al., 1995; Williamson, 1995; Baumgartner et al., 1996; Ikeda et al., 2001; Ikeda et al., 2002). The profound connectivity and size of the frontal lobes probably explain the plethora of aura and seizure descriptions in the frontal lobe epilepsies. A relative dearth of systematic, standardized reporting suggests that matters currently remain unclear although overall, there is a plethora of generic frontal lobe epilepsy semiological literature (Geier et al., 1977; Stores et al., 1991; 1992; Bancaud & Talairach, 1992; Chauvel et al., 1992; Dreifuss, 1992; Quesney, Constain et al., 1992; Quesney, Constain et al., 1992; Roger & Bureau, 1992; Saygi et al., 1992; Veilleux et al., 1992; Wieser et al., 1992; Williamson, 1992; Harvey et al., 1993; Cascino, 1995; Chauvel et al., 1995; Laskowitz et al., 1995; Salanova et al., 1995; Wieser & Hajek, 1995; Williamson, 1995; Kramer et al., 1997; Gawel et al., 1998; Kotagal & Arunkumar, 1998; Swartz et al., 1998; Ferrier et al., 1999; Janszky et al., 2000; Mosewich et al., 2000; Provini et al., 2000; Williamson & Jobst, 2000; Fogarasi et al., 2001; Wetjen et al., 2002; Zaatreh et al., 2002; Kotagal et al., 2003; Kellinghaus & Luders, 2004; Prevost et al., 2006; Battaglia et al., 2007; Bonelli et al., 2007; Jeha et al., 2007; Lee et al., 2008; O'Brien et al., 2008).

In analyzing available literature, a clear distinction needs to be drawn between frontal lobe epilepsy and frontal lobe seizures (Dreifuss, 1992). The gold standard by which an epilepsy is determined to be frontal has to be enduring seizure freedom following frontal lobe resection. This exacting standard, whilst necessary, unfortunately renders the derivation of meaningful semiological information from many studies of frontal lobe epilepsy difficult. Equally, frontal lobe seizure semiology can be seen in some extra-frontal epilepsies (Blume et al., 1991; Chauvel, 1992; Williamson et al., 1992a; Williamson et al., 1992b; Chauvel, 1995; Salanova et al., 1995; Williamson, 1995; Baumgartner et al., 1996; Ikeda et al., 2001; Ikeda et al., 2002). By extension, unless curative surgical resection in a seizure free patient has been exquisitely restricted to a subdivision of the frontal lobe, calling an epilepsy prefrontal or orbito-frontal, for example, may not be accurate. In practice, frontal lobe resections often involve contiguous subdivisions – both because of the nature of the epilepsy and because wider resections probably improve chances of seizure freedom. Accordingly, surgeries that meticulously respect these boundaries are relatively infrequent.

■ Prefrontal epilepsy and prefrontal seizure semiology

In 1992, Bancaud and Talairach analyzed semiological characteristics in 210 patients with 648 frontal lobe seizures (Bancaud, 1992). They used a predominantly anatomical classification system of analysis (*Table I*). It is reasonable to assume that the intermediate dorsolateral frontal and the frontopolar regions in this classification would correspond closely to the prefrontal cortex.

Bancaud found that in the dorsolateral intermediate frontal group where 25 patients had 61 seizures, a variety of phenomena were observed. These included tonic adversive eye turning followed by contralateral head turning, face and motor disorders, visual hallucinations and illusions, forced thinking, complex postural manifestations, autonomic disorders and tonic-clonic generalization. However, they concluded that the most significant and frequent early sign was one of contralateral tonic deviation of the eyes, preceding head version. This was not the case with seizures arising from Brodmann areas 4 and 6. They held that the visual disturbances in this group, also a prominent feature, differed from those of occipital origin although overall, other authors have not made similar observations.

In 65 seizures arising in 14 patients of the frontopolar group, an equally diverse range of semiological features were noted. These included eye opening, staring, loss of contact, head and trunk anteflexion, complex gestural behavior, drops, tonic-clonic generalization, tonic axial seizure, bilateral clonic "complex" absences and "generalized" postural movements. Interestingly, they noted, as had Penfield, that there was early alteration of consciousness although this was not a statistically tested observation.

However, it is important to understand that Bancaud and Talairach identified patients for study through recorded ictal onsets in intra-operative or chronically implanted stereo-EEG electrodes. Furthermore, some of these were induced by megimide. Most importantly, cases were not identified according to surgical outcomes and so extra-frontal epileptogenic zones were therefore not conclusively excluded. In essence, this was a study examining frontal lobe seizures rather than frontal lobe epilepsy, a distinction that is not always heeded in literature and in clinical practice.

Table I. Topographic distribution of 648 frontal lobe seizures in 210 patients

Area of seizure onset	Seizures (n)	Patients (n)	Patients (%)
Areas 4 and 6	154	53	25
Inferior frontal gyrus	33	18	8
Intermediate medial frontal region	161	39	19
Intermediate dorsolateral frontal region	61	25	12
Anterior cingulate gyrus (area 24)	66	16	8
Frontopolar region	65	14	7
Orbitofrontal region	37	18	8
Operculo-insular region	71	27	13
Total	648	210	100

Another case series analyzed 40 patients, diagnosed with frontal lobe epilepsy on the basis of successful epilepsy surgery, the majority of whom would now be considered to have an Engel Class 1 outcome today (Quesney, Constain et al., 1992 [**1992a ou 1992b?**]). It would be reasonable to suppose that in these patients, the epileptogenic zones would have lain wholly or at least in part, within the frontal lobe. This was therefore a study of frontal lobe epilepsy rather than frontal lobe seizures. On the anatomical basis of their resections, they were classified into anterofrontal, parasagittal and fronto-opercular groups. Although varying amounts of prefrontal cortex may have been included within the resection margins of all three groups, the antero-frontal group, comprising 21 patients, is probably most representative of prefrontal epilepsy.

As can be seen in *Table II*, there is considerable semiological overlap between the three groups, the exceptions being an absence of SMA features in the fronto-opercular group and an absence of automatisms in the parasagittal group. The authors speculated on the connectivity of the anterofrontal and fronto-opercular areas to the temporal lobe via the uncinate fasciculus and cingulum as an explanation for automatisms in this group. Auras, as the initial clinical manifestations of seizures and most likely to indicate proximity to the epileptogenic zone, also overlapped between the different groups *(Table III)*. Contra-lateral head version, accounting for 80% of all versions, was seen in 44% (4 patients) of the fronto-opercular group as opposed to 30% (3 patients) and 19% (4 patients) of the parasagittal and antero-frontal groups respectively. In the fronto-opercular group, the dis-tribution of conscious and unconscious version was approximately equal – a finding that did not confirm Penfield's observations. Unfortunately, the numbers analyzed are so small that firm conclusions cannot really be drawn from them.

■ Prefrontal epilepsy and version

Penfield, in 1954, described a simple distinction between seizures arising from the anterior dorsolateral frontal cortex (prefrontal areas) and those arising from the intermediate dor-solateral frontal cortex (premotor areas) (Penfield, 1954). He held that the anterior seizure discharge produced the "unconscious adversive seizure" where the patient lost conscious-ness before version. In distinction, he believed that seizures arising from the more posterior discharge from within the premotor areas produced the conscious or "simple adversive seizure" where the patient not only remained aware of version, but sometimes tried to correct it with his own hand.

Table II. Behavioral (semiological) manifestations in patients with frontal lobe epilepsy

Region	N	Aura	PMC	PMT	Head/eye Turning	SMA	Arrest of Activity	Aphasia	Automatism
AF	21	9 (42%)	6 (29%)	2 (9.5%)	5 (20%)	1 (5%)	5 (24%)	5 (24%)	7 (33%)
PS	10	9 (90%)	6 (60%)	5 (50%)	4 (40%)	2 (20%)	2 (20%)	3 (30%)	0
FO	9	6 (67%)	4 (44%)	2 (22%)	4 (44%)	0	1 (11%)	1 (11%)	2 (22%)

AF: anterior frontal; PS: parasagittal; FO: fronto-opercular; PMC: partial motor clonic; PMT: partial motor tonic; SMA: supplementary motor area seizures.

Table III. Warnings (auras) in frontal lobe epilepsy

Type of aura	Region of surgical removal		
	PS	AF	FO
Cephalic	2	1	1
Somatosensory	6	-	-
Dizziness	-	3	-
Epigastric	-	1	2
Fear	-	1	-
Auditory	1	-	-
Visual	-	-	2
Dreamlike	-	-	-
Other	-	3	1

AF: anterior frontal; PS: parasagittal; FO: fronto-opercular.

His observations were based on a study of 222 cases published in 1951 where 7 patients had conscious version and 16 had unconscious version (Penfield, 1951). The premise for this lay in the hypothesis that anatomical distance between the premotor cortex and the motor cortex, where version was actually produced, was short. The seizure discharge therefore spread to this contiguous symptomatogenic area before it spread widely enough to bilateral cortex and/or to diencephalic and brainstem structures to produce loss of consciousness. On the other hand, the seizure discharge, if it arose from the anterior, prefrontal areas, had the opportunity to spread widely enough to produce loss or alteration of consciousness even before it spread to the version producing motor cortex. He did not identify any other semiological features that distinguished the two regions.

Whilst this distinction may be useful in determining prefrontal from premotor epilepsy, "unconscious" version can be seen commonly in temporal lobe epilepsy and indeed a variety of other epilepsies and so would appear not to be a useful semiological feature in determining prefrontal from extra-frontal epilepsy.

■ Statistical analysis of seizure semiology

In an attempt to systematically analyze seizure semiology, cluster analysis has been used to subdivide psychomotor seizures into frontobasal cingulate, temporal polar, temporal basal limbic, posterior temporal neocortical and opercular insular seizures (Wieser, 1983; Salanova et al., 1995). The same as been done with frontal lobe seizures in order to distinguish them from temporal lobe seizures separating frontal seizures into peri-rolandic, SMA and psychomotor seizure groups (Kotagal et al., 1995; Salanova et al., 1995). These studies have reported on relatively small sample sizes although one other study utilized the cluster analysis technique to look at seizure patterns in 252 patients with frontal and temporal lobe epilepsies (Manford et al., 1996). A combination of history, semiology, neuro-imaging and EEG were used to analyze 346 seizure descriptions in 252 patients. 14 different seizure types were identified. Version/posturing, focal somatosensory, Jacksonian motor and motor agitation were identified as seizure types typical of extratemporal epilepsies. In 7/29 (25%) of the "motor agitation" (hypermotor) group, the fronto-polar cortex was affected although most of these patients also had orbitofrontal cortex involvement. In the version/posturing group, 18 of the 29 lesional cases (62%), the lateral premotor cortex was involved and only 4/29 (14%) had fronto-polar, orbito-frontal or "rostral" frontal cortex involvement. Deriving any specific information on prefrontal epilepsy is therefore difficult in this study which falls short in a number of other areas as well. For example, there was no proof of the epileptogenic zone as surgical outcome was not a requisite; only a minority of patients had video-EEG monitoring and some of the information was questionnaire derived. However, there may be some merit in the statistical approach used although there is a requirement for much larger patient numbers and a very stringent scrutiny of aura descriptions, video-EEG analysis and a reasonable period of post-surgical seizure freedom to ensure identification of the epileptogenic zone. These are exacting requirements that are not easily met.

■ Case illustrations

We found 4 recent patients with surgical resections restricted to the dorsal pre-frontal cortex as ascertained by post-operative MRI scans in the database of the Bristol Complex Epilepsy Surgery Service who were seizure free after surgery at last follow-up. Three of these patients underwent invasive monitoring with subdural grids + depth electrodes.

Case 1

A 25 year old right-handed man with mild learning difficulties presented to the surgery program with a history of epilepsy from the age of 7 years without a background of epilepsy risk factors or family history. He reported a non-specific aura comprising a pressure like sensation in the head followed by bilateral asymmetric tonic seizures. Rarely, these went on to secondarily generalize. His interictal EEG showed sharp waves in the left frontal region, maximum in the F3 electrode. He underwent video-EEG monitoring which showed the ictal onsets to arise from the left frontal region although some of these could not be lateralized, appearing centrally. The clinical seizures were confirmed to be his habitual bilateral asymmetric tonic seizures. PET imaging was negative. Since no MRI lesion was demonstrable with high resolution 3T epilepsy protocol MRI scans, he underwent invasive monitoring for identification of the ictal onset zone and for cortical mapping of eloquent tissue. Invasive studies with a combination of subdural grids (4 x 8 lateral frontal, 4 × 4 orbitofrontal, 2 × 6 mesial frontal, 2 × 6 frontopolar) and frontal/cingulate depth electrodes confirmed ictal EEG onset of his habitual seizures from the left anterior lateral pre-frontal cortex *(Figure 1)*. After cortical mapping, he underwent a tailored resection of this area to include the ictal onset and irritative zones. He had ongoing seizure freedom at 6 months of follow-up on medication. Histopathology revealed cortical dysplasia.

Case 2

A 22 year old right handed woman was assessed for epilepsy surgery. Her habitual seizures had started at the age of 17 years without any prior history or family history of seizure risk factors. They were characterized by a right face somato-sensory aura followed by a right face tonic seizure and then secondary generalization. Routine interictal EEGs showed continuous slowing in the left fronto-central region with sharp transients in the same area. Video-EEG monitoring captured several typical seizures, with onset in the left frontal

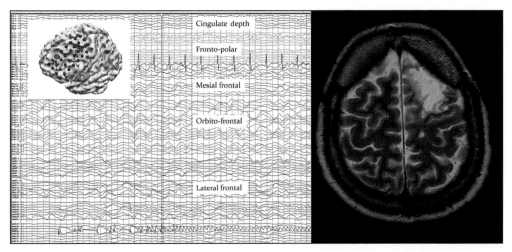

Figure 1. Anterior left lateral prefrontal cortex seizure onset in the 8 x 4 lateral frontal subdural grid and resection in Case 1.

region, maximum at the F7 electrode. Initial MRI scans were negative but high resolution 3T MRI frontal lobe protocol scans showed a trans-mantle cortical dysplasia in the left frontal lobe. She underwent invasive monitoring with a combination of frontal depth electrodes and subdural grids (8 × 8 lateral frontal, 2 × 6 mesial frontal, 2 × 8 frontopolar and orbitofrontal) which captured several of her habitual partial seizures. These consistently arose from the left posterior lateral prefrontal cortex. After mapping of eloquent cortex, she underwent a tailored resection to include the ictal onset and irritative zones. She was left with subtle, but resolving language difficulties after resection and was seizure free at 3 month follow-up on medication. Histopathology confirmed the presence of cortical dysplasia.

Case 3

A 32 year old right handed woman was assessed for epilepsy surgery after presenting with two generalized tonic clonic seizures 5 years previously followed by very frequent partial seizures. These were characterized by a non-specific aura of a funny feeling in the head followed by left face clonic seizures and left hemi-clonic seizures. High resolution 3T MRIs were consistently negative but interictal PET images showed extensive right frontal and right temporal hypometabolism. Interictal EEGs showed only continuous slowing in the right frontal region. Video-EEG monitoring showed that her typical clinical seizures began in the right frontal region, maximally in the F8 and F4 electrodes. Invasive monitoring was carried out with a combination of depth electrodes and subdural grids targeting the right frontal and temporal lobes in order to identify the ictal onset zone and to map eloquent cortex. Seizures were found to consistently arise from the posterior lateral prefrontal cortex. A tailored resection of the ictal onset and part of the irritative zones was carried out. At 3 month follow-up, the patient was deficit free and seizure free on medication.

Case 4

A 46 year old right handed man was referred for epilepsy surgery for intractable seizures arising from the age of 29 years. He suffered a seizure frequency of 3-4 seizures per week, each characterized by a feeling of dizziness and light headedness, followed by bilateral asymmetric tonic seizures. On two occasions, these had gone on to secondarily generalize. MRI scans showed a small DNET situated in the right anterior lateral prefrontal cortex, occupying the proximal end of the middle frontal gyrus. Video-EEG confirmed seizures arising from this area with ictal onsets maximum at the right frontal F8/F4/Fp2 electrodes. A decision to carry out a resection of the anterior lateral prefrontal cortex with a wide margin around the lesion without invasive studies was made. The patient became completely seizure free following surgery and remained so at 12 months of follow-up.

■ Conclusions

In this small sample of cases with lateral prefrontal epilepsy, no consistent pattern of aura onset and seizure progression can be observed that would distinguish them from premotor or any other kind of frontal epilepsy. In each case, the first clinical lateralization and localization features are provided by the most proximate eloquent cortex. In Case 1, this is evidenced by the proximity of the seizure onset electrode to the SSMA in the mesial frontal lobe. Here the patient became seizure free with resection of the ictal onset and irritative zones in the lateral prefrontal cortex without SSMA removal. In Case 2, the right face somatosensory aura is likely to have been a "motor" aura where the initial face tonicity was perceived as a "sensation" particularly since invasive studies did not reveal any activity at seizure onset in the face sensory cortex as identified by stimulation. However, the symptomatogenic area closest to the ictal onset electrodes was the face motor cortex. Case 3 had almost identical features. Thus Penfield's observation about seizures arising from the posterior lateral frontal areas and early symptom reporting in the absence of altered consciousness could be logically applied to the posterior lateral prefrontal cortex although this would not provide reliable distinction from premotor epilepsy. Further exploration of prefrontal epilepsy semiology can only be carried out through study of a large number of patients who have undergone frontal lobe resection cleanly restricted to the prefrontal cortex, are seizure as well as aura free and have undergone comprehensive, preferably intracranial electrophysiological studies that provide information and ultimately an understanding of seizure networks involved in seizure initiation and propagation.

References

- Bancaud J, Talairach J. Clinical semiology of frontal lobe seizures. *Adv Neurol* 1992; 57: 3-58.
- Battaglia D, Lettori D, *et al*. Seizure semiology of lesional frontal lobe epilepsies in children. *Neuropediatrics* 2007; 38 (6): 287-91.
- Baumgartner C, Flint R, *et al*. Supplementary motor area seizures: propagation pathways as studied with invasive recordings. *Neurology* 1996; 46 (2): 508-14.
- Bleasel AF, Morris HH 3rd. Supplementary sensorimotor area in adults. Supplementary sensorimotor area. *Adv Neurol* 1996; 70: 271-84.
- Blume WT, Whiting SE, *et al*. Epilepsy surgery in the posterior cortex. *Ann Neurol* 1991; 29 (6): 638-45.

- Bonelli SB, Lurger S, et al. Clinical seizure lateralization in frontal lobe epilepsy. *Epilepsia* 2007; 48 (3): 517-23.
- Cascino GD. Magnetic resonance imaging in frontal lobe epilepsy. *Adv Neurol* 1995; 66: 199-207; discussion 207-111.
- Chauvel P, Trottier S, et al. Somatomotor seizures of frontal lobe origin. *Adv Neurol* 1992; 57: 185-232.
- Chauvel P, Kliemann F, Vignal JP, Chodkiewicz JP, Talairach J, Bancaud J. The clinical signs and symptoms of frontal lobe seizures. Phenomenology and classification. *Adv Neurol* 1995; 66: 115-25; discussion 125-6.
- Dreifuss FE. From frontal lobe seizures to frontal lobe epilepsies. *Adv Neurol* 1992; 57: 391-8.
- Ferrier CH, Engelsman J, et al. Prognostic factors in presurgical assessment of frontal lobe epilepsy. *J Neurol Neurosurg Psychiatry* 1999; 66 (3): 350-6.
- Fogarasi A, Janszky J, et al. A detailed analysis of frontal lobe seizure semiology in children younger than 7 years. *Epilepsia* 2001; 42 (1): 80-5.
- Gawel M, Bidzinski J, et al. Frontal lobe epilepsy: symptomatology and results of surgical treatment. *Neurol Neurochir Pol* 1998; 32 (Suppl 2): 107-17.
- Geier S, Bancaud J, et al. The seizures of frontal lobe epilepsy. A study of clinical manifestations. *Neurology* 1977; 27 (10): 951-8.
- Green JR, Angevine JB, et al. Significance of the supplementary motor area in partial seizures and in cerebral localization. *Neurosurgery* 1980; 6 (1): 66-75.
- Harvey AS, Hopkins IJ, et al. Frontal lobe epilepsy: clinical seizure characteristics and localization with ictal 99mTc-HMPAO SPECT. *Neurology* 1993; 43 (10): 1966-80.
- Ikeda A, Matsumoto R, et al. Asymmetric tonic seizures with bilateral parietal lesions resembling frontal lobe epilepsy. *Epileptic Disord* 2001; 3 (1): 17-22.
- Ikeda A, Sato T, et al. "Supplementary motor area (SMA) seizure" rather than "SMA epilepsy" in optimal surgical candidates: a document of subdural mapping. *J Neurol Sci* 2002; 202 (1-2): 43-52.
- Janszky J, Fogarasi A, et al. Are ictal vocalisations related to the lateralisation of frontal lobe epilepsy? *J Neurol Neurosurg Psychiatry* 2000; 69 (2): 244-7.
- Jeha LE, Najm I, et al. Surgical outcome and prognostic factors of frontal lobe epilepsy surgery. *Brain* 2007; 130 (Pt 2): 574-84.
- Kellinghaus C, Luders HO. Frontal lobe epilepsy. *Epileptic Disord* 2004; 6 (4): 223-39.
- Kotagal P, Arunkumar G, et al. Complex partial seizures of frontal lobe onset statistical analysis of ictal semiology. *Seizure* 2003; 12 (5): 268-81.
- Kotagal P, Arunkumar GS. Lateral frontal lobe seizures. *Epilepsia* 1998; 39 (Suppl 4): S62-68.
- Kotagal P, Luders HO, et al. Psychomotor seizures of temporal lobe onset: analysis of symptom clusters and sequences. *Epilepsy Res* 1995; 20 (1): 49-67.
- Kramer U, Riviello JJ Jr, et al. Clinical characteristics of complex partial seizures: a temporal versus a frontal lobe onset. *Seizure* 1997; 6 (1): 57-61.
- Laskowitz DT, Sperling MR, et al. The syndrome of frontal lobe epilepsy: characteristics and surgical management. *Neurology* 1995; 45 (4): 780-7.
- Lee JJ, Lee SK, et al. Frontal lobe epilepsy: clinical characteristics, surgical outcomes and diagnostic modalities. *Seizure* 2008; 17 (6): 514-23.
- Manford M, Fish DR, et al. An analysis of clinical seizure patterns and their localizing value in frontal and temporal lobe epilepsies. *Brain* 1996; 119 (Pt 1): 17-40.
- Morris HH 3rd, Dinner DS, et al. Supplementary motor seizures: clinical and electroencephalographic findings. *Neurology* 1988; 38 (7): 1075-82.

- Mosewich RK, So EL, *et al.* Factors predictive of the outcome of frontal lobe epilepsy surgery. *Epilepsia* 2000; 41 (7): 843-9.
- O'Brien TJ, Mosewich RK, *et al.* History and seizure semiology in distinguishing frontal lobe seizures and temporal lobe seizures. *Epilepsy Res* 2008; 82 (2-3): 177-82.
- Ohara S, Ikeda A, *et al.* Propagation of tonic posturing in supplementary motor area (SMA) seizures. *Epilepsy Res* 2004; 62 (2-3): 179-87.
- Penfield W, Jasper H. *Epilepsy and the functional anatomy of the human brain.* London: J&A Churchill, 1954.
- Penfield WG, Kristiansen K. *Epileptic seizure patterns.* Springfield, 1951.
- Prevost J, Lortie A, *et al.* Nonlesional frontal lobe epilepsy (FLE) of childhood: clinical presentation, response to treatment and comorbidity. *Epilepsia* 2006; 47 (12): 2198-201.
- Provini F, Plazzi G, *et al.* The wide clinical spectrum of nocturnal frontal lobe epilepsy. *Sleep Med Rev* 2000; 4 (4): 375-86.
- Quesney LF, Constain M, *et al.* Seizures from the dorsolateral frontal lobe. *Adv Neurol* 1992; 57: 233-43.
- Quesney LF, Constain M, *et al.* Presurgical EEG investigation in frontal lobe epilepsy. *Epilepsy Res* 1992; (Suppl 5): 55-69.
- Roger J, Bureau M. Distinctive characteristics of frontal lobe epilepsy versus idiopathic generalized epilepsy. *Adv Neurol* 1992; 57: 399-410.
- Rosenow FL, Luders HO. *Presurgical Assessment of the epilepsies with clinical neurophysiology and functional imaging.* Amsterdam: Elsevier, *Handbook of Clinical Neurophysiology*, 2004; 3: 3-7.
- Salanova V, Morris HH, *et al.* Frontal lobe seizures: electroclinical syndromes. *Epilepsia* 1995; 36 (1): 16-24.
- Saygi S, Katz A, *et al.* Frontal lobe partial seizures and psychogenic seizures: comparison of clinical and ictal characteristics. *Neurology* 1992; 42 (7): 1274-7.
- So N. Supplementary motor area epilepsy: the clinical syndrome. In: P. Wolf, ed. *Epileptic seizures and syndromes.* London: John Libbey, 1994: 299-317.
- Stores G, Zaiwalla Z, *et al.* Frontal lobe complex partial seizures in children: a form of epilepsy at particular risk of misdiagnosis. *Dev Med Child Neurol* 1991; 33 (11): 998-1009.
- Swartz BE, Delgado-Escueta AV, *et al.* Surgical outcomes in pure frontal lobe epilepsy and foci that mimic them. *Epilepsy Res* 1998; 29 (2): 97-108.
- Veilleux F, Saint-Hilaire JM, *et al.* Seizures of the human medial frontal lobe. *Adv Neurol* 1992; 57: 245-55.
- Wetjen NM, Cohen-Gadol AA, *et al.* Frontal lobe epilepsy: diagnosis and surgical treatment. *Neurosurg Rev* 2002; 25 (3): 119-38; discussion 139-40.
- Wieser HG. *Electroclinical features of the psychomotor seizure.* Stuttgart; Fisher, London: Butterworths, 1983.
- Wieser HG, Hajek M. Frontal lobe epilepsy. Compartmentalization, presurgical evaluation, and operative results. *Adv Neurol* 1995; 66: 297-318; discussion 318-299.
- Wieser HG, Swartz BE, *et al.* Differentiating frontal lobe seizures from temporal lobe seizures. *Adv Neurol* 1992; 57: 267-85.
- Williamson PD. Frontal lobe seizures. Problems of diagnosis and classification. *Adv Neurol* 1992; 57: 289-309.
- Williamson PD. Frontal lobe epilepsy. Some clinical characteristics. *Adv Neurol* 1995; 66: 127-50; discussion 150-22.
- Williamson PD, Boon PA, *et al.* Parietal lobe epilepsy: diagnostic considerations and results of surgery. *Ann Neurol* 1992; 31 (2): 193-201.
- Williamson PD, Jobst BC. Frontal lobe epilepsy. *Adv Neurol* 2000; 84: 215-42.

- Williamson PD, Thadani VM, *et al*. Occipital lobe epilepsy: clinical characteristics, seizure spread patterns, and results of surgery. *Ann Neurol* 1992; 31 (1): 3-13.
- Zaatreh MM, Spencer DD, *et al*. Frontal lobe tumoral epilepsy: clinical, neurophysiologic features and predictors of surgical outcome. *Epilepsia* 2002; 43 (7): 727-33.

Semiology of mesial frontal and parietal lobe epilepsy

Bassel Abou-Khalil

Vanderbilt University Medical Center, Department of Neurology, Nashville, USA

The description of seizure semiology based on anatomic localization of the epileptogenic zone is derived mainly from epilepsy surgery centers, with different levels of ascertainment. The most definitive proof of relationship between semiology and localization is derived from seizure freedom following focal resection. Less definitive evidence is derived from MRI localization of an epileptogenic lesion, from ictal single photon emission tomography, and from EEG localization with implanted intracranial or with scalp electrodes. Even with the most definitive anatomic localization of the epileptogenic zone, it is important to note that seizure manifestations do not only depend on the region of seizure origin, but also on the path of seizure propagation. Thus, seizures originating in the mesial frontal or parietal cortex could manifest with lateral frontal or even temporal semiology if seizures rapidly propagate to these regions, and seizures propagating to the mesial frontal cortex from other regions could manifest with semiology typical of mesial frontal involvement. While there are several clinical seizure patterns described with mesial frontal or parietal epileptogenic zones, most are not specific.

Seizures originating in the mesial frontal and parietal regions *(Figure 1)* often present with unusual or bizarre manifestations that result in misdiagnosis as psychogenic non-epileptic events. The recognition of these clinical patterns is made even more important because the depth and unfavorable orientation of electrical dipoles may make abnormal electrical activity invisible on EEG. Interictal epileptiform activity may be absent and ictal activity may be subtle and masked with muscle and motion artifact.

The two main seizure patterns recognized to originate in the mesial fronto-parietal region are supplementary motor area seizures and frontal lobe hypermotor seizures. There are also other seizure types that are less frequently reported, including frontal lobe absence seizures, focal clonic or myoclonic and focal sensory seizures affecting the lower extremity, frontal lobe akinetic or atonic seizures, startle induced seizures and frontal lobe gelastic seizures. Each seizure type will be described individually.

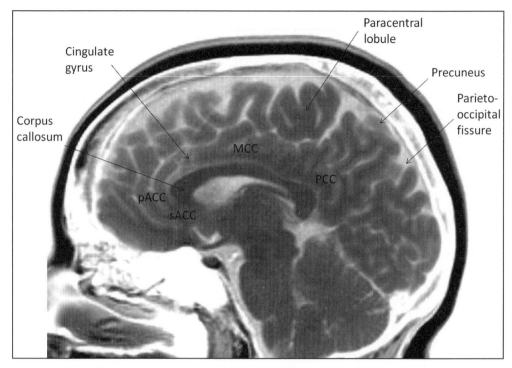

Figure I. Sagital MRI image demonstrating key anatomical structures and landmarks. The figure also shows some subdivisions of the cingulate cortex as suggested by Vogt (Vogt, 2005). ACC: anterior cingulate cortex; sACC: subgenu ACC; pACC: pregenu ACC; MCC: mid-cingulate cortex; PCC: posterior cingulate cortex.

■ Supplementary motor area seizures

The supplementary motor area (SMA) was first identified in the human mesial frontal region by Penfield and Welch (Penfield, 1949). It is located anterior to the primary motor area for the lower extremity, above the cingulate sulcus. It is distinguished from the primary motor area in that its stimulation produces simultaneous contraction of several muscle groups with tonic contraction and posturing rather than clonic activity (Lim, 1994). The classical supplementary motor area (SMA) seizures are brief asymmetrical tonic seizures not associated with loss of consciousness (Video 1). However, the motor activity may be preceded in by sensory symptoms in a large minority of patients. The sensory symptoms may be unusual and may be described as pulling, pulsing, heaviness, numbness, or tingling (Morris, 1988). These sensations can be contralateral, ipsilateral, or bilateral. They may even be cephalic (Bleasel, 1996; Canuet, 2008). One peculiar feature is that the sensory aura may involve a very focal body area, and one with a small cortical representation that is not typically involved with primary sensory area seizures. For example the sensory aura may be in the thigh, the shoulder, the axilla or a small region of the trunk (Morris, 1988; Reutens, 1996). When there is no sensory aura, the onset is abrupt, usually with tonic posturing of one or more extremities (Morris, 1988). If only one arm or one arm and one leg are involved, the tonic posturing is generally contralateral to the epileptogenic zone. Most often, more than one extremity is involved, and there may be tonic posturing on both sides. In the Cleveland Clinic series of Morris *et al.*, all four extremities were involved in two out of 11 patients (Morris, 1988). Supplementary motor seizures are an important exception to the rule that consciousness is lost with bilateral motor activity. The upper extremity posturing typically involves abduction at the shoulder, and there may also be external rotation. The posturing of the extremities is predominately proximal while the hands and fingers or feet and toes may seem to be free and the patient may wiggle them. The lower extremity posturing may involve extension or there may be some flexion at the hip and knee (Williamson, 2008). Towards the end of the seizure there may be a few rhythmic clonic movements before relaxation occurs. When only the contralateral side is involved, there may be thrashing, flailing or writhing movements of the ipsilateral side. The tonic posturing may spread sequentially from one body part to another (Ohara, 2004). Despite the variability of motor manifestations between patients, the seizure pattern is typically stereotyped with a particular patient.

In the classical description of the "fencing posture", the head is deviated to look at the extended arm (Penfield, 1954). However, head turning is not a common feature of SMA seizures that do not progress to secondary generalization (Bleasel, 1996; Morris, 1988), and head deviation without secondary generalization may be either contralateral or ipsilateral (Bleasel, 1996; Green, 1980). Thus, head deviation is not lateralizing, but if there is secondary generalization, the direction of versive head deviation in transition to generalization is usually contralateral (Wyllie, 1986).

The tonic posturing is commonly associated with speech arrest but also variably associated with vocalizations. The patient may emit loud moaning, groaning or gasping sounds, or repeated vowel sounds or syllables (Cho, 2009; Morris, 1988; Williamson, 2008). Some patients may report difficulty breathing during attacks.

Seizures most often predominate out of sleep, but they may also occur in waking. The seizure duration is typically 10-30 seconds, and it is rare for seizures to last longer than one minute. However, seizures often recur in clusters that can last up to an hour or more.

Consciousness is typically preserved during seizures (Morris, 1988). Even though the patients may not be able to respond, they are able to recall words given to them during the tonic contraction. However, consciousness may be impaired with more severe seizures associated with medication withdrawal, particularly when there is secondary generalization (Reutens, 1996). Postictal recovery is very fast, and the seizures seem to stop as fast as they start.

Precipitation by startle has been occasionally reported in SMA seizures (Aguglia, 1984; Serles, 1999), and it has even been suggested that startle epilepsy is an epilepsy of the supplementary motor area (Bancaud, 1968; Garcia-Morales, 2009). However, startle-induced tonic seizures have also been reported with parietal lobe foci (Kanemoto, 2001), as well as with generalized tonic seizures (Tibussek, 2006).

It is important to recognize that typical SMA seizure semiology is not specific for seizures originating in the supplementary motor area, and is not uncommonly seen with seizures presumably propagating to the SMA from outside the SMA (Aghakhani, 2004; Ikeda, 2001). The possibility also exists that the same tonic manifestations may arise outside the SMA (Geier, 1977; Williamson, 1992a; Williamson, 1992b).

The differential diagnosis of SMA seizures includes psychogenic non-epileptic seizures and generalized tonic seizures. Patients with supplementary motor seizures are often misdiagnosed with non-epileptic psychogenic seizures based on the absence of interictal or recognized ictal activity in association with events. In addition the report of bilateral motor activity without altered consciousness and the very high seizure frequency elicit a suspicion of psychogenic origin. The key features that distinguish SMA seizures from psychogenic seizures are that they are short in duration, are stereotypic, and typically occur in sleep, while psychogenic seizures tend to be long in duration, non-stereotypic, and occur in the awake state (Kanner, 1990). In addition, the tonic contraction of the upper extremities in abduction was specific for SMA seizures (Kanner, 1990). The development of secondary generalization after withdrawal of antiepileptic drugs in the epilepsy monitoring unit may be the most definitive criterion to distinguish SMA seizures from psychogenic seizures. Generalized tonic seizures tend to be symmetrical (but SMA seizures may also be symmetrical at times) and tend to involve the axial muscles with flexion. They usually occur in the setting of symptomatic generalized epilepsy, in patients with evidence of diffuse cognitive dysfunction, in the company of other seizure types including atypical absence seizures, atonic seizures, and generalized tonic-clonic seizures. The EEG is very helpful to distinguish the two seizure types. Patients with symptomatic generalized epilepsy usually have generalized slow spike-and-wave discharges in waking and generalized paroxysmal fast activity in sleep. Finally, SMA seizures may be misdiagnosed as paroxysmal movement disorder or sleep disorder. The preponderance of evidence now suggests that the entity of paroxysmal nocturnal dystonia is actually a form of frontal lobe epilepsy (Hirsch, 1994; Meierkord, 1992; Montagna, 1992; Tinuper, 1990).

Other seizure semiologies have been described with seizure onset in the SMA, including seizures with inhibitory manifestation, but these will be described under a separate heading.

■ Frontal lobe hypermotor seizures

Hypermotor seizures, characterized by prominent agitated motor activity have been variably named frontal lobe "hyperkinetic" seizures, frontal lobe seizures with bizarre behaviors, and frontal lobe complex partial seizures. Hypermotor seizures were first reported with orbitofrontal epileptogenic foci (Tharp, 1972), but they may also arise from the cingulate cortex. The most prominent clinical feature is abrupt prominent agitated frenetic motor activity at onset (Williamson, 1985; Williamson, 1986). Such activity could include back and forth rocking, vigorous flailing or thrashing movements of all extremities, kicking or bicycling movements, side-to-side head motions, and pelvic thrusting (Video 2). Sexual automatisms have been described, including genital manipulation, masturbatory activity, and sexually suggestive motions (Spencer, 1983; Williamson, 1985). Vocalizations are common and may include screaming, yelling, uttering expletives, or even producing animal sounds such as barking, growling or howling. Mild seizures may be less pronounced and may just be characterized by arousal from sleep and a little thrashing in bed. The seizures are usually brief, shorter than 30 seconds, and have minimal if any postictal manifestations (Williamson, 1985). They tend to occur out of sleep, and they tend to be frequent and to cluster. Due to their brief duration and their tendency to occur out of sleep, it is often difficult to assess if they have an associated loss of awareness. Some patients claim to remain aware of their environment, but to be unable to control their motor activity or to respond during attacks.

Some peculiar automatisms noted in mesial frontal seizures have been reproduced with electrical stimulation (Chassagnon, 2008). Irrepressible groping, reaching and grasping were elicited at the vicinity of the cingulate sulcus anterior to the supplementary motor area (Chassagnon, 2008).

Frontal lobe complex partial hypermotor seizures do not usually include oroalimentary automatisms such as lip smacking and chewing that are so typical of mesial temporal seizures. However, they may spread to the temporal lobe at which point they may resemble typical temporal lobe seizures (Williamson, 2000). When they do, they are longer in duration and they may have more pronounced postictal manifestations such as confusion and aphasia than seizures remaining confined to the frontal lobe.

It was initially noted that the clinical manifestations of frontal lobe hypermotor complex partial seizures do not usually allow localization within the frontal lobe, and often do not allow lateralization either (Williamson, 2000), unless they progress to tonic or clonic motor manifestations. They are most likely to arise in either the mesial frontal cortex, particularly cingulate gyrus or the orbitofrontal cortex, but can also arise elsewhere in the frontal lobe (Chauvel, 1995; Jobst, 2000). Hypermotor seizures have also been reported to arise occasionally in the temporal lobe and in the insula (Holthausen, 2000; Ryvlin, 2006). One report found that hypermotor manifestations are particularly common in patients with temporal pole lesions (Wang, 2008). However, the hypermotor manifestations usually reflect seizure spread to the frontal lobe, particularly orbitofrontal region (Vaugier, 2009; Wang, 2008).

Attempts at sub-classifying hypermotor seizures have suggested that certain clinical features may have localizing value. Some hypermotor seizures may include posturing which is otherwise characteristic of supplementary motor seizures, and that component is helpful in suggesting a mesial frontal origin. One retrospective study classified hypermotor behavior in 11 patients who became seizure free following epilepsy surgery. Two types of hypermotor seizures were noted. One type characterized by marked agitation with body rocking, kicking, or boxing, and a facial expression of fear tended to arise from the orbitofrontal region or anterior cingulate region (Rheims, 2008). The other type which consisted of mild agitation with either horizontal movements or rotation of trunk and pelvis usually associated with tonic or dystonic posturing tended to arise within the mesial premotor cortex (Rheims, 2008). The observation that asymmetrical posturing was more likely with mild than marked agitation was also noted in another study, but this was not clearly associated with a mesial origin (Tao, 2010). In another study of patients who have become seizure-free with focal resection, one sign stood out as prevalent in mesial frontal lobe epilepsy and useful in distinguishing it from lateral and orbitofrontal epilepsy. Ictal body turning along the horizontal axis occurred in 57% of patients with mesial frontal lobe epileptogenic foci (28 patients) but only 6.3% of those with lateral frontal (48 patients) and 0% of those with orbitofrontal (8 patients) foci (Leung, 2008). The direction of turning did not have a relationship to the side of the epileptogenic zone, and at times was in opposite directions in the same patient. Cluster analysis of signs in mesial frontal epilepsy demonstrated that the most strongly clustered syndrome was ictal body turning along the horizontal axis, restlessness, facial expression of anxiety and fear, and barking vocalizations, present in 21.5% of patients (Leung, 2008).

The main differential diagnosis of hypermotor seizures is non-epileptic psychogenic seizures. Because of their bizarre manifestations it is not unusual for hypermotor seizures to be misdiagnosed as psychogenic. The problem is compounded by that the interictal EEG is often normal and ictal EEG recordings are masked with artifact and show limited if any changes. One study comparing frontal lobe partial seizures and psychogenic seizures found no difference between the two with respect to ictal pelvic thrusting, rocking of body, side-to-side head movements, or rapid postictal recovery, all reported to be features characteristic of psychogenic non-epileptic seizures (Saygi, 1992). The main distinguishing semiological features were ictal duration with longer duration favoring psychogenic seizures (mean of 51 seconds in frontal lobe seizures versus 176 seconds in psychogenic seizures), and nocturnal occurrence and stereotyped pattern which favored frontal lobe partial seizures (Saygi, 1992). One interesting feature that occurred in frontal lobe seizures but not in psychogenic seizures was turning to a prone position. Five out of 11 patients with frontal lobe epilepsy turned to a prone position as part of hypermotor behavior that included rocking, thrashing, hitting the pillow, and in two patients making wild noises. Turning prone is most probably the consequence of ictal body turning along the horizontal axis, described as a feature of mesial frontal lobe origin (Leung, 2008). The quality of vocalization was different between frontal lobe epilepsy and psychogenic seizure patients. Vocalizations had an emotional character in patients with psychogenic seizures, while vocalizations in frontal lobe epilepsy were described as continuous, often monotonous with moaning or grunting, sometimes resembling animal noises, and occasionally with wild loud noises (Saygi, 1992).

Mild hypermotor seizures could be difficult to distinguish from arousals from sleep, particularly when the EEG failed to show ictal or interictal changes. However, this is not an issue with the more severe attacks, particularly when multiple stereotyped attacks have been recorded.

■ Other seizure types of mesial frontal and parietal origin

Frontal absence seizures

Absence seizures also referred to as "dialeptic seizures" are most often seen in idiopathic and in symptomatic generalized epilepsy, and are clinically characterized by altered responsiveness and arrest of activity for a few seconds with almost immediate return to baseline at the end of the seizure. At times there is partial preservation of awareness with inability to respond during the ictal discharge (Gloor, 1986). The seizures are usually associated with rhythmic generalized spike-and-wave activity. The possibility has been raised that generalized absence seizures may be of frontal origin (Craiu, 2006; Kubota, 1997). Some absence seizures have been documented to originate in the frontal lobe, particularly in the mesial frontal region (So, 1998). Niedermeyer *et al.* reported a deep right frontal seizure onset in one patient with typical generalized 3 Hz spike-and-wave discharges who underwent monitoring with depth electrodes. There was almost complete disappearance of absence seizures with a medial frontal lobectomy (Niedermeyer, 1969). Bancaud and colleagues reproduced bursts of generalized 3-Hz spike-and-wave activity as well as clinical absence seizures with stimulation of one frontal lobe with depth electrodes (Bancaud, 1974). The electrodes that produced absence seizures were almost always located in the mesial frontal cortex, extending from the rolandic region to the frontal pole, sometimes in the cingulate gyrus (Bancaud, 1974). In another study increased sporadic and rhythmic spike-and-wave activity was reported with electrical stimulation of the anterior cingulate, in four out of 10 patients who had interictal spike-and-wave discharges, but clinical absence seizures did not occur (Mazars, 1970). On the other hand, the author reported that the first seizures of all of 36 patients with cingulate epilepsy consisted of "absences" that did not differ much from the short attacks of loss of consciousness of "petit mal" seizures. However, some patients had a brief associated head dropping or nodding, some had blushing, and occasionally there was contralateral head turning. In addition,

are occasionally precipitated by unexpected somatosensory stimuli, or even sudden visual stimuli. Unusual precipitating stimuli in patients with startle-induced seizures include gait (Saeki, 2009; Toledano, 2010). Most patients also have spontaneous seizures, usually preceding the onset of startle-induced seizures (Rosenow, 2000). Epilepsy with startle-induced seizures can be focal or generalized. If it is focal, it is often localized to the supplementary motor area or neighboring regions (Bancaud, 1968; Cokar, 2001; Garcia-Morales, 2009; Manford, 1996; Nolan, 2005; Serles, 1999). It is also well-recognized that supplementary motor seizures can be provoked by startle (Reutens, 1996).

Frontal lobe akinetic or atonic seizures

Seizures characterized by focal weakness or loss of tone or focal motor inhibition have been variably named inhibitory motor seizures, negative motor seizures, seizures with ictal paralysis, focal atonic seizures, or focal akinetic seizures (Abou-Khalil, 1995; Noachtar, 1999; Noachtar, 2000). These seizures are usually simple partial or start as simple partial seizures with later evolution to altered awareness. The ictal paralysis may be seen in isolation, may be followed by positive motor (tonic or clonic) activity in the same affected extremity, or may be accompanied by positive motor activity in a different body part on the same side (Noachtar, 2000). These seizures are usually of frontal or parietal origin and the epileptogenic zone may be localized to the mesial frontoparietal cortex in some patients. The ictal paralysis is presumed due to involvement of a negative motor area, the electrical stimulation of which may cause arrest of movement or weakness (Lüders, 1995; Lüders, 1992). One of the two main negative motor areas identified with electrical stimulation is in the mesial frontal region, near the supplementary motor area, while the other is close to Broca's language area in the inferior frontal cortex (Ikeda, 2009).

Generalized atonic seizures are usually a seizure type in some forms of symptomatic generalized epilepsy (such as Lennox-Gastaut syndrome) and myoclonic-astatic epilepsy. However, there are reports of apparently generalized atonic seizures arising focally from the frontal or parietal region, with some evidence favoring mesial or parasagittal involvement (Levin, 1991; Satow, 2002). The falls in these patients tended to be slow in contrast to the falls in Lennox-Gastaut syndrome, which tended to be abrupt (Satow, 2002).

One recent series suggested mesial frontal localization in ten patients with bilateral akinetic seizures without weakness and without altered consciousness (Toledano, 2010). During the seizures most patients were unable to move or speak, and appeared frozen. Subtle upper limb myoclonus was seen at times. There was no postictal deficit. In two patients, there was abrupt gait interruption, but the patients could still talk. In these two patients, the seizures were precipitated by standing up, starting to walk, or turning, and at times by startle. The seizures were short, usually less than 20 seconds in duration, but prolonged seizures or seizure clusters occurred at times (Toledano, 2010). Interictal and ictal EEG discharges were in the midline frontal region. This localization was supported by imaging abnormalities in some patients. However, this localization was not confirmed with invasive EEG or seizure remission with focal resection.

Frontal lobe gelastic seizures

Gelastic seizures are characterized by sudden onset of laughter unrelated to external stimuli. The attacks are typically short in duration, usually lasting less than 30 seconds. The similarity to natural laughter can result in diagnostic delay until other seizure types prompt a diagnostic evaluation. Gelastic seizures are most commonly reported in association with hypothalamic hamartomas (Berkovic, 2003; Cascino, 1993a). There may be other associated seizure types, and the laughter itself may progress to motor manifestations. However, patients are usually aware during the laughter. Gelastic seizures can be reproduced with electrical stimulation of hypothalamic hamartomas and do not require spread of the ictal discharge to other structures (Kahane, 2003; Kuzniecky, 1997). However, gelastic seizures may occur with both temporal and frontal lobe epilepsy (Arroyo, 1993; Battaglia, 2007; Chassagnon, 2003; Cheung, 2007; Iwasa, 2002; Kurle, 2000; McConachie, 1997; Mohamed, 2007; Oehl, 2009; Sartori, 1999; Umeoka, 2008; Unnwongse, 2010). Laughter was also induced by electrical stimulation of cingulate cortex and basal temporal cortex (Arroyo, 1993; Oehl, 2009; Unnwongse, 2010). It is interesting that an associated sense of mirth is typical of temporal gelastic seizures, while frontal and hypothalamic gelastic seizures are not generally associated with emotion (Arroyo, 1993; Iwasa, 2002). Gelastic seizures of frontal origin may have preserved awareness, while temporal lobe gelastic seizures are most often a component of complex partial seizures with altered awareness and responsiveness (but often preceded by a sense of mirth). On the other hand, gelastic manifestations in mesial frontal seizures may also be accompanied by other semiology such as hypermotor manifestations or tonic posturing.

Complex partial seizures resembling temporal lobe complex partial ("automotor" or "psychomotor") seizures

Some mesial frontoparietal seizures may first manifest with clinical manifestation typical of temporal lobe epilepsy, including staring, altered awareness and responsiveness, oroalimentary automatisms, manipulative distal extremity automatisms, and postictal confusion. This is a common occurrence in seizures originating in the posterior cingulate region (Garzon, 2008; Nadkarni, 2009). There is evidence that the posterior cingulate is clinically silent and that its seizure semiology is related to seizure propagation to the mesial temporal structures (Fujii, 1999; Koubeissi, 2009).

Cingulate seizures

Seizures arising from the cingulate cortex are not homogeneous, and may include hypermotor seizures, asymmetrical tonic seizures, and other seizure types. However, some specific semiologic features have been suggested in relation to seizures arising in sub regions of the cingulate cortex (Figure 1), related to the functions of these regions (Nadkarni, 2009). This is particularly the case with the smallest seizures that have limited spread to other regions. For example, autonomic manifestations may be seen with seizures arising in the subgenu anterior cingulate cortex, including tachycardia, papillary dilation, changes in respiratory frequency, warmth, pallor or blushing, urge to void, or even piloerection (Bancaud, 1992; Madhavan, 2007; Mazars, 1970; Nadkarni, 2009; Seo, 2003). Seizures arising in the pre-genu anterior cingulate may include altered motivation and fear and often progress to altered awareness and responsiveness through bilateral seizure spread (Nadkarni, 2009). It is suspected that ictal feeling of impending danger may be a result of involvement of that region (Romeo,

2008). Seizures arising in or involving the mid-cingulate cortex can cause emotional expressions such as laughter, or fragments of these expressions, devoid of associated emotion (Nadkarni, 2009). However, seizure spread to the adjacent supplementary motor area is common. The posterior cingulate cortex appears silent with electrical stimulation (Nadkarni, 2009). Seizures arising there often manifest only after spread to the mesial temporal lobe, with manifestations such as altered consciousness, lip smacking, distal manipulative automatisms, and postictal confusion, which are typical of mesial temporal lobe epilepsy (Garzon, 2008; Koubeissi, 2009). Interestingly, the posterior cingulate and precuneus are tonically active in the baseline state, part of the "default mode of the brain" (Raichle, 2001). These structures are presumed to continuously gather information about the environment, as part of consciousness, and they are deactivated in association with tasks that divert attention, and also in association with generalized spike-and-wave discharges and absence seizures (Archer, 2003; Gotman, 2005). Deactivation of bilateral posterior cingulate may be related to altered consciousness seen with absence seizures.

Mesial parietal seizures

Parietal lobe seizures are best recognized when they have a somatosensory aura, particularly if the sensation has a jacksonian march (see above). Other auras recognized to be of parietal origin include vertigo, a sensation that a body part is moving or is absent, or difficulty localizing position in space (Salanova, 1995a). Some patients report inability to move one extremity or of a feeling of weakness in the contralateral upper extremity (Abou-Khalil, 1995; Salanova, 1995a). However, several studies found that parietal lobe symptoms are absent in the majority of patients with parietal lobe epilepsy, and the seizure manifestations result from seizure spread to other lobes, particularly frontal, temporal, or occipital (Geier, 1977; Ikeda, 2001; Kim, 2004; Siegel, 2000; Williamson, 1992a). Seizures spreading anteriorly may manifest with tonic posturing or hypermotor manifestations, seizures spreading to the mesial temporal lobe may present with altered consciousness, oroalimentary automatisms and distal extremity automatisms, and those spreading to the occipital lobe may manifest with visual hallucinations or amaurosis (Siegel, 2000).

Some patient series included patients with mesial parietal foci (Akimura, 2003; Cascino, 1993b; Salanova, 1995b; Williamson, 1992a), but there are very few studies that specifically evaluated the semiology of seizures originating in the mesial parietal region. The manifestations were usually related to seizure spread to temporal or frontal regions (Fujii, 1999; Koubeissi, 2009; Umeoka, 2007). One case report described linear self-motion perception with seizures originating in the paramedian precuneus (Wiest, 2004). Symptoms were reproduced by electrical stimulation of the same region (Wiest, 2004).

■ Conclusion

Seizures arising in the mesial frontal and parietal regions can manifest with a variety of semiological patterns, some of which reflect seizure propagation rather that site of seizure origin. Although no seizure pattern is totally specific for mesial frontal localization, some seizure semiologies such as asymmetric tonic seizures and hypermotor seizures should prompt a search for mesial frontoparietal epileptogenic lesions and epileptogenic zones.

Case presentation

A 15 year old right-handed boy first presented to the Vanderbilt Epilepsy Clinic with seizures that started at age 7. He reported that 20% of seizures started with a feeling of numbness in the left leg and immediately in the left foot. Sometimes, the left hand was also involved. This warning lasted 1-2 minutes and then he had painful stiffening of the left foot followed immediately by stiffening of the whole left side and then jerking of the left side. About one year before presentation, the motor activity with the seizures became bilateral. Even then, he insisted that he was completely conscious during the whole attack. The seizure duration was usually 10 seconds, but it lasted up to 2 minutes after which he felt weak on the left side, and to a lesser extent, weak all over. He also experienced numbness in the left leg and left hand. He reported more than 15 seizures each night throughout the night, and between 4 and 15 seizures during the day while he was awake. Seizures tended to occur in clusters, with up to eight seizures in a row. He denied isolated auras but reported having single jerks of the left side as the smallest seizure type. He reported secondary generalized tonic-clonic seizures only five or six times ever.

Past medical history offered no definite risk factors for epilepsy. He was born of a full-term pregnancy and a normal delivery. He had normal developmental milestones and no febrile convulsions. He did have a mild head injury at around age 7, preceding the onset of seizures, when he fell off his bike, and may have been knocked out for a moment. There was no family history of epilepsy in first or second degree relatives.

At an outside institution he had an EEG at age 8 that recorded rare vertex spikes. He had normal MRI scans and a fluorodeoxyglucose (FDG) PET scan that reported focal 40% decrease in FDG activity involving the superior, medial and posterior aspects of the right temporal lobe, not corresponding to any MRI anatomic abnormality. EEG-video monitoring recorded 28 habitual seizures, most of which arose out of stage II sleep with EEG activity obscured by muscle artifact. Interictally there was polymorphic delta activity at the vertex and central regions, occasionally more prominent on the right. An attempt at ictal SPECT was not successful, because of the short seizure duration. Because of suspicion of Rasmussen syndrome, he had brain biopsy from the right superior parasagittal region, but this revealed no pathology.

The review of systems indicated difficulty with short-term memory and a decline in school performance. His sleep was disrupted by frequent seizures and he reported excessive tiredness and fatigue.

Neurological examination revealed normal strength, but slower rapid fine movements on the left, and associated mirror movements of the right hand. He had a slight left hyperreflexia and a left upgoing toe. Sensory examination was normal. He had three seizures during his clinic visit. The seizures were characterized by a brief aura and then sudden tonic posturing of the left lower extremity and then the left upper extremity. The right side remained free during that time, and he was able to follow commands with his right hand during the seizure. The seizure duration was less than 30 seconds and it was clear that he had preserved consciousness throughout the seizure.

The patient and the family were not initially interested in surgical therapy. A trial of various medical therapies and vagus nerve stimulation failed to have sufficient impact. Medications that were helpful reduced or even eliminated daytime seizures, but seizures out of sleep never stopped, and he had at least 6-9 every night. Some medications or medication combinations that were helpful also caused unacceptable adverse effects.

Seizures became more frequent when these medications were removed, and some days he reported more than 50 seizures per day. He eventually expressed interest in epilepsy surgery at age 19.

A 2-day video-EEG study recorded 24 seizures characterized by abduction and tonic extension of left arm and leg, sometimes with fanning of left hand fingers, followed by flexion of the right elbow, back arching, and neck extension (video 1). He turned to the left with some seizures. He clearly remained conscious during his seizures and was able to recall words and speak clearly at the cessation of motor activity. The EEG ictal discharge was most often masked by muscle artifact. Just before the onset of the artifact there was at times brief bifrontocentral rhythmic alpha-theta activity, maximal in the midline (at FCz), but sometimes with slight right predominance (*Figure 2*). There were no interictal epileptiform discharges.

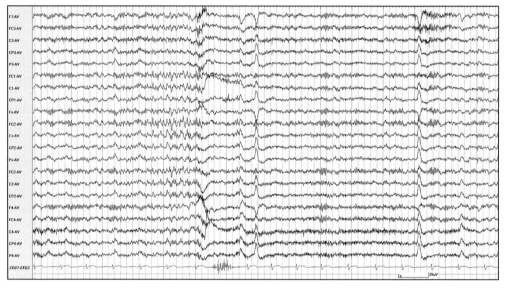

Figure 2. Ictal EEG on scalp recording. The clinical onset (six seconds from beginning of sample) was preceded by brief rhythmic sharp alpha-theta activity maximal at FCz.

Brain MRI only showed the old biopsy. Positron emission tomography with fluorodeoxyglucose (FDG) suggested decreased FDG uptake in the right parasagittal region, corresponding to the region of previous biopsy. Ictal SPECT suggested increased tracer uptake in the midline frontal region.

Neuropsychological testing supported generalized cognitive dysfunction. His full scale IQ was 64, verbal IQ 70, and performance IQ 63. Visual and verbal memory skills were also impaired, visual worse than verbal.

He underwent implantation of subdural grid electrodes. One 64(8 x 8)-electrode grid array was placed over the right frontal and parietal convexity. A 20(2 × 5 bi-sided)-electrode grid was then placed in the interhemispheric fissure overlying the central sulcus. Another 10(2 × 5)-electrode grid was placed in the interhemispheric fissure to record from the right anterior frontal region (*Figure 3*). Thirteen typical seizures were recorded out of sleep. The ictal EEG onset was focal in the right mesial posterior frontal subdural electrodes (*Figure 4*). Numerous subclinical seizures also suggested the same localization. The

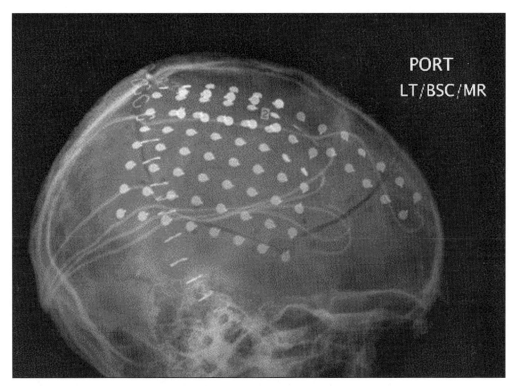

Figure 3. Skull film demonstrating implanted subdural electrode grids.

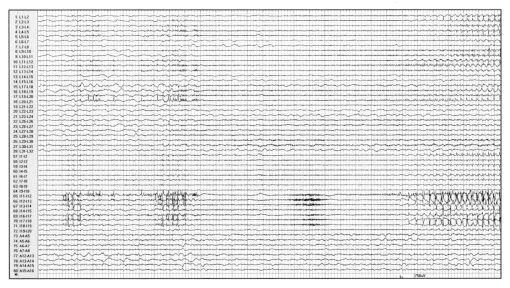

Figure 4. Ictal EEG from subdural electrodes (see *Figure 5*). The discharges to the left of the image were extremely frequent "interictal" bursts. The ictal onset was with the burst of fast activity that was maximal at 111 at the end of the second burst. The posturing started immediately after that.

predominant interictal epileptiform activity was also overwhelmingly right mesial posterior frontal, although some epileptiform discharges were also recorded from the lateral convexity. The cortical mapping suggested that the ictal onset zone was immediately anterior to the supplementary motor area (stimulation produced entire left lower extremity posturing) (*Figure 5*). Stimulation of the ictal onset zone produced typical clinical seizures even with very low stimulation parameters (*Figure 6*).

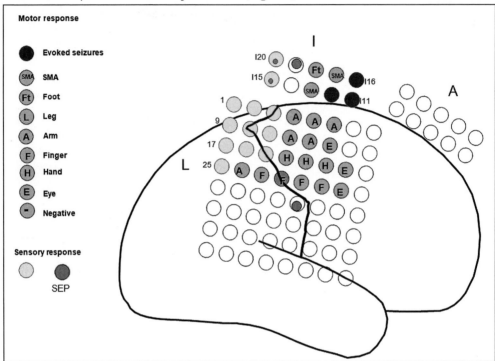

Figure 5. Results of electrical stimulation mapping. Electrode grids I and A are recording from the right mesial frontal cortex. The line estimating the rolandic fissure is based on reversal of polarity of somatosensory evoked potentials. Left leg posturing was elicited with stimulation of I13 and I17. Stimulation of I18 produced left foot dorsiflexion. The bottom 4 rows of the lateral convexity grid were not stimulated.

After removal of subdural grid electrodes, a mesial frontal cortical area measuring 2 × 3 cm was initially removed, including supplementary motor cortex. However, the resection was extended inferiorly and anteriorly based on residual spiking on electrocorticography. The final resection area measured about 4 ×5 cm in the mesial frontal region. Postoperatively he had mild left lower extremity weakness that gradually recovered to baseline at 3 months postoperatively.

He was completely seizure-free postoperatively. His seizure medications were reduced from 4 to 2 antiepileptic drugs and the doses of the antiepileptic drugs were also reduced. About 14 months after surgery, after missing all his seizure medications for two days he reported feeling that he might have a seizure. This did not recur, but resulted in the decision to continue his two seizure medications for several years. He was still seizure-free on seizure medications more than 3 years postoperatively.

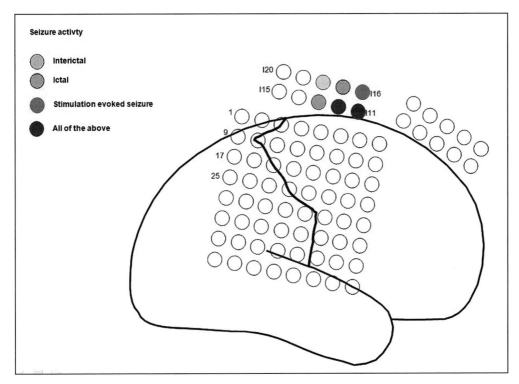

Figure 6. Summary of interictal and ictal seizure activity from the I Grid contacts.

References

- Abou-Khalil B, Fakhoury T, Jennings M, Moots P, Warner J, Kessler RM. Inhibitory motor seizures: correlation with centroparietal structural and functional abnormalities. *Acta Neurol Scand* 1995; 91: 103-8.
- Aghakhani Y, Rosati A, Olivier A, Gotman J, Andermann F, Dubeau F. The predictive localizing value of tonic limb posturing in supplementary sensorimotor seizures. *Neurology* 2004; 62: 2256-61.
- Aguglia U, Tinuper P, Gastaut H. Startle-induced epileptic seizures. *Epilepsia* 1984; 25: 712-20.
- Akimura T, Fujii M, Ideguchi M, Yoshikawa K, Suzuki M. Ictal onset and spreading of seizures of parietal lobe origin. *Neurol Med Chir (Tokyo)* 2003; 43: 534-40.
- Archer JS, Briellmann RS, Syngeniotis A, Abbott DF, Jackson GD. Spike-triggered fMRI in reading epilepsy: involvement of left frontal cortex working memory area. *Neurology* 2003; 60: 415-21.
- Arroyo S, Lesser RP, Gordon B, Uematsu S, Hart J, Schwerdt P, *et al*. Mirth, laughter and gelastic seizures. *Brain* 1993; 116 (Pt 4): 757-80.
- Bancaud J, Talairach J. Clinical semiology of frontal lobe seizures. *Adv Neurol* 1992; 57: 3-58.
- Bancaud J, Talairach J, Bonis A. Physiopathogenesis of startle epilepsy (an epilepsy of the supplementary motor area). *Electroencephalogr Clin Neurophysiol* 1968; 24: 490.
- Bancaud J, Talairach J, Morel P, Bresson M, Bonis A, Geier S, *et al*. "Generalized" epileptic seizures elicited by electrical stimulation of the frontal lobe in man. *Electroencephalogr Clin Neurophysiol* 1974; 37: 275-82.

- Battaglia D, Lettori D, Contaldo I, Veredice C, Sacco A, Vasco J, et al. Seizure semiology of lesional frontal lobe epilepsies in children. *Neuropediatrics* 2007; 38: 287-91.

- Bauer G, Dobesberger J, Bauer R, Embacher N, Benke T, Unterberger I, et al. Prefrontal disturbances as the sole manifestation of simple partial nonconvulsive status epilepticus. *Epilepsy Behav* 2006; 8: 331-5.

- Berkovic SF, Arzimanoglou A, Kuzniecky R, Harvey AS, Palmini A, Andermann F. Hypothalamic hamartoma and seizures: a treatable epileptic encephalopathy. *Epilepsia* 2003; 44: 969-73.

- Bleasel A, Dinner D. Mesial Frontal Epilepsy. In: Lüders HO (ed.). *Textbook of Epilepsy Surgery*. London: Informa Healthcare, 2008, pp. 274-284.

- Bleasel AF, Morris HH, 3rd. Supplementary sensorimotor area epilepsy in adults. *Adv Neurol* 1996; 70: 271-84.

- Blume WT, Jones DC, Young GB, Girvin JP, McLachlan RS. Seizures involving secondary sensory and related areas. *Brain* 1992; 115 (Pt 5): 1509-20.

- Bolay H, Ay H, Saygi S, Ciger A, Saribas O. Late onset absence seizures in multiple sclerosis: a case report. *Clin Electroencephalogr* 1995; 26: 124-30.

- Canuet L, Ishii R, Iwase M, Kurimoto R, Ikezawa K, Azechi M, et al. Cephalic auras of supplementary motor area origin: an ictal MEG and SAM(g2) study. *Epilepsy Behav* 2008; 13: 570-4.

- Cascino GD, Andermann F, Berkovic SF, Kuzniecky RI, Sharbrough FW, Keene DL, et al. Gelastic seizures and hypothalamic hamartomas: evaluation of patients undergoing chronic intracranial EEG monitoring and outcome of surgical treatment. *Neurology* 1993a; 43: 747-50.

- Cascino GD, Hulihan JF, Sharbrough FW, Kelly PJ. Parietal lobe lesional epilepsy: electroclinical correlation and operative outcome. *Epilepsia* 1993b; 34: 522-7.

- Chassagnon S, Hawko CS, Bernasconi A, Gotman J, Dubeau F. Coexistence of symptomatic focal and absence seizures: Video-EEG and EEG-fMRI evidence of overlapping but independent epileptogenic networks. *Epilepsia* 2009; 50: 1821-6.

- Chassagnon S, Minotti L, Kremer S, Hoffmann D, Kahane P. Somatosensory, motor, and reaching/grasping responses to direct electrical stimulation of the human cingulate motor areas. *J Neurosurg* 2008; 109: 593-604.

- Chassagnon S, Minotti L, Kremer S, Verceuil L, Hoffmann D, Benabid AL, Kahane P. Restricted frontomesial epileptogenic focus generating dyskinetic behavior and laughter. *Epilepsia* 2003; 44: 859-63.

- Chauvel P, Kliemann F, Vignal JP, Chodkiewicz JP, Talairach J, Bancaud J. The clinical signs and symptoms of frontal lobe seizures. Phenomenology and classification. *Adv Neurol* 1995; 66: 115-25; discussion 125-6.

- Chauvel P, Trottier S, Vignal JP, Bancaud J. Somatomotor seizures of frontal lobe origin. *Adv Neurol* 1992; 57: 185-232.

- Cheung CS, Parrent AG, Burneo JG. Gelastic seizures: not always hypothalamic hamartoma. *Epileptic Disord* 2007; 9: 453-8.

- Cho YJ, Han SD, Song SK, Lee BI, Heo K. Palilalia, echolalia, and echopraxia-palipraxia as ictal manifestations in a patient with left frontal lobe epilepsy. *Epilepsia* 2009; 50: 1616-9.

- Cokar O, Gelisse P, Livet MO, Bureau M, Habib M, Genton P. Startle response: epileptic or non-epileptic? The case for "flash" SMA reflex seizures. *Epileptic Disord* 2001; 3: 7-12.

- Craiu D, Magureanu S, van Emde Boas W. Are absences truly generalized seizures or partial seizures originating from or predominantly involving the pre-motor areas? Some clinical and theoretical observations and their implications for seizure classification. *Epilepsy Res* 2006; 70 (Suppl 1): S141-55.

- Feindel W. Osler vindicated: glioma of the leg center with Jacksonian epilepsy; removal and cure, with a 50-year follow-up. Historical vignette. *J Neurosurg* 2009; 111: 293-300.

• Fujii M, Akimura T, Ozaki S, Kato S, Ito H, Neshige R. An angiographically occult arteriovenous malformation in the medial parietal lobe presenting as seizures of medial temporal lobe origin. *Epilepsia* 1999; 40: 377-81.

• Garcia-Morales I, Maestu F, Perez-Jimenez MA, Elices E, Ortiz T, Alvarez-Linera J, Gil-Nagel A. A clinical and magnetoencephalography study of MRI-negative startle epilepsy. *Epilepsy Behav* 2009; 16: 166-71.

• Garzon E, Lüders HO. Cingulate Epilepsy. In: Lüders HO (ed.). *Textbook of Epilepsy Surgery*. London: Informa Healthcare, 2008, pp. 334-53.

• Gasparini E, Benuzzi F, Pugnaghi M, Ariatti A, Sola P, Nichelli P, Meletti S. Focal sensory-motor status epilepticus in multiple sclerosis due to a new cortical lesion. An EEG-fMRI co-registration study. *Seizure* 2010; 19: 525-8.

• Geier S, Bancaud J, Talairach J, Bonis A, Hossard-Bouchaud H, Enjelvin M. Ictal tonic postural changes and automatisms of the upper limb during epileptic parietal lobe discharges. *Epilepsia* 1977; 18: 517-24.

• Gloor P. Consciousness as a neurological concept in epileptology: a critical review. *Epilepsia* 1986; 27 (Suppl 2): S14-26.

• Gotman J, Grova C, Bagshaw A, Kobayashi E, Aghakhani Y, Dubeau F. Generalized epileptic discharges show thalamocortical activation and suspension of the default state of the brain. *Proc Natl Acad Sci USA* 2005; 102: 15236-40.

• Green JR, Angevine JB, White JC, Jr., Edes AD, Smith RD. Significance of the supplementary motor area in partial seizures and in cerebral localization. *Neurosurgery* 1980; 6: 66-75.

• Hirsch E, Sellal F, Maton B, Rumbach L, Marescaux C. Nocturnal paroxysmal dystonia: a clinical form of focal epilepsy. *Neurophysiol Clin* 1994; 24: 207-17.

• Holthausen H, Hoppe M. Hypermotor Seizures. In Lüders HO, Noachtar S, (eds) *Epileptic Seizures- Pathophysiology and Clinical Semiology*. Churchill Livingstone, Philadelphia, 2000, pp. 439-448.

• Ikeda A, Hirasawa K, Kinoshita M, Hitomi T, Matsumoto R, Mitsueda T, Taki JY, Inouch M, Mikuni N, Hori T, Fukuyama H, Hashimoto N, Shibasaki H, Takahashi R. Negative motor seizure arising from the negative motor area: is it ictal apraxia? *Epilepsia* 2009; 50: 2072-84.

• Ikeda A, Matsumoto R, Ohara S, Kunieda T, Shirakashi Y, Kaji R, Fukuyama H, Shibasaki H. Asymmetric tonic seizures with bilateral parietal lesions resembling frontal lobe epilepsy. *Epileptic Disord* 2001; 3: 17-22.

• Ikeda A, Nagamine T, Kunieda T, Yazawa S, Ohara S, Taki W, *et al*. Clonic convulsion caused by epileptic discharges arising from the human supplementary motor area as studied by subdural recording. *Epileptic Disord* 1999; 1: 21-6.

• Ikeda A, Ohara S, Matsumoto R, Kunieda T, Nagamine T, Miyamoto S, *et al*. Role of primary sensorimotor cortices in generating inhibitory motor response in humans. *Brain* 2000; 123 (Pt 8): 1710-21.

• Iwasa H, Shibata T, Mine S, Koseki K, Yasuda K, Kasagi Y, *et al*. Different patterns of dipole source localization in gelastic seizure with or without a sense of mirth. *Neurosci Res* 2002; 43: 23-9.

• Jobst BC, Siegel AM, Thadani VM, Roberts DW, Rhodes HC, Williamson PD. Intractable seizures of frontal lobe origin: clinical characteristics, localizing signs, and results of surgery. *Epilepsia* 2000; 41: 1139-52.

• Kahane P, Ryvlin P, Hoffmann D, Minotti L, Benabid AL. From hypothalamic hamartoma to cortex: what can be learnt from depth recordings and stimulation? *Epileptic Disord* 2003; 5: 205-17.

• Kanemoto K, Watanabe Y, Tsuji T, Fukami M, Kawasaki J. Rub epilepsy: a somatosensory evoked reflex epilepsy induced by prolonged cutaneous stimulation. *J Neurol Neurosurg Psychiatry* 2001; 70: 541-3.

- Kanner AM, Morris HH, Luders H, Dinner DS, Wyllie E, Medendorp SV, Rowan AJ. Supplementary motor seizures mimicking pseudoseizures: some clinical differences. *Neurology* 1990 ; 40: 1404-7.

- Kim DW, Lee SK, Yun CH, Kim KK, Lee DS, Chung CK, Chang KH. Parietal lobe epilepsy: the semiology, yield of diagnostic workup, and surgical outcome. *Epilepsia* 2004; 45: 641-9.

- Koubeissi MZ, Jouny CC, Blakeley JO, Bergey GK. Analysis of dynamics and propagation of parietal cingulate seizures with secondary mesial temporal involvement. *Epilepsy Behav* 2009; 14: 108-12.

- Kubota F, Shibata N, Shiihara Y, Takahashi S, Ohsuka T. Frontal lobe epilepsy with secondarily generalized 3 Hz spike-waves: a case report. *Clin Electroencephalogr* 1997; 28: 166-71.

- Kudo T, Sato K, Yagi K, Seino M. Can absence status epilepticus be of frontal lobe origin? *Acta Neurol Scand* 1995; 92: 472-7.

- Kurle PJ, Sheth RD. Gelastic seizures of neocortical origin confirmed by resective surgery. *J Child Neurol* 2000; 15: 835-8.

- Kuzniecky R, Guthrie B, Mountz J, Bebin M, Faught E, Gilliam F, Liu HG. Intrinsic epileptogenesis of hypothalamic hamartomas in gelastic epilepsy. *Ann Neurol* 1997; 42: 60-7.

- Lende RA, Popp AJ. Sensory Jacksonian seizures. *J Neurosurg* 1976 ; 44: 706-11.

- Leung H, Schindler K, Clusmann H, Bien CG, Popel A, Schramm J, *et al*. Mesial frontal epilepsy and ictal body turning along the horizontal body axis. *Arch Neurol* 2008; 65: 71-7.

- Levin B, Duchowny M. Childhood obsessive-compulsive disorder and cingulate epilepsy. *Biol Psychiatry* 1991; 30: 1049-55.

- Lim SH, Dinner DS, Pillay PK, Luders H, Morris HH, Klem G, *et al*. Functional anatomy of the human supplementary sensorimotor area: results of extraoperative electrical stimulation. *Electroencephalogr Clin Neurophysiol* 1994; 91: 179-93.

- Lüders HO, Dinner DS, Morris HH, Wyllie E, Comair YG. Cortical electrical stimulation in humans. The negative motor areas. *Adv Neurol* 1995; 67: 115-29.

- Lüders HO, Lesser RP, Dinner DS, Morris HH, Wyllie E, Godoy J, Hahn JH. A negative motor response elicited by electrical stimulation of the human frontal cortex. *Adv Neurol* 1992; 57: 149-57.

- Madhavan D, Liebman T, Nadkarni S, Devinsky O. Anterior cingulate epilepsy in an 18-year-old woman. *Rev Neurol Dis* 2007; 4: 39-42.

- Manford MR, Fish DR, Shorvon SD. Startle provoked epileptic seizures: features in 19 patients. *J Neurol Neurosurg Psychiatry* 1996; 61: 151-6.

- Mazars G. Criteria for identifying cingulate epilepsies. *Epilepsia* 1970; 11: 41-7.

- McConachie NS, King MD. Gelastic seizures in a child with focal cortical dysplasia of the cingulate gyrus. *Neuroradiology* 1997; 39: 44-5.

- Meierkord H, Fish DR, Smith SJ, Scott CA, Shorvon SD, Marsden CD. Is nocturnal paroxysmal dystonia a form of frontal lobe epilepsy? *Mov Disord* 1992; 7: 38-42.

- Mohamed IS, Otsubo H, Shroff M, Donner E, Drake J, Snead OC, 3rd. Magnetoencephalography and diffusion tensor imaging in gelastic seizures secondary to a cingulate gyrus lesion. *Clin Neurol Neurosurg* 2007; 109: 182-7.

- Montagna P. Nocturnal paroxysmal dystonia and nocturnal wandering. *Neurology* 1992; 42: 61-7.

- Morris HH, 3rd, Dinner DS, Luders H, Wyllie E, Kramer R. Supplementary motor seizures: clinical and electroencephalographic findings. *Neurology* 1988; 38: 1075-82.

- Nadkarni S, Devinsky O. Cingulate Cortex Seizures. In Vogt B, (ed) *Cingulate Neurobiology and Disease*. London: Oxford University Press, 2009, pp. 633-651.

- Niedermeyer E, Laws ER, Jr., Walker EA. Depth EEG findings in epileptics with generalized spike-wave complexes. *Arch Neurol* 1969; 21: 51-8.

- Noachtar S, Holthausen H, Luders HO. Epileptic negative myoclonus. Subdural EEG recordings indicate a postcentral generator. *Neurology* 1997; 49: 1534-7.
- Noachtar S, Luders HO. Focal akinetic seizures as documented by electroencephalography and video recordings. *Neurology* 1999; 53: 427-9.
- Noachtar S, Lüders HO. Akinetic seizures. In Lüders HO, Noachtar S, (eds) *Epileptic Seizures- Pathophysiology and Clinical Semiology*. Philadelphia: Churchill Livingstone, 2000, pp. 489-500.
- Nolan MA, Otsubo H, Iida K, Minassian BA. Startle-induced seizures associated with infantile hemiplegia: implication of the supplementary motor area. *Epileptic Disord* 2005; 7: 49-52.
- Oehl B, Biethahn S, Schulze-Bonhage A. Mirthful gelastic seizures with ictal involvement of temporobasal regions. *Epileptic Disord* 2009; 11: 82-6.
- Ohara S, Ikeda A, Kunieda T, Yazawa S, Taki J, Nagamine T, *et al*. Propagation of tonic posturing in supplementary motor area (SMA) seizures. *Epilepsy Res* 2004; 62: 179-87.
- Penfield W, Jasper H. *Epilepsy and the Functional Anatomy of the Brain*. Boston: Little, Brown, 1954.
- Penfield W, Welch K. The supplementary motor area in the cerebral cortex of man. *Trans Am Neural Assoc* 1949; 74: 179-84.
- Raichle ME, MacLeod AM, Snyder AZ, Powers WJ, Gusnard DA, Shulman GL. A default mode of brain function. *Proc Natl Acad Sci USA* 2001; 98: 676-82.
- Reutens DC, Andermann F, Olivier A, Andermann E, Dubeau F. Unusual features of supplementary sensorimotor area epilepsy: cyclic pattern, unusual sensory aura, startle sensitivity, anoxic encephalopathy, and spontaneous remission. *Adv Neurol* 1996; 70: 293-300.
- Rheims S, Ryvlin P, Scherer C, Minotti L, Hoffmann D, Guenot M, *et al*. Analysis of clinical patterns and underlying epileptogenic zones of hypermotor seizures. *Epilepsia* 2008; 49: 2030-40.
- Romeo A, Chifari R, Capovilla G, Viri M, Lodi M, Dell'Oglio V, *et al*. Ictal impending danger "sixth sense seizures" in patients with benign focal epileptic seizures of adolescence. *Epilepsy Res* 2008; 79: 90-6.
- Rosenow F, Lüders HO. (2000) Startle-Induced Seizures. In Lüders HO, Noachtar S, (eds) *Epileptic Seizures- Pathophysiology and Clinical Semiology*. Churchill Livingstone, Philadelphia, pp. 585-592.
- Ryvlin P, Minotti L, Demarquay G, Hirsch E, Arzimanoglou A, Hoffman D, *et al*. Nocturnal hypermotor seizures, suggesting frontal lobe epilepsy, can originate in the insula. *Epilepsia* 2006; 47: 755-65.
- Saeki K, Saito Y, Sugai K, Nakagawa E, Komaki H, Sakuma H, *et al*. Startle epilepsy associated with gait-induced seizures: Pathomechanism analysis using EEG, MEG, and PET studies. *Epilepsia* 2009; 50: 1274-9.
- Salanova V, Andermann F, Rasmussen T, Olivier A, Quesney LF. Parietal lobe epilepsy. Clinical manifestations and outcome in 82 patients treated surgically between 1929 and 1988. *Brain* 1995a; 118 (Pt 3): 607-27.
- Salanova V, Andermann F, Rasmussen T, Olivier A, Quesney LF. Tumoural parietal lobe epilepsy. Clinical manifestations and outcome in 34 patients treated between 1934 and 1988. *Brain* 1995b; 118 (Pt 5): 1289-304.
- Sartori E, Biraben A, Taussig D, Bernard AM, Scarabin JM. Gelastic seizures: video-EEG and scintigraphic analysis of a case with a frontal focus; review of the literature and pathophysiological hypotheses. *Epileptic Disord* 1999; 1: 221-8.
- Satow T, Ikeda A, Yamamoto J, Takayama M, Matsuhashi M, Ohara S, *et al*. Partial epilepsy manifesting atonic seizure: report of two cases. *Epilepsia* 2002; 43: 1425-31.
- Saygi S, Katz A, Marks DA, Spencer SS. Frontal lobe partial seizures and psychogenic seizures: comparison of clinical and ictal characteristics. *Neurology* 1992; 42: 1274-7.
- Seo DW, Lee HS, Hong SB, Hong SC, Lee EK. Pilomotor seizures in frontal lobe epilepsy: case report. *Seizure* 2003; 12: 241-4.

- Serles W, Leutmezer F, Pataraia E, Olbrich A, Groppel G, Czech T, Baumgartner C. A case of startle epilepsy and SSMA seizures documented with subdural recordings. *Epilepsia* 1999; 40: 1031-5.

- Siegel AM, Williamson PD. Parietal lobe epilepsy. *Adv Neurol* 2000; 84: 189-99.

- Siegel AM, Williamson PD, Roberts DW, Thadani VM, Darcey TM. Localized pain associated with seizures originating in the parietal lobe. *Epilepsia* 1999; 40: 845-55.

- So NK. Mesial frontal epilepsy. *Epilepsia* 1998; 39 (Suppl 4): S49-61.

- Spencer SS, Spencer DD, Williamson PD, Mattson RH. Sexual automatisms in complex partial seizures. *Neurology* 1983; 33: 527-33.

- Tao Y, Guojun Z, Yuping W, Lixin C, Wei D, Yongjie L. Surgical treatment of patients with drug-resistant hypermotor seizures. *Epilepsia* 2010; 51: 2124-30.

- Tharp BR. Orbital frontal seizures. An unique electroencephalographic and clinical syndrome. *Epilepsia* 1972; 13: 627-42.

- Thomas P, Zifkin B, Migneco O, Lebrun C, Darcourt J, Andermann F. Nonconvulsive status epilepticus of frontal origin. *Neurology* 1999; 52: 1174-83.

- Tibussek D, Wohlrab G, Boltshauser E, Schmitt B. Proven startle-provoked epileptic seizures in childhood: semiologic and electrophysiologic variability. *Epilepsia* 2006; 47: 1050-8.

- Tinuper P, Cerullo A, Cirignotta F, Cortelli P, Lugaresi E, Montagna P. Nocturnal paroxysmal dystonia with short-lasting attacks: three cases with evidence for an epileptic frontal lobe origin of seizures. *Epilepsia* 1990; 31: 549-56.

- Toledano R, Garcia-Morales I, Kurtis MM, Perez-Sempere A, Ciordia R, Gil-Nagel A. Bilateral akinetic seizures: A clinical and electroencephalographic description. *Epilepsia* 2010 [in press].

- Tuxhorn IE. Somatosensory auras in focal epilepsy: a clinical, video EEG and MRI study. *Seizure* 2005; 14: 262-8.

- Umeoka S, Baba K, Mihara T. Symptomatic laughter in a patient with orbitofrontal seizure: A surgical case with intracranial electroencephalographic study: case report. *Neurosurgery* 2008; 63: E1205-6; discussion E1206.

- Umeoka S, Baba K, Terada K, Matsuda K, Tottori T, Usui N, *et al.* Bilateral symmetric tonic posturing suggesting propagation to the supplementary motor area in a patient with precuneate cortical dysplasia. *Epileptic Disord* 2007; 9: 443-8.

- Unnwongse K, Wehner T, Bingaman W, Foldvary-Schaefer N. Gelastic seizures and the anteromesial frontal lobe: A case report and review of intracranial EEG recording and electrocortical stimulation case studies. *Epilepsia* 2010 [in press].

- Vaugier L, Aubert S, McGonigal A, Trebuchon A, Guye M, Gavaret M, *et al.* Neural networks underlying hyperkinetic seizures of "temporal lobe" origin. *Epilepsy Res* 2009; 86: 200-8.

- Vogt BA. Pain and emotion interactions in subregions of the cingulate gyrus. *Nat Rev Neurosci* 2005; 6: 533-44.

- Wang L, Mathews GC, Whetsell WO, Abou-Khalil B. Hypermotor seizures in patients with temporal pole lesions. *Epilepsy Res* 2008; 82: 93-8.

- Wiest G, Zimprich F, Prayer D, Czech T, Serles W, Baumgartner C. Vestibular processing in human paramedian precuneus as shown by electrical cortical stimulation. *Neurology* 2004; 62: 473-5.

- Williamson PD, Boon PA, Thadani VM, Darcey TM, Spencer DD, Spencer SS, *et al.* Parietal lobe epilepsy: diagnostic considerations and results of surgery. *Ann Neurol* 1992a; 31: 193-201.

- Williamson PD, Engel J, Jr. Anatomic Classification of Focal Epilepsies. In: Engel JJ, Pedley TA (eds.). *Epilepsy: A Comprehensive Textbook.* Philadelphia: Lippincott Williams & Wilkins, 2008, pp. 2465-2477.

- Williamson PD, Jobst BC. Frontal lobe epilepsy. *Adv Neurol* 2000; 84: 215-42.

- Williamson PD, Spencer DD, Spencer SS, Novelly RA, Mattson RH. Complex partial seizures of frontal lobe origin. *Ann Neurol* 1985; 18: 497-504.
- Williamson PD, Spencer SS. Clinical and EEG features of complex partial seizures of extratemporal origin. *Epilepsia* 1986; 27 (Suppl 2): S46-63.
- Williamson PD, Thadani VM, Darcey TM, Spencer DD, Spencer SS, Mattson RH. Occipital lobe epilepsy: clinical characteristics, seizure spread patterns, and results of surgery. *Ann Neurol* 1992b; 31: 3-13.
- Wyllie E, Luders H, Morris HH, Lesser RP, Dinner DS. The lateralizing significance of versive head and eye movements during epileptic seizures. *Neurology* 1986; 36: 606-11.

Videos of this chapter available at: www.etle.surgery.jle.com

Video I legend. Typical seizure with initial left upper and lower extremity posturing. There is later posturing of the right upper extremity with flexion at the elbow.

Video 2 legend. Hypermotor seizure in a 27 year old woman with mesial frontal cortical dysplasia.

Ictal semiology
of parieto-occipital lobe epilepsies

Tonicarlo R. Velasco, Americo C. Sakamoto

Epilepsy Surgery Center, Department of Neurosciences and Behavioral Sciences, Ribeirão Preto School of Medicine, University of São Paulo, Brazil

In this chapter we will review the relevant functional anatomy of the parietal and the occipital lobes, followed, respectively by the description of the main ictal characteristics of the seizures involving these areas.

■ Parietal lobe seizures

Functional anatomy of parietal lobe

The parietal lobe is largely concerned with somatic sensation, with forming a body image, and with relating one's body image with extrapersonal space. Sensory information can be classified in mechanoreceptive somatic senses (tactile and position), thermoreceptive senses (heat and cold); and pain. The data captured by different receptors enter the spinal cord through the dorsal roots of the spinal nerves and are conducted through one of two sensory pathways: i) the dorsal column-medial lemniscal system which conveys information from touch, vibratory, movement, position, and fine judgment of pressure intensity; ii) the anterolateral system which conveys information related to pain, thermal sensations, tickle and itch, and sexual sensations. Both systems have second-order neurons that form parallel pathways that decussate to the opposite side of the brain and continue upward to the thalamus. In the sensory relay area of the thalamus, third-order neurons project mainly to the postcentral gyrus of the parietal cortex known as somatic sensory area I, but also to a smaller area in the lateral parietal cortex called somatic sensory area II (Guyton & Hall, 2006; Saper *et al.*, 2000).

The primary sensory area (S1)

The S1 somatosensory area lies in Brodmann's areas 3, 1, and 2 and receives sensory information almost exclusively from the contralateral side of the body. The S1 cortex is spatially organized in representations of the different parts of the body, with some areas represented by large areas (lips, face, and thumbs), whereas the trunk and lower parts of the body are represented by smaller areas. The S1 cortex is related to: i) discrete locali-zation of different sensations in different parts of the body; ii) judgment of pressure degrees; iii) judgment of weight of objects; and iv) judgment of shape, form, and texture of objects. Appreciation of pain and temperature is preserved in the absence of S1, but the informa-tion is poorly localized, suggesting that localization of pain and temperature depends on the topographical map of S1.

The somatosensory association area (S2)

The S2 somatosensory association cortex lies in Brodmann's areas 5 and 7 located in the parietal cortex behind the S1 area, and plays important roles in deciphering more complex meanings of sensation. Sensory information of different modalities processed in S1 converges to adjacent unimodal association cortex in S2, which integrates it in polysensory events. S2 also receives information from ventrobasal nuclei of the thalamus, visual cortex, and auditory cortex. The somatosensory association area is related to i) recognition of complex objects and forms felt on the opposite side of the body, and ii) sense of form of his or her body parts. Finally, the posterior association areas are heavily connected to frontal association areas located in premotor and prefrontal cortex, which are responsible for planning motor actions in response to sensory information. Then, motor planning is translated into concrete motor responses through processing of motor pathways (Guyton & Hall, 2006; Saper et al., 2000).

The supramarginal and angular gyrus

The supramarginal and angular gyrus (Brodmann's areas 39 and 40) located in the inferior parietal lobe integrate the language system in the dominant hemisphere. Individuals with lesions of these areas develop conduction aphasia which is characterized by comprehension of simple sentences and production of intelligible speech but inability to repeat sentences, to assemble phonemes effectively, and impairment in the ability to name pictures and objects. Speech production and auditory comprehension are less compromised in conduc-tion aphasia than in the two other major types of aphasias.

Ictal semiology of parietal lobe seizures

Signs and symptoms of seizures originating from the parietal lobe will be divided in two types: i) signs and symptoms resulting from discharges in the parietal lobe itself, and ii) signs and symptoms resulting from seizure propagation outside the parietal lobe.

Signals and symptoms resulting from parietal lobe discharges

Typically, patients with seizures arising from parietal lobe present paresthetic and dyses-thetic sensations in the contralateral side of seizure onset. The most common symptoms are elementary disturbances of sensation, such as numbness and tingling. Pain and distur-bances of temperature sensation are uncommon, as well as disturbances of body image or position. Table I shows the clinical features of parietal lobe seizures from case series of patients with refractory parietal lobe epilepsy published since 1992 (Williamson et al., 1992a; Kim et al., 2004; Ho et al., 1994; Cascino et al., 1993; Salanova et al., 1995a; 1995b). A total of six studies were included in the analysis, totaling 189 patients. Most patients (82%) had auras at the time of presurgical evaluation or had had auras in some period of their epilepsy history. The studies were reviewed and the somatosensory symp-toms were divided in 3 types: i) tactile sensation (numbness, tingling); ii) pain and tem-perature; and iii) complex somatosensory symptoms, such as disturbances of body image or position and falling sensation. The most common somatosensory symptom was tactile, described in 71 (47%) out of 151 patients. Pain and disturbances of temperature sensation was uncommon, present in only 11 patients (7%). More elaborate somatosensory symptoms were also less frequent, described in only 15 (8%) out of 189 patients. Only 4 (2%) out of 189 patients described difficulty to speak or to understand speech as an initial manifestation of parietal lobe epilepsy (See *Table I* for more details).

Signs and symptoms resulting from ictal propagation

Due to its close proximity to the primary motor area and the dense connections with the frontal lobe, a sizable proportion of patients with parietal seizures have motor symptoms. However, as the parietal lobe has also connections with the temporal and occipital lobes, objective manifestations of parietal seizures may reflect seizure spread inferiorly to the temporal lobe and posteriorly to the occipital lobe. *Table I* shows signs and symptoms resulting from seizure spread in parietal lobe series published since 1992. The most common motor phenomena were clonic seizures, described in 89 (48%) out of 184 patients. Tonic bilateral asymmetric seizures were described in 45 (23%) out of 195 patients, resembling frontal lobe seizures arising from the supplementary motor area. Temporal lobe-like symptoms such as fear, affective aura, and autonomic sensations were described in 18 (10%) out of 189 patients, but epigastric sensation was rarely reported. Finally, visual symptoms (simple or complex) were described in 28 (15%) out of 189 patients.

Lateralizing value of somatosensory auras

As the somatosensory area I in Brodmann's areas 3, 1, and 2 receives sensory informations almost exclusively from the opposite side, it is expected that sensorimotor auras are perceived contralaterally to the side of the epileptogenic lesion. In fact, the presence of lateralizing symptoms has been recognized since the 1900s, and was frequently used to guide epilepsy surgery in the parietal lobe before the neuroimaging era. *Table II* shows the results of a review of the lateralizing value of somatosensory auras in patients with parietal epilepsy (Williamson *et al.*, 1992a; Kim *et al.*, 2004; Ho *et al.*, 1994; Cascino *et al.*, 1993; Salanova *et al.*, 1995 a; 1995b). The articles were reviewed, and the somatosensory symptoms were classified as contralateral or ipsilateral to the side of surgery and bilateral. The studies were pooled together to obtain a better estimate of lateralizing value of somatosensory symptoms. As shown in *Table I*, somatosensory symptoms were present in only 97 (50%) out of 189 patients with parietal epilepsy. However, when lateralized (93/97 patients, 96%), they were contralateral to the side of surgery in 89 (96%) and ipsilateral in only 4 patients (4%). In other words, although the sensitivity is relatively low, unilateral somatosensory symptoms are a reliable lateralizing symptom, occurring contralateral to the side of epileptogenic lesion in 96% of cases (high specificity).

■ Semiology of occipital lobe seizures

Functional anatomy of occipital lobe

The occipital lobe lies posterior to the parieto-occipital sulcus. Occupying the posterior pole of the brain, the occipital lobe totalizes 10% of its mass and embraces the visual cortex. Like the cortical representations of the other sensory systems, the visual cortex is divided into primary and secondary visual areas. The primary visual cortex is the terminus of direct visual signals from the retina, also called striate cortex because this area has a

Table I. Clinical features of patients with parietal epilepsy

Study, year (n of patients)	No Aura	Tactile localizing[a]	Pain temperature	Somato-sensory special[b]	Language	Visual	Temporal lobe-like	Tonic bilat. seizures	Clonic seizures
Kim, 2004 (38)	13 (32%)	–	–	0	0	4 (10%)	10 (25%)	5 (15%)	7 (21%)
Salanova, 1995 (34)	7 (21%)	17 (50%)	4 (12%)	2 (6%)	1 (3%)	2 (6%)	2 (6%)	7 (21%)	28 (82%)
Salanova, 1995 (82)	5 (6%)	39 (48%)	13 (16%)	10 (11%)	3 (4%)	19 (23%)	1 (1%)	23 (28%)	47 (57%)
Ho, 1994 (14)	2 (14%)	7 (50%)	0	1 (7%)	0	0	3 (21%)	6 (43%)	3 (21%)
Cascino, 1993 (10)	3 (30%)	4 (40%)	0	0	0	2 (20%)	1 (10&)	0	4 (40)
Williamson, 1992 (11)	4 (36%)	4 (36%)	0	2 (18%)	0	1 (9%)	1 (9%)	4 (36%)	–
Pooled (189)	34/189 (18%)	71/151 (47%)	11/151 (7%)	15/189 (8%)	4/189 (2%)	28/189 (15%)	18/189 (10%)	45/189 (24%)	89/173 (51%)

[a] Numbness, tingling, itching, pins and needles; [b] disturbances of body image or position.

Table II. Lateralizing value of somatosensory aura in patients with parietal epilepsy

Study, year	Contralateral	Bilateral	Ipsilateral
Kim, 2004	10	2	1
Salanova, 1995	16	0	1
Salanova, 1995	49	1	1
Ho, 1994	7	0	0
Cascino, 1993	3	1	0
Williamson, 1992	4	0	1
Pooled	89/97 (92%)	4/97 (4%)	4/97 (4%)

grossly striated appearance. The secondary visual areas, also called visual association areas, lie lateral, anterior, superior, and inferior to the primary visual cortex. As we shall see, the primary and secondary visual areas have multisynaptic projections to other brain regions involved in processing visual information.

The visual cortex is highly connected to the parietal and inferior temporal lobes

The photoreceptors of the retina project onto bipolar cells, which have synapses on retinal ganglion cells, the efferent cells of the retina. Its axons form the optic nerve, which projects to the lateral geniculate nucleus in the thalamus. Then, visual information is conveyed from the lateral geniculate to the primary visual cortex (Brodmann's area 17 or V1, also called the striate cortex). Because these projections are orderly, the striate cortex contains a complete neural map of the retina. Beyond the striate cortex, lie the extrastriate areas, a group of higher-order visual areas also containing representations of the retina. It is well-known that each extrastriate area is specialized for processing a different type of visual information, such as motion, form, and color. For example, clinical studies have shown that visual orientation is disrupted in humans with lesions in the parietal cortex. In particular, some patients demonstrate a visual neglect. Although they do not have a blind spot or scotoma, as would result from damage to the striate cortex, they do not respond to objects presented in the visual field contralateral to the parietal lesions. In contrast, patients with lesions in the temporal cortex frequently have difficulty in discriminating different forms and have poor visual memory for forms, including an inability to identify faces. These clinical observations have suggested that the parietal cortex is specialized for spatial representation, whereas the temporal cortex is specialized for object recognition (Saper et al., 2000; Kandel & Wurtz, 2000).

In fact, since different regions of extrastriate visual cortex appear to have different functions, these different areas receive different inputs from the pathways emanating from the retina. Two types of retinal ganglion cells – large M cells and small P cells – transmit different information to geniculate nucleus of the thalamus (M pathway and P pathway). These two pathways continue separately from the geniculate nucleus to separate layers in the visual cortex (V1). Then, the P pathway projects to V2 and V4, and next to the inferior temporal cortex, forming the ventral pathway (*Figure 1*). Neurons from the ventral pathway are more sensitive to outline, orientation, and boundaries; being more concerned with object recognition. The M pathway extends from V1 to V2, then to the middle temporal area and posterior parietal cortex, forming the dorsal pathway (*Figure 2*). Neurons

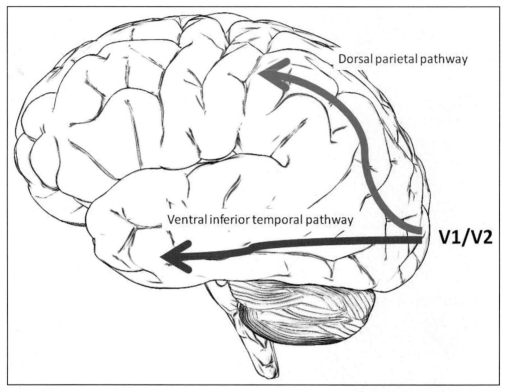

Figure I. Two major systems connect the primary visual areas of occipital with the parietal and temporal lobes. Separate pathways to the parietal (dorsal parietal pathway) and temporal (ventral inferior temporal pathway) cortices through the visual cortex (VI and V2). The magnocellular cells from the retina contribute mostly to the dorsal parietal pathway are more sensitive to motion and depth, being concerned with visuospatial recognition. The parvocellular cells projects to the inferior temporal cortex and are more sensitive to outline, orientation, and boundaries; being more concerned with object recognition.

from the dorsal pathway are more sensitive to motion and depth, being concerned with visuospatial recognition. As a result of such specificity, lesions in the dorsal pathway or in the transition between temporal and parietal areas impair movement control and perception of motion, while lesions in the ventral pathway or the inferior temporal areas impair object vision and face recognition (Saper *et al.*, 2000; Kandel & Wurtz, 2000).

The implications of functional anatomy of occipital lobe to the study of epileptic seizures originating in this region are twofold. First, seizures originating from the striate cortex (V1) should initially manifest as simple, unformed visual phenomena, such as flashes of light and shadows. On the other hand, seizures originating in extrastriate areas (V2-V4) should initially manifest with more complex, structured visual symptoms, such as illusions and hallucinations. Second, due to the parallel pathways arising both from the striate occipital cortex to parietal (dorsal parietal pathway) and temporal lobes (ventral inferior temporal pathway), seizures originating from striate cortex may give origin to different seizure types. Those propagating via dorsal pathway would reach the extrastriate areas of the parietal lobe and the frontal lobe, given origin to disturbances of movement control and perception of motion, or sensorimotor symptoms, such as disturbances or body perception, version, and clonic movement. Seizures propagating via ventral pathway would

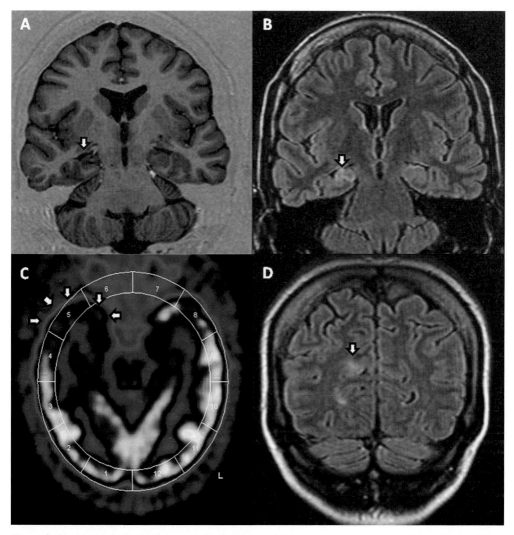

Figure 2. Occipito-temporal dual pathology. Typical images of right hippocampal atrophy and increased signal intensity are seen in inversion recovery **(A)** and FLAIR **(B)** coronal sequences, respectively. PET imaging corroborated the hypothesis of TLE, showing hypometabolism in right anterior temporal lobe (**C**, arrows). However, a complementary MRI sequence cutting the occipital lobe all the way to the pole revealed an area of cortical thickening with increased signal on FLAIR sequence **(D)**.

reach the temporal lobe, given origin to more elaborate visual hallucinations as well as seizures with symptoms resembling temporal lobe seizures, such as visceral, dysmnestic, and affective sensations. In the next section, we will review aspects of the semiology of occipital lobe seizures from studies reporting series of patients with refractory occipital epilepsy.

Ictal semiology of occipital lobe seizures

Signals and symptoms of seizures originating from the occipital lobe can be divided in two types: i) signals and symptoms resulting from discharges in the occipital lobe itself, and ii) signals and symptoms resulting from seizure propagation outside the occipital lobe.

Signals and symptoms resulting from occipital lobe discharges

Neuronal discharges in the striate cortex of occipital lobe generally give origin to simples (unformed) visual symptoms. The simple visual symptoms may be negative, such as ictal amaurosis (black-out), hemianopsia, quadrantanopsia, and uniocular amaurosis; or positive symptoms, such as flashes, bright lights, wheels, colored disks, lines, and sparks. Positive symptoms may appear together with negative ones and may evolve to complete amaurosis as the seizure progresses. Complex (formed) visual symptoms origin from seizures involving the secondary visual areas, and include visual hallucinations of faces or formed scenes, as well as visual illusions, such as macropsia, micropsia, micro or macroteleopsia, palinopsia, and loss of stereoscopic vision. Seizures arising from the occipital lobe may also present with ocular motor signals and symptoms, such as forced eye blinking, eyelid flutter, nistagmus, sensation of ocular movement without noticeable movement, and ocular deviation (with or without head deviation). Finally, patients with occipital lobe seizures may also report no visual aura.

In *Table II* we review the clinical features of occipital lobe seizures from case series of patients with occipital lobe epilepsy published since 1992. Studies were included in the analysis if they had more than 10 patients and included exclusively patients with symptomatic or probably symptomatic occipital lobe epilepsy. One study separated symptomatic from idiopathic patients and only the symptomatic patients were included in the analysis (Van den Hout et al., 1997). The data were reviewed, integrated, and pooled together to obtain a more accurate picture of occipital lobe seizures. Seven studies summing up 202 patients with occipital lobe epilepsy were included (Williamson et al., 1992b; Blume et al., 2005; Jobst et al., 2010; Van den Hout et al., 1997; Tandon et al., 2009; Kun et al., 2005; Salanova et al., 1992). The number of patients per study ranged from 14 to 42 (mean = 28.8).

The prevalence of visual auras in occipital lobe epilepsy is high. Six out of seven studies reported a prevalence higher than 50%. One study including only children with symptomatic occipital lobe epilepsy reported that only 15% of patients had visual auras (Van den Hout et al., 1997). Pooled data showed that 127 out of 202 patients with occipital lobe epilepsy had visual auras (63%). The prevalence of simple visual symptoms is higher than complex visual symptoms. Six studies that separated simple from complex visual symptoms showed that, out of 169 patients, 97 (57%) had simple visual symptoms and 43 (25%) had complex visual symptoms. Six studies reported the presence of ocular motor symptoms, such as forced blinking, nistagmus, or ocular movement sensation in 38 (22%) out of 169 patients.

Signals and symptoms resulting from ictal propagation

As stressed before, although occipital seizures may remain confined to the occipital lobe, seizures generally propagate to other brain regions, especially those highly connected to the occipital lobe. For example, due to integration of sensory (visual) and motor function, seizures propagating by the dorsal parietal pathway may spread directly to premotor frontal association areas, given origin to asymmetric postural tonic seizures. Spread to the somatosensory cortex may give origin to contralateral paresthesias, clonic, and tonic motor phenomena. Seizures propagating by the ventral inferior temporal pathway may give origin to visceral symptoms, such as epigastric sensation, nausea and vomits, gustative and olfactory sensations (temporal lobe like auras), as well as complex partial seizures impossible to differentiate from temporal lobe seizures.

Table III shows that non-visual auras (sensorimotor or visceral symptoms) occurred in 45 (31%) out of 144 patients with occipital lobe seizures. Headache and vomiting appear to be more frequent in series reporting only children with occipital epilepsy than series reporting both adults and children (12% versus 6%, respectively). Clonic and tonic eye or head deviation were frequent, reported in 142 out of 176 patients (47%), generally contralateral to the side of seizure origin. Six studies reported the presence of temporal lobe-like symptoms, which occurred in 31 out of 169 patients (18%).

Localizing value of visual epileptic auras

In occipital lobe epilepsy, the presence of abundant projections from the occipitales cortex to temporal structures facilitates the spread of occipital seizures to the ipsilateral or contralateral temporal lobe, making the differentiation between occipital and temporal lobe epilepsy difficult. This can be particularly challenging in MRI-negative patients with refractory focal epilepsy. In the absence of an MRI lesion, the proportion of patients submitted to surgery and the proportion of seizure-free patients after surgery are lower when compared to MRI-positive cases (Berg *et al.*, 2009). Therefore, in such patients a careful assessment of seizure semiology, interictal and ictal EEG is warranted to avoid false localization of epileptogenic zone. Studies have shown that visual auras are not specific for occipital lobe epilepsy. A study reported 20 patients experiencing visual auras from a series of 878 surgically treated patients suffering from intractable focal seizures. They found that elementary hallucinations, illusions, and visual loss – although considered typical for occipital lobe epilepsy – can also occur in anteromedial temporal and occipitotemporal seizures and are therefore not a discordant feature in presurgical evaluation of patients with suspected temporal lobe epilepsy (Bien *et al.*, 2000). However, the study did not provide the proportion of patients with occipital epilepsy had visual auras in comparison with non-occipital epilepsy patients. In our review of occipital lobe epilepsy series, 63% of 202 patients had visual areas compared with 2.9% in a study with 290 patients with temporal lobe epilepsy (Gupta *et al.*, 1983). On the other hand, whether patients with temporal lobe epilepsy may present with occipital-like (visual) auras, approximately 20% of occipital lobe epilepsy patients disclose temporal lobe-like auras. A recent study assessing the contribution of ictal semiology in determining the epileptogenic region within an occipital lobe found that no aspect of ictal semiology distinguished lateral from mesially occipital originating seizures (Blume *et al.*, 2005). *Figure 1* shows a MRI of a patient with a previous history of febrile seizures and complex partial seizures preceded by fear since 8 years of age. The MRI shows hippocampal atrophy and increased signal intensity. The EEG revealed interictal spikes over the right temporal region and the ictal EEG a typical theta rhythm at the same region. However, a careful analysis of MRI also revealed an abnormal area of signal intensity in supracalcarine region on FLAIR sequence, as well as indistinct white-gray matter junction on inversion recovery. An invasive investigation covering both epileptogenic lesions was indicated. This case is an example of the need for a careful analysis of occipitotemporal region at the MRI in patients with suspected temporal lobe epilepsy (Berg *et al.*, 2009; Palmini *et al.*, 1993; 1999).

Table III. Clinical features of patients with occipital epilepsy

Study (n of patients)	Visual aura	Simple visual symptoms	Complex visual symptoms	Non-visual	Ocular motor	Eye/head deviation	Headache/vomiting	TL-like auras
Jobst, 2010 (14)	7 (50%)	4 (29%)	3 (21%)	7 (50%)	1 (7%)	5 (36%)	0	3 (21%)
Tandon, 2009 (21)	11 (52%)	9 (43%)	2 (10%)	10 (48%)	2 (10%)	6 (29%)	0	2 (10%)
Blume, 2005 (41)	35 (85%)	31 (75%)	19 (46%)	6 (15%)	6 (15%)	15 (37%)	3 (7%)	11 (27%)
Lee, 2005 (26)	16 (62%)	9 (35%)	7 (27%)	6 (23%)	4 (15%)	–	–	2 (8%)
Van den Hout, 1997 (33)[a]	5 (15%)	–	–	–	–	19 (46%)	5 (12%)	–
Salanova, 1992 (42)	31 (73%)	29 (69%)	9 (21%)	16 (38%)	11 (26%)	21 (50%)	2 (5%)	6 (24%)
Williamson, 1992 (25)	22 (88%)	15 (60%)	3 (7%)	–	14 (56%)	16 (64%)	–	7 (28%)
Pooled data (202)	127/202 (63%)	97/169 (57%)	43/169 (25%)	45/144 (31%)	38/169 (22%)	142/176 (47%)	10/116 (9%)	31/169 (18%)

TL: temporal lobe.

References

- Berg AT, Mathern GW, Bronen RA, Fulbright RK, DiMario F, Testa FM, Levy SR. Frequency, prognosis and surgical treatment of structural abnormalities seen with magnetic resonance imaging in childhood epilepsy. *Brain* 2009; 132: 2785-97.
- Bien CG, Benninger FO, Urbach H, Schramm J, Kurthen M, Elger CE. Localizing value of epileptic visual auras. *Brain* 2000; 123 (Pt 2): 244-53.
- Blume WT, Wiebe S, Tapsell LM. Occipital epilepsy: lateral versus mesial. *Brain* 2005; 128, 1209-25.
- Cascino GD, Hulihan JF, Sharbrough FW, Kelly PJ. Parietal lobe lesional epilepsy: electroclinical correlation and operative outcome. *Epilepsia* 1993; 34: 522-7.
- Gupta AK, Jeavons PM, Hughes RC, Covanis A. Aura in temporal lobe epilepsy: clinical and electroencephalographic correlation. *J Neurol Neurosurg Psychiatry* 1983; 46: 1079-83.
- Guyton AC, Hall JE. Somatic sensations: I. General organization, the tactile and position senses. In: Guyton AC, Hall JE, eds. *Medical Physiology*. Jackson (Mississippi): Elsevier Sauders, 2006, 585-97.
- Ho SS, Berkovic SF, Newton MR, Austin MC, McKay WJ, Bladin PF. Parietal lobe epilepsy: clinical features and seizure localization by ictal SPECT. *Neurology* 1994: 44: 2277-84.
- Jobst BC, Williamson PD, Thadani VM, Gilbert KL, Holmes GL, Morse RP, *et al.* Intractable occipital lobe epilepsy: Clinical characteristics and surgical treatment. *Epilepsia* 2010; 51: 2334-7.
- Kandel E, Wurtz ER. Central Visual Pathways. In: Kandel E, Schwartz JH, Jessell TM, eds. *Principles of Neuroscience*. New York: McGraw-Hill, 2000.
- Kim DW, Lee SK, Yun CH, Kim KK, Lee DS, Chung CK, Chang KH. Parietal lobe epilepsy: the semiology, yield of diagnostic workup, and surgical outcome. *Epilepsia* 2004; 45: 641-9.

- Kun LS, Young LS, Kim DW, Soo LD, Chung CK. Occipital lobe epilepsy: clinical characteristics, surgical outcome, and role of diagnostic modalities. *Epilepsia* 2005; 46: 688-95.
- Palmini A, Andermann F, Dubeau F, da Costa JC, Calcagnotto ME, Gloor P, *et al*. Occipito-temporal relations: evidence for secondary epileptogenesis. *Adv Neurol* 1999; 81: 115-29.
- Palmini A, Andermann F, Dubeau F, Gloor P, Olivier A, Quesney LF, Salanova V. Occipito-temporal epilepsies: evaluation of selected patients requiring depth electrodes studies and rationale for surgical approaches. *Epilepsia* 1993; 34: 84-96.
- Salanova V, Andermann F, Olivier A, Rasmussen T, Quesney LF. Occipital lobe epilepsy: electroclinical manifestations, electrocorticography, cortical stimulation and outcome in 42 patients treated between 1930 and 1991. Surgery of occipital lobe epilepsy. *Brain* 1992; 115 (Pt 6): 1655-80.
- Salanova V, Andermann F, Rasmussen T, Olivier A, Quesney LF. Parietal lobe epilepsy. Clinical manifestations and outcome in 82 patients treated surgically between 1929 and 1988. *Brain* 1995a; 118 (Pt 3): 607-27.
- Salanova V, Andermann F, Rasmussen T, Olivier A, Quesney LF. Tumoural parietal lobe epilepsy. Clinical manifestations and outcome in 34 patients treated between 1934 and 1988. *Brain* 1995b; 118 (Pt 5): 1289-304.
- Saper CB, Iversen S, Frackowiak R. Integration of sensory and motor function: the association areas of the cerebral cortex and the cognitive capabilities of the brain. In: Kandel E, Schwartz JH, Jessell TM, eds. *Principles of Neuroscience*. New York: McGraw-Hill, 2000.
- Tandon N, Alexopoulos AV, Warbel A, Najm IM, Bingaman WE. Occipital epilepsy: spatial categorization and surgical management. *J Neurosurg* 2009; 110: 306-18.
- Van den Hout BM, Van der Meij W, Wieneke GH, Van Huffelen AC, Van Nieuwenhuizen O. Seizure semiology of occipital lobe epilepsy in children. *Epilepsia* 1997; 38: 1188-91.
- Williamson PD, Boon PA, Thadani VM, Darcey TM, Spencer DD, Spencer SS, *et al*. Parietal lobe epilepsy: diagnostic considerations and results of surgery. *Ann Neurol* 1992a; 31: 193-201.
- Williamson PD, Thadani VM, Darcey TM, Spencer DD, Spencer SS, Mattson RH. Occipital lobe epilepsy: clinical characteristics, seizure spread patterns, and results of surgery. *Ann Neurol* 1992b; 31: 3-13.

Ictal semiology
of hypothalamic hamartomas

Andre Palmini

*Neurology Service & Epilepsy Surgery Program, Hospital São Lucas
Faculty of Medicine and the Brain Institute (InsCer), Pontificia
Universidade Católica do Rio Grande do Sul (PUCRS),
Porto Alegre, Brazil*

A combination of neurophysiologic techniques, imaging studies and basic science research is uncovering the mechanisms of epileptogenesis of many epileptic syndromes (Chen *et al.*, 2009; Escayg & Goldin, 2010). Some entities, however, still challenge our understanding, a major prototype being the epilepsy associated with hypothalamic hamartomas (HH). A thorough comprehension of the mechanisms of ictal generation in this syndrome is still lacking, rendering both the large variation of semiological features and the wide spectrum of severity of the epilepsies in need of a coherent explanation. This notwithstanding, a surge of interest in the HH-epilepsy syndrome has been observed in recent years, driven by the possibility to identify even very small HH with high-resolution MRI (*Figure 1*) and by the discovery that the HH itself is intrinsically epileptogenic (Lokovic *et al.*, 2009; Munari *et al.*, 1995). In fact, invasive EEG recordings, functional imaging studies and post-operative evolution have demonstrated the pivotal role of the HH in epileptogenesis (Kuzniecky *et al.*, 1997; Palmini *et al.*, 2002): this lesion has been shown both to directly generate some of the seizures and to "control" the cortical generation of other, more severe types. In this regard, the HH-epilepsy syndrome challenges the classical "cortical" tenet of epileptogenesis, in the sense that for some of the seizures in a given patient there is a *subcortical* epileptogenic zone, whereas for other seizures there may exist *cortical* epileptogenic zones yet most likely within a "dependent" stage of secondary epileptogenesis. Although these "dependent" cortical epileptogenic zones (which also function as symptomatogenic zones, as discussed later) generate both the more severe seizures and the cognitive dysfunction some of these patients have (Kahane *et al.*, 2003), their resection is not needed to bring seizures under control and to reverse the encephalopathic disorder. Resection of the diencephalic hamartoma is the required surgical strategy, often leading to the control of the cortically-generated seizures (Palmini *et al.*, 2002; Berkovic *et al.*, 2003; Freeman *et al.*, 2003; Palmini *et al.*, 2003; Striano *et al.*, 2009). Furthermore, as discussed below, many patients with the HH-epilepsy syndrome progress over the years from a mild to a severe epileptic and cognitive disorder. Therefore, the evidences that a mechanism of subcortical-to-cortex secondary epileptogenesis operates to shape the

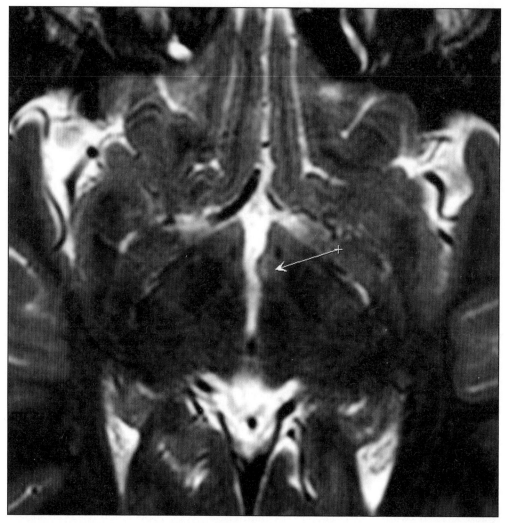

Figure 1. Axial 3T T2-weighted MRI. A very small hypothalamic hamartoma, which passed unnoticed in 4 previous MRI examinations, minimally protrudes into the third ventricle.

epilepsy syndrome are quite convincing (Freeman *et al.*, 2003; Berkovic *et al.*, 1997; Oehl *et al.*, 2010). In this chapter, the HH-epilepsy syndrome will be revisited through the "lens of semiology". In other words, the major aspects of this disorder will be highlighted having ictal semiology as the common denominator of several pressing epileptological issues.

■ Seizure types in patients with hypothalamic hamartomas: hypothalamic hamartoma as the "great pretender"

Any educational text has to integrate common knowledge with broader views and new data on the subject at hand. In regard to the suspicion of a HH in the origin of an epileptic disorder, it should be stated that there is one single seizure type which is *characteristic of*

HH, namely, gelastic attacks. These are sudden, usually brief episodes of laughter, which can be quite "natural" or present an almost "mechanical" quality (Oehl *et al.*, 2010; Arzimanoglou *et al.*, 2003). There are, however, several deviations from the more typical presentations of gelastic attacks, which must be actively sought in clinical history and video recordings. These include a loud laughter, a subtle smile and even a subjective sensation of a "pressure to laugh", which patients may try to voluntarily suppress (Oehl *et al.*, 2010; Sturm *et al.*, 2000). Further variation is the inconsistent reporting of a feeling of mirth associated with the laughing spells (Arroyo *et al.*, 1993).

Beyond gelastic seizures, ictal semiology in patients with HH often depends i) upon propagation routes outside the hypothalamus via the stria terminalis or the mammilo-thalamic tract, and ii) to the progression of the epileptic condition, ie, secondary epileptogenesis in overlying cortical structures. Here comes the necessary understanding of the HH-epilepsy entity as a "great pretender" in that it can mimic a number of other more common epilepsy syndromes. For instance, a significant majority of patients with HH also have seizures virtually indistinguishable from temporal or frontal lobe attacks (Kahane *et al.*, 2003; Oehl *et al.*, 2010; Leal *et al.*, 2003). Disconnection, gestural and oral automatisms as well as hypermotor features with thrashing, rocking and versive movements can all be part of the semiology of seizures associated with HH. Furthermore, EEGs often show temporal, frontal or fronto-temporal epileptic discharges (*Figure 2*). In fact, these cortical regions act both as "dependent" epileptogenic zones and also symptomatogenic zones, which is a unique feature of the HH-epilepsy syndrome. In this strict sense, the notion of this entity as leading to "pseudo-temporal" or "pseudo-frontal" epilepsies may not be totally correct because at least some of these partial seizures with disconnection and automatisms probably truly originate in these cortical regions (Kahane *et al.*, 2003). Thus, they would be truly temporal or frontal lobe-generated seizures, yet because they are in a state of "dependent" stage of secondary epileptogenesis, resection of these regions does not control seizures (which, conversely, are usually controlled by resection of the subcortical hamartoma [Palmini *et al.*, 2003; Berkovic *et al.*, 1997]). Thus, taking into account that HH can be quite small (*Figure 1*), epileptologists must have a high degree of suspicion

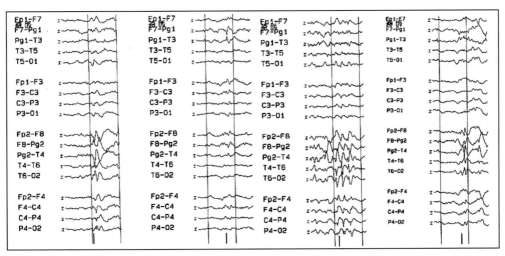

Figure 2. Bitemporal interictal spikes with right side predominance in a patient with a small HH and preserved cognition.

and i) pay attention to the presence of atypical features of temporal lobe attacks, such as dilatation of the pupils, facial twitching and urination, ii) always ask about a past history of laughing attacks, a current history of a "pressure to laugh" and review videos looking for subtle laughing or smiling features at the onset of current "temporal" or "frontal" lobe seizures and iii) carefully look at the regions surrounding the third ventricle in the MRIs of patients with apparently cryptogenic, medically refractory temporal or frontal lobe epilepsies.

Finally, in the most severe forms of epilepsy associated with HH, more malignant seizure types, commonly seen in epileptic encephalopathies, dominate the picture (Palmini *et al.*, 2002; Freeman *et al.*, 2003; Palmini *et al.*, 2003). These patients have drop attacks, prolonged atypical absences and generalized tonic or tonic-clonic seizures, as well as a deteriorating course. Semiology is a marker of this evolution. Patients may initially present only gelastic attacks but over the years progress to these other types of more malignant seizures (Striano *et al.*, 2009; Oehl *et al.*, 2010). Therefore, the HH-epilepsy syndrome may masquerade as a cryptogenic Lennox-Gastaut-like syndrome if the lesion is not carefully searched and the gelastic components are not actively searched in history or video examinations.

■ EEG in relation to semiology

Ictal and interictal EEG in patients with HH is variable and relates to semiology. In fact, semiology and EEG mirror the epilepsy syndrome associated with HH (Freeman *et al.*, 2003; Striano *et al.*, 2009; Arzimanoglou *et al.*, 2003). When only gelastic seizures are present the interictal EEG may be normal and ictal recordings may not show epileptiform activity at all; instead, attenuation of the electrical activity associated with muscle artifacts is the most common finding. On the other hand, patients in the more catastrophic side of the spectrum have EEG features indistinguishable from those of symptomatic generalized epilepsy, the Lennox-Gastaut-like syndromes (*Figure 3*). Multifocal spikes are intermingled with slow spike and wave complexes and these patients have a predominance of prolonged bouts of atypical absences, atonic and tonic seizures, drop attacks, and variable types of complex and motor partial seizures (Striano *et al.*, 2009; Oehl *et al.*, 2010). Some of these patients still have pure gelastic attacks or gelastic components in the beginning of the more severe seizures, but the predominant clinical picture is that of more malignant seizures. However, in pace with the general concept of this chapter, it should be stressed that even though more severe seizures dominate the clinical picture in this catastrophic end of the HH-epilepsy spectrum (Palmini *et al.*, 2002; Freeman *et al.*, 2003), gelastic components should be actively sought. These may have been present at epilepsy onset and not be spontaneously reported by relatives or may still be present in at least some of the current, more malignant seizures, and because they are mild, they may be missed. Interictal scalp EEG in other patients shows spikes at any cortical lobe (*Figure 2*), or may be multilobar. In some patients spikes are unilateral or bilateral frontal, in other they are unilateral or bilateral temporal and in still others they cluster in the posterior quadrants. Several aspects related to EEG findings are of utmost importance: i) in situ and in vitro recordings from hypothalamic hamartoma cells confirm the intrinsic epileptogenicity of these lesions, and the fact that they can generate spikes and seizures – gelastic seizures (Lokovic *et al.*, 2009; Waldau *et al.*, 2009); ii) in many situations – and probably even more so in the less severe cases, in whom gelastic seizures are associated or followed years later by partial seizures with motor, dialeptic, hypo or hypermotor automatisms and relative

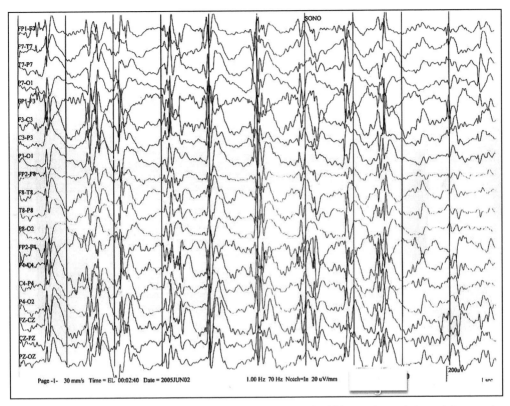

Figure 3. Generalized discharges as the main EEG feature of a girl with a HH, mental retardation and drop attacks.

cognitive sparing – spikes most likely relate to one of the propagation pathways from the hypothalamus (Leal *et al.*, 2003). Because of the richness of hypothalamic connectivity, spikes can be virtually seen everywhere in the brain; iii) in other situations, interictal and ictal (intracranial) data suggest that spikes are indeed generated in the cortex (Kahane *et al.*, 2003); however, because many of these cortical spikes and most of these "cortically generated seizures" usually disappear after resection of the diencephalic lesion, they most likely represent instances of "dependent" stage secondary epileptogenesis (Palmini *et al.*, 2002; Berkovic *et al.*, 1997; 2003; Striano *et al.*, 2009); iv) finally, there is a clear evolution of the EEG abnormalities over the years in selected patients. Why some patients (but not all) progress from focal spikes with reasonably preserved background activity to diffuse slowing and generalized slow spike wave complexes is unclear (Freeman *et al.*, 2003).

■ The bi-axial view of the HH-epilepsy syndrome: electro-clinical and imaging aspects

There are two distinct but intersecting axes, which must be considered when approaching patients with the HH-epilepsy syndrome. Axis 1 concerns the *presentation of the epilepsy syndrome* at any given point in time, which intersects with axis 2, related to *disease progression over time*. Thus, presentation and prognosis are distributed along these 2 axes.

Axis I. The presentation of the epileptic disease

In the mildest end of this spectrum are patients who, despite having seizures for years, are not easily diagnosed as "epileptics", because the only seizures they have are a subjective "pressure to laugh" or brief giggling episodes. Some of these patients may successfully control the impending laughter and their subjective manifestation may not be correctly interpreted as a simple partial seizure or the brief laughter may be seen as normal. Hamartomas are often small. Some of these patients may have had in the past a few more characteristic seizures (dialeptic seizures, partial motor attacks or isolated generalized tonic clonic seizures) who were easily controlled and replaced by the "pressure to laugh", the brief giggling or a sudden "smile" (Oehl et al., 2010). Later on, more obvious seizure phenomena may resume and the diagnosis of these mild gelastic features as true seizure is then made retrospectively.

Then there are patients who have partial seizures, which only infrequently generalize, and relatively preserved cognition, although neuropsychological deficits in some domains are seen. Children and adolescents are able to attend normal schools and adults may work, marry and raise children. The hamartoma is usually small and does not protrude into the interpeduncular cistern. There may be, however, significant morbidity because the attacks are usually refractory to medication. In addition to gelastic seizures, these patients often present partial seizures with autonomic, dialeptic, hypomotor or hypermotor components, as well as focal features such as peri-oral twitching or unilateral clonic or tonic features (Oehl et al., 2010; Olivieri et al., 2010). In fact, ictal semiology is strongly suggestive of temporal or frontal lobe seizures, and because epileptic discharges are also often focally recorded from these regions, cortical resections were attempted in the past, disregarding the HH. These resections uniformly failed to control these seizures (Cascino et al., 1993) and, in this respect, the frontal and temporal lobes must be regarded as "symptomatogenic zones". Thus, a crucial electroclinical fact in the HH-epilepsy syndrome is its presentation as "pseudo-temporal" or "pseudo-frontal" epilepsies (also, see above). A high index of suspicion must be kept to both seek for gelastic elements in the past history or at present seizure onset and to carefully examine the MRI around the third ventricle. Some HH may be so small as to be missed by thick sections around the diencephalon.

Toward the more severe end of this first axis or spectrum are patients with partial and secondarily generalized seizures *without* an overt encephalopathic, "Lennox-Gastaut-like" picture, although with variable degrees of mental retardation. These are usually children with sessile or pedunculated HH who present with uncontrolled seizures, learning disabilities, behavioral abnormalities and variable features of precocious puberty. The gelastic component is usually clearly mentioned, either as part of current seizures or as isolated seizures in the past. Although these patients often lack malignant drop attacks, prolonged bouts of atypical absences and autistic features, they are severely disabled and the diagnosis and resection of the HH is critical to promote major improvements in long-term prognosis.

In the far end of the spectrum of presentation of the epilepsy syndrome are patients with unequivocal epileptic encephalopathies in that they have severe mental retardation with autistic features, multifocal or generalized, very frequent epileptic discharges, multiple refractory seizure types, including drop attacks and generalized tonic seizures and progressive cognitive deterioration (Palmini et al., 2002; 2003; Berkovic et al., 2003; Freeman et al., 2003). These were the patients initially identified as presenting this syndrome when high resolution neuroimaging was in its infancy, because the HH is of moderate to large size, with variable protrusion into the interpeduncular cistern or deformation of the third ventricle (Berkovic *et al.*, 1988). A major distinguishing feature of the epileptic encephalopathy when the etiology is a HH stems exactly from ictal semiology, namely, the occurrence of gelastic seizures either at the very beginning of the current seizures or when epilepsy began, usually years before presentation.

Axis 2. Disease progression over time

Importantly, the epileptic disorder in patients with the HH-epilepsy syndrome often progresses toward more severe seizure types, EEG abnormalities and overall neurological dysfunction (Freeman *et al.*, 2003; Oehl *et al.*, 2010). The fact such progression is not uniformly seen is one of the persisting puzzles of the HH epilepsy syndrome and leads to this second axis of variation in disease activity: i) patients who have an epileptic encephalopathy when they are first seen and have evidence for severe disease from very early in the epilepsy history, ii) patients who begin with partial seizures and reasonably preserved cognition who later progress to a diffuse epileptic encephalopathy and iii) patients who have partial seizures and preserved cognition who do not progress to more severe epileptological and cognitive dysfunction.

This second axis intersects with the presentation of the disorder because the latter depends partially on whether patients progress to more severe epilepsy presentations. The three-tiered classification depicted in the paragraph above is somewhat simplistic but reflects what is seen in clinical practice. Most likely, those patients who have evidence for severe epilepsy very early in their epilepsy history and who are already very compromised when first seen, may also have progressed to this more severe picture, except that such progression took place very early and in a faster pace than others. This is illustrated by the fact that many children have delayed acquisition of some developmental milestones (*e.g.*, language), but may initially develop normally in other spheres. Seizure recurrence and other mechanisms underlying secondary epileptogenesis may then lead to more diffuse and severe cognitive, behavioral and motor abnormalities, unless successful treatment is entertained.

A demonstration of the relevance of axis 2 was provided by Freeman and colleagues in a study comparing seizure types and EEG abnormalities early in the history of epilepsy and many years later, when patients were admitted to surgical treatment of the HH. They showed a semiological progression over the years from gelastic to partial to generalized tonic seizures, which parallels a progression from normal or moderately abnormal EEG to severe EEG abnormalities in the form of generalized slow spike and waves, polyspikes and epochs of low voltage fast activity (Freeman *et al.*, 2003). A detailed semiological review recently published from Freiburg confirms the progression toward more severe and generalized seizure types according to patient age (Oehl *et al.*, 2010).

■ Illustrative cases highlighting important issues

Case I

An adolescent with early gelastic seizures controlled for 10 years and later appearance of partial seizures with disconnection and motor features. Atypical brief gelastic elements (a broad smile, and not laughter) were still present at the beginning of the attacks but were easily overlooked.

MRIs were read as normal because the lesion was very small. There was progression toward more severe epilepsy over the years although cognition was not significantly impaired, except for sedation associated with antiepileptic drug polytherapy.

IM is a 16 year-old boy without perinatal complications, born from non-consanguineous parents, who started with ictal episodes consisting of labial twitching, a cry and a brief laugh at 1 month of life. No etiological diagnosis was possible and, after a few months on phenobarbital, the boy was seizure free without antiepileptic medication for the next 10 years. At age 10 he had a generalized tonic-clonic seizure and then recurrent partial seizures. He resumed antiepileptic medication, however with inconsistent seizure control. Development was normal and the boy loves to skate, surf and play soccer. For the last 3 years, however, he has been barely able to engage in these activities because of frequent seizures, characterized by head turning accompanied by a "smile", then disconnection "as if he was in a prolonged absence spell", followed by gestural automatisms and limb dystonia. At times, these episodes recurred several times in a single day and would only be arrested by intravenous diazepam or midazolam. The many attempts to control his seizures led to a hardly rational 5-drug polytherapy consisting of lamotrigine, oxcarbazepine, clonazepam, ethosuximide and valproic acid. Despite this regimen, he had several clusters of seizures each month and major somnolence. His interictal scalp EEGs showed independent bilateral frontal and temporal lobe discharges, at times predominating on the left side. Ictal recordings showed only diffuse attenuation of electrical activity. Four 1.5 T MRIs were read as normal. However, upon close review of "home-made" videos of many seizures it was clear that there was a broad smile at very beginning of all attacks, just before and accompanying the turning of the head. This prompted a detailed review of the MRIs and the request for a study with very thin sections through the diencephalon and this led to the discovery of a tiny, 5 mm HH (*Figure 1*), recently operated through an endoscopic route.

Case 2

A man with unrecognized gelastic seizures since childhood, temporal lobe attacks and an unrecognized hypothalamic hamartoma at the time of presurgical evaluation for the refractory temporal lobe seizures. Sudden onset of status gelasticus with clusters of classical gelastic seizures following temporal lobectomy. Ictal PET, ictal SPECT and MRI showed a HH involved with the status gelasticus.

This 35 year-old man reported epilepsy since age 10. There was no presumed etiology and some of his seizures manifested only with rising epigastric sensation and nausea. Infrequently, he would have secondary generalization. At age 32 he started with medically refractory seizures in which he would stare and then have hypomotor gestural automatisms. He was referred to preoperative evaluation, which showed left temporal lobe discharges and 4 seizures with left temporal onset on scalp EEG. MRI showed a left temporal lobe subarachnoid cyst, which was resected in conjunction with a left anterior temporal lobectomy. In the immediate post-operative period he developed status gelasticus, characterized by uncontrollable laughing spells lasting 10-20 sec and recurring every 1-5 min, for up to an hour. He was again evaluated and the post-operative MRI showed a small HH with increased metabolism on "ictal" PET. Review of the MRI showed a small, previously unidentified hypothalamic lesion and, upon specific questioning, the patient described 'pressure to laugh' and brief laughing episodes for as long as he could remember. However, he never paid attention to those episodes.

Case 3

Gelastic, "smiley", seizures in the first few months of life, temporarily controlled and followed by pressure to laugh, disconnection, gestural automatisms and falls from age 4. Deterioration in behavior with severe aggressiveness and depression. A small, previously overlooked HH was seen protruding into the third ventricle.

This 14 year-old boy started with seizures at 4 months, characterized by a sudden smile and disconnection. These episodes were completely controlled with phenobarbital for 4 years, when medication was discontinued. Seizures resumed 2 months later, characterized by a 'pressure to laugh' or unmotivated laughter, disconnection, orofacial automatisms and falls. Although seizures were refracrtory to medication, he continued to develop normally and achieved good grades at school. However, his behavior progressively deteriorated and he became extremely aggressive, to the point that his parents wanted to institutionalize him. A school report at age 10 stated that ..."he is a very intelligent boy, fully aware of what he says or does. However, he cannot control his rude expressions and threats. Recently, he said to a colleague that he would get a knife and stick it through the boy's head". He had long periods of depression, only partially alleviated by medication. EEGs had a combination of partial and generalized features *(Figure 4)* and the MRI showed a small, previously overlooked HH *(Figure 5)*.

Case 4

Early onset of typical laughing attacks and precocious puberty progressing to partial and generalized seizures and severe behavior abnormalities, including sexual misconduct.

Following normal delivery and early development, this 20 year-old patient started with sudden laughing attacks at 9 months of age. Seizures were frequent and characterized by gelastic attacks associated with episodes of disconnection, hypomotor automatisms, face twitching and secondary generalization. Somatic and psychomotor developments were clearly precocious. At 9 months he was said to have "all teeth", at 12 months he walked and had body hair and at 1.5 years started to speak full sentences. However, in the context of 6 to 8 seizures a day his cognition and behavior deteriorated and he was aggressive, hypersexual and still went to kindergarten at age 10. When first evaluated, at age 11, he could not read or write, counted only up to 20 and had very low scores and poor cooperation when evaluated with the Wechsler Intelligence Scale for Children (WISC). Furthermore, he expressed overt verbal and physical aggression against children and adults. A few months before admission he had hanged his bird and attacked his dog. He was highly hyperactive and had an awkward hypersexual conduct with obscene gestures and verbal content toward staff. EEGs showed generalized, 3-5 Hz irregular discharges and multifocal spikes, involving independently both frontal and temporal lobes. Background activity, however, was reasonably preserved. Ictal recordings did not localize the ictal onset zone. MRI showed a hypothalamic hamartoma protruding into the interpeduncular cistern *(Figure 6)*. He underwent subtotal resection and complete disconnection of the lesion through a pterional approach and has not had any seizures in the last 10 years. One year after operation he began reading and had such a dramatic behavioral improvement that his mother would repeatedly utter that he was not the same child; he was completely transformed'. At age 20 he lives with his mother and continues to make progress.

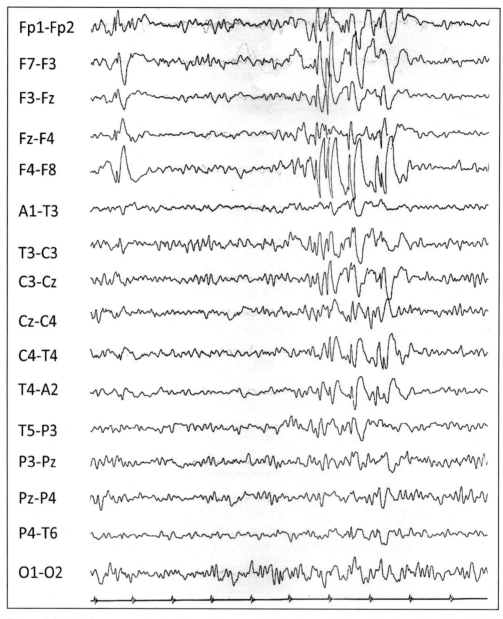

Figure 4. Bilateral fronto-central epileptiform discharges with left side predominance in a boy with a left sided HH (Figure 5).

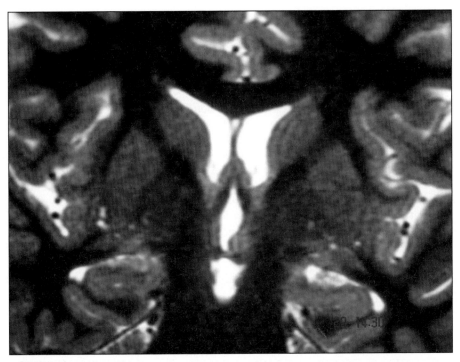

Figure 5. Axial T2-weighted MRI shows a small hamartoma protruding into the third ventricle from the left hypothalamus.

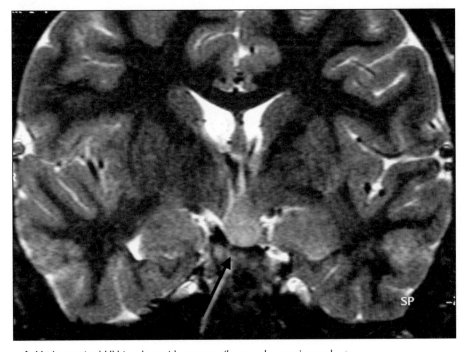

Figure 6. Moderate sized HH in a boy with severe epilepsy and precocious puberty.

Case 5

A boy with gelastic, partial and generalized seizures with important developmental delay and behavioral abnormalities. Despite control of the severe seizures and a dramatic improvement in behavior with surgery, there is lingering cortical EEG discharges and inability to read or write.

This 18 year-old boy started with frequent seizures at age 1. At age 5 he had 3 to 5 episodes of sudden, mechanical laughter accompanied by left facial twitching, 1-2 drop attacks and more than 10 episodes of disconnection every day. Seizures were poorly responsive to medication and the boy made poor contact with others, was highly hyperactive, aggressive and had short attention span and delayed speech acquisition. He would cry loudly, present recurrent temper tantrums and needed constant supervision because of the combination of agitation and sudden epileptic falls. Presurgical evaluation showed independent left frontal and left temporo-parieto-occipital discharges. Ictal EEG had a diffuse left hemisphere onset. Interictal FDG PET showed a left posterior quadrant hypomatabolism and MRI showed a medium-sized, left-sided hypothalamic hamartoma, protruding into the interpeduncular cistern.

The lesion was sub-totally resected through a pterional approach, which largely controlled seizures *(Figure 7)*. He never fell again and for the last 13 years has been having weekly brief episodes of left facial twitching and disconnection. His behavior improved markedly. However, despite excellent vocabulary and oral language skills, he cannot read or write, and needs special education. Recent EEG evaluation shows an intense epileptic focus in the left fronto-temporal region *(Figure 8)*.

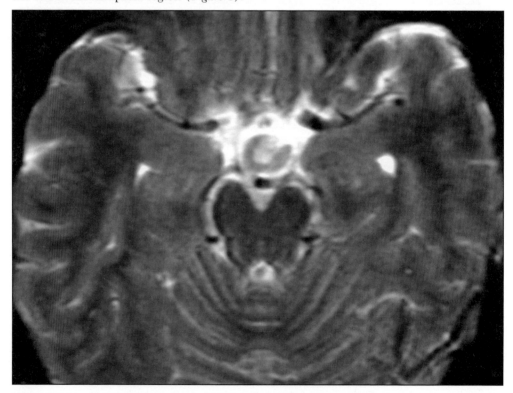

Figure 7. Subtotal resection/disconnection of a HH, fully controlling major attacks.

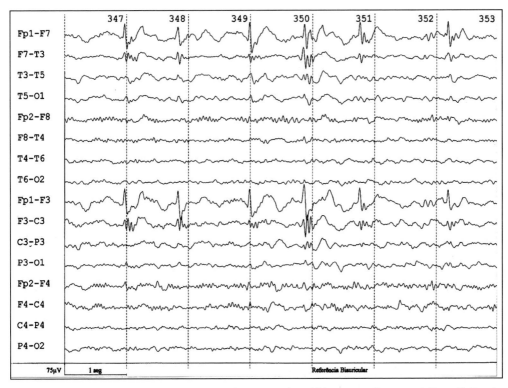

Figure 8. Persistent left frontal lobe discharges in the patient whose HH was partially resected *(Figure 7)*. Despite full control of major attacks, a significant learning disability persisted over the years, which may be related to the persisting discharges.

Case 6

Retrospective diagnosis of gelastic seizures accompanied by autonomic features since childhood in a cognitively preserved man who works and is popular with girlfriends, who had presented with generalized and then partial seizures at age 17.

This 30 year-old right handed man working as an office clerk had uneventful pregnancy and early development. There was no family history of epilepsy and he was able to complete secondary school, although with some difficulties. He has always been impulsive and often loses temper and reacts aggressively. Seizures started in the form of a single generalized tonic-clonic attack at age 17, and progressed as complex partial seizures, occurring 2 to 3 times per week. There is no generalization or drop attacks. Seizures may be controlled for weeks and then return for several days, despite the use of several different antiepileptic drug regimens. The attacks do not incapacitate the patient for his professional and social activities. He has had many girlfriends and is very popular with his friends. Seizures, however, interfere with his ability to drive. This current situation led him to be admitted for preoperative evaluation at our center. Review of the early history shows that, as a child, the patient had daily episodes of staring, giggling, brief cyanosis and heavy sweating. These were not interpreted as seizures. Neurological examination is normal. Interictal EEG recordings showed frequent, bilateral independent epileptic discharges in the temporal lobes, which were isolated in the left, and occurred in rhythmic trains of spikes and spike-wave complexes in the right side *(Figure 2)*. No seizures were recorded. Immediate and late verbal and nonverbal memory scores were within normal range. Verbal learning was also normal, although language and visuospatial abilities were in the intermediate to inferior level. Attentional abilities were within average, and he achieved 6 categories out of 6 in the Wisconsin Card sorting Test. MRI showed an hamartomatous lesion in the right side of the hypothalamus, posterior to the level of the mammilary bodies, which protruded into the third ventricle and slightly displaced downwards the right mammilary body *(Figure 9)*. The lesion measured 12 mm in the larger axis.

■ Wrapping up: ictal semiology and the crucial role of the epileptologist

Interestingly enough, the HH-epilepsy syndrome can be seen from the perspective of an established and easily identifiable disorder or as a major epileptological challenge. I suggest epileptologists take this second view and realize the challenges begin with semiology. Although "classical" gelastic attacks are highly suggestive (albeit not pathognomonic [Cheung *et al.*, 2007; Dericioglu *et al.*, 2005]) of HH, there are several possible variations both in semiologic presentation and timing of gelastic seizures in these patients. These must be recognized by the epileptologist who then needs to look in detail to the MRI. Small HH may often pass unrecognized and not be mentioned in radiological reports.

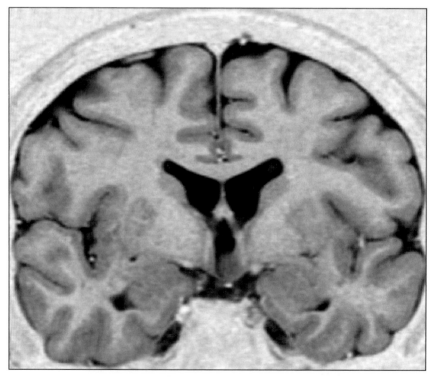

Figure 9. Coronal IR MRI section showing a small HH protruding into the thrid ventricle. This man had a retrospective diagnosis of gelastic seizures and is currently cognitively preserved, despite refractory partial attacks.

Furthermore, HH may disguise as several other, more common epilepsy syndromes. Because fairly typical features of frontal, temporal or symptomatic generalized epilepsies are very frequent semiological elements in patients with HH, a high index of suspicion must be kept in the minds of epileptologists to look at the diencephalon. In fact, a practical lesson thought by experience is that in patients with severe partial or generalized epilepsies and normal "cortical" MRI, a HH must be suspected and carefully searched – and the epileptologist is often in a better position to do this than the neurordiologist. This would spare quite a lot of trouble, including evaluating these patients invasively and resecting cortical regions presumably related to seizure generation without real chances of a good result (Cascino et al., 1993).

Perhaps the best final words for this text come from these honest past experience of failures with cortical resections in patients with HH. Along with the advances in the last 20 years, these initial cases helped us to understand a unique feature of the syndrome of HH-epilepsy, and that is the "dual interference" these lesions have with the cortical regions with which they are connected. When associated with an HH, these cortical areas **behave both** as epileptogenic zones in a dependent stage of secondary epileptogenesis (ie, they generate seizures but do not need to be resected for seizure control) and as symptomatogenic zones (in the sense that they are activated by ictal propagation from the hypothalamus and seizures are controlled by resection or disconnection of the true subcortical epileptogenic zone). Finally, the development of this subcortical-cortical interplay takes time and the passage of time shapes the presentation of the epilepsy syndrome. Therefore, I have proposed here that the epileptologist should look at this syndrome from the perspective of two intersecting axes and takes into account as much the actual clinical presentation at any given point in time but also the progression of the disease over time. Brain plasticity is everywhere and the HH-epilepsy syndrome illustrates it beyond doubt.

References

- Arroyo S, Lesser RP, Gordon B. Mirth, laughter and geleastic seizures. *Brain* 1993; 116: 757-80.

- Arzimanoglou A, Hirsch E, Aicardi J. Hypothalamic hamartoma and epilepsy in children: illustrative cases of possible evolutions. *Epileptic Disord* 2003; 5: 187-99.

- Berkovic S, Andermann F, Melanson D, et al. Hypothalamic hamartomas and ictal laughter: evolution of a characteristic epileptic syndrome and diagnostic value of magnetic resonance imaging. *Ann Neurol* 1988; 23: 429-39.

- Berkovic S, Kuzniecky R, Andermann F. Human epileptogenesis and hypothalamic hamartomas: new lessons from an experiment of nature. *Epilepsia* 1997; 38: 1-3.

- Berkovic SF, Arzimanoglou A, Kuzniecky R, et al. Hypothalamic hamartoma and seizures: a treatable epileptic encephalopathy. *Epilepsia* 2003; 44: 969-73.

- Cascino GD, Andermann F, Berkovic S. Gelastic seizures and hypothalamic hamartomas: evaluation of patients undergoing chronic intracranial EEG monitoring and outcome o surgical treatment. *Neurology* 1993; 43: 747-50.

- Chen Y, Wu L, Fang Y, et al. A novel mutation of the nicotinic acetylcholine receptor gene CHRNA4 in sporadic nocturnal frontal lobe epilepsy. *Epilepsy Res* 2009; 83: 152-6.

- Cheung CS, Parrent AG, Burneo JG. Gelastic seizures: not always hypothalamic hamartoma. *Epileptic Disord* 2007; 9: 453-8.

- Dericioglu N, Cataltepe O, Tezel GG, Saygi S. Gelastic seizures due to right temporal cortical dysplasia. *Epileptic Disord* 2005; 7: 137-41.
- Escayg A, Goldin AL. Sodium channel *SCN1A* and epilepsy: mutations and mechanisms. *Epilepsia* 2010; 51: 1650-8.
- Freeman JL, Harvey AS, Rosenfeld JV, *et al.* Generalized epilepsy in hypothalamic hamartoma: evolution and postoperative resolution. *Neurology* 2003; 60: 762-7.
- Kahane P, Ryvlin P, Hoffmann D, *et al.* From hypothalamic hamartoma to cortex: what can be learnt from depth recordings and stimulation? *Epileptic Disord* 2003; 5: 205-17.
- Kuzniecky R, Guthrie B, Mountz J. Intrinsic epileptogenicity of hypothalamic hamartomas in gelastic epilepsy. *Ann Neurol* 1997; 42: 60-7.
- Leal AJ, Moreira A, Robalo C, Ribeiro C. Different electroclinical manifestations of the epilepsy associated with hamartomas connecting to the middle or posterior hypothalamus. *Epilepsia* 2003; 44: 1191-5.
- Lokovic GP, Kerrigan JE, Waiy S, *et al.* In situ single-unit recording of hypothalamic hamartomas under endoscopic direct visualization. *Neurosurgery* 2009; 65: E1195-E1196.
- Munari C, Kahane P, Francione S, *et al.* Role of the hypothalamic hamartoma in the genesis of gelastic fits (a video-stereo-EEG study). *Electroencephalogr Clin Neurophysiol* 1995; 95: 154-60.
- Oehl B, Brandt A, Fauser S, *et al.* Semiologic aspects of epileptic seizures in 31 patients with hypothalamic hamartoma. *Epilepsia* 2010; 51: 2116-23.
- Olivieri I, Teutonico F, Orcesi S, *et al.* Paroxysmal tonic eye deviation: an atypical presentation of hypothalamic hamartoma. *Epileptic Disord* 2010; 12: 233-5.
- Palmini A, Chandler C, Andermann F, *et al.* Resection of the lesion in patients with hypothalamic hamartomas and catastrophic epilepsy. *Neurology* 2002; 58: 1338-47.
- Palmini A, Paglioli-Neto E, Montes J, Farmer JP. The treatment of patients with hypothalamic hamartomas, epilepsy and behavioural abnormalities: facts and hypotheses. *Epileptic Disord* 2003; 5: 249-55.
- Striano S, Striano P, Coppola A, Romanelli P. The syndrome gelastic seizures-hypoythalamic hamartoma: severe, potentially reversible encephalopathy. *Epilepsia* 2009; 50 (Suppl. 5): 62-5.
- Sturm JW, Andermann F, Berkovic SF. "Pressure to laugh": an unusual epileptic symptom associated with small hypothalamic hamartomas. *Neurology* 2000; 54: 971-3.
- Waldau B, McLendon RE, Fuchs HE, *et al.* Few isolated neurons in hypothalamic hamartomas may cause gelastic seizures. *Pediatr Neurosurg* 2009; 45: 225-9.

Section II:
Non-invasive neurophysiology
of extratemporal lobe epilepsies

Nonivasive neurophysiology of extratemporal lobe epilepsy: interictal epileptiform discharges

Felix Rosenow, Sebastian Bauer, Hajo M. Hamer

Epilepsy Center Hessen, Department of Neurology, UKGM Marburg & Philipps-University of Marburg, Marburg, Germany

■ General considerations

The main goal of the presurgical evaluation in patients with medically intractable epilepsy is the identification of the cortical area capable of generating seizures, and whose removal or disconnection will result in seizure freedom. This area is called the epileptogenic zone. The irritative zone is the area of cortex capable of generating interictal epileptiform discharges (IED, spikes and sharp waves). It does not coincide but frequently overlaps with the usually smaller epileptogenic zone (Rosenow & Lüders, 2001; Carreno & Lüders, 2001). Extensive experience with routine extracranial EEG shows that in general the location of IED is a good indicator of the area of cortex from which seizures are originating (Binnie & Stefan, 1999; Hamer, 2008).

IED have a pointed peak and are usually of negative polarity because they are generated by depolarization of vertically oriented neurons (Pedley & Traub, 1997; Celesia & Chen, 1976). Spikes and sharp waves convey an increased risk of epilepsy and must be differentiated from benign variants resembling IED (Binnie & Stefan, 1999; Foldvary, 2000; Hamer *et al.*, 2010). Cerebral activity is attenuated by the impedance of the cerebrospinal fluid, meninges, skull and scalp. Therefore, scalp EEG fails to show a great number of IED recorded by depth or subdural electrodes and interictal activity arising from sulci (*Figure 1*), deep or midline structures and from small generators of less than 10 cm^2 of cortex (*Figure 1*) is usually not reflected in surface EEG (Carreno & Lüders, 2001, see also the chapter on subdural EEG recordings in this book). The distribution of IED on the scalp depends on the conductive properties of the surrounding tissue, the spatial characteristics of the generator, propagation pathways and on the spatial resolution of the surface EEG. Consequently, the distribution of interictal epileptic discharges in the scalp EEG can fail to localize or even mislocalize the region or hemisphere of seizure origin (Foldvary, 2000). Patients with an epileptogenic zone in the frontal, occipital, insular-opercular and orbitofrontal regions may show falsely localizing temporal IED (Kutsy, 1999; Aykut-Bingol *et al.*, 1998; Kellinghaus & Luders, 2004).

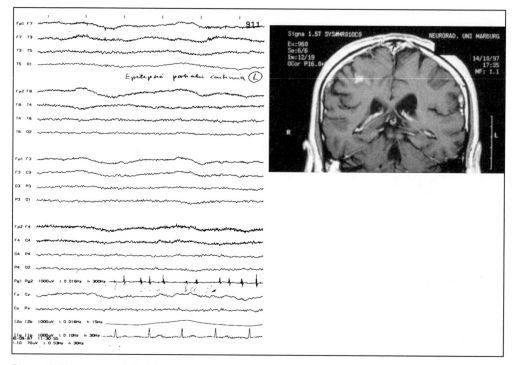

Figure 1. Clonic status of the left thumb - no EEG change. **A.** The normal EEG and the EMG from left forearm (channel 17) correlated with repetitive twitching of the left thumb observed clinically in this patient with an acute right central sulcus infarction shown in **B.** The coronal T1-weighted MRI with contrast media. This illustrates that epileptiform discharges generated by deeply seated small lesions are frequently missed by non-invasive surface EEG even if localized on the fronto-lateral convexity.

The first EEG will uncover IED in about 30%-50% of the patients with epilepsy and the yield increases to 60%-90% by the fourth EEG (Marsan & Zivin, 1970, Salinsky et al., 1987; Binnie & Stefan, 1999). This contrasts with the frequency of IED in non-epileptic patients ranging from 0.5% in healthy young men (Gregory et al., 1993) to 12% in a study including all age groups and patients with cerebral disorders (Sam & So, 2001).

Closely spaced scalp electrodes can improve the yield of spike detection and localization over the standard 10-20 system (Morris HH et al., 1986). The yield from a single EEG is substantially increased in patients investigated within one or two days after a seizure, and is greater in patients with monthly seizures than in those who had been seizure-free for a year (Marsan & Zivin, 1970; Sundaram et al., 1990, King et al. 1998). The duration of recording may also affect the detection rate of interictal spiking (Gotman & Koffler 1989).

Moreover, the yield can be significantly increased and new abnormalities found, if the EEG includes sleep recordings (Binnie & Stefan, 1999; King et al., 1998, Dinner et al., 2002, Bazil & Walczak 1997). IED are seen more commonly during sleep, with the greatest activation during non-REM sleep (Dinner et al., 2002; Malow et al., 1998; Samaritano et al., 1991). On the other hand many sharp transients of unknown significance, e.g. benign epileptiform transients of sleep (also referred to small sharp spikes, Hamer et al., 2010) and normal sleep transient such as vertex sharp waves are recorded, which can be difficult to discern from IED occurring with a similar distribution (for example see *Figure 2*).

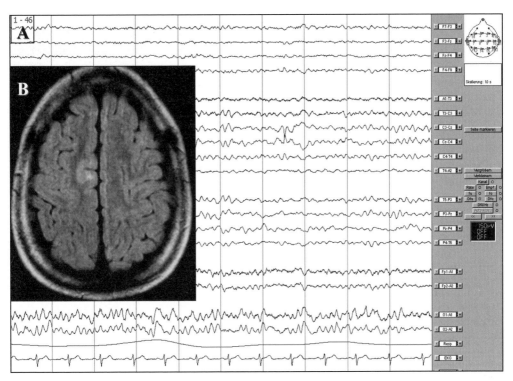

Figure 2. Sharp wave at the vertex or "vertex sharp wave" as a normal sleep transient? **A.** The EEG shows an interictal epileptiform discharge at the vertex, likely related to the mesiofrontal focal cortical dysplasia shown in **B.** The FLAIR-MRI in this patient with drug refractory mesial frontal lobe epilepsy. As the patient is in sleep stage I this discharge could also represent a physiological vertex sharp wave, from which it cannot be clearly discerned. Only the MRI and the facts that such discharges did also occur in the awake state and an EEG-seizure pattern started with an equally distributed sharp wave argue for its epileptic nature.

Hyperventilation or photic stimulation rarely activate IED in patients with focal epilepsies (Klein *et al.*, 2003; Celesia & Chen, 1976; Kasteleijn-Nolst Trenite, 1989; Shiraishi *et al.*, 2001).

Specificity of IED is probably lower and sensitivity higher in children as compared to adults (Binnie & Stefan, 1999). Overall, it can be expected that around 10% of the patients with epilepsy, more with extratemporal than with temporal epilepsy, will show no IED in scalp EEG during wakefulness or sleep in spite of prolonged or repeated recordings (Salinsky *et al.*, 1987; Binnie & Stefan, 1999; Adachi *et al.*, 1998).

Multichannel whole-head MEG has a similar sensitivity to detect IED as compared to non-invasive EEG (Barkley & Baumgartner, 2003; Barkley, 2004; Baumgartner, 2004) and the combination of both provide complementary and confirmatory information for the localization IED which cannot be obtained with either technique alone. In a study on 70 surgical candidates, MEG identified IED in one third of EEG negative patients, especially in cases of lateral neocortical epilepsies and epilepsies due to cortical dysplasia. Conversely, IED were seen only in the EEG in a subset of patients with mesial frontal lobe epilepsy (Knake *et al.*, 2006).

In general, the frequency, repetition rate, morphologic characteristics and state dependence of interictal epileptiform activity cannot be used to predict the etiology or severity of the disorder (Foldvary, 2000). However, rhythmic spiking on a slow background activity and not associated with behavioral changes and polyspike burst (*Figure 3*) have been found to be characteristic for focal cortical dysplasia (Palmini *et al.*, 1995; Noachtar *et al.*, 2008). Tumors tended to cause wider distributed IED as compared to developmental abnormalities or hippocampal sclerosis (Hamer *et al.*, 1999).

In both, temporal and extratemporal epilepsy, the presence of unifocal IED preoperatively (Holmes *et al.*, 2000) and the absence of IED 6-month or 1-year postoperative scalp EEG was associated with superior postoperative outcome (Godoy *et al.*, 1992; Patrick *et al.*, 1995; Hildebrandt *et al.*, 2005). The prognostic value of a 3-month postoperative EEG remains controversial (Radhakrishnan *et al.*, 1998; Tuunainen *et al.*, 1994). The presence of IED in the early extracranial postoperative EEG (within one or two weeks) were not found to be of prognostic value in most of the studies (Salanova *et al.*, 1992; Mintzer *et al.*, 2005; Radhakrishnan *et al.*, 1998).

■ Extratemporal lobe epilepsies

The yield of surface EEG is lower in extratemporal lobe epilepsy (ETLE) as compared to temporal lobe epilepsy (TLE). More than a third of patients with frontal lobe epilepsy may not show any IED in extracranial EEG so that absence of interictal spikes with

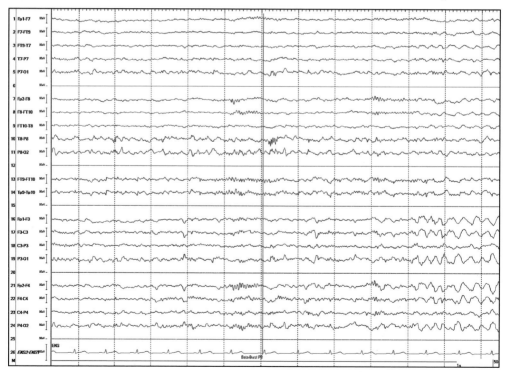

Figure 3. Occipital polyspike burst. The EEG (bipolar longitudinal montage) shows a continuous slowing, and polyspike burst regional right occipital (P8 maximum), clearly indicative of right occipital or parieto-occipital lobe epilepsy. Furthermore, polyspike burst are characteristic of but not specific for focal cortical dysplasia.

documented seizures suggests extratemporal epilepsy (So, 2000; Provini *et al.*, 1999; Stuve *et al.*, 2001). If IED are recorded in extratemporal epilepsy, especially in FLE, they tend to be less well-localized, multifocal, generalized, or even mislateralized (Stuve *et al.*, 2001; Binder *et al.*, 2009; Westmoreland, 1998; Quesney, 1991; Laskowitz *et al.*, 1995; Garzon & Lüders, 2008). In ETLE with irritative zones localized parasagitally near the midline two typical phenomena can occur: a) secondary bilateral synchrony initially reported by Tükel and Jasper (1952) and b) paradoxical lateralization.

Secondary bilateral synchrony *(Figure 4)* refers to bilaterally synchronously generalized IED which can be observed in up to 40% of such patients (Tükel & Jasper, 1952; Blume & Pillay, 1985; Cukiert *et al.*, 1999; Ferrier *et al.*, 1999; Williamson *et al.*, 1986). Fifty percent of the cases were related to FLE in one study (Blume & Pillay, 1985). Bilateral synchronous spikes were more frequently associated with a thalamic fMRI bold response as compared to focal discharges in the same patient suggesting a role of the thalamus in the pathophysiology of secondary bilateral synchrony (Aghakhani *et al.*, 2006). The presence of unilateral focal discharges (for $\geq$ 2 seconds) prior to the occurrence of generalized IED and additional focal or at least lateralized epileptiform or non-epileptiform abnormalities seen strictly on the same side differentiate secondary bilateral synchrony from generalized IED (Blume & Pillay, 1985; Tükel & Jasper, 1952; Bautista *et al.*, 1998; Vadlamudi *et al.*, 2004).

Paradoxical lateralization refers to a situation when IEDs are recorded with the highest amplitudes in the scalp electrodes contralateral to the generator of an EEG discharge (Blume, 2001; Garzon *et al.*, 2009; Adelman *et al.*, 1982). This occurs if the compound vector of an IED is directed in such a way that contralateral electrodes best record the discharge (Cruse *et al.*, 1982; Rosenow & Lüders, 2001) *(Figure 5)*. Paradoxical lateralization can be suspected if IED appear ipsilateral to more normal background activity or contralateral to an epileptogenic lesion and does not predict a poor postoperative outcome (Garzon *et al.*, 2009).

■ Frontal lobe epilepsy

As the value of ictal recordings is restricted in frontal lobe epilepsy (FLE) due to movement and muscle artefact, rapid spread and short seizure duration (Lee *et al.*, 2000), careful analysis of the interictal EEG is of special importance. Because of the inaccessibility of much of the frontal lobe to surface electrodes the interictal EEG reveals spikes or sharp waves in only 60-80% of patients with frontal lobe epilepsies. These epileptiform discharges are of less localizing value than in temporal lobe epilepsy because they can be bilateral, lateralized or even generalized (Salanova *et al.*, 1993; Laskowitz *et al.*, 1995; Mosewich *et al.*, 2000; Wetjen *et al.*, 2002; Kellinghaus & Luders, 2004; Beleza *et al.*, 2009). The localizing value of both interictal and ictal EEG findings is higher if the epileptogenic zone is located in the dorso-lateral frontal lobe as compared to mesial or basal frontal lobe (Bautista *et al.*, 1998). Concordance of the epileptogenic zone with the irritative zone was found in 72% of the patients with lateral FLE compared to 33% with mesial FLE (Vadlamudi *et al.*, 2004). Possible reasons for this difference are the smaller distance between lateral cortex areas and scalp electrodes and the fact that tangential dipoles in mesial FLE cannot be detected by EEG. The use of closely spaced surface electrodes (according to the 10-10 system) can improve localization of the irritative zone but did neither increased EEG sensitivity in 23 patients with frontal or central lobe epilepsy nor did it help in

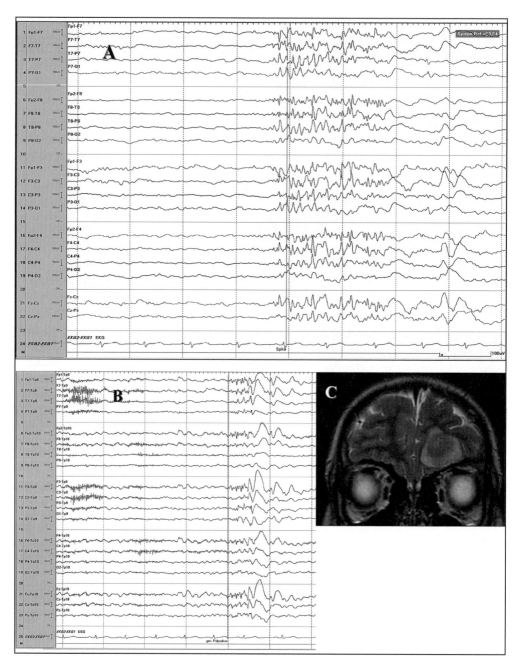

Figure 4. (Secondary) bilateral synchrony – left frontal lesion. **A.** The EEG (bipolar longitudinal montage) shows an interictal group of bilaterally synchronous spikes and sharp waves, generalized maximum bifrontal. **B.** At other times more clearly (left) lateralized discharges were recorded (referential montage against ipsilateral mastoids). **C.** Shows the epileptogenic lesion which was a left fronto-baso-polar tumor (PNET WHO °IV) localized near the midline.

lateralizing the irritative zone in those patients who had bilateral epileptic discharges in conventional EEG (Gross et al., 2000). Generalized IED in FLE are associated with poor postoperative outcome while unifocal IED were highly predictive of successful outcome (Janszky et al., 2000; Holmes et al., 2000).

Interictal rhythmic midline theta (RMT) during wake state (5-7 Hz, duration 3-12 sec, located over vertex (Cz) or fronto-central midline (Fz), occurrence 2-10 times per day) could be found in about 50% of FLE patients, but only in 4% of TLE patients (Beleza et al., 2009). Moreover, RMT appeared more often in patients with mesial FLE and in patients without interictal epileptiform discharges. Thus, RMT can be helpful to distinguish FLE from TLE and adds to the localization of the epileptogenic zone. However, drowsiness and mental activation are other causes for the appearance of RMT and have to be excluded.

■ Cingulate epilepsy

The cingulated gyrus, while formally localized in the frontal and parietal lobes is part of the limbic system and has extensive connections to the mesial temporal and other limbic structures (Garzon & Lüders, 2008; Vogt & Pandya, 1987; Devinsky et al., 1995). In a recent case series (n = 8) including a review of the literature 75% of the patients had mainly ipsilateral IED which were localized to the vertex or temporal area. Only 2 of 4 patients with anterior (frontal) cingulate lesion had any IED, one at the vertex and one bitemporally. In the posterior (parietal) cingulated lesion group (n = 4) three had temporal IED and one showed vertex spikes (Garzon & Lüders, 2008). Therefore, localization of the irritative zone to one ore both temporal lobes appears to frequent in patients with cingulated gyrus epilepsies.

■ Parietal lobe epilepsy

The relative frequency of parietal lobe epilepsy (PLE) is generally considered low and the data concerning this patient group are limited (Sveinbjornsdottir & Duncan, 1993, Kim et al., 2004). The majority of patients with PLE shows IED. The IED are usually widespread and multifocal and can be bilateral suggesting an extent of the irritative zone far beyond the epileptogenic zone (Blume et al., 1991; Binder et al., 2009; Bösebeck et al., 2002; Cascino et al., 1993; Salanova et al., 1995; Sveinbjornsdottir & Duncan, 1993). In a recent study all 26/26 patients with adequate interictal recordings had IED. IED were unilateral and unifocal in 7/26, unilateral multifocal in 11/26 and 8/26 patients had additional contralateral foci (Binder et al., 2009). Secondary bilateral synchrony can be recorded in up to 30% of the cases especially with parasagittal lesions (Salanova et al., 1995; Bösebeck et al., 2002). In general, extracranial interictal EEG findings are an unreliable indicator of parietal lobe epilepsy and should be carefully addressed if there is disagreement between scalp-recorded EEG and neuroimaging (Cascino et al., 1993; Williamson, 1992a).

■ Occipital lobe epilepsy (OLE)

A great majority of patients with occipital lobe epilepsy (OLE) have abnormal interictal or ictal EEG findings but scalp EEG may fail to detect epileptiform activity generated by an irritative zone on the inferior and mesial occipital surfaces. The most frequent interictal

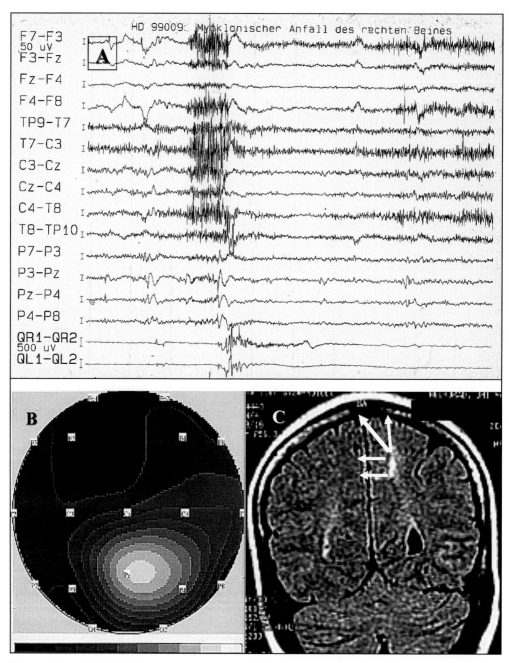

Figure 5. Paradoxical lateralization (modified from Rosenow & Lüders 2001). **A.** The EEG (bipolar transverse montage) shows a regional spike followed by a slow wave, maximum Pz followed by P4 and associated with a tonic contraction of the quadriceps muscles bilaterally (EMG: lowest two channels) and clinically by a myoclonic seizure. **B.** Spike amplitude field seen from the top showing the maximum more to the right (Pz > P4). **C.** A left parietal focal cortical dysplasia type IIB is shown with the direction of single (green) vectors likely generated by the discharges in the gyri overlying the FCD and the resulting sum vector (yellow) pointing to the contralateral side (paradox lateralization).

epileptiform discharges (IED) in OLE are spikes and sharp waves in temporal or temporo-occipital regions with shifting maximums in some patients (Aykut-Bingol et al., 1998; Sveinbjornsdottir & Duncan, 1993; Taylor et al., 2003; Williamson et al., 1992b). Widespread and bilateral IED including secondary bilateral synchrony are common and isolated epileptiform activity restricted to the occipital lobe is infrequent (Aykut-Bingol et al., 1998; Salanova et al., 1992; Williamson & Spencer, 1986; Williamson et al., 1992b).

Rarely, IED can be recorded with highest amplitudes in the contralateral occipital region in the sense of a paradoxical lateralization if their dipole is oriented in such a way that contralateral occipital electrodes best detect it (Blume, 2001; Blume & Wiebe, 2000).

In a recent study of 54 patients with OLE 49 had adequate interictal EEG samples for review. Of these 20 (41%) had unilateral IED which were restricted to posterior leads in on three patients. Nine patients had IED extending beyond the posterior leads and eight had unilateral IED not including posterior leads. Sixteen patients (22%) had bilateral or contralateral (paradoxically lateralized) IED and in 13 patients (27%) no IED were recorded (Binder et al., 2008).

A preponderance of focal IED may reflect the underlying pathology because the incidence of focal occipital IED was much higher in occipital epilepsies caused by malformations than in those due to tumors (Kutsy, 1999). Patients with focal epilepsies generally have a low incidence of photosensitivity of 0.7% to 3.0% (Wolf & Goosses, 1986; Kasteleijn-Nolst Trenite, 1989; Shiraishi et al., 2001). Among these patients, however, patients with OLE have the highest incidence ranging from 6% to 13% (Ludwig & Marsan, 1975; Shiraishi et al., 2001; Taylor et al., 2003).

In contrast to temporal lobe epilepsies, where the lack of contralateral IED is predictive for a seizure-free postoperative outcome (Schulz et al., 2000), this correlation is under discussion in posterior epilepsies (Aykut-Bingol et al., 1998; Binder et al., 2008; Bösebeck et al., 2002; Kun et al., 2005). Moreover, location of IED in any cortical region was not associated with the outcome in 42 surgical candidates suffering from occipital or parietal lobe epilepsy (Bösebeck et al., 2002). Similarly in two other studies of 35 and 54 patients who underwent surgery for intractable OLE, there was no relation between occipital and extraoccipital interictal surface EEG findings and seizure characteristics, postoperative outcome, or lesion location on MRI (Aykut-Bingol et al., 1998; Binder et al., 2008).

∎ Conclusion

The value of IEDs in the scalp-recorded EEG is more limited in extratemporal epilepsy as compared to temporal lobe epilepsy. Many of the patients with extratemporal epilepsy show either no or widespread, multifocal and even contralateral discharges. Mesial frontal and parieto-occipital lesions facilitate secondary bilateral synchrony and paradoxical lateralization. In contrast to temporal and frontal lobe epilepsy, no association could be found between poor postoperative outcome and preoperatively recorded multifocal or bilateral IED in occipital or parietal lobe epilepsies.

References

- Adachi N, Alarcon G, Binnie CD, *et al*. Predictive value of interictal epileptiform discharges during non-REM sleep on scalp EEG recordings for the lateralization of epileptogenesis. *Epilepsia* 1998; 39: 628-32.

- Adelman S, Lueders H, Dinner DS, Lesser RP. Paradoxical lateralization of parasagittal sharp waves in a patient with epilepsia partialis continua. *Epilepsia* 1982; 23: 291-5.

- Aghakhani Y, Kobayashi E, Bagshaw AP, Hawco C, Bénar CG, Dubeau F, Gotman J. Cortical and thalamic fMRI responses in partial epilepsy with focal and bilateral synchronous spikes. *Clin Neurophysiol* 2006; 117: 177-91.

- Aykut-Bingol C, Bronen RA, Kim JH, Spencer DD, Spencer SS. Surgical outcome in occipital lobe epilepsy: implications for pathophysiology. *Ann Neurol* 1998; 44: 60-9.

- Barkley GL. Controversies in neurophysiology. MEG is superior to EEG in localization of interictal epileptiform activity: Pro. *Clin Neurophysiol* 2004; 115: 1001-9.

- Barkley GL, Baumgartner C. MEG and EEG in epilepsy. *J Clin Neurophysiol* 2003; 20: 163-78.

- Baumgartner C. Controversies in clinical neurophysiology. MEG is superior to EEG in the localization of interictal epileptiform activity: Con. *Clin Neurophysiol* 2004; 115: 1010-20.

- Bautista RE, Spencer DD, Spencer SS. EEG findings in frontal lobe epilepsies. *Neurology* 1998; 50: 1765-71.

- Bazil CW, Walczak TS. Effects of sleep and sleep stage on epileptic and nonepileptic seizures. *Epilepsia* 1997; 38: 56-62.

- Beleza P, Bilgin O, Noachtar S. Interictal rhythmical midline theta differentiates frontal from temporal lobe epilepsies. *Epilepsia* 2009; 50: 550-5.

- Binder DK, Podlogar M, Clusmann H, Bien C, Urbach H, Schramm J, Kral T. Surgical treatment of parietal lobe epilepsy. *J Neurosurg* 2009; 110: 1170-8.

- Binder DK, Von Lehe M, Kral T, Bien CG, Urbach H, Schramm J, Clusmann H. Surgical treatment of occipital lobe epilepsy. *J Neurosurg* 2008; 109: 57-69.

- Binnie CD, Stefan H. Modern electroencephalography: its role in epilepsy management. *Clin Neurophysiol* 1999; 110: 1671-97.

- Blume WT. Interictal electroencephalography in neocortical epilepsy. In: Lüders HO, Comair Y, eds. *Epilepsy Surgery*. Philadelphia: Lipppincott Williams & Wilkins, 2001, 403-12.

- Blume WT, Pillay N. Electrographic and clinical correlates of secondary bilateral synchrony. *Epilepsia* 1985; 26: 636-41.

- Blume WT, Whiting SE, Girvin JP. Epilepsy surgery in the posterior cortex. *Ann Neurol* 1991; 29: 638-45.

- Blume WT, Wiebe S. Occipital lobe epilepsies. *Adv Neurol* 2000; 84: 173-87.

- Bösebeck F, Schulz R, May T, Ebner A. Lateralizing semiology predicts the seizure outcome after epilepsy surgery in the posterior cortex. *Brain* 2002; 125: 2320-31.

- Carreno M, Lüders HO. General principles of presurgical evaluation. In: Lüders HO, Comair YG, eds. Epilepsy Surgery. Philadelphia: Lippincott Williams & Wilkins, 2001, 185-99.

- Cascino GD, Hulihan JF, Sharbrough FW, Kelly PJ. Parietal lobe lesional epilepsy: electroclinical correlation and operative outcome. *Epilepsia* 1993; 34: 522-7.

- Celesia GG, Chen RC. Parameters of spikes in human epilepsy. *Dis Nerv Syst* 1976; 37: 277-81.

- Cruse R, Klem G, Lesser RP, Leuders H. Paradoxical lateralization of cortical potentials evoked by stimulation of posterior tibial nerve. *Arch Neurol* 1982; 39: 222-5.

- Cukiert A, Forster C, Buratini JA, *et al*. Secondary bilateral synchrony due to fronto-mesial lesions. An invasive recording study. *Arq Neuropsiquiatr* 1999; 57: 636-42.

- Devinsky O, Morrell MJ, Vogt BA. Contributions of anterior cingulate cortex to behaviour. *Brain* 1995; 118: 279-306.
- Dinner DS. Effect of sleep on epilepsy. *J Clin Neurophysiol* 2002: 19: 504-13.
- Ferrier CH, Engelsman J, Alarcon G, Binnie CD, Polkey CE. Prognostic factors in presurgical assessment of frontal lobe epilepsy. *J Neurol Neurosurg Psychiatry* 1999; 66: 350-6.
- Foldvary N. Focal epilepsy and surgical evaluation. In: Levin KH, Lüders HO, eds. *Comprehensive Clinical Neurophysiology*. Saunders Company: Philadelphia, 2000, 481-96.
- Garzon E, Gupta A, Bingaman W, Sakamoto AC, Lüders H. Paradoxical ictal EEG lateralization in children with unilateral encephaloclastic lesions. *Epileptic Disord* 2009; 11: 215-21.
- Garzon E, Lüders HO. Cingulate epilepsy. In Lüders HO, ed. *Textbook of Epilepsy Surgery*. Informa: 2008, 334-53.
- Godoy J, Luders H, Dinner DS, *et al*. Significance of sharp waves in routine EEGs after epilepsy surgery. *Epilepsia* 1992; 33: 285-8.
- Gotman J, Koffler DJ. Interictal spiking increases after seizures but does not after decrease in medication. *Electroencephalogr Clin Neurophysiol* 1989; 72: 7-15.
- Gregory RP, Oates T, Merry RT. Electroencephalogram epileptiform abnormalities in candidates for aircrew training. *Electroencephalogr Clin Neurophysiol* 1993; 86: 75-7.
- Gross DW, Dubeau F, Quesney LF, Gotman J. EEG telemetry with closely spaced electrodes in frontal lobe epilepsy. *J Clin Neurophysiol* 2000; 17: 414-8.
- Hamer HM, Najm I, Mohamed A, *et al*. Interictal epileptiform discharges in temporal lobe epilepsy due to hippocampal sclerosis versus medial temporal lobe tumors. *Epilepsia* 1999; 40: 1261-8.
- Hamer HM, Rosenow F, v. Stuckrad-Barre S. EEG Pocketflyer. Börm: Bruckmeier Verlag, 2010.
- Hamer HM. Non-invasive EEG evaluation of the irritative zone. In: Lüders HO, ed: *Textbook of Epilepsy Surgery*. Informa 2008, 512-20
- Hildebrandt M, Schulz R, Hoppe M, *et al*. Postoperative routine EEG correlates with long-term seizure outcome after epilepsy surgery. *Seizure* 2005; 14: 446-51.
- Holmes MD, Kutsy RL, Ojemann GA, *et al*. Interictal, unifocal spikes in refractory extratemporal epilepsy predict ictal origin and postsurgical outcome. *Clin Neurophysiol* 2000; 111: 1802-8.
- Janszky J, Jokeit H, Schulz R, Hoppe M, Ebner A. EEG predicts surgical outcome in lesional frontal lobe epilepsy. *Neurology* 2000; 54: 1470-6.
- Kasteleijn-Nolst Trenite DG. Photosensitivity in epilepsy. Electrophysiological and clinical correlates. *Acta Neurol Scand* 1989; 125 (Suppl): 3-149.
- Kellinghaus C, Lüders HO. Frontal lobe epilepsy. *Epileptic Disord* 2004; 6: 223-39.
- Kim DW, Lee SK, Yun CH, Kim KK, Lee DS, Chung CK, Chang KH. Parietal lobe epilepsy: the semiology, yield of diagnostic workup, and surgical outcome. *Epilepsia* 2004; 45: 641-9.
- King MA, Newton MR, Jackson GD, *et al*. Epileptology of the first-seizure presentation: a clinical, electroencephalographic, and magnetic resonance imaging study of 300 consecutive patients. *Lancet* 1998; 352:1007-11.
- Klein KM, Knake S, Hamer HM, Ziegler A, Oertel WH, Rosenow F. Sleep but not hyperventilation increases the sensitivity of the EEG in patients with temporal lobe epilepsy. *Epilepsy Res* 2003; 56: 43-9.
- Knake S, Halgren E, Shiraishi H, *et al*. The value of multichannel MEG and EEG in the presurgical evaluation of 70 epilepsy patients. *Epilepsy Res* 2006; 69: 80-6.
- Kutsy RL. Focal extratemporal epilepsy: clinical features, EEG patterns, and surgical approach. *J Neurol Sci* 1999; 166: 1-15.
- Laskowitz DT, Sperling MR, French JA, O'Connor MJ. The syndrome of frontal lobe epilepsy: characteristics and surgical management. *Neurology* 1995; 45: 780-7.

- Lee SK, Kim JY, Hong KS, Nam HW, Park SH, Chung CK. The clinical usefulness of ictal surface EEG in neocortical epilepsy. *Epilepsia* 2000; 41: 1450-5.

- Ludwig BI, Marsan CA. Clinical ictal patterns in epileptic patients with occipital electroencephalographic foci. *Neurology* 1975; 25: 463-71.

- Malow BA, Lin X, Kushwaha R, *et al*. Interictal spiking increases with sleep depth in temporal lobe epilepsy. *Epilepsia* 1998; 39: 1309-16.

- Marsan CA, Zivin LS. Factors related to the occurrence of typical paroxysmal abnormalities in the EEG records of epileptic patients. *Epilepsia* 1970; 11: 361-81.

- Mintzer S, Nasreddine W, Passaro E, *et al*. Predictive value of early EEG after epilepsy surgery. *J Clin Neurophysiol* 2005; 22: 410-4.

- Morris HH 3rd, Lüders H, Lesser RP, Dinner DS, Klem GH. The value of closely spaced scalp electrodes in the localization of epileptiform foci: a study of 26 patients with complex partial seizures. *Electroencephalogr Clin Neurophysiol* 1986; 63: 107-11.

- Mosewich RK, So EL, O'Brien TJ, Cascino GD, Sharbrough FW, Marsh WR, *et al*. Factors predictive of the outcome of frontal lobe epilepsy surgery. *Epilepsia* 2000; 41: 843-9.

- Noachtar S, Bilgin O, Rémi J, Chang N, Midi I, Vollmar C, Feddersen B. Interictal regional polyspikes in noninvasive EEG suggest cortical dysplasia as etiology of focal epilepsies. *Epilepsia* 2008; 49: 1011-7.

- Palmini A, Gambardella A, Andermann F, *et al*. Intrinsic epileptogenicity of human dysplastic cortex as suggested by corticography and surgical results. *Ann Neurol* 1995; 37: 476-87.

- Patrick S, Berg A, Spencer SS. EEG and seizure outcome after epilepsy surgery. *Epilepsia* 1995; 36: 236-40.

- Pedley TA, Traub RD. Physiological basis of the EEG. In: Daly DD, Pedley TA, eds. *Current Practice of Clinical Electroencephalography*. Lippincott-Raven: Philadelphia, 1997, 107-38.

- Provini F, Plazzi G, Tinuper P, *et al*. Nocturnal frontal lobe epilepsy. A clinical and polygraphic overview of 100 consecutive cases. *Brain* 1999; 122: 1017-31.

- Quesney LF. Preoperative electroencephalographic investigation in frontal lobe epilepsy: electroencephalographic and electrocorticographic recordings. *Can J Neurol Sci* 1991; 18: 559-63.

- Radhakrishnan K, So EL, Silbert PL, *et al*. Predictors of outcome of anterior temporal lobectomy for intractable epilepsy: a multivariate study. *Neurology* 1998; 51: 465-71.

- Rosenow F, Lüders H. Presurgical evaluation of epilepsy. *Brain* 2001; 124: 1683-700.

- Salanova V, Andermann F, Olivier A, Rasmussen T, Quesney LF. Occipital lobe epilepsy: electroclinical manifestations, electrocorticography, cortical stimulation and outcome in 42 patients treated between 1930 and 1991.

- Surgery of occipital lobe epilepsy. *Brain* 1992; 115 (Pt 6): 1655-80.

- Salanova V, Andermann F, Rasmussen T, Olivier A, Quesney LF. Parietal lobe epilepsy. Clinical manifestations and outcome in 82 patients treated surgically between 1929 and 1988. *Brain* 1995; 118 (Pt 3): 607-27.

- Salanova V, Morris HH, III, Van Ness PC, Luders H, Dinner D, Wyllie E. Comparison of scalp electroencephalogram with subdural electrocorticogram recordings and functional mapping in frontal lobe epilepsy. *Arch Neurol* 1993; 50: 294-9.

- Salinsky M, Kanter R, Dasheiff RM. Effectiveness of multiple EEGs in supporting the diagnosis of epilepsy: an operational curve. *Epilepsia* 1987; 28: 331-4.

- Sam MC, So EL. Significance of epileptiform discharges in patients without epilepsy in the community. *Epilepsia* 2001; 42: 1273-8.

- Sammaritano M, Gigli GL, Gotman J. Interictal spiking during wakefulness and sleep and the localization of foci in temporal lobe epilepsy. *Neurology* 1991; 41: 290-7.

- Schulz R, Luders HO, Hoppe M, Tuxhorn I, May T, Ebner A. Interictal EEG and ictal scalp EEG propagation are highly predictive of surgical outcome in mesial temporal lobe epilepsy. *Epilepsia* 2000; 41: 564-70.
- Shiraishi H, Fujiwara T, Inoue Y, Yagi K. Photosensitivity in relation to epileptic syndromes: a survey from an epilepsy center in Japan. *Epilepsia* 2001; 42: 393-7.
- So EL. Integration of EEG, MRI, and SPECT in localizing the seizure focus for epilepsy surgery. *Epilepsia* 2000; 41 (Suppl 3): S48-S54.
- Stuve O, Dodrill CB, Holmes MD, *et al*. The absence of interictal spikes with documented seizures suggests extratemporal epilepsy. *Epilepsia* 2001; 42: 778-81.
- Sundaram M, Hogan T, Hiscock M, *et al*. Factors affecting interictal spike discharges in adults with epilepsy. *Electroencephalogr Clin Neurophysiol* 1990; 75: 358-60.
- Sveinbjornsdottir S, Duncan JS. Parietal and occipital lobe epilepsy: a review. *Epilepsia* 1993; 34: 493-521.
- Taylor I, Scheffer IE, Berkovic SF. Occipital epilepsies: identification of specific and newly recognized syndromes. *Brain* 2003; 126: 753-69.
- Tükel K, Jasper H. The electroencephalogram in parasagittal lesions. *Electroencephalogr Clin Neurophysiol* 1952; 4: 481-94.
- Tuunainen A, Nousiainen U, Mervaala E, *et al*. Postoperative EEG and electrocorticography: Relation to clinical outcome in patients with temporal lobe surgery. *Epilepsia* 1994; 35: 1165-73.
- Vadlamudi L, So EL, Worrell GA, Mosewich RK, Cascino GD, Meyer FB, Lesnick TG. Factors underlying scalp-EEG interictal epileptiform discharges in intractable frontal lobe epilepsy. *Epileptic Disord* 2004; 6: 89-95.
- Vogt BA, Pandya DN. Cingulate cortex of the rhesus monkey: II. Cortical afferents. *J Comp Neurol* 1987; 262: 271-89.
- Westmoreland BF. The EEG findings in extratemporal seizures. *Epilepsia* 1998; 39 (Suppl 4): S1-S8.
- Wetjen NM, Cohen-Gadol AA, Maher CO, Marsh WR, Meyer FB, Cascino GD. Frontal lobe epilepsy: diagnosis and surgical treatment. *Neurosurg Rev* 2002; 25: 119-38.
- Williamson PD, Boon PA, Thadani VM, Darcey TM, Spencer DD, Spencer SS, *et al*. Parietal lobe epilepsy: diagnostic considerations and results of surgery. *Ann Neurol* 1992a; 31: 193-201.
- Williamson PD, Spencer SS. Clinical and EEG features of complex partial seizures of extratemporal origin. *Epilepsia* 1986; 27 (Suppl 2): S46-S63.
- Williamson PD, Thadani VM, Darcey TM, Spencer DD, Spencer SS, Mattson RH. Occipital lobe epilepsy: clinical characteristics, seizure spread patterns, and results of surgery. *Ann Neurol* 1992b; 31: 3-13.
- Wolf P, Goosses R. Relation of photosensitivity to epileptic syndromes. *J Neurol Neurosurg Psychiatry* 1986; 49: 1386-91.

Source localization
of extratemporal spikes

John P. Turnbull

University Hospitals of Cleveland, Case Medical Center, Institute of Neurology, Epilepsy Center, Cleveland, USA

▪ Introduction

One important part of the diagnosis and treatment planning for patients with epilepsy is the localization of interictal spikes and seizures. To this end we employ various source imaging techniques such as dipole source localization. In contrast, the customary method of identifying the epileptogenic source assumes the source is beneath the scalp surface of maximum electro-negativity as observed on the electroencephalogram (EEG). However, this can produce misleading results because: i) the orientation of the neuronal generators may not be perpendicular to the surface, as when the generator is in a cortical fissure. This produces oblique projections such that the source and point of maximum surface negativity do not coincide and therefore produce a false localization; ii) surface negativity does not give radial information concerning the depth of the source; and iii) differences in intervening tissue conductivities can also produce inaccurate results. The motivation for using source dipole localization is to control for these factors and give a more accurate localization of the epileptogenic source. The physics of dipole localization is the same regardless of the brain lobe under study. However, there are certain anatomical considerations that make temporal source localization different from extratemporal source localizations. We present here a discussion of these differences.

The problem of spike source localization is often referred to as the inverse problem. This is because we know how to solve the following problem known as the forward problem: given a distribution of electrical charges throughout the volume inside the head and given a complete knowledge of intervening conductivities, determine the electric field potentials distributed over the surface of the head and in particular at each of the EEG electrodes. However, the problem as it presents itself to us is the inverse (given a distribution of electric field potentials distributed over the surface of the head and knowledge of intervening conductivities, determine the distributions of the electrical charges throughout the volume of the head). Unfortunately, although the forward solution is unique, the inverse solution is not. There are infinitely many different charge distributions that result in the same identical surface potential distribution. It is for this reason that we must impose certain assumptions to constrain the solution so that it will be unique and thus solvable.

Fortunately, for the special case of a spike, we can assume that the charge distribution is reasonably modeled as a point dipole source (discussed below). We then can use various methods to determine its location. These methods still rely on certain assumptions and in this article, we will discuss these assumptions and how sensitive our localizing estimates are with respect to each of these factors and methods for controlling – as best we can – for these sources of error in our estimations.

■ Theory

If the region of the cortex involved in the generation of a spike is comparatively small, then we assume that the spike can be modeled as a single equivalent dipole. We can then apply the theory of electric fields to estimate the source of the dipole from information provided by the surface electrodes. A dipole is a pair of equal but oppositely charged particles in very close proximity. The dipole produces an electric field like that in *figure 1*.

The source of the potentials recorded by the EEG on the surface of the head is the result of electrochemical processes that occurs in the neurons. A single neuron, which has opposite charges at the base and top, forms a small dipole.

The source of the charges can come from excitatory post synaptic potentials (EPSPs) or inhibitory post synaptic potentials (IPSPs) and have the following effect on the formation of a neuronal dipole in *figure 2*.

When a local collection of neurons synchronously have the same dipole orientation, the summation potential becomes strong enough to be detected on the surface of the head (*Figure 3*).

Although normal EEG is the result of a large distribution of neuronal dipoles over the cortical surface, individual paroxysmal spikes have an electric potential sufficient in strength to make all other background activity negligible. For this reason, we can model the brain activity of the spike as a single dipole. The standard methods of localization assume that the spike is directly under the point on the surface with the most electronegative field potential. However, this assumes that the neuronal dipoles generating the spike are oriented perpendicular to the surface of the head. For most cases, this is true. But because of the convolutions in the cortical sulci and gyri, the field projections may not be perpendicular and may be at some other angle resulting in a surface negativity that is not directly above the spike. This is called false or paradoxical localization. *Figure 4* illustrates this condition when the spike is in a deep fissure, such as the sagittal fissure, compared with a spike that projects perpendicularly to the scalp surface.

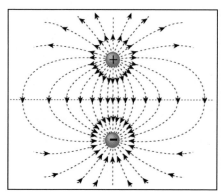

Figure I.

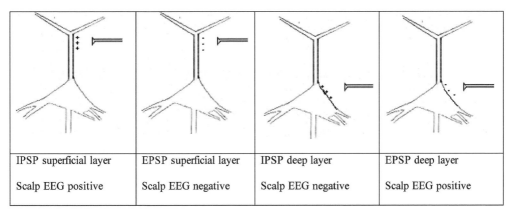

IPSP superficial layer	EPSP superficial layer	IPSP deep layer	EPSP deep layer
Scalp EEG positive	Scalp EEG negative	Scalp EEG negative	Scalp EEG positive

Figure 2.

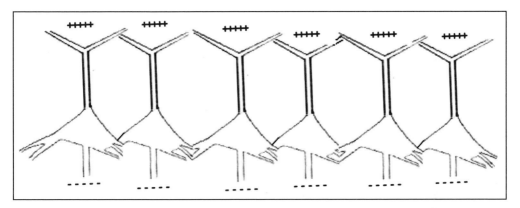

Figure 3.

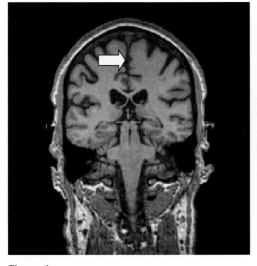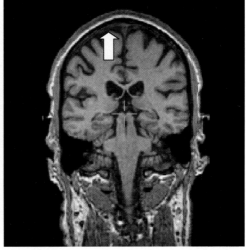

Figure 4.

■ Methods

The search algorithm for identifying the location of the equivalent dipole of a spike successively approximates the strength, location and orientation of the dipole by comparing the forward solution computed by standard formulas from electrostatic field theory with a resulting surface electric field. The algorithm searches for parameters of a dipole with a resulting field that best matches – in a least squares sense – the observed field as measured by the EEG electrodes. There are various search strategies. The most common of which are the gradient search methods used in optimization theory. If the match is good (very low total square error) and all assumptions about the nature of the source and intervening conductivities, then the location and orientation of the source is found. The least squares problem is stated mathematically as follows:

Minimize χ^2

$$\chi^2 (\vec{p}) = \sum_{i=1}^{n} [V (\vec{r}_i) - \phi (\vec{p}, \vec{r}_i)]^2$$

$V (\vec{p}_i)$ is the potential at tje i^{th} electrode

$\phi (\vec{p}, \vec{r}_i)$ is the theoretical potential estimated from the forward solution of the dipole

$\vec{p}$ has 6 components :

$x, y, z, \theta_1, \theta_2, s$

Where :

x, y, z are the Cartesian coordinates

θ_1, θ_2 are the orientation (asthmith and elevation)

s is the dipole strength

$\vec{r}_i$ is the position of the ith electrode

n is the number of electrodes

Thus, the position, orientation and strength of the theoretical dipole are successively approximated until the forward solution of the dipole best matches the observed surface potentials, in the least square sense. The following figures demonstrate by example the results of the method in localizing a given spike *(Figures 5 and 6)*.

■ Techniques for improving results

Filters

The method of source localization requires an accurate estimate of the surface potential produced by the spike at each electrode. This spike is superimposed on other EEG activity from local generators as well as noise processes. This corruption of the data can reduce the accuracy of the estimate. A simple method to eliminate some of the background noise and non-spike activity is the application of simple band pass filters. Spikes and sharp waves are generally between 20-200 milliseconds in duration and this corresponds to a band pass filter setting 2.5-25 Hz. Of course these filters settings may need to be adjusted depending on the nature of each of spike. But in general, this will remove much of the background while preserving most of the spike.

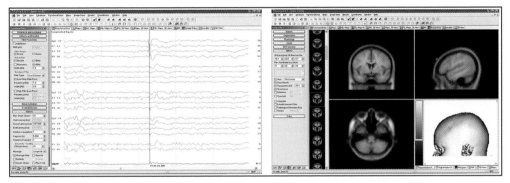

Figure 5.

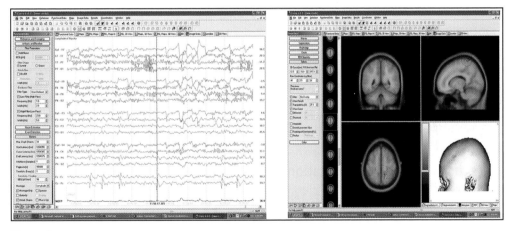

Figure 6.

PCA/ICA

A more advanced method than time domain filters is the application of spatial domain filters. These filters approximate the EEG channels as a sum of uncorrelated local generators derived from a method called eigen-decomposition of the covariance matrix. Applications of this technique include those circumstances in which a spike occurs concurrently with some other uncorrelated activity, such as an eye blink. The technique is able to express the signals as a summation of uncorrelated generators and this permits the separation of spikes from other unrelated activity. *Figure 7* illustrates the technique. Note that the activity between the red markers is decomposed into its various components so that it will be possible to measure the field distribution of a single generator with other uncorrelated activity nulled out.

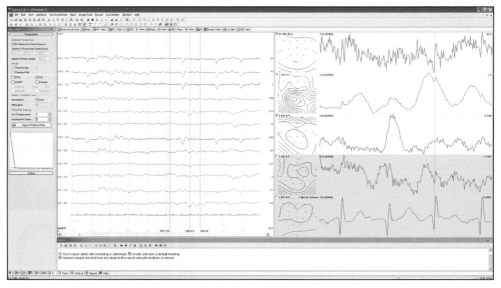

Figure 7.

Conduction models

Local conductivities of intervening tissues greatly affect the observed surface potentials. To this end, we can compensate by computing the forward solution with respect to a reasonable estimate of these conductivities. The first level approximation involves the use of concentric spherical shells with known conductivities of brain parenchyma, meninges, skull bone, skin, etc. A better method is to compute the forward solution from conductivities estimated from the MRI data.

■ Methods for results verification

The method of least squares always yields a result regardless if the source is a spike or not. It is therefore imperative that the model matches the processes.

Statistical analysis

The application of statistical analysis such as the normalized Goodness of fit of a fitted dipole will help to evaluate the hypothesis that the observed EEG signals were created by a single dipole source. The normalized Goodness of Fit ranges from 0 to 1 with 1 representing a perfect fit.

Visual inspection of field distribution plots

After computing the source location, one can check the results by computing the topographical field distribution of the theoretical dipole and visually comparing this with the topographical field distribution estimated from the EEG data. If the source is nearly a dipole, these plots should match very well. In *figure 8* the top row represents a sequence of the actual EEG topographical field distribution as measured from the EEG electrodes,

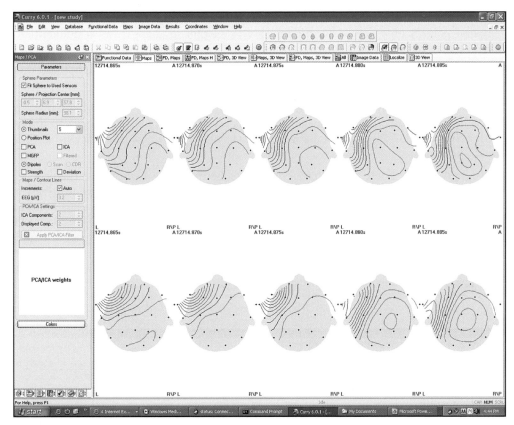

Figure 8.

and the bottom row represents the field distribution computed from the theoretical equivalent dipole fitted to the electric field from de EEG electrodes. The better this correspondence between upper and lower plots the higher the confidence is in the source localization results.

Clustering of the dipoles

The more the dipoles of spikes from a stable focus cluster, the higher the confidence in the results.

■ Localization from extratemporal sources

The physics of source localization is the same throughout the brain. However, there are regional considerations based on the anatomy of the brain.

Frontal. Frontal pole, sagittal fissure. Functional zones like Broca's area straddle frontal and temporal.

There are instances when the EEG surface negativity is at a maximum in the facial cheek area and is therefore beyond the longitudinal bipolar chain of the scalp electrodes. This usually manifests as an increase in signal from posterior to anterior but having no phase reversal. These spikes are generally caused by spikes in the frontal or at times from the temporal pole. Source dipole localization is very helpful in these cases to differentially diagnose between these two potential sources.

Parietal and occipital. localization of the sources in this area must be precise because they are highly functional.

Insular. Insular spikes can be difficult because they connect to so many other structures in the brain. The dipole source imaging methods are useful here because they can distinguish between spikes from the insular and spikes from the cortical surface that are directly above the insular.

Inter-hemispherical. There are different structures between the hemisphere that can be epiletogenic, including the supplementary motor area (SMA) and the cingulate gyrus. In some cases it is necessary to include invasive electrodes such as subdural grids between the hemispheres of the brain. In these circumstances, source dipole localization can be useful in surgical planning to determine which side of the dura mater to place the grids and where to place the grids with respect to the cortical mass. If the orientation of an interhemispherical dipole is longitudinal (left to right or right to left) the spike is lateralized to the side that is dipole positive.

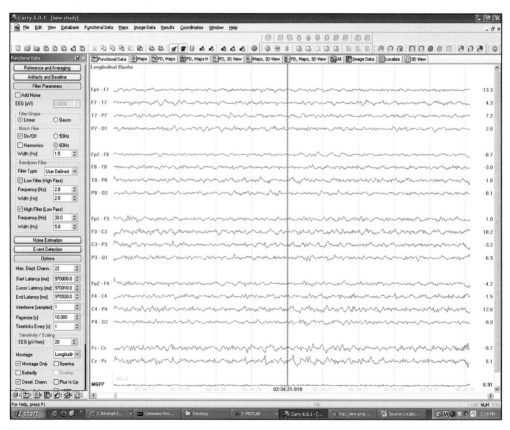

Figure 9.

Mid-line. Spikes near the midline can be very difficult to localize and indeed at times they are very difficult to lateralize. In these cases, source dipole localization can be useful. The following case study in *figure 9* demonstrates how source dipole localization may be useful. The location of the dipoles in *figure 10* demonstrates the source is left sided near the mid-line. The orientation of the dipoles is from posterior to anterior and the dipoles are almost parallel to the scalp (not perpendicular). This suggests that the source is in a longitudinal sulcus (the posterior side of the central sulcus in this case).

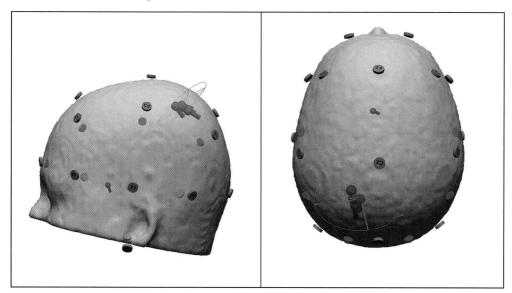

Figure 10.

■ Conclusion

There are several imaging technologies that assist the epileptologist in localizing the source of focal epilepsy. These include structural imaging methods such as CT and MRI, functional imaging such as PET, SPECT and fMRI, and source imaging such as EEG source localization and MEG source localization. Most of these methods provide indirect evidence imaging methods that show regions of high (or low) metabolism or blood flow; only the EEG and MEG use methods that localize with respect to the actual electrical chemical activity of the brain. Although the MEG generally provides more accurate estimates, the EEG source methods provide very good estimates at a much lower cost and with improved volume conductivity methods; the accuracy of EEG source localization can approach that of MEG. In Addition, the MEG detection is specific to the orientation of the field of the source. It cannot detect electrical activity that is tangential to the surface of the head. It is most sensitive to fields that are perpendicular to the surface of the head. Together, all of these modalities provide complimentary information that gives a fuller profile of the epileptic zone.

References

- Boon P, D'Have M, Van Hoey G, Vanrumste B, Vonck K, Adam C, Vandekerchove T. Interictal and ictal source localization in neocortical versus medial temporal lobe epilepsy, *Adv Neurology* 2000; 84: 365-75.
- Plummer C, Simon Harvey A, Cook M. EEG Source localization in focal epilepsy: Where are we now? *Epilepsia* 2008; 49 (2): 201-18.
- Cuffin BN. EEG localization accuracy improvements using realistically shaped head models. *IEEE Trans Biomed Eng* 1996; 43: 299-303.
- Ebersole J, Wade P. Spike voltage topography and equivalent dipole localization in complex partial epilepsy. *Brain Topography* 1990; 3: 21-34.
- Scherg M, Bast T, Berg P. Multiple source analysis of interictal spikes; goals, requirements, and clinical value, *J Clin Neurophysiol* 1999; 16: 214-24.

Magnetoencephalography in extratemporal lobe epilepsy

Richard C. Burgess

Cleveland Clinic Epilepsy Center, Cleveland, USA

Magnetoencephalography (MEG) measures the minute magnetic fields that are generated within the brain and that can be recorded from outside the head, unimpeded by tissue boundaries, such as meninges, skull, and scalp. Synchronous activation of about 10^7 synapses produces a detectable field outside head, and the skull and other extracerebral tissues are essentially transparent to the magnetic fields emanating from these neuronal networks. While other modalities *infer* brain function indirectly by measuring changes in blood flow, metabolism, oxygenation, etc., MEG, as well as EEG, measures neuronal and synaptic function directly; and, like EEG, MEG enjoys sub-millisecond temporal resolution. As the signal travels from the brain source to the external sensors, it is not distorted by anatomy, because magnetic susceptibility is the same for all the tissues – including the skull. Hence, MEG allows for a more accurate measurement and localization of brain activities than EEG. Because one of its primary strengths is the ability to precisely localize electromagnetic activity within brain areas, MEG results are always co-registered to the patient's MRI. When combined in this way with structural imaging, it has been called magnetic source imaging (MSI), but MEG is best understood as a clinical neurophysiological diagnostic test.

A current dipole generated in the cerebral cortex produces not only electric, but also magnetic fields (Barth, 1988; Barth, 1991; Okada, 1997). MEG is a non-invasive tool which provides precise localization of the epileptic activity generating these fields – both interictal and sometimes ictal (as shown in one of the examples below) – as well as mapping of functional cortex. Clinical whole head systems currently have 200–300 magnetic sensors, thereby offering very high resolution. The measurement of magnetic fields provides information not only about the amplitude of the current, but also its orientation (Hari, 1999).

Dipole sources in sulci or fissures generate tangential currents and are the likely major contributors to the activity recorded by MEG, resulting in several favorable brain areas for MEG source localization. Theoretically, the opercular area, mesial fronto-parietal cortex and deep sulci, such as the central sulcus are optimal areas for MEG source generators, because these regions include large volumes of cortical area that are perpendicular to the surface of the head. Another reason that regions outside the temporal lobe are most probably *more* accessible to MEG than temporal sources is because the magnetic field originating from the lowest part of the brain, *e.g.* basal temporal cortex, may not always be adequately recorded (Leijten, 2003), and therefore MEG's recording and localization abilities are better in extratemporal lobe epilepsy (ETLE) than in TLE (Oishi, 2002, Papanicolau, 2005). A recently published small series comparing intracranial recordings to MEG found that MEG detected and localized 95% of the neocortical spikes, but only 25% - 60% of mesial spikes (Santiuste, 2008). Thirdly, the *spherical* head model, typically employed for calculation of epileptic spike location, is a better approximation in the extratemporal regions.

The two primary indications for magnetoencephalography are well established (and confirmed specifically by the applicable CPT codes issued in 2003) – namely epilepsy localization and mapping prior to neurosurgical lesion resection. In the evaluation of patients with ETLE, the role of MEG can be further defined:

- Identification of epileptogenic areas that are difficult or impossible to identify on scalp EEG.
- Confirmation of the ictal onset zone established by other tests.
- Demonstration of widespread or multi-focal discharges suggesting an unfavorable prognosis for epilepsy surgery.
- Identification of eloquent areas of cortex and their proximity to planned areas of resection.

The recent (2009) MEG policy by the American Academy of Neurology specifically highlights the value of MEG "when discordance or continuing questions arise from amongst other techniques designed to localize the focus". In non-lesional cases, or in patients where the EEG is non-localizing, MEG can be particularly helpful. Even when it picks up no new areas of epileptic activity, MEG provides more precise localization than scalp EEG (Shibasaki, 2007). Many patients with ETLE, especially non-lesional cases, will require invasive recording prior to resective surgery, and MEG is of crucial assistance in determining the placement of the intracranial electrodes. In MRI-positive cases, MEG is especially helpful in pinpointing the source of epileptic activity when lesions are extensive or multiple.

■ Background

The advantages of MEG for recording brain signals have a strong theoretical basis, and are well known in practice:

- No exposure to radiation, magnetic field, or other active device.
- Inherently higher source resolution.
- Reference-free.
- Easy to obtain multichannel, whole-head, high spatial-density recordings.
- No direct connection to patient required.
- Signals not attenuated or distorted by bone and scalp, or other inhomogeneities that exist between brain and surface.
- Therefore for source analysis, the head modeling problem is significantly simpler.

Nevertheless, few studies exist that compare MEG localization with direct intracranial electrode recording (ICEEG), and the patient numbers have been small (Mikuni, 1997; Oishi, 2002; Santiuste, 2008; Shigeto, 2002).

One of a handful of studies that has demonstrated true clinical value for MEG in a prospective, blinded crossover-controlled, single treatment case series of 69 sequential patients was published by Sutherling in 2008. Although the effect on outcome was not studied, they looked at the decisions made at patient management conference before and after presentation of MEG results. They found that MEG provided entirely new information in 33%, altered the intra-cranial EEG (ICEEG) examination (phase 2) in 23%, and changed the surgical decision in 20%. All of the patients in this study were extratemporal, and the post-operative outcome results demonstrated clear benefit from MEG in 21% of the patients who went to resection (9% of the patients in the study).

In an important 2006 publication, Knowlton el al studied the effect of MEG on the subsequent placement of ICEEG electrodes in a prospective study of 115 patients, 43% of whom were ETLE. By the design of the study, MEG could only affect the addition of supplemental electrodes after an initial decision was made without MEG. Forty-nine patients proceeded to intracranial evaluation, where this study investigated the concordance between ICEEG and MEG localization to the sublobar level, with a view towards the practicality of eventually substituting MEG for ICEEG in some patients. MEG and ICEEG had about the same success in localizing the epileptic source, 65% and 69% respectively. Agreement at a sublobar level between tests was good; 55% were localized and concordant for site. There were 7 cases (14%) who were localized by ICEEG but not by MEG and 3 cases (6%) localized by MEG but not by ICEEG. MEG's positive predictive value for seizure localization was 82 to 90%, depending on whether computed against ICEEG alone or in combination with surgical outcome. A notable conclusion from this study is that the absence of ictal recordings (usually the situation in MEG) did not affect the results.

MEG evaluation has even been advocated as the *screening* tool of choice for frontal lobe epilepsy by a group in the Netherlands. Simultaneous MEG and EEG were recorded in 24 patients; in 18 at least 6 spikes per hour were recorded. Not only were spikes much more frequent on MEG than EEG, but localization via MEG was successful in twice as many patients as EEG (14 vs. 7 patients). Although the use of MEG differs somewhat from that in the USA because of differences in insurance reimbursement, the higher yield per minute of recording of MEG makes this proposition thought-provoking.

■ Recording technique

Whole head MEG systems have a cylinder-shaped dewar (container vessel) with a helmet-shaped concavity on one end, into which the subject's head is placed for measurement (Hamalainen, 1993; Hari, 1999). Typically, 100-300 channels of magnetic sensors coupled to SQUIDs (super-conducting quantum interference devices) are arrayed over the inner surface of the concavity, immersed in the liquid helium within the dewar, and maintained at a temperature of 4.2 kelvin. The equipment containing the dewar with the MEG sensors (*Figure 1*) is housed in a magnetically shielded room (MSR) in order to block magnetic interference coming from the environment. Active noise cancellation, *i.e.* real-time feedback compensation, helps to counteract any residual interference which penetrates into the MSR. Implanted devices such as vagal nerve stimulators (VNS), pacemakers, and responsive neural stimulators (RNS) do not preclude MEG recording, but post-processing to eliminate extra-cranial interference is required (*e.g.* spatiotemporal signal space separation (tSSS; Taulu, 2006).

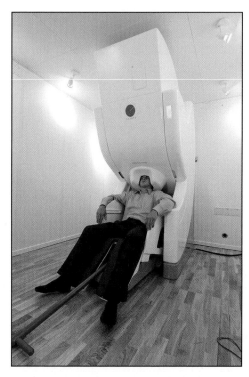

Figure 1. The apparatus for recording brain magnetic signals resides inside of a housing which bathes the sensors in liquid helium in order to maintain a super-conducting state. The machine shown in the figure, from Elekta Neuromag, can record from a patient in a sitting position, as shown, in order to facilitate presentation of visual stimuli, or on a bed in a supine position to promote sleep. Recording is done inside of a magnetically shielded room in order to block environmental interference which is several orders of magnitude larger than the signal from the patient's brain.

At the Cleveland Clinic, our recording procedures have been optimized to maximize the information obtained from each patient appointment, in a high-volume clinical epilepsy center. All of our studies include simultaneous EEG recording with at least the standard 10-20 electrode derivations, applied with collodion. The EEG channels can sometimes provide complementary information, and help clinicians to understand the results by confirming that the abnormalities seen in the MEG channels are consistent with the patient's previous EEG abnormalities. In addition to application of EEG electrodes, our preparation includes patient degaussing to remove any remnant magnetization.

In contrast to electroencephalography, where the electrodes are in fixed positions on the scalp, the MEG sensors bear only a vague relationship to brain regions. In addition, the location of the head within the dewar varies from patient to patient, and it changes even during a recording session on an individual patient. The spatial relationships of the sensor locations to the brain are obtained indirectly based on three-dimensional digitization of several anatomical landmarks, *e.g.* nasion and pre-auricular points, and by "head position indicating" (HPI) coils that are affixed to the head with collodion. The locations of the HPI coils, as well as the locations of the anatomical fiducials, are carefully digitized so that their positions can be co-registered with the same landmarks ascertained from the patient's MRI. Because we continuously track and correct for charges in head-position with 5 HPI coils, general anesthesia or conscious sedation has not been required in our first 100 patients (Burgess, 2010). Because the patient must remain relatively still during MEG recording, duration is limited and generally confined to the interictal state (Barkley, 2003). Typical MEG monitoring times for epilepsy patients range from 35 minutes to a few hours.

We also routinely carry out somatosensory evoked fields (SEF) on all patients. SEF from left and right electrical stimulation of the median nerves helps not only to identify the central sulcus, but also provides a system integrity check. Satisfactory localization of the SEF responses to the primary sensory cortex provides reassurance that the localization of epileptiform activity is also proceeding correctly. Our typical parameters are ~ 3/sec stimuli, pulse duration 0.2 msec, ~200 satisfactory trials. The stimulus amplitude is titrated to the patient to achieve supra-motor threshold, starting at 4-5 ma and increasing to create a thumb twitch.

■ Analysis and interpretation

It is important to review the raw MEG waveforms, and to realize that these "brain waves" are analogous to the familiar EEG waveforms, as shown in *figure 2*. Experience as an electroencephalographer can be applied to MEG, and the fundamental concepts of field determination and source localization, previously established for EEG, are also similarly applied to MEG interpretation (Iwasaki, 2005). Review of the recorded data, averaging 50 minutes per patient, is accomplished by paging through 10 second pages in a process quite similar to the traditional electro-encephlographic review of high-density EEG, employing several "montages" of MEG sensors. In contrast to EEG, MEG is inherently reference-free (Lopes da Silva, 1999).

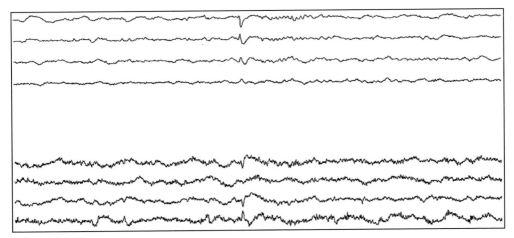

Figure 2. The top four channels are bipolar EEG derivations from the left temporal lobe. At the bottom are four sequential channels from the left temporal MEG sensors recorded at the same time. Notice that the morphological characteristics of the sharp wave shown in the middle of the tracing are quite similar on EEG and MEG. Although MEG "montages" have far more channels than traditional scalp EEG and differing sensitivities to certain brain activities, visual identification of epileptiform discharges relies on customary neurophysiological skills learned in electroencephalography.

Although there are some differences between normal variants seen in MEG and EEG, identification of MEG spikes essentially follows traditional EEG criteria: Sharp contour, standing out from the surrounding background, following a physiological distribution, often with an aftergoing slow-wave. The EEG can be viewed separately (blindly if desired) or simultaneously (*Figure 3*), but in the majority of patients, spikes and sharp waves are more copious on the MEG channels than on the EEG (Iwasaki, 2005; Ossenblok, 2007). Since EEG and MEG record the same phenomenon, *e.g.* epileptic spiking, reports should include the results of MEG localization along with interpretation of the simultaneous EEG.

After identifying and marking candidate spikes in the raw waveforms, the next step is to ascertain what part of the brain is generating these epileptiform discharges. Magnetic field distribution is usually displayed as an iso-field contour map with the aid of computerized calculation. The field distribution produced by a single current dipole is observed as a pair of influx and outflux field maxima distributed on each side of the dipole location (Hari, 1999). Assuming a single dipolar generator for a typical "dipolar" field distribution, an equivalent current dipole is localized below the middle point of both influx and outflux field maxima. The reason that the term "single equivalent current dipole" (or SECD) is encountered frequently in magnetoencephalography is often misunderstood. We look for a "dipolar field" distribution for reassurance that employment of the single equivalent current dipole model is appropriate. Modeling the source of cerebral currents as a SECD offers a convenient and rapid method for finding the location of that source. Dipole models are well established for known regional sources, such as somatosensory evoked responses. However for sources of unknown origin like epileptic spikes, the interpreter must make sure that the SECD is reasonable, as the solution can be significantly biased by the interpreter's assumptions. Several automated approaches have been proposed to avoid such biases (Fuchs, 1999; Jeffs, 1987; Mosher, 1998).

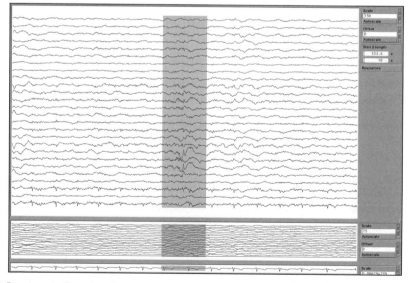

Figure 3. Data is typically reviewed on ten second pages that look like the figure. The top plotting area contains MEG, the middle EEG, and the bottom EKG. Both the MEG and EEG plotting areas can display any desired montage or channel layout, and the relative size of each area is controlled by sliders. In this example, the sliders have been positioned to view primarily MEG, with the EEG area much smaller, and only a small window for the EKG. The epoch highlighted in gray has been selected by the operator for source localization and will be automatically transferred to the dipole-fitting algorithm.

Computerized source estimation is more feasible in MEG than in EEG, because of the relatively simpler source and volume conductor models. Employing the vendor's software (Elekta Neuromag, Helsinki, Finland) epileptic spikes can be localized using an equivalent current source dipole model, on an interactive basis as each spike is encountered, in order to continuously build and test a hypothesis. Alternatively, spike identification can be carried out in a first pass, then source localization as a second pass. Our process is to carry out localization of individual spikes, and never to average spikes, because of the well known pitfalls of spike averaging (Rose, 1987). Whether the localization of *each* spike is considered acceptable is based on:

- presence of a dipolar appearing magnetic field pattern;
- no simultaneously occurring artifact;
- stability of the localization with time (*i.e.* within a window of ~5-50 msec);
- acceptable goodness of fit/confidence volume (usually a function of SNR).

Figure 4 illustrates the selection of a time point to localize, the magnetic field potential at the scalp surface, and SECD-modeled source of the sharp wave in the left frontal region.

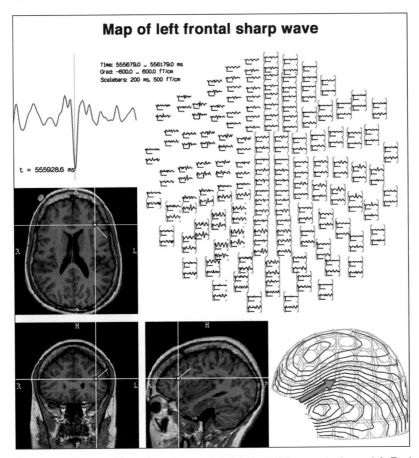

Map of left frontal sharp wave

Time: 555679.0 – 556179.0 ms
Grad: -600.0 – 600.0 fT/cm
Scalebars: 200 ms, 500 fT/cm

t = 555928.6 ms

Figure 4. The time course of a spike is shown for a single left frontal MEG sensor in the top left. To the right is a whole-head gradiometer display of the same epoch. At the bottom right, the topography of the magnetic field shows a dipolar pattern. At the bottom left, the location of the ECD source for this spike is co registered to the patient's MRI, showing the irritative zone in the left frontal lobe.

Sources deemed to be acceptable are co-registered to the patient's own MRI, primarily based on three spatial fiducials, the nasion and both pre-auricular points. Using these digitized landmarks and continuous monitoring of the position of the HPI coils during the recording, the location and orientation of the equivalent current dipole solution can be co-registered with the anatomy and displayed graphically. Typically for epileptiform discharges, dipole locations of several representative spikes are shown (Baumgartner, 2000; Knowlton, 1997; Leijten, 2003; Otsubo, 2001; Stefan, 2003). Some magnetoencephalographers try to superimpose as many as 100 dipoles on one image, in an effort to convey the extent or variability of spike distribution (Iwasaki, 2002).

Whether the localizations of *all* detected spikes are diagnostically significant is determined from:
- number of acceptable dipoles;
- tightness of the dipole cluster;
- orientation of the dipoles;
- plausibility of the location.

Studies of the localization accuracy of MEG have shown variable results, primarily dependent on the phenomenon under study (*e.g.* epileptic spikes *vs.* SEF), the location of the activity (*e.g.* dorsal, inferior, mesial), signal to noise ratio (which is dependent on room shielding, noise cancellation methods, etc), localization technique (ECD *vs.* linear methods), and types of subjects (highly motivated volunteers *vs.* clinical patients). Certainly sublobar precision is expected, and the consensus is that for the usual epileptiform activity, a localization accuracy of 4-6 mm can be obtained. Because of the better sensor coverage, and higher signal to noise ratio ETLE sources can be expected to be more precisely localized than TLE focii.

■ Example cases

Because of the complexity of their evaluation and the difficulties encountered while trying to develop a treatment plan, ETLE referrals to the MEG lab constitute the vast majority of cases. The following three cases typify the challenges and results obtained in ETLE magnetoencephalography.

Poorly defined on EEG

The example shown in *figure 5* is a typical case where the EEG discharges show a broad distribution and inconsistent morphology which made confident localization by EEG impossible. On the MEG, the discharges are clearly seen and consistently localized to the right frontal lobe. The tightness of the clusters and uniform dipole orientation (along with the objective parameters of goodness of fit and confidence volume) provide assurance that the MEG localization can be relied upon.

Ictal MEG recording

Although seizures in the MEG are relatively uncommon, they can be serendipitously captured. During the first 100 MEG recordings at the Cleveland Clinic, 10 included ictal activity (Burgess, 2010). Scalp EEG is often obscured by movement-associated artifacts accompanying seizures, which MEG is not plagued by, as shown in *figure 6*. In addition, MEG's greater ability to detect epileptiform activity means that the ictal electrical activity

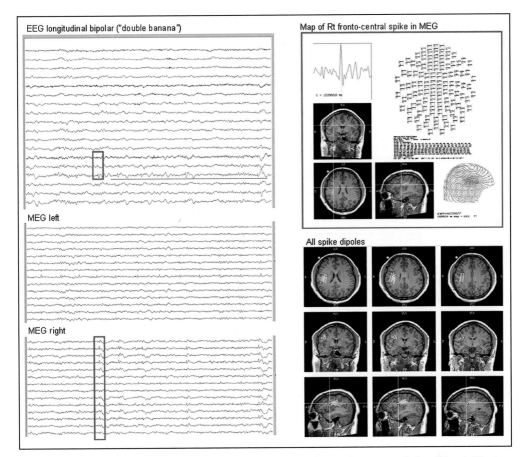

Figure 5. The upper left panel shows an example of inter-ictal discharges that are poorly formed and difficult to localize on EEG, seen best on the 15th channel (C3-P3). The left and right frontal MEG recordings from the same 8 second page are shown below the EEG. In the top right panel, MEG localization of the spike outlined in magenta is shown with the MEG waveforms from 204 sensors in upper left and the corresponding field distribution in the lower right. The bottom right panel shows source localization of all acceptable spikes recorded during this MEG test, co-registered to the patient's MRI. The yellow spheres represent the location of the sources, and their tails show the orientation of the dipoles.

may actually be picked up *earlier* in the MEG. For the patient whose MEG result is seen in figure 6, these advantages permitted localization of a seizure to the right parietal lobe by MEG that was non-localizable by EEG. Sequential localization of repetitive waves that occur during seizure onset allows MEG to study seizure propagation.

Non-lateralized, variable EEG manifestations fit to consistent unilateral MEG focus

There are a substantial number of patients with generalized or midline EEG abnormalities in whom the clinical semiology or other information suggests a focal origin. In the 30 year old patient shown in *figures 7 and 8*, MEG demonstrates a consistent left mesial frontal location despite highly variable – and mostly midline – EEG manifestations.

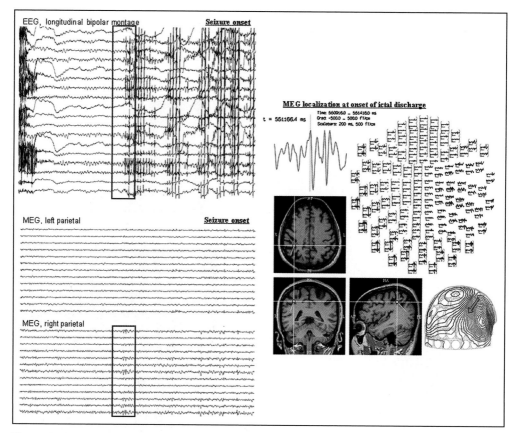

Figure 6. The upper left panel shows 8 seconds of EEG capturing the onset of a seizure in this adult patient. The EEG montage order is left temporal (4 ch), right temporal (4 ch), left parasagittal (4 ch), right parasagittal (4 ch), and midline (2 ch). The blue box marks the same time-period recorded on EEG and MEG. The lower left panel demonstrates the relative immunity of MEG to artifact from muscle and electrodes, as compared to the EEG. The clear changes in the MEG parietal sensors are localized using a single equivalent current dipole in the panel on the right. The magnetic field distribution shows a typical dipolar pattern, and the seizure onset is localized to the right parietal region.

How sensitive is MEG and what does MEG not see? MEG has a different spatial sensitivity than EEG and generally does show more spikes than scalp EEG (Yoshinaga, 2002; Iwasaki, 2005). The strength of the magnetic field decreases in proportion to the square of the distance from the current dipole, according to the Bio-Savart's law. Therefore the sensitivity of MEG to deep sources is similar to scalp EEG (Malmivuo, 1997). In 85 patients studied with intracranial EEG at the Cleveland Clinic after our MEG system first became operational, 19% also underwent MEG, and 67% of those were ETLE (Bulacio, 2009). Concordance between MEG and ICEEG was evaluated based on the criteria published by Knowlton *et al.* (2006). Forty percent were concordant at the sublobar level, 30% were concordant for the same lobe, and in 10% neither ICEEG nor MEG were able to localize a possible epileptogenic zone. In only 20% of patients, there was no concordance between the two modalities.

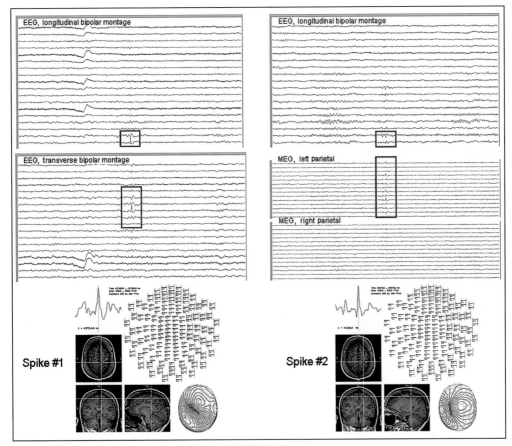

Figure 7. The panels on the left show a spike, which on EEG was easily seen but appeared localized to the midline, phase reversing at Cz on both longitudinal and transverse montages. Using MEG to localize spike #1 placed it in the left mesial frontal region. On the right side, a second spike is less clearly seen on EEG but appears to be maximal around C3. MEG localization also places spike #2 in the left mesial frontal area.

■ Conclusion

MEG has distinct advantages over EEG for the purposes of precise localization, especially in patients with skull defects or when a focal abnormality is suspected but the EEG appears to show bilateral synchrony. Because the head coverage by sensors superior to the inferior temporal regions is more complete, MEG is generally of even greater benefit in ETLE patients. Although MEG cannot completely replace invasive EEG recordings, its use may guide the placement and tailor the design of intracranial investigations, and in some patients obviate unnecessary invasive evaluations.

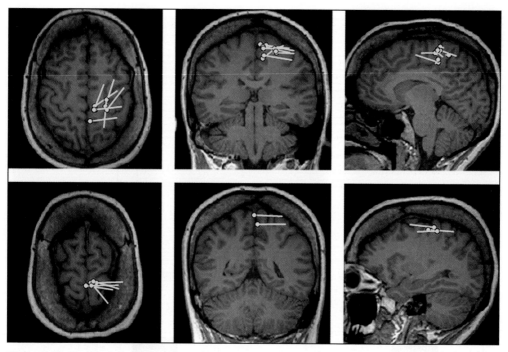

Figure 8. The locations of all sources obtained during the MEG test are shown with a fairly consistent left mesial frontal location, despite a wide variety of EEG manifestations.

References

- Barkley GL, Baumgartner C. MEG and EEG in epilepsy. *J Clin Neurophysiol* 2003; 20: 163-78.
- Barth DS. Empirical comparison of the MEG and EEG: animal models of the direct cortical response and epileptiform activity in neocortex. *Brain Topogr* 1991; 4: 85-93.
- Barth DS, Sutherling W. Current source-density and neuromagnetic analysis of the direct cortical response in rat cortex. *Brain Res* 1988; 450: 280-94.
- Baumgartner C, Pataraia E, Lindinger G, Deecke L. Neuromagnetic recordings in temporal lobe epilepsy. *J Clin Neurophysiol* 2000; 17: 177-89.
- Bulacio JC, Jin K, Alexopoulos AV, Nair D, O'Connor T, Gonzalez-Martinez J, et al. Concordance between magnetoencephalography and intracranial electrocorticographic findings. *Epilepsia* 2000; 50 (Suppl 11): 183.
- Burgess RC, Jin K, Mosher JC, Alexopoulos AV. Notable interictal and ictal findings during MEG testing in patients with epilepsy: The first 100 MEG studies at the Cleveland Clinic Epilepsy Center. *Proceedings of the American Clinical Neurophysiology Annual Meeting*, February 2010.
- Fuchs M, Wagner M, Köhler T, Wischmann HA. Linear and nonlinear current density reconstructions. *J Clin Neurophysiol* 1999; 16: 267-95.
- Hamalainen M, Hari R, Ilmoneimi RJ. Magnetoencephalography-theory, instrumentation, and applications to noninvasive studies of the working brain. *Rev Mod Phys* 1993; 65: 413-97.
- Hari R. Magnetoencephalography as a tool of clinical neurophysiology. In: Niedermeyer E. *Electroencephalography. Basic Principles, Clinical Applications and Related Fields*, 4th edition. Baltimore: Lippincott Williams & Wilkins, 1999, 1107.

- Iwasaki M, Nakasato N, Shamoto H, Nagamatsu K, Kanno A, Hatanaka K, Yoshimoto T. Surgical implications of neuromagnetic spike localization in temporal lobe epilepsy. *Epilepsia* 2002; 43: 415-24.

- Iwasaki M, Pestana E, Burgess RC, Luders HO, Shamoto H, Nakasato N. Detection of epileptiform activity by human interpreters: blinded comparison between electroencephalography and magnetoncephalography. *Epilepsia* 2005; 46: 59-68.

- Jeffs B, Leahy R, Singh M. An evaluation of methods for neuromagnetic image reconstruction. *IEEE Trans Biomed Eng* 1987; 34: 713-23.

- Knowlton RC. Can magnetoencephalography aid epilepsy surgery? *Epilepsy Currents* 2008; 8: 1-5.

- Knowlton RC, Laxer KD, Aminoff MJ, Roberts TP, Wong ST, Rowley HA. Magnetoencephalography in partial epilepsy: clinical yield and localization accuracy. *Ann Neurol* 1997; 42: 622-31.

- Knowlton RC, Elgavish R, Howell J, Blount J, Burneo JG, Faught E, *et al.* Magnetic source imaging versus intracranial electroencephalogram in epilepsy surgery: a prospective study. *Ann Neurol* 2006; 59: 835-42.

- Leijten FS, Huiskamp GJ, Hilgersom I, Van Huffelen AC. High-resolution source imaging in mesiotemporal lobe epilepsy: a comparison between MEG and simultaneous EEG. *J Clin Neurophysiol* 2003; 20: 227-38.

- Lopes da Silava FH, van Rotterdam A. Biophysical Aspects of EEG and magnetoencephalogram generation. In: Niedermeyer E, ed. *Electroencephalography. Basic Principles, Clinical Applications and Related Fields*, 4th edition, Baltimore, MD: Lippincott, Williams & Wilkins, 1999, pp. 93-109.

- Malmivuo J, Suihko V, Eskola H. Sensitivity distributions of EEG and MEG measurements. *IEEE Trans Biomed Eng* 1997; 44: 196-208.

- Mikuni N, Nagamine T, Ikeda A, Terada K, Taki W, Kimura J, *et al.* Simultaneous recording of epileptiform discharges by MEG and subdural electrodes in temporal lobe epilepsy. *Neuroimage* 1997; 5 (Pt 1): 298-306.

- Mosher JC, Leahy RM. Recursive MUSIC: a framework for EEG and MEG source localization. *IEEE Trans Biomed Eng* 1998; 45: 1342-54.

- Oishi M, Otsubo H, Kameyama S, Morota N, Masuda H, Kitayama M, Tanaka R. Epileptic spikes: magnetoencephalography versus simultaneous electrocorticography. *Epilepsia* 2002; 43: 1390-5.

- Okada YC, Wu J, Kyuhou S. Genesis of MEG signals in a mammalian CNS structure. *Electroencephalogr Clin Neurophysiol* 1997; 103: 474-85.

- Olivier A, Gloor P, Andermann F, Ives J. Occipitotemporal epilepsy studied with stereotaxically implanted depth electrodes and successfully treated by temporal resection. *Ann Neurol* 1982; 11: 428-32.

- Ossenblok P, deMunck JC, Colon A, Droisbach W, Boon P. Magnetoencephalography is more successful for screening and localizing frontal lobe epilepsy than electroencephalography. *Epilepsia* 2007; 48: 2139-49.

- Otsubo H, Ochi A, Elliott I, Chuang SH, Rutka JT, Jay V, *et al.* MEG predicts epileptic zone in lesional extrahippocampal epilepsy: 12 pediatric surgery cases. *Epilepsia* 2001; 42: 1523-30.

- Papanicolaou AC, Castillo EM, Billingsley-Marshall R, Pataraia E, Simos PG. A review of clinical applications of magnetoencephalography. *Int Rev Neurobiol* 2005; 68: 223-47.

- Rose DF, Smith PD, Sato S. Magnetoencephalography and epilepsy research. *Science* 1987; 238 (4825): 329-35.

- Santiuste M, Nowak R, Russi A, Tarancon T, Oliver B, Ayats E, *et al.* Simultaneous magnetoencephalography and intracranial EEG registration: technical and clinical aspects. *J Clin Neurophysiol* 2008; 25: 331-9.

- Shibasaki H, Ikeda A, Nagamine T. Use of magnetoencephalography in the presurgical evaluation of epilepsy patients. *Clin Neurophysiol* 2007; 118: 1438-48.

- Shigeto H, Morioka T, Hisada K, Nishio S, Ishibashi H, Kira D, *et al.* Feasibility and limitations of magnetoencephalographic detection of epileptic discharges: simultaneous recording of magnetic fields and electrocorticography. *Neurol Res* 2002; 24: 531-6.
- Stefan H, Hummel C, Scheler G, Genow A, Druschky K, Tilz C, *et al.* Magnetic brain source imaging of focal epileptic activity: a synopsis of 455 cases. *Brain* 2003; 126: 2396-405.
- Sutherling WW, Mamelak AN, Thyerlei D, Maleeva T, Minazad Y, Philpott L, Lopez N. Influence of magnetic source imaging for planning intracranial EEG in epilepsy. *Neurology* 2008; 71: 990-6.
- Taulu S, Simola J. Spatiotemporal signal space separation method for rejecting nearby interference in MEG measurements. *Phys Med Biol* 2006; 51: 1759-68.
- Yoshinaga H, Nakahori T, Ohtsuka Y, Oka E, Kitamura Y, Kiriyama H, *et al.* Benefit of simultaneous recording of EEG and MEG in dipole localization. *Epilepsia* 2002; 43: 924-8.

Section III:
Neuroimaging of extratemporal lobe epilepsies

Imaging in extratemporal lobe epilepsy Overview

Fergus J. Rugg-Gunn, John S. Duncan

Department of Clinical and Experimental Epilepsy, Institute of Neurology, University College London, National Hospital for Neurology and Neurosurgery and Epilepsy Society, UCLH NHS Foundation Trust, Queen Square, London, United Kingdom

Over the last 15 years, advances in structural and functional imaging of the brain have revolutionised the investigation and management of patients with epilepsy. The integration of anatomical, physiological and functional information is now possible and the ability to discern epileptic networks is being realised. This is of particular importance in patients with extratemporal lobe epilepsy, who are being considered for surgery more frequently than previously, as the relationship between eloquent cortical function and the epileptogenic zone is frequently more complicated and challenging than in temporal lobe epilepsy. This chapter reviews the evolution and recent advances in structural MRI, tractography, functional MRI, PET and SPECT imaging and attempts to address the specific challenges posed by extratemporal lobe epilepsy.

Regarding MRI, advances have been made as a result of improvements in imaging hardware and analysis methods, and although initially, this was financially and computationally expensive, 3 Tesla MRI scanners and imaging sequences such as functional MRI and diffusion tensor imaging for tractography are now becoming commonplace. With increasing resolution and improved detection of subtle abnormalities, the challenge in focal epilepsy is to avoid attributing significance to normal variations, incidental findings or co-morbidity.

In patients with extratemporal lobe epilepsy being considered for epilepsy surgery the identification of a structural lesion is associated with improved prognosis post-operatively and frequently obviates the need for intracranial EEG recordings which possess a small but significant risk of morbidity and mortality. Despite technological advances, up to 25% of patients with refractory extratemporal lobe epilepsy have normal optimal MRI. However, in addition to standard, visual, qualitative inspection of images, structural MR data can also be analysed on a voxel-wise basis against a cohort of healthy control subjects to look for subtle variations at a group or individual level. This is a more objective method for analysing data and may be more sensitive in identifying occult abnormalities.

An intuitive development of diffusion tensor imaging is tractography which provides high-resolution anatomical detail of brain white matter and detailed definition of structural connectivity between brain regions. This may provide information on seizure propagation pathways or probe the relationship between structure and function by correlating tractographic parameters with cognitive deficit and motor and visual function. Tractography has already been shown to be of use in tumour surgery by delineating major white matter tracts and thereby informing the surgical approach and defining resection margins. This can be combined with functional MRI which is able to localise primary sensorimotor cortex and confidently lateralise language function using simple expressive and receptive language paradigms. Functional MRI has largely replaced the intracarotid sodium amytal (Wada) test in lateralising language dominance and may provide prognostic information regarding postoperative verbal memory outcome. Anatomical localisation of interictal epileptic discharges using functional MRI with simultaneous EEG recordings is possible and may be useful in patients being considered for epilepsy surgery although obtaining a meaningful result is entirely dependent on the presence of an epileptic discharge during the recording period. Ictal EEG-fMRI is also possible in well-selected patients and exploratory safety and feasibility studies in patients with intracranial EEG electrodes are ongoing.

Single photon emission computed tomography (SPECT) visualises cerebral perfusion and, due to neurovascular coupling, brain metabolism. Comparison of interictal and ictal perfusion images will thereby provide a snapshot of cerebral activity during seizures and thereby localise the ictal focus. In extratemporal lobe epilepsies there are specific logistical concerns, for example, the short duration of frontal lobe seizures, presence of motor activity during the injection of the tracer and rapid seizure propagation. Nevertheless, ictal SPECT is a sensitive imaging technique in localising the ictal onset zone and surgical resection which includes the area of SPECT hyperperfusion is associated with a good postoperative outcome.

The most widely utilised tracer in positron emission tomography (PET) is 2-deoxy-18F fluoro-D-glucose (FDG) which reflects cellular energy demand. Unlike SPECT, (18F) FDG PET imaging is performed interictally and regions of interictal glucose hypometabolism are associated with seizure foci. Other PET ligands may provide additional information on the in-vivo neurochemistry of epilepsies and seizures and the functional anatomy of abnormalities, for example, flumazenil or 11C-alpha-methyl-L- tryptophan, which may be specific for the epileptic focus in patients with multiple lesions, such as tuberous sclerosis. Larger validation studies are required before these techniques become more widely utilised.

In summary, there have been major advances in a number of structural and functional imaging modalities over the last 15-20 years and individually they have shown promise in identifying epileptic foci, major nerve fibre pathways and eloquent cortex, often prior to epilepsy surgery. Of paramount importance in future is the fusion of these multi-modality data to comprehensively inform the surgical planning process and provide information on post-operative seizure, cognitive and neurological outcomes and possibly the redundancy of investigations.

High resolution magnetic resonance imaging in extratemporal lobe epilepsy

Neel Madan[1], Douglas L. Teich[2], David B. Hackney[3]

[1] Tufts Medical Center, Tufts University School of Medicine, Department of Radiology, Boston, USA
[2] Dept. of Radiology, Beth Israel Deaconess Medical Center, Instructor, Harvard Medical School, Boston, USA
[3] Harvard Medical School, Chief of Neuroradiology, Beth Israel Deaconess Medical Center, Boston, USA

■ Introduction

Identifying and delineating a structural lesion on magnetic resonance imaging (MRI) in patients with extratemporal lobe epilepsy (ETLE) remains one of the most important factors in determining surgical outcomes (Krsek *et al.*, 2009; Téllez-Zenteno *et al.*, 2010). As MRI technology continues to advance, so too has our ability to identify the underlying structural substrate of an epileptogenic focus. However, given how subtle these lesions can be, it is imperative in the presurgical workup of extratemporal lobe epilepsy to optimize MRI protocols to increase the probability of identifying this structural substrate.

In order to increase sensitivity and specificity, the MR imaging must be targeted towards the suspected epileptogenic zone based on the semiology (Colombo *et al.*, 2009), reviewed with a complete understanding of the MR appearance of structural lesions and ideally, in collaboration with all available data including PET, SPECT, and fMRI. This requires a close collaboration between all members of the team, including the neurologist, neurosurgeon, neuropsychologist and neuroradiologist.

The following chapter will describe technical considerations in obtaining MR imaging in patients with ETLE as well as review common structural etiologies of extratemporal lobe epilepsy with an emphasis on cortical dysplasias, detailing imaging findings of these lesions.

■ Imaging techniques

Given the multiple pulse sequences, multi-planar capability and capacity for both structural and functional imaging, MRI is a robust instrument. However, in order to increase sensitivity, it is important that the imaging protocol be targeted towards the specific clinical concerns. Thus, a routine seizure protocol at most hospitals in a patient being initially worked up for epilepsy is different than a more targeted protocol based on the semiology in the work-up of a patient being considered for surgery. While the basic MRI technology is reproducible between scanners from different manufacturers, newer technology and sequences may be available only from one vendor, or may be implemented in a different manner. Thus, in developing a seizure protocol, it is important to work with the neuroradiologist, physicist and/or technologists to maximize image quality on the specific scanner being used. The following section will discuss MR equipment considerations, routine and targeted MRI protocols in the evaluation of epilepsy, as well as review advanced sequences to consider in the evaluation of epilepsy.

MR equipment considerations

With the continuing progression of magnetic resonance imaging technology over the last 40 years since it was initially introduced for clinical applications, there has been constant improvement in the detection, definition, and delineation of malformations of cortical development and other epileptogenic lesions. While the routine clinical MRI scanner in most radiology departments has a field strength of 1.5 Tesla (T), 3T MRI scanners are becoming more prevalent, especially at academic centers. And in a few research centers around the world, even higher field strength (7T and higher) scanners are now being employed in human imaging (Figure 1). For epilepsy imaging, the major advantage from the higher field strength is increased signal to noise (SNR). This provides increased signal of the brain parenchyma, increasing sensitivity for detection of cortical dysplasia (CD) (Knake et al., 2005; Phal et al., 2008; Zijlmans et al., 2009; Madan & Grant, 2009), although larger prospective studies are needed to verify these findings.

In addition to MRI magnetic field strength, phased array (PA) surface coils with larger arrays have also tremendously increased signal to noise. Compared to the older quadrature head coil technology, PA coils are closer to the brain with the produced imaging being a summation of the many individual coils, resulting in a dramatic increase in SNR, again improving diagnostic yield (Grant et al., 1997). This is especially apparent at the cortical surface, with a less but still substantial increase in signal in the central parts of the brain (Wald et al., 1995). However, given that most epileptogenic lesions, especially cortical dysplasias are seen in the peripheral cortex, this improvement in image quality dramatically improves sensitivity for detection of CDs (Figure 2). This increase in the number of channels has also allowed parallel imaging techniques to be utilized, improving imaging time, with improvement in the brain coverage, or improving spatial and temporal resolution (although this concurrently decreases SNR). While 32 channel PA coils are the highest number of channels available commercially, 96 and 128 channel PA coils are currently under development, and will hopefully continue to improve image quality and diagnostic sensitivity.

While there are distinct benefits from imaging at higher field strengths with improved coil technology, it is important to note that in transitioning from one field strength to the next, imaging parameters must be optimized. This is due to a decrease in T1 relaxivity, resulting in different time to repetition (TR) and time to echo (TE) than at lower field strengths as well as inherent disadvantages of the higher field strength such as susceptibility artifacts (related to bone, air in the sinuses, dental hardware, etc.), and increased radiofrequency energy needed to cause magnetization displacement resulting in higher specific

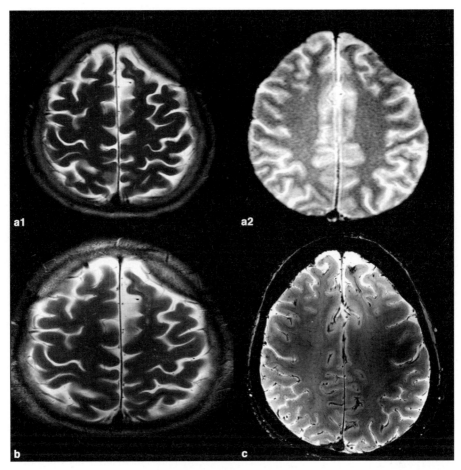

Figure 1. Comparison of 1.5, 3 and 7 Tesla field strengths. A 44 year old male who presented with aphemia. **A.** An initial 1.5 Tesla MRI with T2 and T2* images demonstrates non specific areas of T2 white matter abnormality. **B.** 3 Tesla T2 and **C.** 7 Tesla T2* images are better able to characterize the extent of T2 signal abnormality and demonstrate an area of susceptibility involving the right superior frontal gyrus with extension to involve the underlying white matter, in a distribution consistent with an old venous infarct.

absorption rates (Briellmann et al., 2003). At ultra high field strengths (7 Tesla and beyond), inhomogeneous magnetic fields becomes a greater issue, and currently requires manual manipulation in order to image accurately.

While the advantages discussed here for improved image quality and faster imaging apply to the structural MRI imaging described below, there is potentially even greater impact on fMRI and DTI imaging (discussed in subsequent chapters) given the improved SNR in these inherently low SNR imaging paradigms.

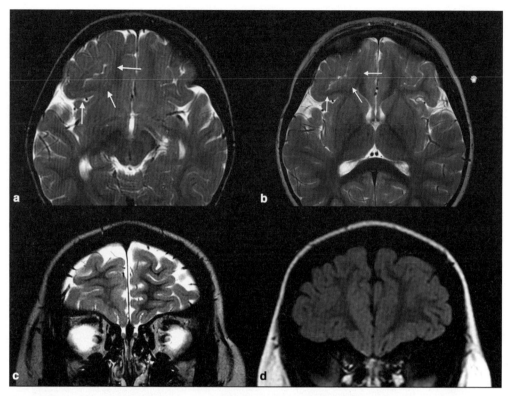

Figure 2. Comparison of 12 and 32 channel phased array coils. A 4 year old female with drug-resistant epilepsy with an focal cortical dysplasia Type I. Axial T2 image at 3T with a **A.** 12 channel and **B.** 32 channel phased array coil demonstrates an area of abnormal cortical gyration involving the right supraorbital gyrus with extension to the inferior frontal gyrus with associated abnormal signal in the underlying subcortical white matter and apparent blurring of the gray-white matter junction. Additional **C.** coronal T2 and **D.** coronal FLAIR images using the 32 channel phased array coil depict areas of signal abnormality in the underlying white matter.

MRI imaging protocol in ETLE

Given the myriad of neurologic disorders that can result in seizures (as discussed in the following section), the initial evaluation of patient's with seizures is oftentimes a survey.

Routine imaging protocols (*Figure 3*) should include T1 weighted spin echo (SE) sequences for structural anatomy evaluation. A volumetric T1 weighted acquistion (MPRAGE, SPGR, T1 3D TFE depending on the manufacturer) depicts structural detail beautifully, and when optimized (especially at 3T) with isotropic voxels (ideally 1 mm^3 or less), provides diagnostic quality reformatted images. These sequences are important in identifying subtle malformations of cortical development (heterotopia, polymicrogyria, cortical dysplasias) by depicting gray white matter differentiation, as well as allowing detailed anatomical evaluation that can be used in correlation with the semiology. Because of the reduced imaging time, this sequence is often acquired in the sagittal plane and reformatted into axial and coronal planes, although if reformatted images are inadequate, a direct coronal acquisition may be more useful. Additionally, when acquired in the sagittal plane, in order to prevent wrap artifact on the reformatted images (including in the temporal lobes), care must be taken such that the image excursion extend through both the entirely of both ears.

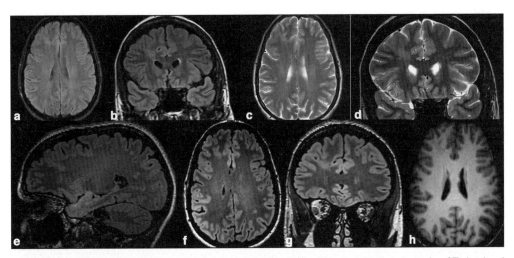

Figure 3. Multiple images in a 46 year old female with a Type IIb focal cortical dysplasia imaged at 3T. Axial and coronal FLAIR **(A-B)** and T2 **(C-D)** images demonstrate a transmantle sign with FLAIR /T2 hyperintensity fanning out from the ependymal surface with apparent abnormal cortical thickness and blurring of the gray-white matter junction. A volumetric FLAIR sequence was also performed **(E-F)** in the sagittal plane and reformatted into the axial and coronal plane. The multiple thin cut images (1 mm) through the lesion allow improved characterization and in subtle abnormalities, improved detection. An MPRAGE sequence was also performed with the axial reformat showing vague T1 hypointensity corresponding to the abnormal T2/FLAIR signal abnormality.

T2 fast spin echo (FSE) and T2 weighted fluid attenuation inversion recovery (FLAIR) sequences are vital in detection of pathophysiology, as most pathologic processes result in edema or gliosis which can be identified as bright signal on these sequences. Because of the suppression of background CSF bright signal on FLAIR images, subtle areas of signal abnormality are more conspicuous on this sequence than on a T2 sequence. While FLAIR may be more sensitive, an optimized T2 sequence is more specific with better resolution and SNR, which allows better characterization of underlying lesions as well as improved evaluation of the gray-white matter junction. Imaging should be performed in at least two planes (usually axial and coronal) to maximize the identification of areas of signal abnormality. While optimized protocols for temporal lobe epilepsy imaging will have thin cut (3 mm or less) coronal T2 and FLAIR sequences perpendicular to the hippocampus, in extratemporal lobe epilepsy it is more important that the imaging extends through the entire potentially epileptogenic area (which may be in the posterior parietal or occipital lobes).

T1, T2 and T2 weighted FLAIR sequences are not sensitive for detection of foci of hemorrhage. Given that hemorrhage as the result of injury, vascular malformations, etc., can act as an epileptogenic substrate, T2* susceptibility gradient echo (GRE) images are necessary.

Several considerations are important in determining the utility for post contrast images. In the younger patient, post-contrast images do not usually identify a suspicious area, but rather helps characterize lesions that are seen on other sequences. Thus, post-contrast images may not be necessary in all pediatric patients. In older patients, contrast enhanced imaging also helps characterize lesions, but is more important in potentially identifying occult malignancy, especially metastatic disease, which can be subtle and may not be observed on other sequences without contrast. If the clinical concern is primarily for a malformation of cortical development, scar, or other long standing epileptogenic substrate, high resolution structural imaging is far more important than post-contrast imaging.

Finally, given the concern for dual pathology, while imaging in ETLE may be directed away from the temporal lobe, it still may be vital to assess this region, and specifically the hippocampus, in the presurgical evaluation of patients with intractable epilepsy.

However, a standard MRI (especially when interpreted by a non-epilepsy expert radiologist) fails to detect focal epileptogenic lesions in a majority of patients (Van Oertzen *et al.*, 2002). Thus, the targeted approaches described below in conjunction with interpretation by an experienced neuroradiologist can significantly increase detection rates.

Advanced techniques

A detailed understanding of the electroclinical presentation is paramount to performing a proper, targeted MRI (Colombo *et al.*, 2009). Various techniques can be employed to identify subtle abnormalities, including imaging in multiple planes, using thin slices, increasing the resolution, and improving signal to noise. However, for each sequence that is acquired and for each parameter that is adjusted, there may be a large cost in overall image acquisition time. Because MR imaging is time intensive, sequence optimization depends on balancing the needs of signal to noise (with multiple contributing factors), image resolution (matrix), the area of brain to be imaged (both slice thickness and inter-slice gap), as well as the overall time of image acquisition. This is especially true as patients are more prone to move during a sequence if there is a longer imaging acquisition time, with motion artifact potentially obscuring a suspicious lesion. And as the overall time for the entire study increases, patient motion also increases.

Thin contiguous slices may make it possible to identify and delineate subtle abnormalities, but may require alterations in other imaging parameters in order to compensate for the reduced signal to noise that accompanies the decrease in voxel size. When very thin images (less than 3 mm) are utilized, the number of slices and overall coverage of the brain is limited, and thus, must be targeted towards the suspected epileptogenic zone. Additionally, specialized sequences described below may also be employed to help identify subtle abnormalities. These include:

- Volumetric FLAIR: Several vendors now offer a volumetric FLAIR sequence which allows isotropic acquisitions similar to the volumetric T1 sequence described above. This permits a single acquisition to be reformatted into any imaging plane. Additionally, because of the thin nature of the images (1 mm thin sections with no interslice gap), this sequence is particularly well suited for evaluation of FLAIR hyperintense lesions such as radial glial bands *(Figure 3)*.

- Susceptibility weighted imaging (SWI): A recently described imaging technique, SWI is a T2* weighted sequence which incorporates the phase encoded information that had previously been discarded in order to create a new imaging sequence with its own unique tissue contrast. While SWI is exquisitely sensitive to iron, calcium and hemorrhage, the amount of "blooming" is significantly less than a traditional T2* sequence. This allows for better characterization of structure within cortical layers (especially at ultra high field MRI) as well as blood vessels (Haacke *et al.*, 2009; Mittal *et al.*, 2009). While SWI will be very useful in identifying lesions with hemosiderin or calcification, it remains to be seen if it may help in the detection of CDs *(Figure 4)*.

- Arterial Spin Labeling (ASL): ASL is a noninvasive MRI technique for evaluating cerebral blood flow (CBF). Epileptogenic foci are known to be hyperperfused at ictal perfusion analysis, which is more sensitive in detection of an underlying area of abnormality than interictal evaluations, where the underlying substrate will be hypoperfused. However, MRI is usually performed as an interictal examination (and without EEG monitoring), and thus ASL is usually obtained interictal. The main advantage of ASL is the ease with which the perfusion data can be fused with the anatomical data *(Figure 5)*. A non-invasive manner for detecting hypoperfusion may help increase diagnostic sensitivity and specificity (Wolf *et al.*, 2001).

- Advanced post-processing techniques are being developed for analysis of the acquired data. This may potentially aid detection of subtle abnormalities such as cortical dysplasias, which can be obscured by the complexity and variation in the convolutions of the gyri. Because of the subtlety of the imaging findings, and the sheer number of images produced in a typical 3 Tesla MRI with volumetric acquisitions (with reformats), identifying an epileptogenic zone can be extremely time consuming and challenging. Automated and semi-automated techniques for evaluating volume, signal variation, etc., could potentially aid in detection of an epileptogenic lesion. Two major techniques have been described – voxel based morphometry and segmentation techniques. Voxel based morphometry identifies areas of the brain that may be different (in volume, signal intensity, texture, sharpness of boundaries, etc.) using statistical parametric mapping techniques employed in functional MRI to permit voxel based comparisons between patients and a cohort of control subjects. Segmentation techniques parcellate the brain into multiple different regions, allowing for automated measurements of thickness and volume of gray matter as well as volume of white matter. While there is promise that these techniques may aid in detection of lesions, it remains to be seen whether they will be able to identify cortical dysplasias or other abnormalities that would have otherwise been missed (Madan & Grant, 2009).

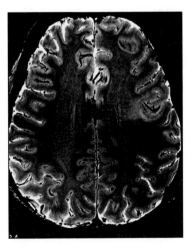

Figure 4. An axial susceptibility weighted image at 7T depicts a probable FCD Type IIb on the left. The normal vessels coursing through the white matter are well depicted on this sequence as areas of tubular hypointensity. Given differences in signal intensity in the cortical layers, there is a sense of cortical lamination, which may in the future allow better detection and characterization of subtle malformations.

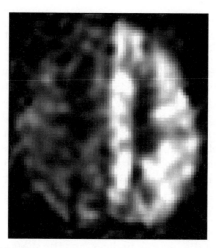

Figure 5. An axial arterial spin labeling image in a patient with tuberous sclerosis complex with poorly controlled seizures demonstrates asymmetric perfusion to the hemispheres, with the area of decreased perfusion corresponding to the hemisphere with significant EEG abnormalities. Focal areas of ictal hyperperfusion or inter-ictal hypoperfusion can also be observed with epilepsy.

In some patients, other factors, such as a vagal nerve stimulator (VNS) or invasive EEG leads in place may affect the ability to image. In order to image in patients with such devices, the compatibility of the device needs to be considered, not just in terms of the effects of the magnetic field itself, but oftentimes more importantly, the specific absorption rate related to radiofrequency power deposition. This may require changes in imaging acquisition such as using a quadrature send/receive coil instead of the standard phased array coil. Caution needs to be taken also in terms of using high field magnets, potentially rapidly shifting gradients in sequences such as diffusion weighted imaging, and SAR, especially with T2 and FLAIR sequences. Modifications in imaging sequences, utilizing three dimensional FSE sequences with a reduced flip angle instead of the traditional FSE or FLAIR sequences can substantially reduce SAR, without significant compromise in image quality (Sarkar *et al.*, 2011). Thus, while it is possible to image patients with invasive EEG leads/depth electrodes (*Figure 6*), VNS (*Figure 7*) and other devices, appropriate care needs to be taken to insure patient safety.

In conclusion, MRI is a robust imaging modality, with multiple tools available to help in identifying potential underlying abnormalities in patients with drug-resistant epilepsy. Despite the many powerful techniques described here, an epileptogenic substrate may not be identified. In these cases, reevaluation of a "negative" MRI in conjunction with other imaging modalities, including PET (potentially co-registered with the MRI), SPECT, MEG, DTI, fMRI and in conjunction with semiology may help identify subtle lesions.

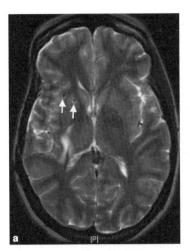
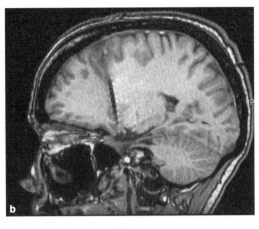

Figure 6. Low SAR axial T2 **(A)** and sagittal MPRAGE **(B)** images in a patient with depth electrodes for evaluation of refractory epilepsy, demonstrating exact location of placement.

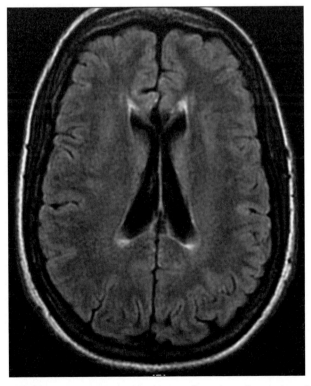

Figure 7. Low SAR axial FLAIR image in a patient with a history of anterior collosectomy and vagal nerve stimulator with persistent treatment related seizures demonstrates areas of gliosis and collosectomy defect.

■ Imaging findings in extratemporal lobe epilepsy

While there is a vast number of different pathologies that can result in extratemporal lobe epilepsy, the largest subtypes include neoplasms, malformations of cortical development, and glial scars. Since neoplasms and glial scars are more apparent on imaging, these are usually identified on the initial MRI. And while some malformations of cortical development are readily identifiable, others, especially cortical dysplasias, represent the largest subgroup of patients with intractable seizures, and are also the subgroup where high resolution, optimized MRI is paramount in order to detect subtle lesions. This section will review the classification and imaging findings of malformations of cortical development, and subsequently discuss other underlying pathology in ETLE.

Malformations of cortical development

Malformations of cortical development (MCD) represent a broad group of disorders resulting from disruption in one of the major steps of cerebral cortical development. The most widely used classification scheme (Barkovich et al., 2005) separates MCDs on the basis of the developmental stage at which it is believed the disruption in normal development occurred: A. abnormal neuronal and glial proliferation or apoptosis; B. abnormal neuronal migration; C. abnormal cortical organization; or D. not otherwise classified. As our understanding of the underlying genetics has rapidly advanced, the classification system has also evolved taking into account the spectrum of disease that can result from the same genetic mutation. However, there are still many malformations where the underlying genetics or embryology is poorly understood, or which are more heterogeneous (with involvement at more than one stage of cortical development). Thus, the current framework will certainly continue to evolve.

While MCDs can be asymptomatic, they frequently are associated with a wide range of symptoms including developmental delay, mental retardation and epilepsy. Many of the entities in this category can result in medically refractory epilepsy; however, a number of them are associated with such diffuse abnormalities that surgical resection with the goal of "cure" is not achievable. In these instances, additional evaluation utilizing the neuroimaging techniques described in subsequent chapters as well as neurophysiologic techniques described in the prior section are necessary to determine if an epileptogenic focus can be identified whereby the patient may benefit from targeted resection. However, the largest subgroup of patients with drug-resistant epilepsy (DRE) have a focal lesion – most commonly a cortical dysplasia - which may be amenable to surgical resection. Thus, in patients with DRE and a negative initial MRI, more targeted imaging needs to be performed, guided by the semiology.

While many malformations of cortical development can be associated with intractable seizures (Figure 8), the most common focal entities to be associated with intractable seizures include cortical dysplasias, nodular heterotopic gray matter (subependymal and subcortical) and polymicrogyria (Russo et al., 2003). While these entities can be focal, they can also be multiple, bilateral and far more extensive than initially perceived; and given that these entities can be difficult to fully define, targeted high-resolution imaging in those being considered for surgery may be helpful in determining whether a patient is a surgical candidate. A full description of the full gamet of malformations of cortical development is beyond the scope of this chapter; the reader is referred to several other pivotal texts for more information (Caruso et al., 2008; Barkovich et al., 2005).

Cortical dysplasias

Cortical dysplasias (CD) are a spectrum of disorders with architectural and cytoarchitectural disturbances. They represent the most common cause of epilepsy in children, and are the most frequent malformation of cortical development found in patients with intractable epilepsy. (Nobili *et al.*, 2007; Russo *et al.*, 2003; Urbach *et al.*, 2002, Tassi *et al.*, 2002; Fauser *et al.*, 2004; Hildebrandt *et al.*, 2005; Krsek *et al.*, 2009).

While cortical dysplasias are the most frequent cause of intractable epilepsy, they can be the most difficult to detect. However, identifying and defining a focal lesion is one of the most important factors in determining surgical outcome, as complete excision is the most powerful variable affecting outcome (Krsek *et al.*, 2009). As imaging is so vital in the detection of cortical dysplasias, the techniques described above for image optimization are vital to increase sensitivity. As technology has and continues to evolve, and as our understanding of these lesions expands, presurgical detection also continues to improve (Madan & Grant, 2009), resulting in improved outcomes (Elshakawry *et al.*, 2008).

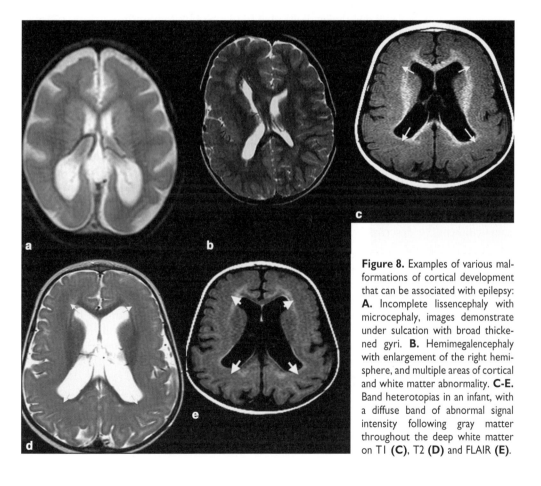

Figure 8. Examples of various malformations of cortical development that can be associated with epilepsy: **A.** Incomplete lissencephaly with microcephaly, images demonstrate under sulcation with broad thickened gyri. **B.** Hemimegalencephaly with enlargement of the right hemisphere, and multiple areas of cortical and white matter abnormality. **C-E.** Band heterotopias in an infant, with a diffuse band of abnormal signal intensity following gray matter throughout the deep white matter on T1 **(C)**, T2 **(D)** and FLAIR **(E)**.

Because cortical dysplasias are difficult to detect, even at autopsy, the true incidence is unknown. While the most common presenting symptom in patient's identified with cortical dysplasias at pathology is seizures, many have hypothesized that cortical dysplasias, especially the more subtle subtypes, may be involved in learning disabilities, cognitive impairment, behavioral disturbances/psychiatric diseases, headaches, etc. This may be partly related to the size of the lesion, the location of the malformation, or the type of malformation (Blümcke et al., 2010).

The pathophysiology of cortical dysplasias is not known, but it may be related to a combination of malformative and disruptive processes (Colombo et al., 2009). With the revised 2010 ILAE classification system described below, some of the cortical dyslamination may be secondary or related to the development of neoplasms, vascular malformations, or prior injuries. Cepeda et al. (2006) suggested that failure of prenatal cell degeneration leads to incomplete cellular maturation in dysplastic tissue, with interactions between these abnormal dysmature cells and normal postnatal neurons resulting in seizures. Another hypothesis is that the insulin-secreting pathway may be hyperactive in FCD, TSC, and hemimegalencephaly, and that the underlying abnormal signaling results in epileptogenicity (Crino, 2009). This may then be secondary to an underlying genetic mutation. Ongoing research will be needed to better understand the different subtypes of cortical dysplasias, and subsequently to understand the underlying pathophysiology.

Classification

Since Taylor et al. (1971) initially described a series of 10 patients with drug-resistant epilepsy whose surgical specimens revealed cortical dysplasia, many classification systems have been espoused. In 2004, a consensus panel used histopathologic, imaging and clinical data to unify the terminology for cortical dysplasias, which has become widely used, referred to as the Palmini classification (Palmini et al., 2004). More recently, an ad hoc Task Force of the International League Against Epilepsy (ILAE) Diagnostic Methods Commission (which included many of those were part of the initial consensus panel and experts throughout the field) has revised the classification scheme for focal cortical dysplasias (Blümcke et al., 2010). As there are some distinctions between these classification systems, they will both be described.

The Palmini classification system *(Table I)* separates cortical dysplasias into mild malformations of cortical development (mMCDs) and focal cortical dysplasias (FCDs). Mild malformations of cortical development represent cortical disorganization resulting from microscopic neuronal heterotopia, and is further subdivided into those where the ectopic neurons are in or adjacent to layer I (Type I), and those where the neuronal heterotopia are outside layer I (Type II). The spectrum of histopathologic findings in focal cortical dysplasias was separated into those without (Type I) and those with (Type II) dysmorphic neurons. Type I FCDs were further broken down into those with dyslamination in cortical organization only (Type Ia) and those with giant/immature neurons (Type Ib). FCD Type II thus represents a Tyalor-type architectural abnormality with dysmorphic neurons, and was further separated into those without (Type IIa) and those with (Type IIb) balloon cells.

Table I. Palmini classification of cortical dysplasias (Palmini *et al.*, 2004)

Mild malformations of cortical development:
    Type I: Ectopic neurons in/adjacent to layer I
    Type II: Ectopic neurons outside layer I

Focal cortical dysplasia:
    Type I: No dysmorphic neurons, no balloon cells
        Type Ia: Architectural abnormality
        Type Ib: Architectural abnormality + giant/immature neurons
    Type II: Taylor-type with dysmorphic neurons
        Type IIa: Achitectural abnormality + dysmorphic neurons
        Type IIb: Architectural abnormality + dysmorphic neurons + balloon cells

The ILAE 2010 Classification (*Table II*) reviewed the current histopathologic, neuroimaging, electrophysiologic and neurodevelopmental understanding of FCDs, and separated isolated FCDs (Type I and II) from those associated with other epileptogenic lesions (Type III). However, they reclassified the subtypes of Type I FCDs into those with abnormal radial microcolumnar organization (Type Ia), abnormal tangential cortical lamination (Type Ib) or both (Type Ic). Reclassification of the subtypes of FCD Type I was in part based on the ambiguity in the Palmini classification in both the pathology as well as the overlapping imaging features, with research showing a lack of a consensus (Chamberlain *et al.*, 2009). The subtypes of Type II FCDs were preserved, with Type IIa representing a cortical dysplasia with dysmorphic neurons and Type IIb representing a cortical dysplasia with both dysmorphic neurons and balloon cells.

Focal cortical dysplasia Type III is defined as a cortical lamination abnormality (without dysmorphic neurons) adjacent to a principal lesion, with the subtypes based on the pathology of the accompanying abnormality. Of note, patients with a type II FCD and another lesion are considered to have dual pathology, and not a Type III FCD. FCD Type IIIa is a cortical lamination abnormality in the temporal lobe associated with hippocampal sclerosis. This subtype does not include patients with mesial temporal sclerosis and is not considered dual pathology; thus patients with hippocampal sclerosis and other pathology such as a glial scar, neoplasm, etc. are not included in this subtype. FCD Type IIIb is a cortical lamination abnormality associated with a glial or glioneuronal neoplasm. A cortical lamination abnormality adjacent to a vascular malformation is classified as FCD Type IIIc. And finally, a cortical lamination abnormality adjacent to any other lesion acquired during early life (*e.g.* trauma, ischemic injury, encephalitis, etc.) is classified as FCD Type IIId.

Of note, the ILAE 2010 Classification did not address or change the classification of mMCDs. They felt there was not enough data yet to critically review mMCDs and there is still not good data to determine if any neuroimaging features exist for this entity.

Imaging findings

Many imaging features have been identified in CDs, including apparent thickening of the cortex and blurring of the gray-white matter junction, abnormal cortical and white matter signal (on T1, T2/FLAIR or both), and a linear or conical T2/FLAIR hyperintense, T1 hypointense signal fanning out from the ependymal surface to the area of abnormal cortical lamination (transmantle sign). Other described features include a deep sulcus (with the malformation at the depth of the sulcus), focal hypoplasia/atrophy, and broadening of the

Table II. 2010 ILA classification of focal cortical dysplasias (Blümcke *et al.*, 2010)

Focal cortical dysplasia Type I (isolated)
    a: Abnormal radial cortical lamination
    b: Abnormal tangential cortical lamination
    c: Abnormal radial and tangential cortical lamination

Focal cortical dysplasia Type II (isolated)
    a: Abnormal cortical lamination + dysmorphic neurons
    b: Abnormal cortical lamination + dysmorphic neurons + balloon cells

Focal cortical dysplasia Type III (associated with principal lesion)
    a: Abnormal cortical lamination in the temporal lobe with hippocampal sclerosis
    b: Abnormal cortical lamination adjacent to a glial or glioneuronal tumor
    c: Abnormal cortical lamination adjacent to vascular malformation
    d: Abnormal cortical lamination adjacent to other lesion acquired during early life
      (trauma, ischemic injury, encephalitis, etc.)

gyri. Lesions can be quite variable in size, from focal to hemispheric (Krsek *et al.*, 2008), and while usually solitary, multifocal cases have been described (Fauser *et al.*, 2009). The form fruste of tuberous sclerosis complex should also be considered.

Usually a few of these imaging features will be observed in a particular CD, but the combination of findings is neither consistent nor reliable in identifying or discriminating between the various subtypes. Studies based on the Palmini classification have shown a large overlap between mMCD and FCD Type I, as well as FCD Type II. In the revised classification, it is hypothesized that this may be related to the non-uniformity of the underlying histopathology. Thus, it remains to be seen whether the 2010 ILAE classification system will allow better discrimination of the various subtypes of FCD based on their imaging appearance (Blümcke *et al.*, 2010; Krsek *et al.*, 2008; Lerner *et al.*, 2009).

While FLAIR images are sensitive for the detection of signal abnormalities, it is more difficult to define lesion boundary on these images as they can overestimate the degree of blurring at the gray white matter interface as well as apparent cortical thickness. Thus, while these images may help identify a lesion, T1 and T2 images will be superior at defining/ delineating lesions, especially for presurgical planning (Madan & Grant, 2009; Colombo *et al.*, 2009). Additionally, because the subcortical white matter involvement may be isointense to cortex on T1 images, this may lead to blurring of the gray white matter junction on these sequences. However, on T2 weighted images, the involved white matter will be T2 hyperintense to cortex, and thus may appear sharper. The blurring at the gray white matter interface identified on MRI likely reflects pathologically a combination of densely heterotopic neurons in the subcortical white matter, dysmyelination and/or reduced number of myelinated fibers. This may be why there is more likely to be blurring of the gray white matter junction in Type 2 rather than Type 1 FCDs (Colombo *et al.*, 2009).

Imaging features will also vary depending on the age of the patient (*Figure 9*), and the underlying extent of myelination. In the immature brain, the background increased T2 signal of the brain may obscure both involvement of the white matter itself as well as blurring at the gray white matter junction (which is actually a normal finding in the neonatal brain). Additionally, because the contrast between gray and white matter in children with incomplete myelination is different, areas of increased signal in the cortex may not be as readily apparent. Finally, because of the small size of the brain, there is decreased signal to noise which can result in decreased conspicuity of lesions. However, in patients presenting with seizures in infancy, it is important to image as early as possible, as maximal contrast is at birth, which is subsequently obscured by the variable pattern of myelination between 6 and 24 months. In any child without a discrete abnormality detected on initial imaging, repeat imaging after 30-36 months may increase sensitivity. Additionally, for patients with a discrete abnormality identified, the extent of the abnormality may be more apparent once complete myelination has occurred.

Focal cortical dysplasia Type I

Under the Palmini classification, heterogeneous imaging features were observed in FCD Type I (*Figure 2 and 10*). The most characteristic feature described is hypoplasia/atrophy, with either lobar or sublobar involvement (Widjaja *et al.*, 2008; Krsek *et al.*, 2008). Abnormal T2/FLAIR hyperintensity can be seen in the subcortical white matter, with corresponding T1 hypointensity, as well as blurring at the gray white matter junction. Abnormal signal is more commonly seen in the white matter than gray matter in these lesions, although pathologically there may actually be cortical thinning. These lesions are more frequently found in the temporal lobe, although they can be extratemporal and mimic FCD Type II (Blümcke *et al.*, 2010).

Previous descriptions have commented on the high association with hippocampal sclerosis, neoplasms, and prior brain injury (Raymond *et al.*, 1994; Ho *et al.*, 1998; Diehl *et al.*, 2004, Krsek *et al.*, 2008). Since this is now recategorized as FCD Type III, it remains to be seen whether this leads to a better definition of electroclinical and imaging findings in these subtypes. Additionally, as discussed above, it remains to be seen if more homogeneous imaging features will be seen under the new classification of FCD Type I under the 2010 ILAE classification.

Focal cortical dysplasia Type II

Since FCD Type II has not been redefined between the Palmini and 2010 ILAE classifications, the features are better understood with multiple studies describing imaging findings (*Figure 3 and 11*). These lesions are more frequently extratemporal, with a predilection for the frontal lobes. The transmantle sign is specific for this subtype, although it is variably present, with a range from 21% (Krsek *et al.*, 2008) to 72% (Widjaja *et al.*, 2009).

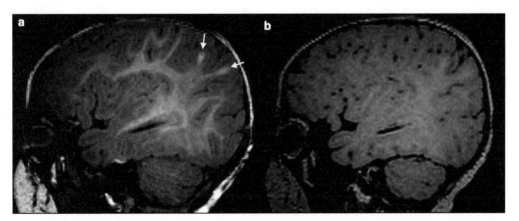

Figure 9. A 5 month old patient with tuberous sclerosis complex. Because of the incomplete myelination, the radial-glial bands associated with the tubers are easily seen on T1 MPRAGE sequence **(A)** as bands of hyperintensity, but are completely obscured on FLAIR **(B)** and T2 (not shown) images.

However, this may in part be due to the imaging acquisition, as identifying the transmantle sign when it is subtle depends on having thin (or volumetric) FLAIR/T2 images, and may be better seen on one plane depending on the orientation of the involved gyrus. Other common features include blurring of the gray-white matter interface, abnormal gyral/ sulcation pattern (best seen on volumetric images) with enlargement of the subarachnoid space, and abnormal gray matter and white matter signal. Many studies have also described increased cortical thickness in FCD Type II, although it is not frequently defined, and some have questioned whether this is due to pseudo-thickening (Colombo *et al.*, 2009).

And while these imaging features help differentiate Type II from Type I FCD, there is still considerable overlap. Even greater overlap exists between Type IIa and Type IIb FCD, and while Type IIa may be more difficult to observe than Type IIb and may be less frequent (making sample sizes small), there are no clear distinguishing features.

Focal cortical dysplasia Type III

As this classification subtype has only recently been created, there is no good data yet as to the imaging findings of this entity as distinct from either FCD type 1 or the accom-

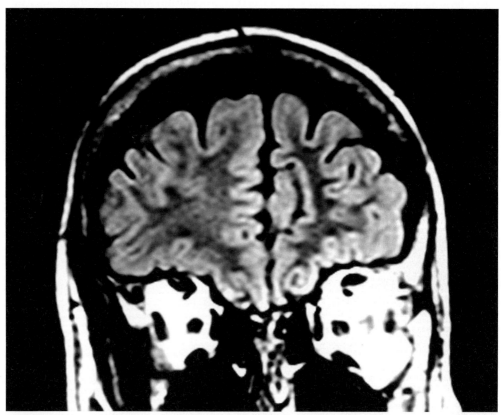

Figure 10. Coronal FLAIR MRI image from a 17 year old with intractable epilepsy demonstrates diffuse FLAIR hyperintensity in the subcortical white matter in the anterior right frontal lobe, without definite cortical signal abnormality, thickening, or loss of gray-white matter differentiation. At pathlogy, cortical lamination abnormalities were seen, with ectopic neurons in the subcortical white matter, but without dysmorphic neurons or balloon cells, consistent with an FCD Type I.

panying lesion. However, hippocampal sclerosis has been commonly observed related to FCD Type I in the temporal lobe, and now is separately classified as Type IIIa.

Neoplasms associated with ETLE are described in detail below, and it remains to be seen whether an FCD associated with a neoplasm can be identified on imaging and fully delineated pre-surgically. The FCDs usually observed are Type I or mMCD (not Type II which by definition would be considered dual pathology and not Type IIIb). Neoplasms usually seen related to areas of cortical dysplasia are gangliogliomas and DNETs, although other glial tumors are also observed. The vast majority are in the temporal lobes, with occipital and parietal lobes less frequently involved (Prayson *et al.*, 2010)

Of note, cases arise where it can be difficult to differentiate pre-surgically between underlying neoplasm and an FCD, including when there is no definite mass effect, the signal abnormality is focal and confined to the cortex, without clear cystic/solid components, enhancement or calcifications. On pathology, it will be important to exclude neoplastic cells in areas of suspected cortical dysplasia, as the tumor may be intermingled with normal cortex.

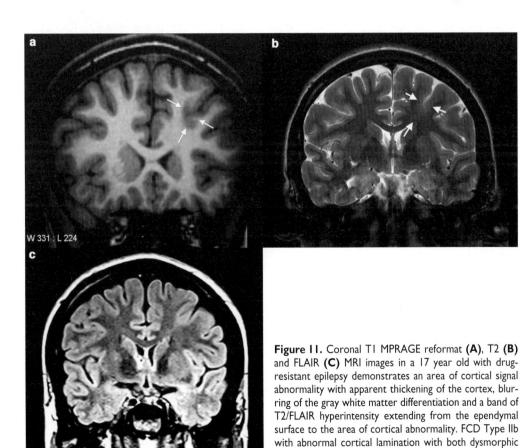

Figure 11. Coronal T1 MPRAGE reformat **(A)**, T2 **(B)** and FLAIR **(C)** MRI images in a 17 year old with drug-resistant epilepsy demonstrates an area of cortical signal abnormality with apparent thickening of the cortex, blurring of the gray white matter differentiation and a band of T2/FLAIR hyperintensity extending from the ependymal surface to the area of cortical abnormality. FCD Type IIb with abnormal cortical lamination with both dysmorphic cells and balloon cells was found at pathology.

While a couple of reports have described vascular malformations associated with FCD, there is no large body of cases which have here to now been described. Thus, the frequency of cortical dysplasias related to vascular malformations is unknown. However, Blümcke *et al.*, (2010) hypothesized that FCD Type IIIc is an acquired process (not dual pathology), related to the vascular malformation itself, be it a cavernous malformations, arteriovenous malformations, leptomeningeal vascular malformations, telangiectasias, or meningioangiomatosis. They also describe an association with abnormal sulcation, with a large single draining vein (that may be misinterpreted as a developmental venous anomaly).

Finally, areas of cytoarchitectural abnormalities have been described in relation to lesions acquired during early life, and are now subdivided as FCD Type IIId, and will likely represent an acquired rather than a primary cortical dysplasia. Underyling etiologies include traumatic brain injury, glial scarring as a sequela of pre- or perinatal brain injury (ischemic, bleeding, etc.), as well as inflammatory/ infectious processes including bacterial/viral encephalitis, limbic encephalitis, and Rasmussen encephalitis.

Mild malformations of cortical development

When Palmini *et al.*, (2004) outlined their classification system, they were uncertain whether mMCDs (and even FCD Type I) would be detectable on imaging. Only one study has specifically described imaging features in mMCD (Krsek *et al.*, 2008), with lobar hypoplasia/atrophy the most common finding, and therefore, it has significant overlap with FCD Type I. But with the redefinition of FCD Type I with clearer subtypes, it remains to be seen whether these would now be reclassified as FCD Type I and whether imaging features then exist for mMCD, or if they will only be detected at pathology.

Heterotopia

Heterotopia are a collection of nerve cells (and thus gray matter) in abnormal locations secondary to an arrest in the radial migration of neurons. While three imaging patterns of heterotopias are commonly described – subependymal, subcortical, and band (double cortex) heterotopias – the last of these is now considered to be a part of the lissencephaly spectrum given the underlying genetic basis of this malformation.

As with other MCDs, heterotopia may be asymptomatic and incidentally identified. For those with symptoms, the most common presentation of subependymal nodular heterotopia is epilepsy, oftentimes intractable, mental retardation and/or developmental delay (in part related to the severity of the malformation). For those with subcortical heterotopia, in addition to seizures, these patients oftentimes present with weakness, spasticity and hyperreflexia in a distribution related to the area of the brain affected (Barkovich, 2000).

The majority of patients with subependymal nodular heterotopia have a few, asymmetric heterotopic foci usually adjacent to the trigones and temporal and occipital horns of the lateral ventricles. These cases are rarely familial, but may be associated with other brain anomalies (including Chiari II, cephaloceles, agenesis of the corpus callosum, etc.). The less frequently seen variant manifests with a large number of heterotopic nodules, often bilateral, which is more widespread and can completely or near completely line the ventricular margin. These cases are more likely to be familial in origin, and associated with other malformations of the brain as well as facial structures. In patients with heterotopia, complete pre-operative evaluation will help determine the epileptogenicity of these foci. Patients with unilateral heterotopia do better than those with bilateral heterotopia postoperatively (Tassi *et al.*, 2005). These patients are also more like to be sporadic whereas patients with bilateral heterotopia are more likely to be familial in nature. The underlying genetics in these cases is still incompletely understood, but likely is heterogeneous with multiple underlying etiologies (Guerrini and Marini, 2006; van Kogelenberg et al., 2010).

On MRI, subependymal heterotopia will follow gray matter signal intensity on all sequences (including T1, T2 and diffusion weighted imaging among others), which allow them to be differentiated from other nodular pathology including tumor and subependymal nodules associated with tuberous sclerosis (*Figure 12*). While heterotopia can be diagnosed in utero on fetal MRI (Mitchell *et al.*, 2000), it may be more difficult to differentiate it from subependymal hemorrhage and subependymal nodules of tuberous sclerosis given that most current uses of fetal MRI are highly dependent on fast T2 weighted imaging (with other sequences needed to differentiate these possibilities).

Focal subcortical heterotopia (Barkovich, 1996) have a more variable appearance, varying in size from 1 to 2 cm to much larger regions involving much of an entire hemisphere. Barkovich (2000) described three different appearances: i) multiple nodules (isointense

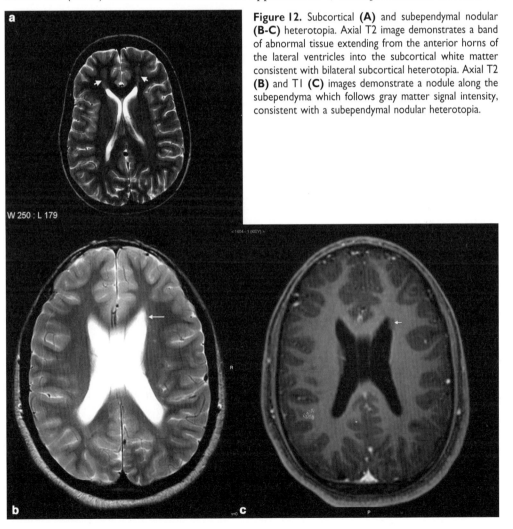

Figure 12. Subcortical **(A)** and subependymal nodular **(B-C)** heterotopia. Axial T2 image demonstrates a band of abnormal tissue extending from the anterior horns of the lateral ventricles into the subcortical white matter consistent with bilateral subcortical heterotopia. Axial T2 **(B)** and T1 **(C)** images demonstrate a nodule along the subependyma which follows gray matter signal intensity, consistent with a subependymal nodular heterotopia.

to gray matter) extending from the ependymal surface into the white matter without involvement of the overlying cortex; ii) a curvilinear appearance with ribbons of abnormal gray matter extending into the white matter with the appearance of enfolded cortex in contiguity with the overlying cortex; and iii) a combination of the two, with deep nodular heterotopia and overlying curvilinear heterotopias. Callosal dysgenesis and dysplasia of the ipsilateral basal ganglia were frequently associated anomalies. On imaging, these lesions appear as isointense to gray matter on all pulse sequences, with the imaging appearance corresponding.

Pathologic review has shown that the heterotopia may also be associated with other abnormalities including dystrophic cortex (Tassi et al., 2005), neoplasms such as gangliogliomas (Meroni et al., 2009), polymicrogyria (Wieck et al., 2005; Leventer et al., 2010) and hippocampal sclerosis (Lopez et al., 2010).

Polymicrogyria

Polymicrogryia (PMG) is a disorder of neuronal organization characterized histologically by abnormal lamination of the cortex with an associated derangement of sulcation and fusion of the molecular layers across sulci (McBride & Kemper, 1982; Barkovich et al., 1992). Patients frequently have extensive areas of involvement, frequently including eloquent cortex, therefore contraindicating surgical intervention. However, this is a heterogeneous group of disorders, with variable clinical presentation, epileptogenicity, imaging appearance, and topographical distribution. Thus, two subgroups of patients may benefit from surgery: 1) those with a more focal area of involvement where complete surgical resection is possible and 2) those where neurophysiologic testing indicates a focal epileptogenic region whereby surgery may help diminish seizure frequency.

While cases of PMG may be incidentally found in patients without any clinical symptoms, the vast majority are seen in patients with varying degrees of developmental delay and epilepsy. Severity of symptoms may be in part related to extent of PMG (Jansen et al., 2005) although this may be in part a secondary phenomenon as these patients were more likely to have severe seizures with an earlier onset, and cognitive issues may then be secondary to seizures. Leventer et al., (2010) report in a retrospective review of 328 patients with PMG that 61% of patients presented before 1 year of age and 87% presented before age 5. They found that patients with a more diffuse pattern of PMG presented earlier. Additionally, patients with bilateral perisylvian PMG presented earlier than those with unilateral involvement.

However, this retrospective review only included patients who presented to a variety of clinical settings which excludes asymptomatic patients and therefore may have a selection bias. Asymptomatic patients may therefore present much later in life (Tezer et al., 2008).

A wide variety of presenting symptoms have been reported, in part related to the regions of brain involved. Symptoms include seizures, global developmental delay and language impairments, hemiparesis or other motor impairment, sensory abnormalities, abnormal feeding, as well as visual impairment (Leventer et al., 2010; Hayashi et al., 2002). Patients are more frequently microcephalic, although normocephalic and macrocephalic patients are also seen. Other associated findings include dysmorphic features and other congenital anomalies (especially in syndromic/genetic forms of PMG).

While the etiology of PMG is frequently unclear, both non-genetic and genetic causes/ associations are seen. PMG can be seen in the setting of in-utero ischemic insults (including related to encephaloceles and Sturge-Weber syndrome) as well as congenital infections, especially cytomegalovirus (CMV), although other TORCH infections including syphllis and varicella have also been described. As our ability to identify genetic abnormalities improves, the number of associated genetic abnormalities associated with PMG has dramatically increased, with multiple described. The most robust association is the GPR56 mutation which is associated with bilateral frontoparietal PMG. Other associated genetic abnormalities include chromosomal deletion and duplication syndromes, familial autosomal and x-linked PMG, as well as multiple syndromic forms (Jansen & Andermann, 2005). The best known of these includes Aicardi syndrome, Delleman syndrome, Digeorge syndrome, Warburg micro syndrome, and d-bifunctional protein deficiency, although many more exist (Barkovich, 2010). Various inborn errors of metabolism have also been associated with PMG as well, the best known of which is Zellweger syndrome, a peroxisomal leukodystrophy (Jansen and Andermann, 2005).

Given the heterogeneous nature of PMG, the MRI findings reflect the pathology (*Figure 13*). The most commonly described findings in PMG include a coarse, irregular, high frequency bumpy cortical surface involving both the inner and outer margins of the cortex, with shallow sulci, broad gyri and apparent cortical thickening without T2 hyperintensity (Haygashi *et al.*, 2002; Leventer *et al.*, 2010; Barkovich *et al.*, 1999; Takanashi & Barkovich, 2003). Given the fusion across the sulci as well as the high frequency nodularity of the cortical surface, there may be a paradoxical smooth appearance of the abnormal areas of brain. Additionally, as the brain develops, PMG may initially have a small, delicate, undulating pattern to the gyri with normal thickness which as the brain develops and as more myelination occurs becomes more thick and bumpy (Takanashi & Barkovich, 2003; Barkovich, 2010), although cases where the delicate pattern persist even after myelination occurs has also been described (Barkovich, 2010). Finally, one other contributing factor to the apparent coarse appearance may be the imaging technique, with thin volumetric T1 weighted images demonstrating the gray-white matter contrast and differentiation to best effect.

While at times, PMG and schizencephaly have been separated into distinct entities, there is overlap between these entitities, and they likely represent appearances along the same spectrum. A cleft like configuration without connection to the ventricle may be seen in approximately 30% of patients (Haygashi *et al.*, 2002) with PMG. As the underlying genetics is better understood, the relationship of some of these entities may become clearer (*e.g.* emx2 gene; Jansen & Andermann, 2005).

Fetal MRI in patients with PMG confirm the evolving nature of these lesions, as a subtle irregularity in utero may be found to be a more far reaching abnormality post-natally. However, the subtle nature of these findings also decreases sensitivity for detection of MCD (Righini *et al.*, 2004).

A number of different patterns of involvement are seen, with the most frequent representing perisylvian involvement, either bilateral or unilateral, followed by a generalized, frontal, parasagittal, and parietal distributions. Most of those that involve the perisylvian region are bilateral and symmetric (Haygashi *et al.*, 2002; Levanter *et al.*, 2010). However, many other patterns have been described with virtually all cortical regions found to be involved. Leventer *et al.*, (2010) observed a severity gradient, such that there was a tapering of the areas of brain involved with distance from the primary area of involvement.

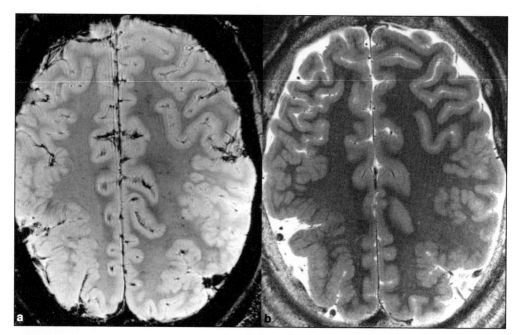

Figure 13. T2 and T2* images in a 19 year old with drug-resistant epilepsy and extensive bilateral perisylvian polymicrogyria imaged at 7 Tesla.

Various associated abnormalities have been described including heterotopia, abnormal decreased volume of subjacent white matter (although a minority are found to have a localized megalencephaly), abnormal morphology of sylvian fissures (Leventer *et al.*, 2010), perivascular space dilatation and large cortical veins, corpus callosum dysgenesis, hippocampal malformation, and absent septum pellucidum (Hayashi *et al.*, 2005).

Other etiologies of extratemporal lobe epilepsies

While malformations of cortical development, especially cortical dysplasias, are the most frequent underlying etiology of drug-resistant extratemporal lobe epilepsy, many other underlying etiologies have also been observed. While it is beyond the scope of this chapter to delineate the neuroimaging findings of each of these entities, the most common entities will be briefly described.

Neoplasms

The relationship of neoplasms, particularly gangliogliomas and DNETs, with focal cortical dysplasias was addressed previously, and is now included as part of the 2010 ILAE FCD classification system. This association with malformations of cortical development may be in over a quarter of all patients with neoplasms (Prayson, 2010). However, neoplasms can also be observed without adjacent cortical dysplasia, and are found more frequently in patients with drug-resistant epilepsy. While the most frequent pathologies observed are gangliogliomas and DNETs, other neoplasms can be identified, including gliomas, gangliogliomas, mixed gangliogliomas/DNETs, oligodendrogliomas, and meningioangiomatosis (Prayson *et al.*, 2010). And while these are most frequently seen in a temporal location, parietal and frontal locations are also seen (Oda *et al.*, 1998).

Gangliogliomas are a slowly growing, well-differentiated neuroepithelial tumor composed of neoplastic ganglion and glial cells. They can have a variable appearance, and while they classically present with a circumscribed cyst with a mural nodule, they can also have a solid appearance with thickening and expansion of the gyri. These lesions commonly calcify, with variable size from 2 to 3 cm to bigger than 4 cm *(Figure 14)*.

Dysembryoplastic neuroepithelial tumors (DNETs) are focal, intracortical masses which are commonly well demarcated, wedge shaped, bubbly lesion, with minimal or no mass effect and no enhancement. While they most commonly occur in the temporal lobe, they can be seen elsewhere in the brain *(Figure 15)*.

Vascular malformations

The most common vascular malformations associated with intractable epilepsy are cavernous malformations and to a lesser extent arteriovenous malformations (AVMs) (Dodick *et al.*, 1994). However, other vascular malformations such as leptomeningeal vascular malformations (including Sturge Weber), or meningioangiomatosis may also be associated with ETLE. While some have described capillary telangiectasias and developmental venous anomalies (DVAs) in the setting of epilepsy as well (Maciunas *et al.*, 2010), it is less clear if this was incidentally found related to another underlying epileptogenic substrate, or if these vascular malformations actually contributed or resulted in seizures, especially given the associate of DVAs and cavernous malformations.

Vascular malformations can frequently be identified by susceptibility on gradient echo sequences corresponding to hemosiderin deposition from remote hemorrhage. Cavernous malformations are classically centrally T2 hyperintense with a popcorn configuration, and surrounding rim of T2 hypointensity *(Figure 16)*. Other vascular malformations can be identified by their flow voids/vascular enhancement (AVMs, DVAs) or enhancement pattern (capillary telengiectasia, leptomeningeal vascular malformations).

While some studies have shown that the duration and frequency of seizures were strong predictors of whether lesionectomy (and removal of surrounding hemosiderin stained brain) will yield a seizure free outcome (Cappabianca *et al.*, 1997), others have indicated that carefully selected patients (based on location, multiplicity and correlation with semiology) regardless of duration and frequency of seizures was more important in predicting seizure outcome (Kraemer *et al.*, 1998; Dodick *et al.*, 1994). While many case studies have

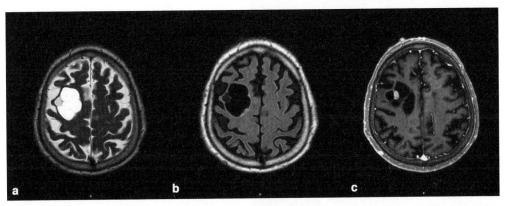

Figure 14. A typical appearance of a ganglioglioma on T2 **(A)**, FLAIR **(B)** and T1 post contrast **(C)** with multiple large cystic components as well as a solid nodule of enhancement.

described the association of cavernous malformations and cortical dysplasias (Maciunas *et al.*, 2010; Giulioni *et al.*, 2007), with the new FCD Type IIIc classification, it remains to be seen to what extent this association may have a distinct electroclinical presentation.

Other

Injury to the brain, regardless of the etiology, can result in neuronal cell loss or astroglial proliferation, resulting in epileptogenicity. This can be the sequela of traumatic brain injury, an infarct, either hemorrhagic or non-hemorrhagic, as well as infection/inflammation (including infectious encephalitis, Rasmussen encephalitis, etc.). This can involve gray matter, white matter or both, manifesting as T2/FLAIR hyperintensity on MR imaging (*Figure 17*). This may be associated with areas of focal encephalomalacia related to the prior injury,

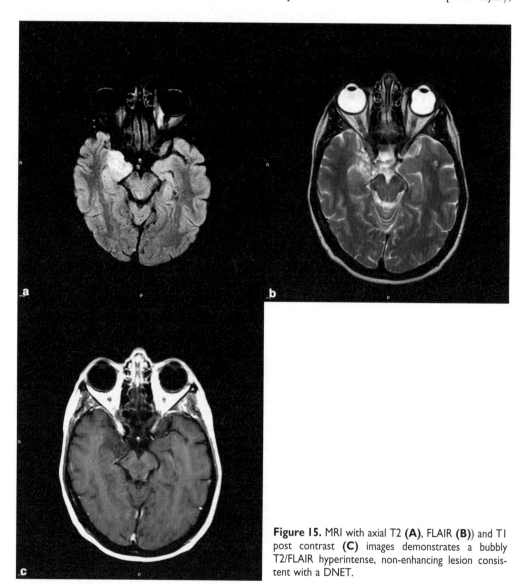

Figure 15. MRI with axial T2 **(A)**, FLAIR **(B)**) and T1 post contrast **(C)** images demonstrates a bubbly T2/FLAIR hyperintense, non-enhancing lesion consistent with a DNET.

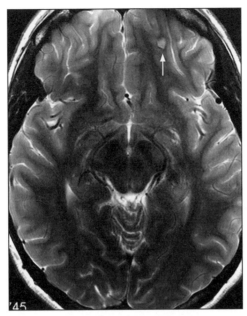

Figure 16. An 18 year old with drug-resistant epilepsy had an initial MRI at 1.5 Tesla (not shown) without a focal abnormality identified. Subsequently, images at 3 Tesla demonstrated an area of central T2 hyperintensity with a rim of hypointensity consistent with a cavernous malformation at the inferior left frontal lobe. Because of the close relationship of this lesion to the skull base, the abnormality was obscured by susceptibility from the adjacent bone on the initial MRI.

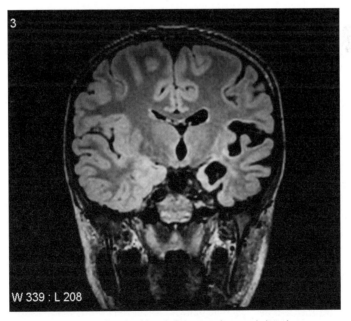

Figure 17. Coronal FLAIR images in an 8 year old with Rassmusen's encephalitis demonstrates extensive areas of atrophy and FLAIR hyperintensity throughout the left hemisphere.

helping differentiate it from other etiologies associated with ETLE. For patients with such injuries, surgical resection may help reduce or eliminate seizure frequency (Chiricozzi, 2005).

■ Dual pathology

In the assessment and presurgical workup of patients suspected to have extratemporal lobe epilepsy, it is important to assess the temporal lobe for any early evidence of mesial temporal (MTS) or hippocampal sclerosis, as surgical seizure free outcome after lesionectomy will depend on removing all epileptogenic tissue. Up to one-third of patients with a malformation of cortical development may have abnormal appearance of the hippocampus (Kuchukhidze et al., 2010). As MTS can be secondary to a primary lesion elsewhere in the brain, in patients with longstanding ETLE, dual pathology must be evaluated as addressing both possible epileptogenic foci will improve outcome (Kim et al., 2010).

However, it is important to note that seizures themselves can present with imaging findings that may subsequently resolve. This includes areas of decreased diffusion (possibly with T2/FLAIR hyperintensity), especially in the hippocampi and if this is observed on initial imaging, follow-up may be needed to determine if these areas of signal abnormality are transient or persist.

References

- Barkovich AJ. Subcortical heterotopia: a distinct clinicoradiologic entity. *AJNR Am J Neuroradiol* 1996; 17: 1315-22.

- Barkovich AJ. MRI analysis of sulcation morphology in polymicrogyria. *Epilepsia* 2010; 51 (Suppl 1): 17-22.

- Barkovich AJ. Current concepts of polymicrogyria. *Neuroradiology* 2010; 52: 479-87.

- Barkovich AJ, Kuzniecky RI. Gray matter heterotopia. *Neurology* 2000; 55: 1603-8.

- Barkovich AJ, Gressens P, Evrard P. Formation, maturation, and disorders of brain neocortex. *AJNR Am J Neuroradiol* 1992; 13: 423-46.

- Barkovich AJ, Hevner R, Guerrini R. Syndromes of bilateral symmetrical polymicrogyria. *AJNR Am J Neuroradiol* 1999; 20: 1814-21.

- Barkovich AJ, Kuzniecky RI, Jackson GD, Guerrini R, Dobyns WB. A developmental and genetic classification for malformations of cortical development. *Neurology* 2005; 65: 1873-87.

- Briellmann RS, Pell GS, Wellard RM, Mitchell LA, Abbott DF, Jackson GD. MR imaging of epilepsy: state of the art at 1.5 T and potential of 3 T. *Epileptic Disord* 2003; 5: 3-20.

- Cappabianca P, Alfieri A, Maiuri F, Mariniello G, Cirillo S, de Divitiis E. Supratentorial cavernous malformations and epilepsy: seizure outcome after lesionectomy on a series of 35 patients. *Clin Neurol Neurosurg* 1997; 99: 179-83.

- Caruso P, Robertson R, Setty B and Grant E. Disorders of brain development. In: Atlas S, ed. *Magnetic Resonance Imaging of the Brain and Spine.* China: Lippincott Williams & Wilkins, 2009, 194-271.

- Cepeda C, André VM, Levine MS, Salamon N, Miyata H, Vinters HV, Mathern GW. Epileptogenesis in pediatric cortical dysplasia: the dysmature cerebral developmental hypothesis. *Epilepsy Behav* 2006; 9: 219-35.

- Chamberlain WA, Cohen ML, Gyure KA, Kleinschmidt-DeMasters BK, Perry A, Powell SZ, *et al*. Interobserver and intraobserver reproducibility in focal cortical dysplasia (malformations of cortical development). *Epilepsia* 2009; 50: 2593-8.

- Chiricozzi F, Chieffo D, Battaglia D, Iuvone L, Acquafondata C, Cesarini L, *et al*. Developmental plasticity after right hemispherectomy in an epileptic adolescent with early brain injury. *Childs Nerv Syst* 2005; 21: 960-9.

- Colombo N, Salamon N, Raybaud C, Ozkara C, Barkovich AJ. Imaging of malformations of cortical development. *Epileptic Disord* 2009; 11: 194-205.

- Crino PB. Focal brain malformations: seizures, signaling, sequencing. *Epilepsia* 2009; 50 (Suppl 9): 3-8.

- Diehl B, Najm I, LaPresto E, Prayson R, Ruggieri P, Mohamed A, *et al*. Temporal lobe volumes in patients with hippocampal sclerosis with or without cortical dysplasia. *Neurology* 2004; 62: 1729-35.

- Dodick DW, Cascino GD, Meyer FB. Vascular malformations and intractable epilepsy: outcome after surgical treatment. *Mayo Clin Proc* 1994; 69: 741-5.

- Elsharkawy AE, Behne F, Oppel F, Pannek H, Schulz R, Hoppe M, *et al*. Long-term outcome of extratemporal epilepsy surgery among 154 adult patients. *J Neurosurg* 2008; 108: 676-86.

- Fauser S, Schulze-Bonhage A, Honegger J, Carmona H, Huppertz H, Pantazis G, *et al*. Focal cortical dysplasias: surgical outcome in 67 patients in relation to histological subtypes and dual pathology. *Brain* 2004; 127 (Pt 11): 2406-18.

- Fauser S, Sisodiya SM, Martinian L, Thom M, Gumbinger C, Huppertz H, *et al*. Multi-focal occurrence of cortical dysplasia in epilepsy patients. *Brain* 2009; 132 (Pt 8): 2079-90.

- Giulioni M, Zucchelli M, Riguzzi P, Marucci G, Tassinari CA, Calbucci F. Co-existence of cavernoma and cortical dysplasia in temporal lobe epilepsy. *J Clin Neurosci* 2007; 14: 1122-4.

- Grant PE, Barkovich AJ, Wald LL, Dillon WP, Laxer KD, Vigneron DB. High-resolution surface-coil MR of cortical lesions in medically refractory epilepsy: a prospective study. *AJNR Am J Neuroradiol* 1997; 18: 291-301.

- Guerrini R, Marini C. Genetic malformations of cortical development. *Exp Brain Res* 2006; 173: 322-33.

- Haacke EM, Mittal S, Wu Z, Neelavalli J, Cheng YN. Susceptibility-weighted imaging: technical aspects and clinical applications, part 1. *AJNR Am J Neuroradiol* 2009; 30: 19-30.

- Hayashi N, Tsutsumi Y, Barkovich AJ. Polymicrogyria without porencephaly/schizencephaly. MRI analysis of the spectrum and the prevalence of macroscopic findings in the clinical population. *Neuroradiology* 2002; 44: 647-55.

- Hildebrandt M, Pieper T, Winkler P, Kolodziejczyk D, Holthausen H, Blümcke I. Neuropathological spectrum of cortical dysplasia in children with severe focal epilepsies. *Acta Neuropathol* 2005; 110: 1-11.

- Ho S, Kuzniecky RI, Gilliam F, Faught E, Morawetz R. Temporal lobe developmental malformations and epilepsy: dual pathology and bilateral hippocampal abnormalities. *Neurology* 1998; 50: 748-54.

- Jansen A, Andermann E. Genetics of the polymicrogyria syndromes. *J Med Genet* 2005; 42: 369-78.

- Jansen AC, Leonard G, Bastos AC, Esposito-Festen JE, Tampieri D, Watkins K, *et al*. Cognitive functioning in bilateral perisylvian polymicrogyria (BPP): clinical and radiological correlations. *Epilepsy Behav* 2005; 6: 393-404.

- Kim DW, Lee SK, Nam H, Chu K, Chung CK, Lee S, *et al*. Epilepsy with dual pathology: surgical treatment of cortical dysplasia accompanied by hippocampal sclerosis. *Epilepsia* 2010; 51: 1429-35.

- Knake S, Triantafyllou C, Wald LL, Wiggins G, Kirk GP, Larsson PG, *et al*. 3T phased array MRI improves the presurgical evaluation in focal epilepsies: a prospective study. *Neurology* 2005; 65: 1026-31.

- Kraemer DL, Griebel ML, Lee N, Friedman AH, Radtke RA. Surgical outcome in patients with epilepsy with occult vascular malformations treated with lesionectomy. *Epilepsia* 1998; 39: 600-7.
- Krsek P, Maton B, Korman B, Pacheco-Jacome E, Jayakar P, Dunoyer C, *et al.* Different features of histopathological subtypes of pediatric focal cortical dysplasia. *Ann Neurol* 2008; 63: 758-69.
- Krsek P, Maton B, Jayakar P, Dean P, Korman B, Rey G, *et al.* Incomplete resection of focal cortical dysplasia is the main predictor of poor postsurgical outcome. *Neurology* 2009; 72: 217-23.
- Lerner JT, Salamon N, Hauptman JS, Velasco TR, Hemb M, Wu JY, *et al.* Assessment and surgical outcomes for mild type I and severe type II cortical dysplasia: a critical review and the UCLA experience. *Epilepsia* 2009; 50: 1310-35.
- Leventer RJ, Jansen A, Pilz DT, Stoodley N, Marini C, Dubeau F, *et al.* Clinical and imaging heterogeneity of polymicrogyria: a study of 328 patients. *Brain* 2010; 133 (Pt 5): 1415-27.
- López HE, Fohlen M, Lelouch-Tubiana A, Robain O, Jalin C, Bulteau C, *et al.* Heterotopia associated with hippocampal sclerosis: an under-recognized cause of early onset epilepsy in children operated on for temporal lobe epilepsy. *Neuropediatrics* 2010; 41: 167-75.
- Maciunas JA, Syed TU, Cohen ML, Werz MA, Maciunas RJ, Koubeissi MZ. Triple pathology in epilepsy: coexistence of cavernous angiomas and cortical dysplasias with other lesions. *Epilepsy Res* 2010; 91: 106-10.
- Madan N, Grant PE. New directions in clinical imaging of cortical dysplasias. *Epilepsia* 2009; 50 (Suppl 9): 9-18.
- McBride MC, Kemper TL. Pathogenesis of four-layered microgyric cortex in man. *Acta Neuropathol* 1982; 57: 93-8.
- Meroni A, Galli C, Bramerio M, Tassi L, Colombo N, Cossu M, *et al.* Nodular heterotopia: a neuropathological study of 24 patients undergoing surgery for drug-resistant epilepsy. *Epilepsia* 2009; 50: 116-24.
- Mitchell LA, Simon EM, Filly RA, Barkovich AJ. Antenatal diagnosis of subependymal heterotopia. *AJNR Am J Neuroradiol* 2000; 21: 296-300.
- Mittal S, Wu Z, Neelavalli J, Haacke EM. Susceptibility-weighted imaging: technical aspects and clinical applications, part 2. *AJNR Am J Neuroradiol* 2009; 30: 232-52.
- Nobili L, Francione S, Mai R, Cardinale F, Castana L, Tassi L, *et al.* Surgical treatment of drug-resistant nocturnal frontal lobe epilepsy. *Brain* 2007; 130 (Pt 2): 561-73.
- Oda M, Arai N, Maehara T, Shimizu H, Kojima H, Yagishita A. Brain tumors in surgical neuropathology of intractable epilepsies, with special reference to cerebral dysplasias. *Brain Tumor Pathol* 1998; 15: 41-51.
- Palmini A, Najm I, Avanzini G, Babb T, Guerrini R, Foldvary-Schaefer N, *et al.* Terminology and classification of the cortical dysplasias. *Neurology* 2004; 62 (6 Suppl 3): S2-8.
- Phal PM, Usmanov A, Nesbit GM, Anderson JC, Spencer D, Wang P, *et al.* Qualitative comparison of 3-T and 1.5-T MRI in the evaluation of epilepsy. *AJR Am J Roentgenol* 2008 Sep; 191: 890-5.
- Prayson RA. Tumours arising in the setting of paediatric chronic epilepsy. *Pathology* 2010; 42: 426-31.
- Prayson RA, Frater JL. Cortical dysplasia in extratemporal lobe intractable epilepsy: a study of 52 cases. *Ann Diagn Pathol* 2003; 7: 139-46.
- Raymond AA, Fish DR, Stevens JM, Cook MJ, Sisodiya SM, Shorvon SD. Association of hippocampal sclerosis with cortical dysgenesis in patients with epilepsy. *Neurology* 1994; 44: 1841-5.
- Righini A, Zirpoli S, Mrakic F, Parazzini C, Pogliani L, Triulzi F. Early prenatal MR imaging diagnosis of polymicrogyria. *AJNR Am J Neuroradiol* 2004; 25: 343-6.
- Russo GL, Tassi L, Cossu M, Cardinale F, Mai R, Castana L, Colombo N, Bramerio M. Focal cortical resection in malformations of cortical development. *Epileptic Disord* 2003; 5 (Suppl 2): S115-23.

- Sarkar SN, Alsop DC, Madhuranthakam AJ, Busse RF, Robson PM, Rofsky NM, Hackney DB. Brain MR Imaging at Ultra-low Radiofrequency Power [Internet]. *Radiology* 2011; [cited 2011 Mar 15] Available from: http://www.ncbi.nlm.nih.gov/pubmed/21357520

- Takanashi J, Barkovich AJ. The changing MR imaging appearance of polymicrogyria: a consequence of myelination. *AJNR Am J Neuroradiol* 2003; 24: 788-93.

- Tassi L, Colombo N, Garbelli R, Francione S, Lo Russo G, Mai R, *et al.* Focal cortical dysplasia: neuropathological subtypes, EEG, neuroimaging and surgical outcome. *Brain* 2002; 125(Pt 8): 1719-32.

- Tassi L, Colombo N, Cossu M, Mai R, Francione S, Lo Russo G, *et al.* Electroclinical, MRI and neuropathological study of 10 patients with nodular heterotopia, with surgical outcomes. *Brain* 2005; 128 (Pt 2): 321-37.

- Taylor DC, Falconer MA, Bruton CJ, Corsellis JA. Focal dysplasia of the cerebral cortex in epilepsy. *J Neurol Neurosurg Psychiatr* 1971; 34: 369-87.

- Téllez-Zenteno JF, Hernández Ronquillo L, Moien-Afshari F, Wiebe S. Surgical outcomes in lesional and non-lesional epilepsy: a systematic review and meta-analysis. *Epilepsy Res* 2010; 89: 310-8.

- Tezer FI, Yildiz G, Oguz KK, Elibol B, Saygi S. Newly diagnosed polymicrogyria in the eighth decade. *Epilepsia* 2008; 49: 181-3.

- Urbach H, Scheffler B, Heinrichsmeier T, von Oertzen J, Kral T, Wellmer J, *et al.* Focal cortical dysplasia of Taylor's balloon cell type: a clinicopathological entity with characteristic neuroimaging and histopathological features, and favorable postsurgical outcome. *Epilepsia* 2002; 43: 33-40.

- van Kogelenberg M, Ghedia S, McGillivray G, Bruno D, Leventer R, Macdermot K, *et al.* Periventricular heterotopia in common microdeletion syndromes. *Mol Syndromol* 2010; 1: 35-41.

- Von Oertzen J, Urbach H, Jungbluth S, Kurthen M, Reuber M, Fernández G, Elger CE. Standard magnetic resonance imaging is inadequate for patients with refractory focal epilepsy. *J Neurol Neurosurg Psychiatr* 2002; 73: 643-7.

- Wald LL, Moyher SE, Day MR, Nelson SJ, Vigneron DB. Proton spectroscopic imaging of the human brain using phased array detectors. *Magn Reson Med* 1995; 34: 440-5.

- Widjaja E, Otsubo H, Raybaud C, Ochi A, Chan D, Rutka JT, *et al.* Characteristics of MEG and MRI between Taylor's focal cortical dysplasia (type II) and other cortical dysplasia: surgical outcome after complete resection of MEG spike source and MR lesion in pediatric cortical dysplasia. *Epilepsy Res* 2008; 82: 147-55.

- Wieck G, Leventer RJ, Squier WM, Jansen A, Andermann E, Dubeau F, *et al.* Periventricular nodular heterotopia with overlying polymicrogyria. *Brain* 2005; 128 (Pt 12): 2811-21.

- Wolf RL, Alsop DC, Levy-Reis I, Meyer PT, Maldjian JA, Gonzalez-Atavales J, *et al.* Detection of mesial temporal lobe hypoperfusion in patients with temporal lobe epilepsy by use of arterial spin labeled perfusion MR imaging. *AJNR Am J Neuroradiol* 2001; 22: 1334-41.

- Zijlmans M, de Kort GAP, Witkamp TD, Huiskamp GM, Seppenwoolde J, van Huffelen AC, Leijten FSS. 3T versus 1.5T phased-array MRI in the presurgical work-up of patients with partial epilepsy of uncertain focus. *J Magn Reson Imaging* 2009; 30: 256-62.

Ictal SPECT in extratemporal lobe epilepsy

Wim Van Paesschen[1], Karolien Goffin[2]

[1] *Department of Neurology, University Hospital Leuven, Leuven, Belgium*
[2] *Division of Nuclear Medicine, University Hospital Leuven, Leuven, Belgium*

Single photon emission computed tomography (SPECT) is an imaging technique that allows the study and visualization of cerebral perfusion during the interictal state and also during epileptic seizures (Juni *et al.*, 1998; Kapucu *et al.*, 2009). The localizing value of ictal SPECT is based on the coupling between cerebral metabolism and perfusion, where seizure activity will result in hyperperfusion on ictal SPECT. Ictal SPECT has a poor time resolution and, therefore, the brain region of ictal hyperperfusion often includes not only the ictal onset zone, but also propagation pathways. Blood perfusion tracers, such as ^{99m}Tc-ECD (ethyl cysteinate dimer) and ^{99m}Tc-HMPAO (hexa-methylpropyleneamine oxime) (stabilized form) are used. These lipophilic tracers are trapped in the brain with a first pass extraction fraction of around 85%. Conversion to a polar metabolite prevents washout or regional redistribution during the first 4 hours. The uptake reflects perfusion during the seizure. This technique offers the unique possibility for ictal imaging 1-3 hours after tracer injection without seizure movement artifacts. Due to the half-life of the tracers, a second ictal SPECT study is possible around 36 hours after a first study.

In extratemporal lobe epilepsies (ETLE), specific logistic issues should be considered. Motor signs are often present and should be taken into consideration when inserting a canula in an arm vein of the patient, which will be used to inject the tracer. It is possible that the ictal SPECT injection is not possible because the arm in which the canula is inserted is held in a dystonic flexion during the seizure or due to other motor activity. Frontal and parietal lobe seizures often are nocturnal seizures. Since nocturnal ictal SPECT studies are logistically difficult, it is common practice to switch the patient's day-night rhythm, and have the patient sleep during the day. Frontal lobe seizures are often of short duration. In these cases, it may be necessary to have a person, who will perform the ictal SPECT injection, sit at the bedside, ready to inject as soon as possible after seizure onset. In our hands, less than 0.3% of patients had habitual seizures that were consistently too short in duration in order to obtain a localizing ictal SPECT study.

Ictal SPECT images can be analyzed in different ways (Van Paesschen *et al.*, 2007) *(Figure 1)*. Co-registered interictal and ictal SPECT images can be visually analyzed side-by-side *(Figure 1A-1C)*. Subtraction ictal SPECT co-registered with MRI (SISCOM) is a sensitive and most commonly used method to detect regions of ictal hyperperfusion, and requires registration, normalization, smoothing and subtraction of interictal and ictal images, and thresholding (Zubal *et al.*, 1995; O'Brien *et al.*, 1998) *(Figure 1E-F, 1I-J)*. Composite ictal SPECT (Kaiboriboon *et al.*, 2005) is a new method of analysis which is particularly useful in ETLEs, since ictal propagation is often present *(Figure 1G, K)*. The technique requires two or more ictal SPECT scans in an individual patient. Regions of ictal hyperperfusion which are common in two or more ictal SPECT studies are more likely to represent the ictal onset zone, while other regions are more likely to represent propagated epileptic activity.

Postsurgical correlation in seizure free patients allows an unambiguous distinction between the ictal onset zone and propagated seizure activity. In seizure free patients, the region of resection by definition contains the epileptogenic zone (Rosenow & Lüders, 2001). Ictal SPECT hyperperfusion within the region of resection contains the ictal onset zone and hyperperfusion outside the region of resection represents propagated activity in seizure free patients. Ictal SPECT hyperperfusion fully confined to the region of resection represents the ictal onset zone with no propagation. This pattern is more likely with early injections during simple and complex partial seizures, and can be conclusively localized on blinded assessment (Lee, *et al.*, 2006). Propagated seizure activity is characterized by several hyperperfusion clusters, often connected with each other through small trails of hyperperfusion, which gives the pattern an "hourglass" appearance. The largest hyperperfusion cluster with highest z-score may be the ictal onset zone, but is often observed in brain regions of propagated activity (Dupont *et al.*, 2006) *(Figure 2)*. Propagation may be towards another lobe, ipsi- and contralateral. These patterns may not be conclusively localized on blinded assessment.

In view of these propagation patterns, interpretation of ictal SPECT is optimal with knowledge of the data of a full presurgical evaluation. Injection time with respect to seizure onset should be known, since early injections are more likely to represent the ictal onset zone without propagation. Knowledge of injected seizure type is important. Simple partial seizures have no obvious regions of hyperperfusion in around 40%. Complex partial seizures give the best results, and secondarily generalized seizures often give a correct lateralization, but not a good localization. A transit time of tracer to the brain of around 30 seconds should be taken into account: seizures should last at least 10-15 seconds after injection in order to give localizing information (Van Paesschen, 2004).

Ictal SPECT propagation patterns can be studied in focal dysplastic lesions (FDL), which are often present in ETLE (Dupont *et al.*, 2006). Since these lesions are intrinsically epileptogenic, ictal SPECT shows a hyperperfusion cluster overlapping with the FDL. No propagation, *i.e.* the largest hyperperfusion cluster with highest z-score overlapping with the FDL, was observed in around 30% of cases. Propagated ictal activity with the largest hyperperfusion cluster with highest z-score at a distance from the FDL was seen in around 70%, most often in frontal lobe epilepsy. Ictal SPECT plays an important role in the non-invasive presurgical evaluation of patients with refractory ETLE due to FDLs. Removal of the FDL and the surrounding hyperperfusion cluster in patients with concordant electroclinical data is a good surgical strategy which renders around 80% of these patients seizure-free *(Figure 2)*.

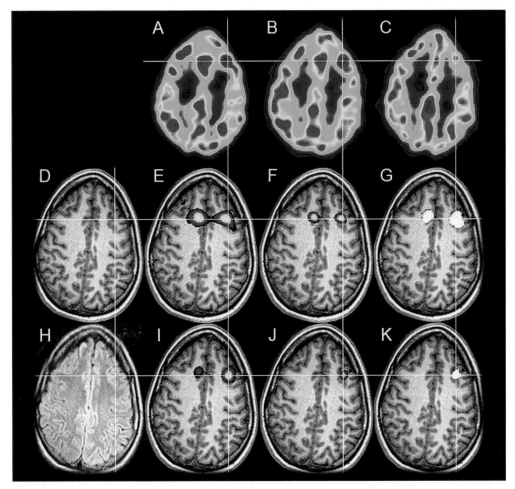

Figure 1. A. First ictal SPECT scan; **B.** Second ictal SPECT scan; **C.** Interictal SPECT scan. Visual assessment showed areas of hyperfusion in the left frontal lobe and at the midline of the frontal lobes. **E.** SISCOM of ictal SPECT 1 thresholded at 2 standard deviation (SD) showed two hyperperfusion clusters of equal intensity connected with a small trail of hyper-fusion; **F.** SISCOM of ictal SPECT 2 thresholded at 2 SD showed two separate hyperfusion clusters; **G.** The composite image of the two ictal SPECT images thresholded at 2 SD (**E** and **F**) confirmed that the frontal lobes had two regions in common displaying ictal hyperperfusion in two different seizures; **I.** SISCOM of ictal SPECT 1 thresholded at 3 SD showed two separate hyperperfusion clusters. The hyperperfusion cluster in the left frontal lobe had a higher z-score than the one in the right frontal lobe; **J.** SISCOM of ictal SPECT 2 thresholded at 3 SD showed one hyperfusion cluster in the left frontal lobe; **K.** The composite ictal SPECT of the two ictal SPECT images thresholded at 3 SD (**I** and **J**) showed that the frontal lobes had one region in common displaying ictal hyperperfusion in two different seizures. Although this region did not reveal an epileptic lesion on a T1-weighted MR image (**D**) and FLAIR (**H**), surgical resection of this region has rendered the patient seziure free for more than 2 years. Pathology revealed a small area of dysplastic neurons.

The epileptogenic zone is often difficult to determine in MR-negative refractory ETLE, and only around 40% of patients with MR-negative refractory ETLE are rendered seizure free after epilepsy surgery. Reevaluation of the MRI, guided by the ictal SPECT reveals small FDLs in around 15%. Also, ictal SPECT may confirm non-invasively that small lesions detected using morphometric MR analysis (Huppertz *et al.*, 2005) are epileptic lesions (*Figure 3*).

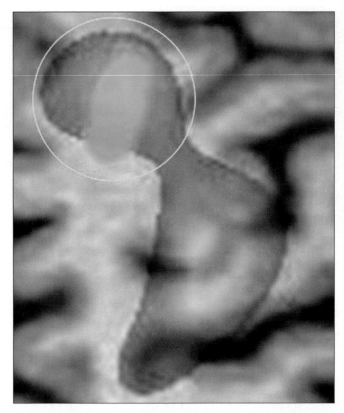

Figure 2. Non-invasive surgical strategy for refractory partial epilepsy due to small focal dysplastic lesions. A small focal dysplastic lesion is outlined in green. The SISCOM hyperperfusion consists of two clusters connected with a small trail of hyperperfusion. The hyperperfusion cluster overlapping the dysplastic lesion had a lower z-score than the other cluster, which represented propagated ictal activity. Surgical removal of the focal dysplastic lesion including the overlapping cluster of hyperperfusion up to the connecting trail of hyperperfusion has a high chance of rendering the patient seizure-free (Dupont et al., 2006). This strategy rendered the patient seizure free, with a follow-up of several years.

SISCOM can be used to guide placement of intracranial electrodes (Ahnlide et al., 2007) (*Figure 4*). SISCOM may alter and extend the strategy for electrode placement at invasive recording. Favorable surgical outcome has been observed when intracranial EEG was concordant with SISCOM hyperperfusion, but not when discordant. SISCOM localization, therefore, is an independent method with an impact in patients with refractory partial epilepsy scheduled for intracranial EEG studies.

Ictal SPECT is able to detect deep-seated epileptogenic zones non-invasively (*Figure 5*). In comparison with MRI, FDG-PET, magneto-encephalography, and scalp EEG, ictal SPECT is probably the most sensitive technique to localize the ictal onset zone in ETLE, and to predict a seizure free outcome after epilepsy surgery (Knowlton et al., 2008; Kim et al., 2009).

In conclusion, ictal SPECT is a sensitive imaging modality to localize the epileptogenic zone in ETLE, and an independent predictor of good surgical outcome. Interpretation of the pattern of hyperperfusion is optimal in the context of a full presurgical evaluation.

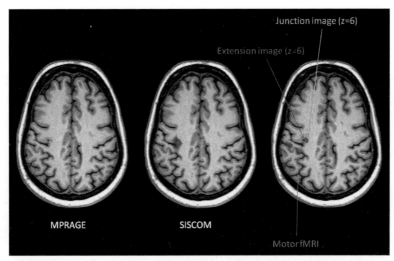

Figure 3. SISCOM is the prototype of multimodal imaging, combining structural with ictal functional information, and allows a confident delineation of the epileptogenic zone in selected patients with small, difficult to visualize dysplastic lesions. SISCOM of a patient with refractory right frontal lobe epilepsy showed a single hyperperfusion cluster. The MRI was read as normal. However, a morphometric analysis program (Huppertz *et al.*, 2005; Wellmer *et al.*, 2010) detected an abnormal grey-white matter transition and abnormal extension of grey matter into white matter, consistent with a focal cortical dysplasia, at the site of ictal SPECT hyperperfusion. Both junction and extension images deviated more than 6 standard deviations compared with a normal control database. Visual re-assessment of the MPRAGE revealed an abnormal gyrus at the site of ictal SPECT hyperperfusion. Motor fMRI suggested that motor cortex was at a small distance from the epileptic lesion and ictal onset zone.

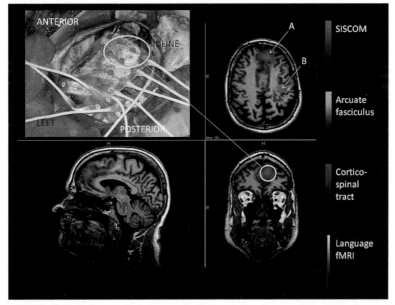

Figure 4. SISCOM-guided placement of subdural grids. Patient had refractory MR-negative frontal lobe epilepsy. SISCOM showed two hyperperfusion clusters that were connected with a small trail of hyperperfusion (not visible in this image). The largest cluster with the highest z-score was in the left frontopolar region **(A)** and the smaller one in the left dorsolateral frontal lobe **(B)**. Both areas were covered with subdural grids. The area covering the left frontopolar region contained the ictal onset zone (yellow circle). Surgical resection rendered the patient seizure free, with a follow-up of more than one year. Pathological examination showed a chronic meningitis.

The highest quality MRI should be used for co-registration. SISCOM allows a non-invasive presurgical evaluation of refractory partial epilepsy due to small focal dysplastic lesions. SISCOM can be used to plan invasive EEG studies.

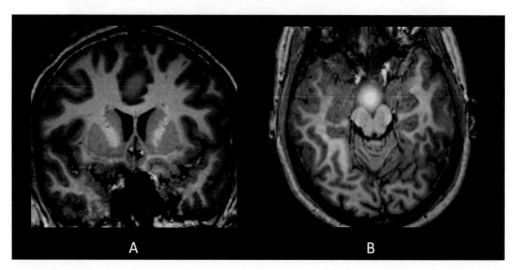

Figure 5. SISCOM is able to visualize a deep-seated ictal onset zone, which may be difficult to localize with scalp-EEG. **A.** Ictal onset zone in the cingulate gyrus. Notice that the hyperperfusion does not allow lateralization. **B.** Ictal hyperperfusion of hypothalamic hamartoma during a gelastic seizure.

References

- Ahnlide JA, Rosen I, Linden-Mickelsson TP, Kallen K. Does SISCOM contribute to favorable seizure outcome after epilepsy surgery? *Epilepsia* 2007; 48: 579-88.

- Dupont P, Van Paesschen W, Palmini A, *et al.* Ictal perfusion patterns associated with single MRI-visible focal dysplastic lesions: implications for the non-invasive delineation of the epileptogenic zone. *Epilepsia* 2006; 47: 1550-7.

- Huppertz HJ, Grimm C, Fauser S, *et al.* Enhanced visualization of blurred gray-white matter junctions in focal cortical dysplasia by voxel-based 3D MRI analysis. *Epilepsy Res* 2005; 67: 35-50.

- Juni JE, Waxman AD, Devous MD, *et al.* Procedure guideline for brain perfusion SPECT using technetium-99m radiopharmaceuticals. *J Nuclear Medicine* 1998; 39: 923-6.

- Kaiboriboon K, Bertrand ME, Osman MM, Hogan RE. Quantitative analysis of cerebral blood flow patterns in mesial temporal lobe epilepsy using composite SISCOM. *J Nucl Med* 2005; 46: 38-43.

- Kapucu OL, Nobili F, Varrone A, *et al.* EANM procedure guideline for brain perfusion SPECT using (99m)Tc-labelled radiopharmaceuticals, version 2. *Eur J Nucl Med Mol Imaging* 2009; 36: 2093-102.

- Kim JT, Bai SJ, Choi KO, *et al.* Comparison of various imaging modalities in localization of epileptogenic lesion using epilepsy surgery outcome in pediatric patients. *Seizure* 2009; 18: 504-10.

- Knowlton RC, Elgavish RA, Bartolucci A, *et al.* Functional imaging: II. Prediction of epilepsy surgery outcome. *Ann Neurol* 2008; 64: 35-41.

- Lee SK, Lee SY, Yun CH, Lee HY, Lee JS, Lee DS. Ictal SPECT in neocortical epilepsies: clinical usefulness and factors affecting the pattern of hyperperfusion. *Neuroradiology* 2006; 48: 678-84.

- O'Brien TJ, So EL, Mullan BP, *et al.* Subtraction ictal SPECT co-registered to MRI improves clinical usefulness of SPECT in localizing the surgical seizure focus. *Neurology* 1998; 50: 445-54.
- Rosenow F, Luders H. Presurgical evaluation of epilepsy. *Brain* 2001; 124: 1683-700.
- Van Paesschen W, Dupont P, Sunaert S, Goffin K, Van Laere K. The use of SPECT and PET in routine clinical practice in epilepsy. *Curr Opin Neurol* 2007; 20: 194-202.
- Van Paesschen W. Ictal SPECT. *Epilepsia* 2004; 45 (Suppl 4): 35-40.
- Wellmer J, Parpaley Y, von LM, Huppertz HJ. Integrating magnetic resonance imaging postprocessing results into neuronavigation for electrode implantation and resection of subtle focal cortical dysplasia in previously cryptogenic epilepsy. *Neurosurgery* 2010; 66:187-94.
- Zubal IG, Spencer SS, Imam K, *et al.* Difference images calculated from ictal and interictal technetium-99m-HMPAO SPECT scans of epilepsy. *J Nucl Med* 1995; 36: 684-9.

Functional MRI in extratemporal lobe epilepsy

Fergus J. Rugg-Gunn, John S. Duncan

*Department of Clinical and Experimental Epilepsy, Institute of
Neurology, University College London, National Hospital for
Neurology and Neurosurgery and Epilepsy Society, UCLH NHS
Foundation Trust, Queen Square, London, United Kingdom*

■ Background

Early studies of fMRI applied to epilepsy used phase mapping techniques (Fish *et al.*, 1988)
and dynamic contrast enhancement with gadolinium (Warach *et al.*, 1994) to demonstrate
abnormal blood flow in epilepsia partialis continua. Technical advances in MRI acquisition and post-processing have enabled cerebral activity, causing changes in regional blood
flow and volume, to be monitored indirectly through the effects of changing deoxyhae-
moglobin concentration (Ogawa *et al.*, 1993). This is termed the blood oxygen level-
dependent (BOLD) effect. BOLD changes are largely determined by cerebral blood flow
and so results are analogous to those obtained with blood flow tracers and PET, but with
improved temporal resolution.

Localisation of ictal blood flow changes using this technique was first described in 1994
in a 4-year-old child with frequent right-sided motor seizures (Jackson *et al.*, 1994). Each
clinical seizure was accompanied by increased MR signal intensity in the left hemisphere.
In addition, abnormal signal was observed in-between clinically apparent seizures suggesting that the method was sensitive to detect subclinical electrical activity. Subsequently,
an fMRI study of a similar patient by Detre *et al.* produced identical results (Detre *et al.*,
1995). Neither of these studies, however, used concurrent EEG monitoring to determine
seizure activity. It has been shown that the EEG can be recorded inside an MR scanner
with sufficient quality to detect high amplitude discharges and to trigger fMRI acquisitions
after these events (Ives *et al.*, 1993; Warach *et al.*, 1996), however, safety issues (Lemieux
et al., 1997) and imaging artefacts on the EEG initially precluded its wider application
(Huang-Hellinger *et al.*, 1995). The on-line subtraction of pulse (Allen *et al.*, 1998) and
scanner artefact (Allen *et al.*, 2000) have allowed continuous fMRI data acquisition
without obscuration of the EEG, thereby permitting accurate temporal correlation of epileptiform abnormality with imaging data (Allen *et al.*, 2000).

Task or epileptic discharge induced fMRI activations are typically analysed using the univariate general linear model. For language, laterality is commonly determined by comparing activation in homologous regions-of-interest in each hemisphere. A variety of approaches have been employed including voxel counting, mean values, and weighted averages (Seghier, 2008). A laterality index is derived from the statistical parametric map of the general linear model analysis. There are a number of limitations of these methods including the inability to control for performance effects or variations in the haemodynamic response function due to underlying pathology. Alternative methods such as coherence laterality may be more appropriate but have not yet been extensively validated and as such, remain in the research domain (Wang et al., 2009).

■ Localisation of the epileptic focus

Early studies of combined EEG and fMRI recordings in epilepsy utilised a "spike-triggered" paradigm, where a whole brain image, using a rapid echo planar sequence, was acquired approximately 3-4 seconds after a spike was detected (Krakow et al., 1999). This method took account of the inherent delay between neuronal activity and a haemodynamic response peak. An equivalent number of "baseline" images also had to be acquired against which the "active" images could be statistically compared. This was problematic in patients with frequent epileptic discharges. Furthermore, this method required continuous monitoring of the EEG recording to ensure optimal triggering of the imaging sequence. More recently, continuous recording of EEG and fMRI has become possible, following the introduction of methods to remove the artefact on the EEG trace caused by the fMRI acquisition, and this result in much a more detailed analysis of the time course of haemodynamic changes (Lemieux et al., 2001). Using either spike-triggered or continuous simultaneous EEG/fMRI recording, focal increases in cerebral blood delivery have been identified in patients with frequent inter-ictal spikes (Krakow et al., 1999; Salek-Haddadi et al., 2006; Al-Asmi et al., 2003). However, even in well-selected patients, approximately 50% do not exhibit interictal epileptiform discharges (IED) during the 40-60 minute EEG/fMRI study. Of the remaining patients, approximately 50%-70% IED are associated with significant BOLD signal changes which are concordant with electro-clinical data (Salek-Haddadi et al., 2006; Al-Asmi et al., 2003). The most recent and largest of these studies reported 76 patients with refractory focal epilepsy, 33 of whom had extratemporal lobe epilepsy. There were no discharges seen during the 35-60-minute acquisition in 64% of the patients. The mean number of discharges during the recording in the remaining patients was 89.3. Ten patients underwent surgical treatment, 7 of whom achieved a Class 1 ILAE outcome (Wieser et al., 2001) In six of these seven patients, the area of resection included the area of maximum BOLD signal increase. Interestingly, in the remaining three patients who continued to have seizures after surgery, the areas of maximal BOLD activation did not overlap with the resected area suggesting that EEG/fMRI may possess a negative predictive value for a good surgical outcome, that is, a lack of concordance with other localising investigations may predict a poor postoperative outcome (Thornton et al., 2010). In addition, the localisation accuracy of EEG/fMRI has been evaluated with other investigative modalities such as electrical source imaging. Distances between dipole localisation and fMRI activations were on average 58 mm apart in one study with 17 patients (Bagshaw et al., 2006) and 33 mm apart in simultaneously acquired EEG/fMRI and ESI datasets from 9 patients (Vulliemoz et al., 2009). The anatomical concordance between ESI and EEG/fMRI for localising the generators of interictal spikes is poorer than with the localisation of evoked potentials where correlations within 10-16 mm are frequently reported. It is possible that this is because of the presence of spatially extended epileptic networks and pathological blood flow changes or neurovascular coupling associated with epileptic activity. Recently, the locations of BOLD signal maxima have been compared to the results of intracranial EEG (iEEG) which is considered the "gold standard" investigation in confirming the location of the irritative and seizure-onset zones. There was judged to be good concordance with active EEG contacts frequently no more than 10-30 mm from an fMRI peak (Benar et al., 2006). The feasibility of combining fMRI with iEEG is being evaluated. The limited spatial sampling of iEEG is of concern in cases in whom the irritative and seizure onset zones are not being sampled directly and are detecting only the propagation of epileptic activity. Whole brain fMRI data can be examined for BOLD changes prior to the first detected EEG changes to ensure against this possibility. There are however a number of safety concerns, including the mechanical forces on electrodes from transient magnetic effects, tissue heating and tissue stimulation (Carmichael et al., 2010).

Malformations of cortical development are frequently the cause of refractory focal epilepsy and there is much debate about the mechanisms that underlie the generation of epileptic activity. EEG/fMRI studies of such patients provide a valuable insight. In nodular and band heterotopia, in addition to maxima within the heterotopia, BOLD changes were frequently observed in the overlying cortex consistent with iEEG findings and supporting theories suggesting that there are significant interconnections between normal and dysgenetic cortex and malformations (Kobayashi et al., 2006; Dubeau & Tyvaert, 2010). iEEG studies of focal cortical dysplasia show that rhythmic spiking activity is generated, and seizures commence, within the abnormality itself and lesional BOLD changes have been seen ictally and interictally (Tyvaert et al., 2008).

Typically, EEG/fMRI studies have focused on IED, but the irritative zone may be different from the ictal onset zone and there is merit therefore in evaluating ictal patterns. There are a number of practical limitations to overcome in studying ictal EEG/fMRI. These include the effects of head movement, the duration of each session due to unpredictable and often infrequent seizures and the complex evolution of clinical and EEG abnormalities during seizures which may be difficult to analyse. Only a relatively small proportion of patients are suitable therefore and ictal recordings are typically the result of serendipity or provocation in reflex epilepsies (Salek-Haddadi et al., 2009). Nevertheless, clinical utility has been demonstrated in a small series of 15 patients with focal epilepsy. Ictal EEG/fMRI findings were correlated with other localising data, including iEEG in four patients, and good agreement was demonstrated (Levan et al., 2010). A number of techniques have been employed to identify seizures during EEG/fMRI data acquisition, such as EEG markers, patient triggers such as button pressing, and synchronous video-recording (Chaudhary et al., 2010).

A number of these studies have reported more widespread BOLD changes, both activations and deactivations, distant to the proposed epileptogenic regions. It has been suggested that these may represent a distributed network of either spike generators or propagation pathways. There is much debate regarding the nature of BOLD deactivations and in particular their relationship to the epileptogenic zone. It has been suggested that these regions are functionally connected to the epileptogenic zone and may represent neuronal inhibition. In this respect, deactivations are predominantly seen in the "default mode network" which are areas of the brain active during rest and suspended during cerebral activity including epileptic events (Thornton *et al.*, 2010). However, in approximately 10% of adult patients, deactivations have been observed in the irritative zone (Rathakrishnan *et al.*, 2010) and approximately 25% of deactivations are preceded by earlier activations suggesting an "undershoot" phenomenon. Most deactivations occur in isolation however. Deactivations are more prevalent in children, occurring in up to 36% of patients (Jacobs *et al.*, 2007). The reason for this difference is not clear.

It is important to note that the spatial extent and number of BOLD maxima is, to some extent, a product of the statistical thresholds used to display the data. As a result, the utility of EEG/fMRI in accurately elucidating the epileptogenic region as a single isolated investigation is limited and suggests that a priori data on the possible location is important in interpreting the results. In reality, this has always been the case and individual investigations are not examined in isolation but integrated to formulate either an intracranial EEG implantation strategy or plan surgical resection. In this respect, EEG/fMRI has an important role, and in particular, in patients with unrewarding or discordant conventional investigations. For example, EEG/fMRI has been used to re-evaluate patients who have been previously rejected for epilepsy surgery due to other investigative modalities being non-localising. In a group of 29 such patients, meaningful and clinically useful EEG/fMRI results were obtained in eight patients, of which four were then considered for surgical treatment (Zijlmans *et al.*, 2007).

Further work in this area includes the careful and critical evaluation of the application, utility and limitations of EEG/fMRI at 3T in defining the irritative zone of the cortex (that generates inter-ictal spikes) and its relationship with the seizure-onset zone (that gives rise to seizures), and correlation with other localising techniques such as magnetoencephalography in patients in whom surgical treatment is being considered.

■ Mapping of eloquent cortex

Sensorimotor

An important application of fMRI in epilepsy is in the delineation of areas of the brain responsible for specific functions, such as the primary motor and sensory cortex. In particular, to identify their anatomical relation with respect to an area of planned neurosurgical resection, thereby allowing a more targeted resection while minimizing postoperative morbidity (Hammeke *et al.*, 1994; Holloway *et al.*, 1999).

Sensorimotor cortex can be reliably delineated with fMRI using relatively simple tasks, such as foot or finger tapping. This permits use in all but the most uncooperative patients. Typically, regions showing activation during such tasks are the contralateral primary motor cortex, ipsilateral cerebellar hemisphere, and in more complex motor tasks, motor association areas including the supplementary motor area, cingulate gyrus and dorsolateral prefrontal cortex (Solodkin *et al.*, 2001). Validation of the spatial accuracy of fMRI in delineating eloquent cortex has been undertaken by directly comparing fMRI results with electrocortical stimulation. For example, in a study of 28 patients undergoing craniotomy, all areas of fMRI activation were 20 mm or less from the intraoperative measurement and in 86% of the comparisons, it was within 10 mm. Word generation, finger, hand and tongue movement co-localised more accurately than lip movement or counting tasks (Yetkin *et al.*, 1997).

Although an estimate of the location of sensorimotor cortex can be made from pre-operative structural imaging, eloquent areas may become displaced by mass lesions or cortical dysgenesis leading to uncertainty about the exact location and increasing the risk of postoperative deficit or an unnecessarily limited resection. In one of the earlier reports of the utility of fMRI, Bookheimer and colleagues reported the postoperative outcomes of six patients with cortical lesions who had preoperative fMRI mapping of motor and visual areas. In three patients, the neurosurgical procedure was modified based on the fMRI results and, in each case, there was no postoperative deficit. In one patient, there was no overlap between the proposed resection and functional activation zone. In two patients, "functional" tissue was resected with the lesions and, as predicted, postoperative deficits were seen in both (Bookheimer et al., 1995). More recently, activations within regions of cerebral dysgenetic tissue have been observed during simple and complex fMRI paradigms. In particular, regions of abnormal cortical organisation, such as polymicrogyria and schizencephaly, showed greater activation during tasks than in MCDs caused by disturbances of early cortical development, such as heterotopia and Type IIB focal cortical dysplasia (FCD). This permits a greater understanding of the functional connectivity of malformations of cortical development and, in particular, their relationship to eloquent cortex (Janszky et al., 2003; Araujo et al., 2006; Barba et al., 2010). Interestingly, in some patients with band heterotopia, activation within the dysplastic band has been seen during motor tasks, consistent with both previous invasive electrophysiological and magnetoencephalographic recordings and the hypothesis that although the pyramidal cells are disorganized, connectivity with subcortical structures is maintained (Jirsch et al., 2006; Toulouse et al., 2003). It has been shown that the presence of a large cerebral lesion, particularly present from an early age, may be associated with abnormal lateralisation of motor cortex, and that fMRI can be useful in characterizing this shift, prior to resective surgery (Macdonell et al., 1999; Pinard et al., 2000). A number of mechanisms for this have been proposed, including the lack of regression of normally transient foetal connections, enhanced development of normally occurring ipsilateral projections, abnormal ipsilateral branching of undamaged corticospinal axons and aberrant ipsilateral projections. Mirror movements may be seen in such patients due to this collateral sprouting. This recruitment of distant cortical sites, demonstrated by motor fMRI can be transient, for example, following subpial transection or stroke, although it is clear that these alternative networks are less efficient than the native, primary pathways (Moo et al., 2002).

Motor fMRI has also demonstrated an atypical pattern of motor cortex activation in a left-handed patient with pharmacoresistant left hemisphere epilepsy without a neocortical lesion, in association with bilateral language dominance and involuntary mirror movements in the contralateral hand. As a child, the patient was considered right-handed, however over a period of time the left hand gradually became dominant. It was hypothesized that habitual left-sided epileptic activity may have disrupted the normal development of the ipsilateral motor cortex and resulted in a shift in handedness (Chlebus et al., 2004). Motor fMRI can be combined with tractography to provide both functional localisation and anatomical connectivity of the motor cortex. Guye and colleagues identified significant differences in connectivity between healthy subjects and a patient with a tumour in the precentral region using motor fMRI activations as "seed" points for the initiation of the tractographic algorithm. This information can be combined with other imaging modalities in order to inform the surgical planning process and avoid intraoperative injury to either the eloquent cortex or major white matter tracts (Guye et al., 2003).

Cognitive function

The intracarotid amytal examination, also known as the Wada test, has traditionally been used to determine lateralisation of speech and adequacy of contralateral memory functions in patients undergoing presurgical evaluation. However, the invasive nature of this examination carries a small risk of morbidity and, in addition, may be hampered by technical limitations, such as incomplete amytal perfusion of the posterior portion of the hippocampus resulting in an inadequate evaluation. Language fMRI is non-invasive and repeatable. Several studies have used fMRI in normal volunteers to demonstrate lateralised language activation with a variety of paradigms (Cuenod et al., 1995; Binder et al., 1995). In patients with epilepsy, a number of studies have compared fMRI with Wada testing and found it to be equally discriminating in determining hemispheric dominance (Hertz-Pannier et al., 1997; Woermann et al., 2003; Adcock et al., 2003). Moreover, preoperative fMRI was as effective as Wada testing in predicting significant language decline postoperatively (Sabsevitz et al., 2003). It is important to note when comparing fMRI to the Wada test that each test obtains information differently and fMRI results do not always accord with carotid amytal data (Worthington et al., 1997). A combination of language tasks may be more reliable than a single task (Rutten et al., 2002a). Artefacts and technical difficulties may adversely affect both methods and false lateralisations may occur (Jayakar et al., 2002). Further, identification of the areas of brain involved in language is not the same as determining if someone can speak when half of the brain is anaesthetised. The Wada test uses inactivation, and therefore provides information only on the functional reserve of the remaining cerebral tissue. Functional MRI identifies regions in a neural network involved in a successful task performance. There is a potential risk therefore, of attributing function to areas that are active in, but not necessarily critical to a particular task performance. Furthermore, there is no evidence that areas that are not activated in fMRI studies are not involved in the performance of the task. Nevertheless, fMRI is safe and repeatable, and simple cognitive and motor paradigms can be used reliably and successfully in children as young as 3 to 4 years of developmental age (Shurtleff et al., 2010).

As well as predicting the lateralisation of language function, fMRI may localise cerebral areas involved in language (Gaillard et al., 2001; Rutten et al., 2002b). For example, in a recent fMRI study of healthy right-handed subjects, tasks of reading comprehension activated the superior temporal gyri, and verbal fluency and verb generation tasks activated the left inferior and middle frontal gyri and left insula (Powell et al., 2006). Verbal fluency typically yields a wider and more intense activation of the left Broca's area than verb generation and may reveal other areas involved in the language network such as the dorsolateral prefrontal cortex and the striatum (Sanjuan et al., 2010). Receptive language paradigms involving the posterior temporal and parietal cortex commonly show bilateral, but asymmetrical, activation. In patients with left hemisphere epilepsy, these functions may become even more widely distributed, recruiting, for example, additional right hemisphere language processing networks, particularly if the functional areas are close to pathology. More distant functions may remain in the ipsilateral hemisphere (Berl et al., 2005). Results of fMRI studies examining anterior language function have been more variable, with no evidence of reorganization in some patients with lesions near Broca's area (Rosenberger et al., 2009) and other patients showing activation within perilesional cortex (Liegeois et al., 2004). It is clear that there is considerable heterogeneity in this regard between individuals. This is most likely dependent on the nature and age of the lesion, and reinforces the importance of interpreting fMRI results with caution when planning surgical treatment. Furthermore, there are concerns over the reliability of language lateralisation in patients with cerebral lesions and the local effect of lesions on neurovascular coupling, which is critical to the analysis of fMRI data. In summary, therefore, although language fMRI has supplanted Wada testing for language lateralisation (Baxendale *et al.*, 2008), currently, fMRI is unable to define language regions accurately enough to obviate the requirement for electrocortical stimulation and/or awake craniotomy.

A more difficult challenge for fMRI is to replace the Wada test in determining memory lateralisation and the prediction of the effects of temporal lobe resection on memory (Cheung *et al.*, 2009). Complex neuroanatomical circuits involving a specific system of related neocortical (frontal and temporal) and medial temporal brain regions mediate memory function and hence the development of a paradigm to specifically activate these regions is complicated. Following anterior temporal lobe resection for temporal lobe epilepsy, patients may experience deterioration in either verbal or visual memory and fMRI paradigms can provide prognostic information in this regard (Bonelli *et al.*, 2010). Memory function in patients with extratemporal lobe epilepsy, has received less attention although there are clearly deficits in a number of memory functions, including, for example, working memory in frontal lobe epilepsy. Nevertheless, despite the suggestion that different subregions serve specific memory functions (Fletcher and Henson 2001), there is much variability and it is unclear whether these will be able to be differentiated using fMRI and importantly whether this will have clinical utility in individual patients with extratemporal lobe epilepsy (Centeno *et al.*, 2010).

References

- Adcock JE, Wise RG, Oxbury JM, Oxbury SM, Matthews PM. Quantitative fMRI assessment of the differences in lateralisation of language-related brain activation in patients with temporal lobe epilepsy. *Neuroimage* 2003; 18: 423-38.

- Al-Asmi A, Benar CG, Gross DW, *et al.* fMRI activation in continuous and spike-triggered EEG-fMRI studies of epileptic spikes. *Epilepsia* 2003; 44: 1328-39.

- Allen PJ, Josephs O, Turner R. A method for removing imaging artifact from continuous EEG recorded during functional MRI. *Neuroimage* 2000; 12: 230-9.

- Allen PJ, Polizzi G, Krakow K, Fish DR, Lemieux L. Identification of EEG events in the MR scanner: the problem of pulse artifact and a method for its subtraction. *Neuroimage* 1998; 8: 229-39.

- Araujo D, de Araujo DB, Pontes-Neto OM, *et al.* Language and motor FMRI activation in polymicrogyric cortex. *Epilepsia* 2006; 47: 589-92.

- Bagshaw AP, Kobayashi E, Dubeau F, Pike GB, Gotman J. Correspondence between EEG-fMRI and EEG dipole localisation of interictal discharges in focal epilepsy. *Neuroimage* 2006; 30: 417-25.

- Barba C, Montanaro D, Cincotta M, Giovannelli F, Guerrini R. An integrated fMRI, SEPs and MEPs approach for assessing functional organization in the malformed sensorimotor cortex. *Epilepsy Res* 2010; 89: 66-71.

- Baxendale SA, Thompson PJ, Duncan JS. Evidence-based practice: a reevaluation of the intracarotid amobarbital procedure (Wada test). *Arch Neurol* 2008; 65: 841-5.

- Benar CG, Grova C, Kobayashi E, *et al.* EEG-fMRI of epileptic spikes: concordance with EEG source localization and intracranial EEG 3. *Neuroimage* 2006; 30: 1161-70.

- Berl MM, Balsamo LM, Xu B, et al. Seizure focus affects regional language networks assessed by fMRI. *Neurology* 2005; 65: 1604-11.

- Binder JR, Rao SM, Hammeke TA, et al. Lateralized human brain language systems demonstrated by task subtraction functional magnetic resonance imaging. *Arch Neurol* 1995; 52: 593-601.

- Bonelli SB, Powell RH, Yogarajah M, et al. Imaging memory in temporal lobe epilepsy: predicting the effects of temporal lobe resection. *Brain* 2010; 133: 1186-99.

- Bookheimer SY, Cohen M, Dapretto M, et al. Functional MRI in surgical planning. *Soc Neurosci Abstr* 1995; 273.

- Carmichael DW, Thornton JS, Rodionov R, et al. Feasibility of simultaneous intracranial EEG-fMRI in humans: a safety study. *Neuroimage* 2010; 49: 379-90.

- Centeno M, Thompson PJ, Koepp MJ, Helmstaedter C, Duncan JS. Memory in frontal lobe epilepsy. *Epilepsy Res* 2010; 91: 123-32.

- Chaudhary UJ, Kokkinos V, Carmichael DW, et al. Implementation and evaluation of simultaneous video-electroencephalography and functional magnetic resonance imaging. *Magn Reson Imaging* 2010; 28: 1192-9.

- Cheung MC, Chan AS, Lam JM, Chan YL. Pre- and postoperative fMRI and clinical memory performance in temporal lobe epilepsy. *J Neurol Neurosurg Psychiatry* 2009; 80: 1099-106.

- Chlebus P, Brazdil M, Hlustik P, Mikl M, Pazourkova M, Krupa P. Handedness shift as a consequence of motor cortex reorganization after early functional impairment in left temporal lobe epilepsy--an fMRI case report. *Neurocase* 2004; 10: 326-9.

- Cuenod CA, Bookheimer SY, Hertz-Pannier L, Zeffiro TA, Theodore WH, Le Bihan D. Functional MRI during word generation, using conventional equipment: a potential tool for language localization in the clinical environment. *Neurology* 1995; 45: 1821-7.

- Detre JA, Sirven JI, Alsop DC, O'Connor MJ, French JA. Localization of subclinical ictal activity by functional magnetic resonance imaging: correlation with invasive monitoring. *Ann Neurol* 1995; 38: 618-24.

- Dubeau F, Tyvaert L. Understanding the epileptogenicity of lesions: a correlation between intracranial EEG and EEG/fMRI. *Epilepsia* 2010; 51 (Suppl 1): 54-8.

- Fish DR, Brooks DJ, Young IR, Bydder GM. Use of magnetic resonance imaging to identify changes in cerebral blood flow in epilepsia partialis continua. *Magn Reson Med* 1988; 8: 238-40.

- Fletcher PC, Henson RN. Frontal lobes and human memory: insights from functional neuroimaging. *Brain* 2001; 124: 849-81.

- Gaillard WD, Pugliese M, Grandin CB, et al. Cortical localization of reading in normal children: an fMRI language study. *Neurology* 2001; 57: 47-54.

- Guye M, Parker GJ, Symms M, et al. Combined functional MRI and tractography to demonstrate the connectivity of the human primary motor cortex in vivo. *Neuroimage* 2003; 19: 1349-60.

- Hammeke TA, Yetkin FZ, Mueller WM, et al. Functional magnetic resonance imaging of somatosensory stimulation. *Neurosurgery* 1994; 35: 677-81.

- Hertz-Pannier L, Gaillard WD, Mott SH, et al. Noninvasive assessment of language dominance in children and adolescents with functional MRI: a preliminary study (see comments). *Neurology* 1997; 48: 1003-12.

- Holloway V, Chong WK, Connelly A, Harkness WH, Gadian DG. Somatomotor fMRI in the pre-surgical evaluation of a case of focal epilepsy. *Clin Radiol* 1999; 54: 301-3.

- Huang-Hellinger F, Breiter HC, McCormack G, Cohen MS, Kwong KK, Sutton JP. Simultaneous functional magnetic resonance imaging and electrophysiological recording. *Human Brain Mapping* 1995; 3: 13-23.

- Ives JR, Warach S, Schmitt F, Edelman RR, Schomer DL. Monitoring the patient's EEG during echo planar MRI. *Electroencephalogr Clin Neurophysiol* 1993; 87: 417-20.

- Jackson GD, Connelly A, Cross JH, Gordon I, Gadian DG. Functional magnetic resonance imaging of focal seizures. *Neurology* 1994; 44: 850-6.
- Jacobs J, Kobayashi E, Boor R, *et al*. Hemodynamic responses to interictal epileptiform discharges in children with symptomatic epilepsy. *Epilepsia* 2007; 48: 2068-78.
- Janszky J, Ebner A, Kruse B, *et al*. Functional organization of the brain with malformations of cortical development. *Ann Neurol* 2003; 53: 759-67.
- Jayakar P, Bernal B, Santiago ML, Altman N. False lateralisation of language cortex on functional MRI after a cluster of focal seizures. *Neurology* 2002; 58: 490-2.
- Jirsch JD, Bernasconi N, Villani F, Vitali P, Avanzini G, Bernasconi A. Sensorimotor organization in double cortex syndrome. *Hum Brain Mapp* 2006; 27: 535-43.
- Kobayashi E, Bagshaw AP, Grova C, Gotman J, Dubeau F. Grey matter heterotopia: what EEG-fMRI can tell us about epileptogenicity of neuronal migration disorders. *Brain* 2006; 129: 366-74.
- Krakow K, Woermann FG, Symms MR, *et al*. EEG-triggered functional MRI of interictal epileptiform activity in patients with partial seizures. *Brain* 1999; 122: 1679-88.
- Lemieux L, Allen PJ, Franconi F, Symms MR, Fish DR. Recording of EEG during fMRI experiments: patient safety. *Magn Reson Med* 1997; 38: 943-52.
- Lemieux L, Salek-Haddadi A, Josephs O, *et al*. Event-related fMRI with simultaneous and continuous EEG: description of the method and initial case report. *Neuroimage* 2001; 14: 780-7.
- Levan P, Tyvaert L, Moeller F, Gotman J. Independent component analysis reveals dynamic ictal BOLD responses in EEG-fMRI data from focal epilepsy patients. *Neuroimage* 2010; 49: 366-78.
- Liegeois F, Connelly A, Cross JH, *et al*. Language reorganization in children with early-onset lesions of the left hemisphere: an fMRI study. *Brain* 2004; 127: 1229-36.
- Macdonell RA, Jackson GD, Curatolo JM, *et al*. Motor cortex localization using functional MRI and transcranial magnetic stimulation. *Neurology* 1999; 53: 1462-7.
- Moo LR, Slotnick SD, Krauss G, Hart J. A prospective study of motor recovery following multiple subpial transections. *Neuroreport* 2002; 13: 665-9.
- Ogawa S, Menon RS, Tank DW, *et al*. Functional brain mapping by blood oxygenation level-dependent contrast magnetic resonance imaging. A comparison of signal characteristics with a biophysical model. *Biophys J* 1993; 64: 803-12.
- Pinard J, Feydy A, Carlier R, Perez N, Pierot L, Burnod Y. Functional MRI in double cortex: functionality of heterotopia. *Neurology* 2000; 54: 1531-3.
- Powell HW, Parker GJ, Alexander DC *et al*. Hemispheric asymmetries in language-related pathways: a combined functional MRI and tractography study. *Neuroimage* 2006; 32: 388-99.
- Rathakrishnan R, Moeller F, Levan P, Dubeau F, Gotman J. BOLD signal changes preceding negative responses in EEG-fMRI in patients with focal epilepsy. *Epilepsia* 2010; 51: 1837-45.
- Rosenberger LR, Zeck J, Berl MM *et al*. Interhemispheric and intrahemispheric language reorganization in complex partial epilepsy. *Neurology* 2009; 72: 1830-6.
- Rutten GJ, Ramsey NF, van Rijen PC, Alpherts WC, Van Veelen CW. FMRI-determined language lateralisation in patients with unilateral or mixed language dominance according to the Wada test. *Neuroimage* 2002a; 17: 447-60.
- Rutten GJ, Ramsey NF, van Rijen PC, Noordmans HJ, Van Veelen CW. Development of a functional magnetic resonance imaging protocol for intraoperative localization of critical temporoparietal language areas. *Ann Neurol* 2002b; 51: 350-60.
- Sabsevitz DS, Swanson SJ, Hammeke TA, *et al*. Use of preoperative functional neuroimaging to predict language deficits from epilepsy surgery. *Neurology* 2003; 60: 1788-92.
- Salek-Haddadi A, Diehl B, Hamandi K, *et al*. Hemodynamic correlates of epileptiform discharges: an EEG-fMRI study of 63 patients with focal epilepsy. *Brain Res* 2006; 1088: 148-66.

- Salek-Haddadi A, Mayer T, Hamandi K, et al. Imaging seizure activity: a combined EEG/EMG-fMRI study in reading epilepsy. *Epilepsia* 2009; 50: 256-64.
- Sanjuan A, Bustamante JC, Forn C, et al. Comparison of two fMRI tasks for the evaluation of the expressive language function. *Neuroradiology* 2010; 52: 407-15.
- Seghier ML. Laterality index in functional MRI: methodological issues. *Magn Reson Imaging* 2008; 26: 594-601.
- Shurtleff H, Warner M, Poliakov A, et al. Functional magnetic resonance imaging for presurgical evaluation of very young pediatric patients with epilepsy. *J Neurosurg Pediatr* 2010; 5: 500-6.
- Solodkin A, Hlustik P, Noll DC, Small SL. Lateralization of motor circuits and handedness during finger movements. *Eur J Neurol* 2001; 8: 425-34.
- Thornton R, Laufs H, Rodionov R, et al. EEG correlated functional MRI and postoperative outcome in focal epilepsy. *J Neurol Neurosurg Psychiatry* 2010; 81: 922-7.
- Toulouse P, Agulhon C, Taussig D, et al. Magnetoencephalographic studies of two cases of diffuse subcortical laminar heterotopia or so-called double cortex. *Neuroimage* 2003; 19: 1251-9.
- Tyvaert L, Hawco C, Kobayashi E, Levan P, Dubeau F, Gotman J. Different structures involved during ictal and interictal epileptic activity in malformations of cortical development: an EEG-fMRI study 3. *Brain* 2008; 131: 2042-60.
- Vulliemoz S, Thornton R, Rodionov R, et al. The spatio-temporal mapping of epileptic networks: combination of EEG-fMRI and EEG source imaging 10. *Neuroimage* 2009; 46: 834-43.
- Wang Z, Mechanic-Hamilton D, Pluta J, Glynn S, Detre JA. Function lateralisation via measuring coherence laterality. *Neuroimage* 2009; 47: 281-8.
- Warach S, Ives JR, Schlaug G, et al. EEG-triggered echo-planar functional MRI in epilepsy. *Neurology* 1996; 47: 89-93.
- Warach S, Levin JM, Schomer DL, Holman BL, Edelman RR. Hyperperfusion of ictal seizure focus demonstrated by MR perfusion imaging. *AJNR Am J Neuroradiol* 1994; 15: 965-8.
- Wieser HG, Blume WT, Fish D, et al. ILAE Commission Report. Proposal for a new classification of outcome with respect to epileptic seizures following epilepsy surgery. *Epilepsia* 2001; 42: 282-6.
- Woermann FG, Jokeit H, Luerding R, et al. Language lateralisation by Wada test and fMRI in 100 patients with epilepsy. *Neurology* 2003; 61: 699-701.
- Worthington C, Vincent DJ, Bryant AE, et al. Comparison of functional magnetic resonance imaging for language localization and intracarotid speech amytal testing in presurgical evaluation for intractable epilepsy. Preliminary results. *Stereotact Funct Neurosurg* 1997; 69: 197-201.
- Yetkin FZ, Mueller WM, Morris GL, et al. Functional MR activation correlated with intraoperative cortical mapping. *AJNR Am J Neuroradiol* 1997; 18: 1311-5.
- Zijlmans M, Huiskamp G, Hersevoort M, Seppenwoolde JH, van Huffelen AC, Leijten FS. EEG-fMRI in the preoperative work-up for epilepsy surgery. *Brain* 2007; 130: 2343-53.

PET in extratemporal epilepsy

Mar Carreño

Epilepsy Unit, Hospital Clínic, Barcelona, Spain

▪ Introduction

Positron emission tomography (PET) is a noninvasive functional neuroimaging technique which can be used to measure regional uptakes and affinity of ligands or metabolic substrates in brain and other organs. In patients with epilepsy, PET has been used in clinical grounds to establish the functional deficit zone in the context of presurgical evaluation of patients with drug-resistant epilepsy. It is also a valuable method to investigate basic mechanisms associated with the process of epileptogenesis, seizure propagation and progression of functional deficits associated to drug-resistant epilepsy.

The most widely available and used PET tracer for presurgical evaluation in children and adults with intractable focal epilepsy is 2-deoxy-18F fluoro-D-glucose (FDG), which is used to measure glucose utilization by the different brain regions. [18F]FDG crosses the blood-brain barrier before phosphorylation in the cell compartment and, unlike glucose-6-phospate, it does not enter into further steps of the Krebs glycolysis cycle, but accumulates in the intracellular compartment and thus directly reflects the energy demand of the brain cells (Mauguiere & Ryvlin, 2004). The mechanisms underlying interictal glucose hypometabolism are not fully understood. Possible mechanisms include: neuronal loss, atrophy, hypometabolic macro or microscopic lesions, decreased synaptic activity, deafferentiation due to reduced number of synapses, postictal metabolic depression, and inhibitory mechanisms of seizures (Mauguiere & Ryvlin, 2004).

Interictal hypometabolism may represent a reversible functional state for several reasons. First, an increase of glucose metabolism can be observed during ictal PET scans in the interictal hypometabolic zone. Second, interictal hypometabolism can be reverted by the application of a specific $GABA_A$ receptor agonist THIP. After THIP injection, the increase of glucose metabolism in the hypometabolic focus was larger than the mean increase in the whole brain. Within the hypometabolic focus, this increase was significantly higher in the regions with the lowest basal metabolic levels. This metabolic response in the hypometabolic focus suggests that $GABA_A$ receptors are upregulated or at least preserved in temporal lobe epilepsy (Baumgartner & Lehner-Baumgartner, 2008). Furthermore, $GABA_A$ receptor mediated inhibition becomes questionable (Hong et al., 2002). In addition, hypometabolic zones surrounding the epileptogenic zone pre-operatively showed a normalization of glucose metabolism after successful surgery. This is usually paralleled by an improvement in neuropsychological functioning (Spanaki et al., 2000; Hajek et al., 1994; Regis et al., 1999).

Although ictal scans may be useful, the long duration for steady-state uptake of glucose (in the order of many minutes compared with partial seizures, which are typically less than 2-3 minutes) often leads to scans that contain a difficult to interpret mixture of interictal, ictal and postictal states. For this reason, it is important to monitor EEG during the PET tracer uptake period, to make sure the state is truly interictal and the patient is not having an active and repetitive discharge which may be associated with a local hyper-metabolism. In this case, it is the opposite side which may look hypometabolic, leading to a false lateralization of the functional deficit zone (Chugani et al., 1993a).

Even in patients with lesions, in whom focal areas of hypometabolism are seen in almost 100% of the cases, this often extends well beyond the lesions. In patients with mesial temporal lobe epilepsy secondary to mesial temporal sclerosis, it is frequent to observe relative hypometabolism extending over the lateral neocortex, temporal pole and even extratemporal, basal ganglia and thalamic regions (Henry et al., 1993).

It is unclear what this more extensive hypometabolism truly represents in relation to the extension of the epileptogenic zone. As explained above, some authors believe it reflects a functional disturbance secondary to the epileptogenic zone. However, how much it should be taken into account when planning the resection remains unclear. And this is especially relevant in extratemporal epilepsies. Unlike temporal lobe epilepsy (in which there is a standard lobectomy procedure), extratemporal resections are quite variable and range from small topectomies to multilobar resections. In most centers, information provided by PET in extratemporal epilepsies (especially when the patient has a "normal" MRI or this shows an ill-defined lesion) is used to plan placement of intracranial electrodes. Resection is finally dependent on the findings in intracranial EEG.

Other receptor ligand PET tracers used in epilepsy are [^{11}C] flumazenil (FMZ) which binds to GABA$_A$ receptors. In clinical studies using FMZ-PET, patients taking benzodiazepines should generally be excluded (Chugani et al., 2008).

Another tracer that has been used is alpha-[^{11}C]methyl-L-tryptophan (AMT), which measures tryptophan metabolism. AMT is an analog of tryptophan (precursor of serotonin) and is converted in the brain to alpha [^{11}C] methyl-serotonin, which is not a substrate for the degradative enzyme monoamine oxidase, and therefore accumulates in serotoninergic terminals. Patients taking medications that affect trypthophan or serotonin metabolism should not undergo AMT-PET scan (Chugani et al., 2008).

■ FDG PET in extratemporal epilepsies

Presurgical evaluation in patients with drug-resistant extratemporal epilepsy is aimed to delineate the location and extent of the epileptogenic region. This may be quite challenging, especially in patients without an apparent lesion on the MRI (non lesional cases). In spite of the advances in structural and fuctional neuroimaging, long term seizure freedom rates after surgery remain modest mainly in frontal lobe epilepsy (around 30% at 5 years), but also in posterior cortex epilepsy (55% at 6 years or more). The outcome seems to be especially poor in patients with normal MRI, with around 50-80% of patients having seizure recurrence (Jehi et al., 2007; Jehi et al., 2009).

FDG-PET results are especially useful in patients with poorly defined or subtle lesions, such as malformations of cortical development (MCD), and also in patients with normal MRI. In patients with MCD, hypometabolic areas may reveal underlying dysplasia that extends beyond the visible lesion on the MRI, or confirm unclear or subtle MRI lesions. In patients with normal MRI, especially if interictal epileptiform abnormalities are diffuse (which is often the case in patiens with frontal or parietal epilepsy) or absent (for example in patients with mesial frontal, mesial parietal or mesial occipital epilepsy), identifying an area with a relative hypometabolism in FDG-PET may be the only way to formulate a reasonable hypothesis about the possible location of the epileptogenic zone, which then will need further confirmation with intracranial monitoring.

However, the clinical value of FDG-PET in extratemporal epilepsy is not completely clear, and this is due in part to the difficulties to interpret small or subtle abnormalities and also to the heterogeneous series of patients that have been published.

Cryptogenic extratemporal epilepsy

When MRI fails to show a focal structural abnormality in extratemporal lobe epilepsy, seizure semiology and scalp EEG findings have to be used by the epileptologist to guide placement of intracranial electrodes. PET often provides important localizing data that, if concordant with EEG, may increase the confidence of the epilepsy surgery team. Frontal lobe "epileptic foci" may be detected by high resolution PET with a sensitivity of 92% and a specificity of 62.5% in pediatric patients (da Silva et al., 1997). In a recent series of children with non lesional epilepsy, hypometabolism was demonstrated in 21 children (78%) in the one region or lobe corresponding to the region considered responsible for seizure origin on subdural EEG (Seo et al., 2009). However, the sensitivity of PET to detect hypometabolic areas related to the epileptogenic zone may be lower in adults with nonlesional neocortical epilepsy, around 43% (Hong et al., 2002).

The sensitivity of the test may also vary depending on the lobe, being highest in temporal lobe epilepsy. In a series of patients with cryptogenic neocortical epilepsy, PET had localizing value in 4/14 patients with frontal lobe epilepsy, 1/3 patients with parietal lobe epilepsy, and 4/7 patients with occipital lobe epilepsy, compared to 14/17 patients with temporal lobe epilepsy (Lee et al., 2005).

Cortical dysplasias

In focal cortical dysplasias (FCD), which are often poorly defined or subtle lesions on the sensitivity of FDG PET to localize these lesions, has been reported to be around 70%, ranging from 60 to 92% (Lerner et al., 2009). Many patients with FCD and normal MRI may have hypometabolic areas on FDG-PET (Kim et al., 2000). In a recent series coming from UCLA, of 22 patients with normal or subtle MRI findings, 14 (64%) showed areas of hypometabolism on FDG-PET scans (Salamon et al., 2008).

Although in most cases the CD visualized by MRI lies within the region of brain responsible for seizure generation (the epileptogenic zone), it may not constitute the entire epileptogenic zone in all cases. This can explain the poor surgical outcome in some cases in which the surgical intervention has been based on MRI alone (Sisodiya, 2000). FDG-PET may help to discover subtle cortical dysplasias and delineate better the peripheral portion of dysplastic lesions that may be unclear on MRI. In FCD, the boundaries of the cortical hypometabolic areas are usually larger on FDG-PET than on MRI (Kim et al., 2000).

Some studies have attempted to correlate the severity of neocortical focal hypometabolism with results of intracranial subdural grid recording. In those studies, the distribution of hypometabolism was often greater in extent, and was more likely to be greatest on the margin of the region of seizure onset (Juhasz et al., 2000a).

■ Correlation with surgical outcome

In several studies, PET localization seems to be related to surgical outcome. Concordance of localization by PET and interictal EEG was associated to a good surgical outcome in a series of patients with cryptogenic neocortical epilepsies including patients with temporal lobe epilepsy (Lee et al., 2005). Similar findings were reported recently in a series of pediatric patients with non lesional epilepsy; 19/21 patients (90%) who had focal hypo-metabolism in the areas considered to be responsible for seizure generation on subdural recordings became seizure free [13]. In a recent series comparing various imaging modalities in the localization of the epileptogenic lesion using surgical outcome in pediatric patients, FDG-PET showed concordance with the epileptic foci in 13/19 patients with extratem-poral epilepsy (concordance rate 68.4%), with precise localization of lesions in 12 cases (12/19 patients, localization rate 63.2%) and discordance in 6/19 cases (31.6%) (Kim et al., 2009).

In addition, a decision tree analysis has concluded that FDG-PET provides useful infor-mation that is cost-effective, particularly if its use is restricted to the evaluation of patients in whom MRI and scalp-video EEG telemetry do not provide a definitive answer (O'Brien et al., 2008).

■ Corregistration with MRI and statistical parametric mapping

PET scan interpretation by visual analysis only carries some inherent difficulties. To address some of these, statistical parametric mapping (SPM) analysis has been used to improve the accuracy of diagnostic imaging, eliminating some of the subjectivity and expertise required with visual analysis (Knowlton, 2006). In one report on 29 frontal lobe epilepsy patients (normal MRI in 15 patients), SPM analysis was compared with visual interpretation (Kim et al., 2002). SPM analysis resulted in a sensitivity of 66% for detec-ting a localized FDG uptake deficit (36% sensitivity in patients without a structural lesion). This result was not statistically different from the sensitivity of visual analysis, but the authors concluded that the possibility of obtaining a precise result comparable to the reading by an expert in epilepsy is encouraging. Another study performed in patients with presumed frontal lobe epilepsy showed that SPM analysis has a better concordance to surface EEG monitoring compared to visual scan analysis and ROI quantification. In comparison with intracranial EEG recordings, the best performance was achieved by combining the ROI based quantification with SPM analysis (Plotkin et al., 2003). For this reason, some centers use this technique when analyzing their results. For example, Lee et al. suggest that the high sensitivity of FDG-PET in their series may be due to the fact of using both statistical parametric and visual analysis (Lee et al., 2005).

■ Corregistration with MRI

The FDG-PET images are fused onto the structural MRI and the degree of hypometabolism is color coded. This technique seems to distinguish subtle lesions not appreciated by MRI or PET alone that often turn out to be CD at histopathology. In a recent study, routine incorporation of this technique into the multimodal presurgical evaluation enhanced the non-invasive identification and successful surgical treatment of patients with CD. In fact, 98% of the patients in their cohort showed true positive FDG-PET/MRI coregistration. The technique was especially useful for the 33% of patients with nonconcordant findings and those with normal MRI scans from mild type I CD [18].

■ FDG-PET and infantile spasms and other epilepsy syndromes

FDG-PET studies in children with drug-resistant cryptogenic infantile spasms have shown unifocal or, more commonly (around 65% of infants) multifocal areas of hypometabolism interictally. The PET hypometabolic areas usually correspond to the EEG localization of focal interictal or ictal abnormalities, or to the focal EEG abnormalities that precede or follow the presence of hypsarrythmia [9]. The discovery of focal cortical metabolic abnormalities on FDG-PET, if concordant with the EEG, has allowed surgical treatment in some patients with subsequent seizure control and at least partial reversal of the associated developmental delay. The most frequent histopathological finding in these patients is cortical dysplasia (Lee et al., 2005; Chugani et al., 1990; Chugani et al., 1993b; Chugani et al., 1996a).

Children with more than one area of cortical hypometabolism on FDG-PET scan are not ideal candidates for cortical resection. Some of these children, usually with bilateral temporal hypometabolism, have a characteristic phenotype with severe developmental delay and autism (Chugani et al., 1996b). Bilateral symmetric or generalized cortical hypometabolism, with or without cerebellar involvement suggests an underlying genetic or metabolic condition (Chugani et al., 2008).

FDG-PET has been used in patients with Sturge Weber syndrome to assess the degree and extent of hemispheric involvement, guide the extent of cortical resection and assess the convenience of early hemispherectomy (Chugani et al., 2008).

In patients with hemimegalencephaly who are potential candidates to hemispherectomy, FDG-PET is useful to assess the functional integrity of the "better hemisphere", which may have prognostic implications (Rintahaka et al., 1993).

FDG-PET has also been used in patients with children with intractable epilepsy and continuous spike and wave during sleep. In some of these patients it shows unilateral metabolic changes, suggesting that the generalized EEG activiy during sleep is a form of secondary bilateral synchrony. If there is concordance with the presumed EEG onset of the EEG discharges, some of these patients may turn out to be surgical candidates (Luat et al., 2005).

■ Progressive changes in FDG-PET during the course of drug-resistant epilepsy

FDG-PET may be used to study the progression of functional deficits associated to chronic epilepsy. Some studies have shown that in patients with an epileptogenic lesion, the extent of perilesional glucose metabolism increases with the number of seizures (Juhasz et al., 2000b). Children with persistent or increasing number of seizures (more than one per day) show extension of the hypometabolic cortex over time, compared to the patients with less than one seizure per day, who show a decrease in the size of the hypometabolic cortex (Benedek et al., 2006). The authors suggest that intractable epilepsy in children is a progressive disorder and that expansion of the cortical hypometabolism may reflect a growing seizure network involving cortical and subcortical areas (Chugani et al., 2008).

In patients with non refractory partial epilepsy and normal MRI, however, the finding of hypometabolic areas does not have predictive value of the future response to antiepileptic drugs. Patients with hypometabolism do not necessarily have a lower likelihood of successful AED treatment (Weitemeyer et al., 2005).

■ Flumazenil PET

Flumazenil binds to $GABA_A$ receptors and is usually labelled with the positron emitting isotope ^{11}C. FMZ PET in neocortical epilepsy has been reported to provide a better indication of the seizure onset zone when compared to FDG-PET, and a better estimation of the perilesional epileptogenic zones (Szelies et al., 2002); it may also detect secondary epileptic foci in patients with chronic drug-resistant epilepsy (Chugani et al., 2008).

In patients with frontal lobe epilepsy, cortical areas of decreased FMZ binding show good correspondence with the locations of seizure onset as determined with subdural electrodes (Savic et al., 1995). When compared to intracranial EEG data, FMZ PET detects at least part of the seizure onset in all patients, whereas FDG PET fails to detect cortex showing seizure onset in 20% of subjects (Muzik et al., 2000). FMZ PET has been shown in some studies to be also more sensitive than FDG-PET in identifying cortical regions showing frequent independent spiking. Neither FDG nor FMZ PET were sensitive to identify cortical areas of rapid seizure spread.

In adult patients with refractory neocortical epilepsy, both increases and decreases in FMZ binding, in gray and white matter, have been described. Some patients showed periventricular increases which the authors believed could represent neuronal migration disorders (Hammers et al., 2003).

As shown in a recent study, almost 50% of patients with refractory neocortical epilepsy and "normal" MRI may show remote cortical areas with decreased FMZ binding outside the lobe of seizure onset. These regions, when covered by subdural electrodes, are often involved in rapid seizure spread on intracranial EEG and are usually associated with high seizure frequency; when they are resected, pathology usually shows gliosis. Higher number of unresected areas with decreased FMZ binding is associated with worse surgical outcome. The authors recommend to evaluate this areas with intracranial EEG prior to resection to improve outcome (Juhasz et al., 2009).

■ Alpha methyl tryptophan PET

PET scanning with alpha-11C-methyl-L-tryptophan (AMT) is used to measure trypophan metabolism and has been used during presurgical evaluation of patients with drug-resistant epilepsy. AMT accumulates in the vicinity of the seizure focus and PET scanning of this radiotracer reveals an increased uptake in the interictal state; FDG and FMZ show, however, decreased uptake in this area. For this reason it has been used in patients with multiple lesions (for example patients with tuberous sclerosis or multifocal cortical dysplasia), to detect those which are epileptogenic (Sood & Chugani, 2006). Several studies have shown that AMT PET may differentiate between epileptogenic and non-epileptogenic tubers in patients with TS, with epileptogenic tubers showing increased AMT uptake interictally, and non-epileptogenic tubers showing decreased uptake, as demonstrated by intracranial EEG. The authors found that there was an excellent correlation between resection of tubers showing increased AMT uptake and good outcome (Kagawa et al., 2005).

AMT PET may be particularly useful to localize epileptogenic tubers that are close to midline and EEG lateralization is difficult (Sood & Chugani, 2006). However, AMT PET fails to show areas of increased uptake in 1/3 of patients with TSC. The reason for this is not clear (Sood & Chugani, 2006).

Increased AMT uptake in epileptic tissue may be seen also in other patients with epilepsy. These uptakes may be seen near the epileptic focus in approximately 50% of the patients with neocortical epilepsy, are less sensitive but more specific than hypometabolism in FDG-PET and frequently correlate with epileptogenic malformations of cortical development (Juhasz et al., 2003). Similar results (focal increases in AMT uptake) have been reported in 57% of patients with cortical dysplasia and 27% of patients with normal MRI (Fedi et al., 2001). Although sensitivity of AMT PET is modest in patients with normal MRI, specificity is very high (100% in some studies) (Wakamoto et al., 2008), suggesting this may be an interesting technique to study patients with occult malformations of cortical development.

■ Other ligands

Other PET tracers with the potential for detecting epileptic brain regions include radio-labeled ligands which bind to opiod recetors, histamine H_1 receptors, monoamine oxidase type B enzyme, N-methyl-D-aspartate receptors and serotonin 1_A receptors. However they have not been used clinically to study drug-resistant neocortical epilepsy.

18F-MPPF (5HT-1A receptor antagonist) PET has been used to study the serotoninergic pathway in patients with epilepsy and depression. Increased binding was found at the raphe nucleus and contralateral insula, ipsilateral hippocampus and bilateral frontal cortex in patients with temporal lobe epilepsy, and there was a correlation with symptoms of depression (Didelot et al., 2008; Lothe et al., 2008).

Alterations in dopamine D2/D3 receptor binding in bilateral posterior putamen studied with 18 F-Fallypride [(18)F]FP have been described in patients with juvenile myoclonic epilepsy, suggesting a specific alteration in the dopaminergic system (Landvogt et al., 2010). Decreased D1 receptor binding has also been described in the striatum in a group of homogeneous patients with autosomal dominant frontal lobe epilepsy and mutations of the acetylcholine receptor.

■ Conclusion

FDG PET has proved to be a valuable tool to evaluate the location and extent of the functional deficit zone in patients with drug-resistant extratemporal epilepsy. In some cases the information provided by FDG-PET may be enough, if concordant with video EEG and other techniques of anatomical and functional neuroimaging, to plan surgical resection. In most patients, however, this information is used to guide placement of invasive electrodes in order to record intracranial EEG and ascertain the location of the seizure onset zone. PET with other ligands, including AMT PET and FMZ PET, have been used during presurgical evaluation with variable results; AMT PET may be useful to detect the epileptogenic zone in patients with multiple, potentially epileptogenic, lesions (such as tubers). FMZ PET is not routinely used in clinical practice, although may provide additional information (such as extension of perilesional epileptogenic zone and secondary epileptic foci). Routine use of new ligands will likely result in increased applicability of this neuroimaging technique for epilepsy surgery.

References

- Baumgartner C, Lehner-Baumgartner E. The functional deficit zone: general principles. In: Lüders H (ed.). *Textbook of Epilepsy Surgery*. London: Informa Healthcare, 2008, pp. 781-791.
- Benedek K, Juhasz C, Chugani DC, Muzik O, Chugani HT. Longitudinal changes in cortical glucose hypometabolism in children with intractable epilepsy. *J Child Neurol* 2006; 21: 26-31.
- Chugani H, Juhász E, Asano E, Sood S. PET in neocortical epilepsies. In: Lüders H (ed.). *Textbook of Epilepsy Surgery*. London: Informa Healthcare, 2008, pp. 803-816.
- Chugani HT, Conti JR. Etiologic classification of infantile spasms in 140 cases: role of positron emission tomography. *J Child Neurol* 1996a; 11: 44-8.
- Chugani HT, Da Silva E, Chugani DC. Infantile spasms: III. Prognostic implications of bitemporal hypometabolism on positron emission tomography. *Ann Neurol* 1996b; 39: 643-9.
- Chugani HT, Shewmon DA, Khanna S, Phelps ME. Interictal and postictal focal hypermetabolism on positron emission tomography. *Pediatr Neurol* 1993a; 9: 10-5.
- Chugani HT, Shewmon DA, Shields WD, Sankar R, Comair Y, Vinters HV, et al. Surgery for intractable infantile spasms: neuroimaging perspectives. *Epilepsia* 1993b; 34: 764-71.
- Chugani HT, Shields WD, Shewmon DA, Olson DM, Phelps ME, Peacock WJ. Infantile spasms: I. PET identifies focal cortical dysgenesis in cryptogenic cases for surgical treatment. *Ann Neurol* 1990; 27: 406-13.
- da Silva EA, Chugani DC, Muzik O, Chugani HT. Identification of frontal lobe epileptic foci in children using positron emission tomography. *Epilepsia* 1997; 38: 1198-1208.
- Didelot A, Ryvlin P, Lothe A, Merlet I, Hammers A, Mauguiere F. PET imaging of brain 5-HT1A receptors in the preoperative evaluation of temporal lobe epilepsy. *Brain* 2008; 131 (Pt 10): 2751-64.
- Fedi M, Reutens D, Okazawa H, Andermann F, Boling W, Dubeau F, et al. Localizing value of alpha-methyl-L-tryptophan PET in intractable epilepsy of neocortical origin. *Neurology* 2001; 57: 1629-36.
- Hajek M, Wieser HG, Khan N, Antonini A, Schrott PR, Maguire P, et al. Preoperative and postoperative glucose consumption in mesiobasal and lateral temporal lobe epilepsy. *Neurology* 1994; 44: 2125-32.

- Hammers A, Koepp MJ, Richardson MP, Hurlemann R, Brooks DJ, Duncan JS. Grey and white matter flumazenil binding in neocortical epilepsy with normal MRI. A PET study of 44 patients. *Brain* 2003; 126 (Pt 6):1300-18.
- Henry TR, Engel J, Jr., Mazziotta JC. Clinical evaluation of interictal fluorine-18-fluorodeoxyglucose PET in partial epilepsy. *J Nucl Med* 1993; 34: 1892-8.
- Hong KS, Lee SK, Kim JY, Lee DS, Chung CK. Pre-surgical evaluation and surgical outcome of 41 patients with non-lesional neocortical epilepsy. *Seizure* 2002; 11: 184-92.
- Hong SB, Han HJ, Roh SY, Seo DW, Kim SE, Kim MH. Hypometabolism and interictal spikes during positron emission tomography scanning in temporal lobe epilepsy. *Eur Neurol* 2002; 48: 65-70.
- Jehi LE, Najm I, Bingaman W, Dinner D, Widdess-Walsh P, Luders H. Surgical outcome and prognostic factors of frontal lobe epilepsy surgery. *Brain* 2007; 130 (Pt 2): 574-84.
- Jehi LE, O'Dwyer R, Najm I, Alexopoulos A, Bingaman W. A longitudinal study of surgical outcome and its determinants following posterior cortex epilepsy surgery. *Epilepsia* 2009; 50: 2040-52.
- Juhasz C, Asano E, Shah A, Chugani DC, Batista CE, Muzik O, et al. Focal decreases of cortical GABAA receptor binding remote from the primary seizure focus: what do they indicate? *Epilepsia* 2009; 50: 240-50.
- Juhasz C, Chugani DC, Muzik O, Shah A, Asano E, Mangner TJ, et al. Alpha-methyl-L-tryptophan PET detects epileptogenic cortex in children with intractable epilepsy. *Neurology* 2003; 60: 960-8.
- Juhasz C, Chugani DC, Muzik O, Watson C, Shah J, Shah A, et al. Is epileptogenic cortex truly hypometabolic on interictal positron emission tomography? *Ann Neurol* 2000a; 48: 88-96.
- Juhasz C, Chugani DC, Muzik O, Watson C, Shah J, Shah A, et al. Electroclinical correlates of flumazenil and fluorodeoxyglucose PET abnormalities in lesional epilepsy. *Neurology* 2000b; 55: 825-35.
- Kagawa K, Chugani DC, Asano E, Juhasz C, Muzik O, Shah A, et al. Epilepsy surgery outcome in children with tuberous sclerosis complex evaluated with alpha-[11C]methyl-L-tryptophan positron emission tomography (PET). *J Child Neurol* 2005; 20: 429-38.
- Kim JT, Bai SJ, Choi KO, Lee YJ, Park HJ, Kim DS, et al. Comparison of various imaging modalities in localization of epileptogenic lesion using epilepsy surgery outcome in pediatric patients. *Seizure* 2009; 18: 504-10.
- Kim SK, Na DG, Byun HS, Kim SE, Suh YL, Choi JY, et al. Focal cortical dysplasia: comparison of MRI and FDG-PET. *J Comput Assist Tomogr* 2000; 24: 296-302.
- Kim YK, Lee DS, Lee SK, Chung CK, Chung JK, Lee MC. (18)F-FDG PET in localization of frontal lobe epilepsy: comparison of visual and SPM analysis. *J Nucl Med* 2002; 43: 1167-74.
- Knowlton RC. The role of FDG-PET, ictal SPECT, and MEG in the epilepsy surgery evaluation. *Epilepsy Behav* 2006; 8: 91-101.
- Landvogt C, Buchholz HG, Bernedo V, Schreckenberger M, Werhahn KJ. Alteration of dopamine D2/D3 receptor binding in patients with juvenile myoclonic epilepsy. *Epilepsia* 2010; 51: 1699-706.
- Lee SK, Lee SY, Kim KK, Hong KS, Lee DS, Chung CK. Surgical outcome and prognostic factors of cryptogenic neocortical epilepsy. *Ann Neurol* 2005; 58: 525-32.
- Lerner JT, Salamon N, Hauptman JS, Velasco TR, Hemb M, Wu JY, et al. Assessment and surgical outcomes for mild type I and severe type II cortical dysplasia: a critical review and the UCLA experience. *Epilepsia* 2009; 50: 1310-35.
- Lothe A, Didelot A, Hammers A, Costes N, Saoud M, Gilliam F, et al. Comorbidity between temporal lobe epilepsy and depression: a [18F]MPPF PET study. *Brain* 2008; 131 (Pt 10): 2765-82.

- Luat AF, Asano E, Juhasz C, Chandana SR, Shah A, Sood S, et al. Relationship between brain glucose metabolism positron emission tomography (PET) and electroencephalography (EEG) in children with continuous spike-and-wave activity during slow-wave sleep. *J Child Neurol* 2005; 20: 682-90.
- Mauguiere F, Ryvlin P. The role of PET in presurgical assessment of partial epilepsies. *Epileptic Disord* 2004; 6: 193-215.
- Muzik O, da Silva EA, Juhasz C, Chugani DC, Shah J, Nagy F, et al. Intracranial EEG versus flumazenil and glucose PET in children with extratemporal lobe epilepsy. *Neurology* 2000; 54: 171-9.
- O'Brien TJ, Miles K, Ware R, Cook MJ, Binns DS, Hicks RJ. The cost-effective use of 18F-FDG PET in the presurgical evaluation of medically refractory focal epilepsy. *J Nucl Med* 2008; 49: 931-7.
- Plotkin M, Amthauer H, Merschhemke M, Ludemann L, Hartkop E, Ruf J, et al. Use of statistical parametric mapping of (18) F-FDG-PET in frontal lobe epilepsy. *Nuklearmedizin* 2003; 42: 190-6.
- Regis J, Semah F, Bryan RN, Levrier O, Rey M, Samson Y, et al. Early and delayed MR and PET changes after selective temporomesial radiosurgery in mesial temporal lobe epilepsy. *AJNR Am J Neuroradiol* 1999; 20: 213-6.
- Rintahaka PJ, Chugani HT, Messa C, Phelps ME. Hemimegalencephaly: evaluation with positron emission tomography. *Pediatr Neurol* 1993; 9: 21-8.
- Salamon N, Kung J, Shaw SJ, Koo J, Koh S, Wu JY, et al. FDG-PET/MRI coregistration improves detection of cortical dysplasia in patients with epilepsy. *Neurology* 2008; 71: 1594-1601.
- Savic I, Thorell JO, Roland P. [11C]flumazenil positron emission tomography visualizes frontal epileptogenic regions. *Epilepsia* 1995; 36: 1225-32.
- Seo JH, Noh BH, Lee JS, Kim DS, Lee SK, Kim TS et al. Outcome of surgical treatment in non-lesional intractable childhood epilepsy. *Seizure* 2009; 18: 625-9.
- Sisodiya SM. Surgery for malformations of cortical development causing epilepsy. *Brain* 2000; 123 (Pt 6): 1075-91.
- Sood S, Chugani HT. Functional neuroimaging in the preoperative evaluation of children with drug-resistant epilepsy. *Childs Nerv Syst* 2006; 22: 810-20.
- Spanaki MV, Kopylev L, DeCarli C, Gaillard WD, Liow K, Fazilat S, et al. Postoperative changes in cerebral metabolism in temporal lobe epilepsy. *Arch Neurol* 2000; 57: 1447-52.
- Szelies B, Sobesky J, Pawlik G, Mielke R, Bauer B, Herholz K, et al. Impaired benzodiazepine receptor binding in peri-lesional cortex of patients with symptomatic epilepsies studied by [(11)C]-flumazenil PET. *Eur J Neurol* 2002; 9: 137-42.
- Wakamoto H, Chugani DC, Juhasz C, Muzik O, Kupsky WJ, Chugani HT. Alpha-methyl-l-tryptophan positron emission tomography in epilepsy with cortical developmental malformations. *Pediatr Neurol* 2008; 39: 181-8.
- Weitemeyer L, Kellinghaus C, Weckesser M, Matheja P, Loddenkemper T, Schuierer G, et al. The prognostic value of [F]FDG-PET in nonrefractory partial epilepsy. *Epilepsia* 2005; 46: 1654-60.

Diffusion tensor tractography in extratemporal lobe epilepsy

Christian Vollmar[1], Beate Diehl[2]

[1] National Hospital for Neurology and Neurosurgery, Queen Square, London, United Kingdom; Department of Neurology, Epilepsy Center, University of Munich, Munich, Germany
[2] Institute of Neurology, University College London and National Hospital for Neurology and Neurosurgery, Queen Square, London, United Kingdom

■ Principles of diffusion imaging and tractography

The principles of diffusion MRI were first developed in vivo in the mid 1980s (Le Bihan et al., 1986; Le Bihan et al., 2001). In diffusion-weighted imaging (DWI), images are sensitized to diffusion by using pulsed magnetic field gradients incorporated into a standard spin echo sequence. By taking measurements in at least three directions it is possible to characterize the mean diffusion properties within a voxel in the image. Diffusion gradients are applied in six or more directions allowing for calculation of the diffusion tensor. The tensor can be diagonalized to give three eigenvectors, $\varepsilon 1$, $\varepsilon 2$, and $\varepsilon 3$ representing the principal directions of diffusion. Each of these eigenvectors has an eigenvalue, $\lambda 1$, $\lambda 2$, and $\lambda 3$ representing the magnitude of diffusion (or the corresponding ADC values) along each of these three main directions. Furthermore, a number of diffusion parameters can be derived in each voxel, which are insensitive to subject positioning and fiber tract alignment within the diffusion gradients of the MRI scanner (Basser & Jones, 2002; Le Bihan & Van Zijl, 2002). Mean diffusivity (MD) is a summary measure of the average diffusion properties of a voxel.

It has been noted that the ADC measurements depended on a subject's orientation relative to the magnet. White matter tracts parallel to an applied gradient had the greatest ADC whereas those at an angle to a gradient had smaller ADC values. Therefore it is important to not only define the mean diffusivity of water molecules within an image voxel, but also their directionality. The fact that diffusion is not the same in the three main spatial directions, but is asymmetric in the brain and restricted in certain directions gave rise to the concept of "anisotropy" (Basser, 1995; Basser & Pierpaoli, 1996). Diffusion tensor imaging (DTI) has been developed to explore this directional information. When more than 5 directions are measured, not only the water molecule diffusion can be characterized, but also the degree and direction of anisotropy (Le Bihan et al., 2001).

Exploring the diffusion information in various directions allows gaining greater insights in the structural changes, possibly on a microscopic level. Fractional anisotropy (FA) is a scalar (unitless) index most commonly used to assess the overall degree of directionality; it ranges from 0 (full isotropy) to 1 (complete anisotropic diffusion). In order to interrogate diffusion changes in the three main directions, parametric maps for the parallel (main direction of diffusion, $\lambda \parallel$) and radial or perpendicular ($\lambda_T = (\lambda_2 + \lambda_3)/2$) directions to the main fiber tract orientation can be studied. Together, these quantitative measures help to characterize the integrity of the underlying white matter.

Such information may allow understanding of the pathophysiologic mechanisms underlying diffusion abnormalities. Furthermore, DTI in combination with tractography has become a powerful opportunity to subdivide compartments of white matter representing different tracts and study their diffusion properties selectively.

Anisotropy information forms the basis of reconstructing tracts. Anisotropy in white matter results from the organization of tissue as bundles of axons and myelin sheaths run in parallel, and the diffusion of water is freer and quicker in the long axis of the fibers, than in the perpendicular direction (Beaulieu, 2001).

By assuming that the largest principal axis of the diffusion tensor aligns with the predominant fiber orientation in an MRI voxel, we can obtain vector fields that represent the fiber orientation at each voxel. The 3 dimensional reconstruction of tract trajectories, or Diffusion Tensor Tractography (DTT), is an extension of such vector fields (Mori & van Zijl, 2002). Various algorithms have been used to reconstruct tracts; some can be easily applied and require little computing time, but may fall short in areas with many "crossing" and "kissing" fibers. Others, such as probabilistic tractography, are very time and computing intense and allow for better reconstruction.

DTI and DTT investigations are of interest from a scientific and practical perspective. They allow insights into microstructural changes in the white matter in patients with (lesional and non lesional) epilepsy, interrogate structural connectivity and allow for structure/function correlations. Finally, explorations are under way to assess DTT as a tool to potentially improve functional outcome following epilepsy surgery.

■ DTI in extratemporal lobe epilepsy

Extratemporal epilepsies represent a growing group being evaluated for epilepsy surgery, and often are challenging as precise localization of the epileptogenic zone in relation to cortical function is mandatory. In general, evidence rapidly accumulated that diffusion changes were seen in a variety of lesions associated with focal epilepsy and often localized outside the temporal lobe, such as cortical dysplasia.

DTI changes have been described in various cortical dysplasias and are mainly characterized by reduced anisotropy and, to a lesser extent, increased diffusivity both within the lesion but also remote to the lesion (Dumas et al., 2005; Eriksson et al., 2001). In addition, distant anisotropic changes can also be observed, possibly due to Wallerian degeneration of WM tracts or gliosis resulting from chronic seizures. Diffusion changes in the white matter surrounding cortical dysplasia and the impact on connectivity and adjacent tracts in children (Widjaja et al., 2007) showed reduced FA, which was found to be a sensitive but nonspecific marker of alteration in microstructure of white matter. Diffusivity was mainly influenced by increased perpendicular diffusivity, which may reflect a dominant effect of abnormal myelin. Furthermore alteration in white matter tracts was observed in most cases of cortical dysplasias, decreased tract size and displacement of tracts occurred in larger dysplasias.

Patients with cryptogenic extratemporal lobe epilepsy are a particularly challenging group. In spite of recent advances in structural imaging, up to 25% of patients in presurgical evaluation still fail to show a structural lesion in conventional MRI. In a series of 30 patients with normal MRI, voxel wise statistical analysis of FA and diffusivity maps showed significant changes in 8 patients (Rugg-Gunn et al., 2001). Interestingly we could replicated these findings nine years later, in a recent series of cryptogenic frontal lobe epilepsy, where voxel wise analysis showed clusters of reduced FA in 6 of 21 patients, 5 of which were consistent with the clinically suspected seizure onset zone. It seems that the progress in structural imaging parallels the advances in DTI, resulting in a similar proportion of newly identified pathologies.

Using DTT can also reveal structural changes in cryptogenic epilepsy. Figure 1b shows all tracts emerging from the frontal lobes of a patient with cryptogenic left FLE. The number of tracts was reduced by 50% on the left side. This indicates severe microstructural changes in spite of normal conventional structural imaging at 3T. Looking at specific fiber bundles, the arcuate fasciculus showed an even higher asymmetry with only 30% of fibers on the left, compared to the right side. This was consistent with complete right language dominance in fMRI.

However, in cryptogenic focal epilepsy, intracranial EEG recording remains the gold standard to identify the epileptogenic zone and findings from DTI and DTT can ultimately be confirmed only in patients undergoing invasive recordings and resective surgery. Nevertheless, the available data indicates the potential role of DTI and DTT as an independent diagnostic tool in cryptogenic cases.

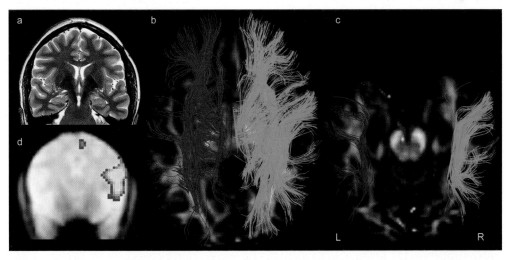

Figure 1. Patient with cryptogenic left frontal lobe epilepsy and normal clinical imaging at 3T (a). Streamline tractography from both frontal lobes showed a reduction of the number of fibers by 50% on the left side (b), indicating microstructural changes in spite of normal conventional imaging. The left arcuate fasciculus showed only 30% of the number of fibers on the right (c). This asymmetry was consistent with right language dominance in fMRI (d).

■ What can diffusion changes tell us about consequences of recurrent seizures?

To date, the pathopysiological mechanism underlying the diffusion changes measured in focal epilepsy is unknown. Diffusion changes are also present in patients with normal conventional MRI. DTI has been increasingly used to gain insight by probing the diffusion changes in all three main directions. Analyzing the pattern of diffusion changes with respect to diffusivities parallel and perpendicular (radial) to the main axonal direction provides in vivo insights into the underlying cause of decreased FA.

Several studies have investigated the mechanisms leading to overall increased diffusivity and reduced FA. The most commonly seen pattern of DTI changes associated with focal epilepsy was unchanged parallel diffusivity and increased perpendicular diffusivity (Concha et al., 2008; Diehl et al., 2008; Govindan et al., 2008; Gross et al., 2006; Kim et al., 2008). As detailed above, such a pattern of FA changes is most consistent with chronic Wallerian degeneration, possibly due to cell loss in the temporal lobe secondary to seizure-induced cell death. There are no comparable studies in ETLE. However, a study in children with recent onset epilepsy showed significant FA reductions and increased perpendicular diffusivity within the first few months after diagnosis. Some of these changes therefore seem to reflect the underlying pathology rather than the secondary consequence of epilepsy (Hutchinson et al., 2010). As with other imaging findings in epilepsy, this overlap can be difficult to disentangle.

■ DTI and ictal onset and irritative zones

One study showed in a small group of patients evaluated with DTI and invasive SEEG recordings that DTI abnormalities correlate better with the irritative zone than the ictal onset zone and may provide accurate data on location and extent of an epileptogenic network in temporal and extratemporal lobe epilepsy (Thivard et al., 2006). Another study investigating FLE confirmed DTI abnormalities in the irriative and epileptogenic zone but also in connected areas. Extend of abnormalities was correlated with epilepsy duration, suggestive of neuroglial injuries (Guye et al., 2007). A recent study used DTT to identify connections between temporal and rolandic irritative zones in children (Bhardwaj et al., 2010). They found connecting tracts through the external capsules that were not present in the contralateral hemisphere or in healthy controls. Such atypical connections may reflect the structural essence of highly active epileptogenic networks and can help understanding the topographic relation of findings within these networks. However, more regional propagation pathways of epileptic activity are more difficult to identify with DTT. Most tractography algorithms are optimized for major anatomical tracts. Also, DTI is currently limited by its spatial resolution of about 2 mm. This results in significant partial volume effects in every DTI voxel and the dominant effect of major descending bundles often overshadow regional U-fibers. *Figure 2* shows the location of intracranial electrodes in a patient with lesional FLE. Ictal onset was recorded at the anterior inferior edge of the lesion and showed non-contiguous propagation to the mesial frontopolar region. After reducing the minimum tract length and increasing the maximum curvature, DTT was able to identify the connection between these two areas and explain the propagation pattern.

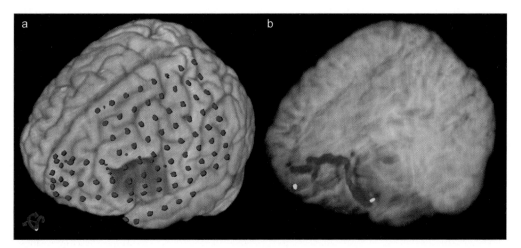

Figure 2. 3D reconstruction of the cortical anatomy and intracranial electrodes in a patient with lesional left FLE (a). Seizure onset was recorded on the lower left electrode of the grid and showed discontinuous propagation to a frontopolar electrode (yellow). Probabilistic tractography, seeded from underneath the grid electrode showed a pathway (blue) to frontopolar cortex, explaining the propagation pattern (b).

■ Correlations with cognitive function

DTI allows new insights in white matter architecture in health and disease. As detailed above, investigations of focal epilepsies revealed diffusion abnormalities in areas of seizure onset and spiking, but also in adjacent and remote and even contralateral areas. In order to understand the meaning of such changes, investigations into structure and function in controls and patients were undertaken. There is mounting evidence that the integrity of white matter tract pathways, as measured by DTI, is systematically related to individual differences in performance across a wide range of cognitive skills (Riley *et al.*, 2010). Furthermore, analysis of WM structure may give insights into the organization of function in individuals, and possibly into reorganization in disease. In addition, studies have explored those structure function correlations in disease and a number of publications have addressed cognitive disability in patients with epilepsy, particularly focusing on language and memory (Diehl *et al.*, 2008; McDonald *et al.*, 2008).

■ Validation of DTT and demonstration of structural connectivity in language or motor systems

Cortical mapping remains the gold standard for functional mapping of eloquent cortex.

Close correlation between invasive recordings, cortical stimulation findings and DTT results may provide in vivo validation in humans. The underlying hypothesis is that the area of cortex that gives rise to a function is also the anchor point of the white matter tract that provides the structural connectivity to other areas of cortex. We examined co localization between anterior and posterior language areas as defined by cortical stimulation in 14 patient undergoing invasive recordings for left hemispheric focal epilepsies and the arcuate fasciculus (AF) as defined by tractography. There was colocalization, defined as less than 1 cm between the AF and the electrode positions delineating language cortex in 84.2% in anterior language areas, and in 55.8% in posterior language areas. This partially supports our hypothesis that fibers defined by DTT as part of the AF tract connect language areas (Diehl et al., 2009).

In patients with FLE, the anatomical connectivity of the functionally active SMA was preserved (Vulliemoz et al., 2010), including patients with mesial seizure onset zone and typical SMA semiology. This documents the potentially greater robustness of the motor system against influences from chronic epilepsy and such preservation of functionally relevant pathways is important when planning resective surgery.

■ DTT – Potential for preserving function in epilepsy surgery

Implementation of DTT has already been shown to benefit in brain tumor surgeries and resections of vascular malformations (Chen et al., 2007; Nimsky et al., 2005; Nimsky et al., 2007b; Wu et al., 2007), and will be increasingly used in epilepsy surgery.

Initial studies in epilepsy have focused on temporal lobectomies and correlations with visual field defects (Powell et al., 2005). The size of temporal lobectomy was systematically correlated with DTT of the optic radiation in 21 postoperative patients (Yogarajah et al., 2009). By applying a linear regression analysis it was shown that the distance from the tip of Meyer's loop to the temporal pole and also the extent of resection predicted the postoperative visual field defects.

Extratemporal surgery carries an even higher risk of postsurgical neurological deficit or incomplete resection due to frequent proximity of epileptogenicity to eloquent cortex.

Figure 3 illustrates the proximity between a focal cortical dysplasia (FCD) and the primary motor cortex. As many FCD extend into the underlying white matter, the topographic relation to functionally relevant tracts is crucial. In the case shown here there was a distance of 1 cm between the inferior extent of the lesion and the descending corticospinal tract. Such information is beneficial in estimating the risk of resective surgery.

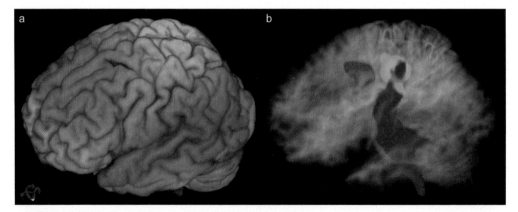

Figure 3. 3D reconstruction of the cortical anatomy and focal cortical dysplasia (red) in the left superior frontal gyrus. The lesion is close to the precentral gyrus, where motor fMRI showed activation in the primary hand motor area (green)(a). Tractography seeded from this functional activation cluster delineated the corticospinal tract (CST, blue) and a distance of more than 1 cm between the lesion and the CST in the semitransparent 3D rendering (b).

However, a great number of difficulties and methodological challenges have yet to be overcome in order to consider using tractography for neuronavigation. Coregistration errors, distortions inherent to EPI sequences are only some of the many technical challenges. In addition, it is unknown how reliably DTT can map the entire tract in health and disease. Intraoperative brain shift after craniotomy is another significant impediment. The availability of intraoperative MR imaging may represent one method to correct for this movement and may improve the accuracy of the data to aid surgical planning.

These data provide evidence that DTT has the potential to inform about risks of epilepsy surgery procedures. Once successfully implemented into neuronavigation systems, this information may also be used intraoperatively to tailor resections (Nimsky *et al.*, 2007a).

To what degree they may improve functional outcome following epilepsy surgery is unknown. The potential however appears great and it is therefore crucial to understand strengths and limitations of DTT in human epilepsy.

References

- Basser PJ. Inferring microstructural features and the physiological state of tissues from diffusion-weighted images. *NMR Biomed* 1995; 8: 333-44.
- Basser PJ, Jones DK. Diffusion-tensor MRI: theory, experimental design and data analysis - a technical review. *NMR Biomed* 2002; 15: 456-67.
- Basser PJ, Pierpaoli C. Microstructural and physiological features of tissues elucidated by quantitative-diffusion-tensor MRI. *J Magn Reson B* 1996; 111, 209-19.
- Bhardwaj RD, Mahmoodabadi SZ, Otsubo H, Snead OC, III, Rutka JT, WidjajaE. Diffusion tensor tractography detection of functional pathway for the spread of epileptiform activity between temporal lobe and Rolandic region. *Childs Nerv Syst* 2010; 26: 185-90.
- Chen X, Weigel D, Ganslandt O, Fahlbusch R, Buchfelder M, Nimsky C. Diffusion tensor-based fiber tracking and intraoperative neuronavigation for the resection of a brainstem cavernous angioma. *Surg Neurol* 2007; 68: 285-91.
- Concha L, Beaulieu C, Collins DL, Gross DW. White matter diffusion abnormalities in temporal lobe epilepsy with and without mesial temporal sclerosis. *J Neurol Neurosurg Psychiatry* 2009; 80: 312-9.
- Diehl B, Busch RM, Duncan JS, Piao Z, Tkach J, Luders HO. Abnormalities in diffusion tensor imaging of the uncinate fasciculus relate to reduced memory in temporal lobe epilepsy. *Epilepsia* 2008; 49: 1409-18.
- Diehl B, Piao Z, Tkach J, Busch RM, LaPresto E, Najm I, *et al.* Cortical stimulation for language mapping in focal epilepsy: Correlations with tractography of the arcuate fasciculus. *Epilepsia* 2010; 51: 639-46.
- Dumas R, Oppenheim C, Chassoux F, Rodrigo S, Beuvon F, *et al.* Diffusion tensor imaging of partial intractable epilepsy. *Eur Radiol* 2005; 15: 279-85.
- Eriksson SH, Rugg-Gunn FJ, Symms MR, Barker GJ, Duncan JS. Diffusion tensor imaging in patients with epilepsy and malformations of cortical development. *Brain* 2001; 124: 617-26.
- Govindan RM, Makki MI, Sundaram SK, JuhaszC, Chugani HT. Diffusion tensor analysis of temporal and extratemporal lobe tracts in temporal lobe epilepsy. *Epilepsy Res* 2008; 80: 30-41.
- Gross DW, Concha L, Beaulieu C. Extratemporal white matter abnormalities in mesial temporal lobe epilepsy demonstrated with diffusion tensor imaging. *Epilepsia* 2006; 47: 1360-3.
- Guye M, Ranjeva JP, Bartolomei F, Confort-Gouny S, McGonigal A, Regis J, *et al.* What is the significance of interictal water diffusion changes in frontal lobe epilepsies? *Neuroimage* 2007; 35: 28-37.

- Hutchinson E, Pulsipher D, Dabbs K, Gutierrez A, Sheth R, Jones J, et al. Children with new-onset epilepsy exhibit diffusion abnormalities in cerebral white matter in the absence of volumetric differences. *Epilepsy Res* 2010; 88: 208-14.
- Kim H, Piao Z, Liu P, Bingaman W, Diehl B. Secondary white matter degeneration of the corpus callosum in patients with intractable temporal lobe epilepsy: a diffusion tensor imaging study. *Epilepsy Res* 2008; 81: 136-42.
- Le Bihan D, Breton E, Lallemand D, Grenier P, Cabanis E, Laval-Jeantet M. MR imaging of intravoxel incoherent motions: application to diffusion and perfusion in neurologic disorders. *Radiology* 1986; 161: 401-7.
- Le Bihan D, Mangin JF, Poupon C, Clark CA, Pappata S, Molko N, Chabriat H. Diffusion tensor imaging: concepts and applications. *J Magn Reson Imaging* 2001; 13: 534-6.
- Le Bihan D, Van Zijl P. From the diffusion coefficient to the diffusion tensor. *NMR Biomed* 2002; 15: 431-4.
- McDonald CR, Ahmadi ME, Hagler DJ, Tecoma ES, Iragui VJ, Gharapetian L, et al. Diffusion tensor imaging correlates of memory and language impairments in temporal lobe epilepsy. *Neurology* 2008; 71: 1869-76.
- Mori S, van Zijl PC. Fiber tracking: principles and strategies - a technical review. *NMR Biomed* 2002; 15: 468-80.
- Nimsky C, Ganslandt O, Fahlbusch R. Implementation of fiber tract navigation. *Neurosurgery* 2007a; 61: 306-17.
- Nimsky C, Ganslandt O, Hastreiter P, Wang R, Benner T, Sorensen AG, Fahlbusch R. Preoperative and intraoperative diffusion tensor imaging-based fiber tracking in glioma surgery. *Neurosurgery* 2007b; 61: 178-85.
- Nimsky C, Grummich P, Sorensen AG, Fahlbusch R, Ganslandt O. Visualization of the pyramidal tract in glioma surgery by integrating diffusion tensor imaging in functional neuronavigation. *Zentralbl Neurochir* 2005; 66: 133-41.
- Powell HW, Parker GJ, Alexander DC, Symms MR, Boulby PA, Wheeler-Kingshott CA, et al. MR tractography predicts visual field defects following temporal lobe resection. *Neurology* 2005; 65: 596-9.
- Riley JD, Franklin DL, Choi V, Kim RC, Binder DK, Cramer SC, Lin JJ. Altered white matter integrity in temporal lobe epilepsy: association with cognitive and clinical profiles. *Epilepsia* 2010; 51: 536-45.
- Rugg-Gunn FJ, Eriksson SH, Symms MR, Barker GJ, Duncan JS. Diffusion tensor imaging of cryptogenic and acquired partial epilepsies. *Brain* 2001; 124: 627-36.
- Thivard L, Adam C, Hasboun D, Clemenceau S, Dezamis E, Lehericy S, et al. Interictal diffusion MRI in partial epilepsies explored with intracerebral electrodes. *Brain* 2006; 129: 375-85.
- Vulliemoz S, Vollmer C, Yogarajah M, Thompson P, Stretton J, Koepp M, et al. Connectivity of the supplementary motor cortex in frontal lobe epilepsies: an fMRI based tractography study. *Epilepsia* 2010; 50 (S11): 87.
- Widjaja E, Blaser S, Miller E, Kassner A, Shannon P, Chuang SH, et al.. Evaluation of subcortical white matter and deep white matter tracts in malformations of cortical development. *Epilepsia* 2007; 48: 1460-9.
- Wu JS, Zhou LF, Tang WJ, Mao Y, Hu J, SongYY, et al. Clinical evaluation and follow-up outcome of diffusion tensor imaging-based functional neuronavigation: a prospective, controlled study in patients with gliomas involving pyramidal tracts. *Neurosurgery* 2007; 61: 935-48.
- Yogarajah M, Focke NK, Bonelli S, Cercignani M, Acheson J, Parker GJ, et al. Defining Meyer's loop-temporal lobe resections, visual field deficits and diffusion tensor tractography. *Brain* 2009; 132: 1656-68.

Section IV:
Invasive evaluation
of extratemporal lobe epilepsies

Subdural EEG recordings in extratemporal lobe epilepsy

Hajo M. Hamer

Epilepsy Center, Department of Neurology, University of Erlangen, Germany

■ Introduction

The goal of diagnosis and treatment of patients with epilepsy is complete seizure freedom but a significant part of epileptic patients will develop medically intractable epilepsy. The majority of these patients have partial epilepsy (Semah *et al.*, 1998). Selected patients are considered for surgical therapy and undergo presurgical evaluation. Epilepsy surgery is based on the principle that resection of an epileptogenic focus can result in seizure freedom. The epileptogenic zone is defined as the area of brain necessary and sufficient to generate seizures the resection of which will result in seizure freedom (Luders *et al.*, 1992). By definition, if surgery fails, the resected area was incorrectly or incompletely removed or was only one of several epileptogenic zones. Accordingly, accurate localization of the epileptogenic zone is crucial for the success of epilepsy surgery.

Data from surface recordings can be concordant with the location of an epileptogenic lesion detected by neuroimaging. In these cases, complementary information of different non-invasive tests may be sufficient to establish an indication for epilepsy surgery (Engel Jr. *et al.*, 1981). In other situations, diverging evidence may appear from neuroimaging and surface EEG or surface EEG may not be able to define the epileptogenic zone or neuroimaging may be normal. In these situations, it can be impossible to intelligently plan a resection and invasive electrodes may aid in the localization of the ictal onset zone. This is especially true for extratemporal lobe epilepsy (ETLE) where seizure semiology is frequently caused by fast propagation of ictal activity and the sensitivity of interictal and ictal EEG is low (Salanova *et al.*, 1993; Laskowitz *et al.*, 1995; Mosewich *et al.*, 2000; Wetjen *et al.*, 2002; Kellinghaus & Luders, 2004; Beleza *et al.*, 2009) as large portions of the frontal, parietal and occipital lobe are "hidden" to scalp electrodes due to the far distance and orientation of the cortex (Williamson & Spencer, 1986; Salanova *et al.*, 1992; Williamson *et al.*, 1992b; Aykut-Bingol *et al.*, 1998; Lee *et al.*, 2000b). While the number of patients with (mesial) temporal lobe epilepsy (TLE) requiring intracranial EEG studies has been markedly reduced over the last decades due to growing experience with this syndrome and better neuroimaging, this was not paralleled by extratemporal epilepsies.

■ General indications and characteristics

Intracranial electrodes are employed when there is evidence that the patient has a resectable epileptogenic focus but the non-invasively obtained information is inadequate and more specific data is needed. In contrast to extracranial recordings, subdural electrodes record directly from the cortex which increases dramatically the sensitivity and allows differentiating smaller pools of neurons (Tao *et al.*, 2005). In addition, artifacts from muscles and electrode movement are rare and impedances tend to remain stable. Indications for invasive video-EEG-monitoring can be divided into four overlapping groups.

Extent and distribution of the epileptogenic zone

In a proportion of individuals with medically intractable partial epilepsy, one may be able to localize the epileptogenic zone in one lobe or area of the brain without precise definition of its extent and distribution. This is frequently the case in "non-lesional frontal lobe patients" in whom imaging clues are missing. Invasive monitoring with multiple strips over the mesial and orbital aspects in combination with grids over the lateral surface may help in the definition of the exact extent and distribution of the ictal onset zone and guide an effective resection (*Figure 1*). In some patients seizures arising from the supplementary sensory-motor area, lateralization of the focus cannot be made which may lead in rare instances to insertion of double-sided electrodes in the interhemispheric fissure to record subdurally from one frontal lobe and epidurally (through the falx) from the other frontal lobe.

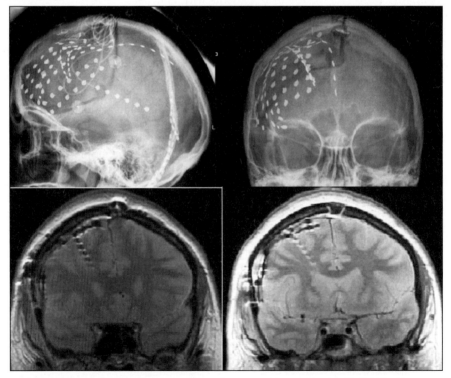

Figure 1. Conventional X-ray (upper left and right) and MRI scans (lower left and right) of a 56yo patient with right frontal lobe epilepsy due to dysplasia. For presurgical evaluation, subdural grid and strips electrodes as well as two depths electrodes were inserted to better define the extent of the epileptogenic zone and its relationship to eloquent cortex.

The comments about frontal lobe seizures also apply for seizures arising from the parietal and occipital lobes. Imaging and primary sensory or visual symptoms may help approximate the epileptogenic zone but are frequently not precise enough for epilepsy surgery and invasive EEG studies must be designed. This is especially true in cases, when asymptomatic seizure onset with rapid propagation into the perirolandic or temporal regions is suspected (Salanova et al., 1992; Williamson et al., 1992a; Williamson et al., 1992b).

At least 20% of all patients who undergo surgical resections for intractable epilepsy do not obtain a significant benefit (Wingkun et al., 1991; Luders et al., 1994; Rosenow & Lüders, 2004). These patients may be candidates for a second surgical procedure. Prolonged video-EEG monitoring with scalp electrodes is necessary to confirm persisting seizures from the initially defined seizure onset zone. However, in some patients, invasive monitoring will also be required to identify the exact location and extent of the residual epileptogenic zone in relationship to remaining tissue. In a study of Awad et al., more than 70% of the candidates for a second operation needed subdural electrodes to accurately localize the ictal onset zone. About 50% of these patients became seizure free after second surgery and 30% had a reduction of greater than 90% in seizure frequency (Awad et al., 1991a).

Epileptogenic zone *versus* structural lesion

Even in "lesional" cases, a resection extending beyond the clearly visualized abnormality on MRI may frequently be advisable since surrounding cortex may include occult pathology and be epileptogenic. This applies especially to dysplastic cortex (Kuzniecky, 1994; Palmini et al., 1995; Rosenow et al., 1998). In these patients, a subdural grid may be placed over the lesion to approximate the extent of the epileptogenic zone (Fish et al., 1993). When multiple lesions are present, as in patients with tuberous sclerosis or multiple cavernomas, successful surgery is still possible, if seizures can be localized to a single or a group of lesions (Bebin et al., 1993; Wyllie et al., 1998). For this purpose, invasive monitoring is frequently necessary. If the resection of the lesion was incomplete but the epileptogenic zone/ictal onset zone defined by invasive recordings was completely removed, 83% of the patients still achieved favorable outcome (Awad et al., 1991b).

Neuroimaging has facilitated presurgical evaluation in many cases but is also responsible for generating a new population of patients for intracranial recordings who may not have been considered before. These patients have so-called "dual pathology", such as bilateral hippocampal sclerosis, tumor and dysplasia or hippocampal sclerosis with a second abnormality. In these settings, invasive monitoring is frequently advisable to clarify which lesion(s) is epileptogenic (Morris, III et al., 1986; Bebin et al., 1993) since MRI demonstration of dual pathology does not imply dual epileptogenesis.

Epileptogenic zone *versus* eloquent cortex

Invasive EEG-studies may become necessary to investigate the epileptogenic zone in the neighborhood of eloquent cortex, such as language, cognitive, motor or sensory areas (Wyllie et al., 1988; Berger et al., 1991). In contrast to depth electrodes, subdural electrodes have the advantage that they allow wide spread mapping of the eloquent cortex by electrical stimulation (Lesser et al., 1986; Lüders et al., 1987; Luders et al., 1989; Hamer

& Morris, 2001). This neurophysiological information permits the surgeon to extend the resection close to eloquent areas without increasing significantly the risk of lasting neurologic sequelae.

■ Different types of subdural monitoring

Certain types of intracranial electrodes are more suited to some locations or questions than others and are indicated under different circumstances. Depth electrodes penetrate brain tissue and are, therefore, used when EEG recordings are needed from buried cortex, such as hippocampus or periventricular heterotopia. Subdural strip electrodes overlie the surface of the brain and multiple strips are most suited for sampling wider neocortical areas of the brain, sometimes bilaterally. Subdural grids are the best choice for functional mapping of the cortex. Many invasive video-EEG-studies require a combination of different types of intracranial electrodes to solve the specific problems formulated during noninvasive testing.

Subdural strip electrodes

Strip electrodes are made from a single row of four to eleven platinum or stainless steel electrode contacts, approximately 2-4 mm in diameter, embedded in flexible materials, such as silastic, at fixed interelectrode distances, typically 10 mm (Hamer & Morris, 2001). One or more strips can be inserted through one burr hole with different planned trajectories through the subdural space. Subdural strips may be inserted bilaterally at roughly corresponding sites, or asymmetrically, when needed. A common reason for multiple subdural strips is localization and extent of the epileptogenic zone in the mesial or orbitofrontal aspects of the frontal lobe, or within the parieto-occipital region. The advantages of subdural strip electrodes over depth electrodes are easier implantation with no stereotactic equipment, coverage of larger cortical areas, and a lesser risk of hemorrhage since they lie on the surface of the brain without direct penetration of brain tissue (Lüders et al., 1986; Eisenschenk et al., 2001). Disadvantages are their relatively inaccurate placement by virtue of the insertion technique and the inability to record from buried structures.

Subdural grid electrodes

Subdural grid electrodes are expanded subdural strips with parallel rows of up to 64 electrodes. Their insertion requires open craniotomy. The main indication is the evaluation of epileptogenic cortex in relationship to functional regions. Although cortical electrical stimulation can also be done using subdural strips, only subdural grid electrodes provide the desired stable and dense array of electrodes for ideal functional mapping (Lesser et al., 2010). Larger arrays of up to 8 x 8 electrodes can be placed over broad areas of the cortex such as the fronto-central or parieto-occipital region. Smaller grids, such as grids with 4 × 4 or 2 × 6 contacts, may be used subfrontally, subtemporally or between the hemispheres. In patients with structural lesions, grids can be placed on the lesion to investigate the surrounding cortex for epileptogenicity and thus, tailor a resective procedure.

The extensive regionalized array of contacts, however, may become a disadvantage when wider areas have to be sampled especially in "non-lesional" patients (Uematsu et al., 1992). Therefore, combined strip and grid studies are frequently applied. Both types of electrodes may be inserted through one open craniotomy.

■ Electrocorticography

A major disadvantage of intraoperative electrocorticography (ECoG) is the usual absence of ictal activity (Stefan *et al.*, 2008). The characteristics of the interictal activity are similar to those seen in chronic subdural recordings although recording time is shorter and spike frequency may be reduced due to general anaesthesia even when barbiturates and benzodiazepines are avoided (Asano *et al.*, 2004). Successful localization of the irritative zone may rely heavily on the selection of the site for electrocorticography which allows only to record with a limited number of electrodes. Intraoperative recording with many electrodes (64 electrodes and more) is challenging to perform because of the long set-up time that such recordings require and the difficulty to maintain synchronously stable impedances in all electrodes. This leads to the conclusion that chronic evaluation techniques may often be preferable to acute intraoperative testing in TLE as well as in ETLE in spite of higher risks of chronic monitoring *versus* acute electrocorticography (Rosenbaum *et al.*, 1986; McBride *et al.*, 1991; Cascino *et al.*, 1995; Schwartz *et al.*, 1997; Hamer *et al.*, 2002; Burneo *et al.*, 2006). An advantage of ECoG is to record after the resection especially in dysplasia although interpretation of the results remain sometimes difficult (Wennberg *et al.*, 1999). Post-resection absence of abundant spikes or sharp waves other than those at the resection borders correlated with a favourable surgical result in frontal lobe epilepsy (Wennberg *et al.*, 1998). However, studies which included patients with TLE due to HS reported contradictory findings regarding the possible association of spikes outside the area of the planned resection and surgical outcome in pre-resection ECoG (Schwartz *et al.*, 1997; Chen *et al.*, 2006). Both studies similarly did not find post-resection ECoG to be helpful.

■ Risks and limitations of chronic subdural electrodes

The advantages of chronic invasive monitoring have to be weighed against their significant costs and risks such as mass effect, hemorrhage, and infection (Wyler *et al.*, 1991). Monitoring with subdural grids was associated with transient complications in 10%-25% of the patients, with more severe complications such as osteomyelitis or infarction in 2% and even with death in rare instances (Hamer *et al.*, 2002; Onal *et al.*, 2003; Burneo *et al.*, 2006; Wong *et al.*, 2009). Risk factors were greater number of electrodes, longer duration of monitoring und older age of patient (Hamer *et al.*, 2002; Burneo *et al.*, 2006; Wong *et al.*, 2009). Transient complications were reported in 0-3% of recordings with strip electrodes (Cohen-Gadol & Spencer, 2003; Burneo *et al.*, 2006).

Because of these adverse effects, it is desirable to limit the number of studies and electrodes to as few as possible without compromising the ability to gain sufficient information for subsequent surgery. Therefore, intracranial electrodes should not be used before the patient's problem is defined. Intracranial electrodes serve a specific need only in the context of a specific question asked of the technology. In any case, a sampling bias remains in invasive monitorings (Salanova *et al.*, 1993) and by the seizure pattern itself, it may be difficult to determine whether the ictal discharge is originating from the area recorded or propagated to it. Recording of a seizure onset in electrodes at the border of a grid makes it impossible to know the exact extent of the seizure onset zone. Another limitation is the inability of subdural electrodes to record from deep, subcortical structures, *e.g.* heterotopias, mesial temporal structures, insula or banks of fissures and sulci. A combination of subdural and depths electrodes, however, may help circumventing this problem.

■ EEG recordings with subdural electrodes

Interictal epileptiform discharges (IED)

The sensitivity to record IED is by far higher with intracranial subdural than with scalp recordings (Tao et al., 2005; Ray et al., 2007). Due to their closer distance to the cortex, subdural electrodes may reveal a smaller extent of the irritative zone in some patients than surface electrodes do although the opposite can also be true. An increased irritative zone was reported after seizures and during AED withdrawal (Rosenow et al., 1998; de Curtis & Avanzini, 2001). The use of subdural grid electrodes in frontal lobe epilepsy that extensively covered broad areas of the cortex were reported to localize the seizure onset zone in the majority of patients even when scalp electrodes showed a widespread seizure onset and the MRI was read as normal or non-localizing (Cukiert et al., 2001; Blume et al., 2001).

The morphology of IED in subdural recordings is frequently more pointed as compared to IED recorded by scalp electrodes. They break the background activity similarly to non-invasive recordings and usually stand out more than three to five times from background EEG. Positive polarity is possible. Interpretational difficulties can pose sharply contoured spindles, mμ or other background activity. There is some evidence that certain patterns of IED, such as repetitive bursting discharges or continuous rhythmic spiking, may be indicative for certain epileptogenic lesions, such as dyplasia or ganglioglioma (Palmini et al., 1995; Rosenow et al., 1998; Rosenow and Luders 2001; Boonyapisit et al., 2003).

It is an ongoing discussion which IED are arising from the epileptogenic zone in contrast to IED which define "only" the irritative zone. IED which appear earliest in a cluster or show the highest amplitude and/or the greatest frequency are considered to be generated in or in the proximity ($\leqslant 2$ cm) of the epileptogenic zone (Hufnagel et al., 2000). In addition, association with abnormal background activity or focal slowing may also identify IED of the epileptogenic zone (Kim et al., 2010).

Complete resection of a focal irritative zone defined by invasive monitoring in mostly non-lesional cases was associated with good surgical outcome as compared to patients where frequent IED extended beyond the area of resection (Bautista et al., 1999; Asano et al., 2009). However, there was a lack of this correlation in studies including different types of pathologies (Paolicchi et al., 2000; Ferrier et al., 2001). Therefore, the importance of complete resection of the irritative zone has still to be established in different settings and is currently less clear than the strong relationship between removal of the seizure onset zone and the epileptogenic lesion and postoperative seizure freedom (Asano et al., 2009).

Seizure patterns

The earliest ictal changes are frequently associated with an electrodecrement which may extend beyond the localized ictal onset. The actual seizure patterns reveal similar characteristics as the ones seen in scalp recordings. They can be of various morphology and are defined as the first (rhythmic) electrical changes detected regardless of their morphology, prior to or with the clinical seizure manifestations (Spencer et al., 1992). Typical seizure onset patterns are low voltage fast activity which is seen especially in ETLE (Lee et al., 2000a) *(Figure 2)*, sinusoidal waves, (ir)regular spike discsharges and the so-called start-stop-start phenomenon defined as a pair of sequential ictal potentials separated by complete or almost complete cessation of seizure activity (Blume & Kaibara 1993). Seizures arising from the extratemporal areas may generate faster frequencies as compared to the temporal lobe (Lee et al., 2000a). Slower frequencies and regional instead of focal onset may indicate propagated activity (Lieb et al., 1981; Schiller et al., 1998). There are also seizure onset patterns beyond the traditional' EEG frequencies, such as intraslow activity < 0.5 Hz (Ikeda et al., 1999) und high frequency oscillations > 80 Hz (Jacobs et al., 2008) which description is beyond the scope of this chapter.

Resection of areas generating ictal low voltage fast activity, rhythmic sinusoidal waves or fast spike trains were related to good postoperative outcome (Weinand et al., 1992; Lee et al., 2000a). These findings, however, could not be confirmed by another study which found only that slow ictal spread predicted favorable outcome in contrast to noncontiguous spread which was associated with unfavorable outcome (Kutsy et al., 1999). Complete removal of the seizure onset zone was the only independent predictor of seizure free outcome in a multivariate logistic regression analysis (Asano et al., 2009).

■ Conclusion

Complete resection of the epileptogenic zone is important for seizure freedom. If non-invasive testing reveals insufficient or diverging information, invasive monitoring with subdural electrodes may be necessary to approximate the location and extent of the epileptogenic zone especially in ETLE. Invasive monitoring is most successful if the patient's individual problem is clearly defined by prior testing. Purely exploratory studies are justified only in exceptional cases. In some patients, a combination of different types of intracranial electrodes best addresses the specific question at hand. In spite of certain risks and costs, intracranial EEG recordings are still necessary in a significant minority of patients because the sensitivity to record IED is usually higher and the precision to define the seizure onset zone is greater than in extracranial recordings.

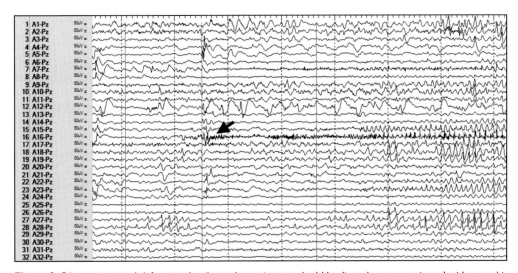

Figure 2. 54 yo patient with left parietal epilepsy due to intracerebral bleeding who was monitored with a combination of subdural grid and strip electrodes to define the extent of the epileptogenic zone. Note the low voltage paroxysmal fast as seizure onset pattern (arrow) in grid electrode A16.

References

- Asano E, Benedek K, Shah A, Juhasz C, Shah J, Chugani DC, *et al*. Is intraoperative electro-corticography reliable in children with intractable neocortical epilepsy? *Epilepsia* 2004; 45: 1091-9.
- Asano E, Juhasz C, Shah A, Sood S, Chugani HT. Role of subdural electrocorticography in prediction of long-term seizure outcome in epilepsy surgery. *Brain* 2009; 132: 1038-47.
- Awad IA, Nayel MH, Luders H. Second operation after the failure of previous resection for epilepsy. *Neurosurgery* 1991a; 28: 510-8.
- Awad IA, Rosenfeld J, Ahl J, Hahn JF, Luders H. Intractable epilepsy and structural lesions of the brain: mapping, resection strategies, and seizure outcome. *Epilepsia* 1991b; 32: 179-86.
- Aykut-Bingol C, Bronen RA, Kim JH, Spencer DD, Spencer SS. Surgical outcome in occipital lobe epilepsy: implications for pathophysiology. *Ann Neurol* 1998; 44: 60-9.
- Bautista RE, Cobbs MA, Spencer DD, Spencer SS. Prediction of surgical outcome by interictal epileptiform abnormalities during intracranial EEG monitoring in patients with extrahippocampal seizures. *Epilepsia* 1999; 40: 880-90.
- Bebin EM, Kelly PJ, Gomez MR. Surgical treatment for epilepsy in cerebral tuberous sclerosis. *Epilepsia* 1993; 34: 651-7.
- Beleza P, Bilgin O, Noachtar S. Interictal rhythmical midline theta differentiates frontal from temporal lobe epilepsies. *Epilepsia* 2009; 50: 550-5.
- Berger MS, Ghatan S, Geyer JR, Keles GE, Ojemann GA. Seizure outcome in children with hemispheric tumors and associated intractable epilepsy: the role of tumor removal combined with seizure foci resection. *Pediatr Neurosurg* 1991; 17: 185-91.
- Blume WT, Kaibara M. The start-stop-start phenomenon of subdurally recorded seizures. *Electroencephalogr Clin Neurophysiol* 1993; 86: 94-9.
- Blume WT, Ociepa D, Kander V. Frontal lobe seizure propagation: scalp and subdural EEG studies. *Epilepsia* 2001; 42: 491-503.
- Boonyapisit K, Najm I, Klem G, Ying Z, Burrier C, LaPresto E, Nair D, Bingaman W, Prayson R, Luders H. Epileptogenicity of focal malformations due to abnormal cortical development: direct electrocorticographic-histopathologic correlations. *Epilepsia* 2003; 44: 69-76.
- Burneo JG, Steven DA, McLachlan RS, Parrent AG. Morbidity associated with the use of intracranial electrodes for epilepsy surgery. *Can J Neurol Sci* 2006; 33: 223-7.
- Cascino GD, Trenerry MR, Jack CR, Jr., Dodick D, Sharbrough FW, So EL, Lagerlund TD, Shin C, Marsh WR. Electrocorticography and temporal lobe epilepsy: relationship to quantitative MRI and operative outcome. *Epilepsia* 1995; 36: 692-6.
- Chen X, Sure U, Haag A, Knake S, Fritsch B, Muller HH, *et al*. Predictive value of electrocorticography in epilepsy patients with unilateral hippocampal sclerosis undergoing selective amygdalohippocampectomy. *Neurosurg Rev* 2006; 29: 108-13.
- Cohen-Gadol AA, Spencer DD. Use of an anteromedial subdural strip electrode in the evaluation of medial temporal lobe epilepsy. Technical note. *J Neurosurg* 2003; 99: 921-3.
- Cukiert A, Buratini JA, Machado E, Sousa A, Vieira JO, Argentoni M, *et al*. Results of surgery in patients with refractory extratemporal epilepsy with normal or nonlocalizing magnetic resonance findings investigated with subdural grids. *Epilepsia* 2001; 42: 889-94.
- De Curtis M, Avanzini G. Interictal spikes in focal epileptogenesis. *Prog Neurobiol* 2001; 63: 541-67.
- Eisenschenk S, Gilmore RL, Cibula JE, Roper SN. Lateralization of temporal lobe foci: depth versus subdural electrodes. *Clin Neurophysiol* 2001; 112: 836-44.
- Engel J, Jr., Rausch R, Lieb JP, Kuhl DE, Crandall PH. Correlation of criteria used for localizing epileptic foci in patients considered for surgical therapy of epilepsy. *Ann Neurol* 1981; 9: 215-24.

- Ferrier CH, Alarcon G, Engelsman J, Binnie CD, Koutroumanidis M, Polkey CE, *et al*. Relevance of residual histologic and electrocorticographic abnormalities for surgical outcome in frontal lobe epilepsy. *Epilepsia* 2001; 42: 363-71.

- Fish DR, Smith SJ, Quesney LF, Andermann F, Rasmussen T. Surgical treatment of children with medically intractable frontal or temporal lobe epilepsy: results and highlights of 40 years' experience. *Epilepsia* 1993; 34: 244-7.

- Hamer HM, Morris HH. Indication of subdural grid electrodes. In: Lüders HO, Comair YG, eds. *Epilepsy surgery*. Philadelphia: Lippincott Williams & Wilkins, 2001: 559-66.

- Hamer HM, Morris HH, Mascha EJ, Karafa MT, Bingaman WE, Bej MD, *et al*. Complications of invasive video-EEG monitoring with subdural grid electrodes. *Neurology* 2002; 58: 97-103.

- Hufnagel A, Dumpelmann M, Zentner J, Schijns O, Elger CE. Clinical relevance of quantified intracranial interictal spike activity in presurgical evaluation of epilepsy. *Epilepsia* 2000; 41: 467-78.

- Ikeda A, Taki W, Kunieda T, Terada K, Mikuni N, Nagamine T, *et al*. Focal ictal direct current shifts in human epilepsy as studied by subdural and scalp recording. *Brain* 1999; 122 (Pt 5): 827-38.

- Jacobs J, LeVan P, Chander R, Hall J, Dubeau F, Gotman J. Interictal high-frequency oscillations (80-500 Hz) are an indicator of seizure onset areas independent of spikes in the human epileptic brain. *Epilepsia* 2008; 49: 1893-907.

- Kellinghaus C, Luders HO. Frontal lobe epilepsy. *Epileptic Disord* 2004; 6: 223-39.

- Kim DW, Kim HK, Lee SK, Chu K, Chung CK. Extent of neocortical resection and surgical outcome of epilepsy: intracranial EEG analysis. *Epilepsia* 2010; 51: 1010-7.

- Kutsy RL, Farrell DF, Ojemann GA. Ictal patterns of neocortical seizures monitored with intracranial electrodes: correlation with surgical outcome. *Epilepsia* 1999; 40: 257-66.

- Kuzniecky RI. Magnetic resonance imaging in developmental disorders of the cerebral cortex. *Epilepsia* 1994; 35 Suppl 6: S44-S56.

- Laskowitz DT, Sperling MR, French JA, O'Connor MJ. The syndrome of frontal lobe epilepsy: characteristics and surgical management. *Neurology* 1995; 45: 780-7.

- Lee SA, Spencer DD, Spencer SS. Intracranial EEG seizure-onset patterns in neocortical epilepsy. *Epilepsia* 2000a; 41: 297-307.

- Lee SK, Kim JY, Hong KS, Nam HW, Park SH, Chung CK. The clinical usefulness of ictal surface EEG in neocortical epilepsy. *Epilepsia* 2000b; 41: 1450-5.

- Lesser RP, Crone NE, Webber WR. Subdural electrodes. *Clin Neurophysiol* 2010; 121: 1376-92.

- Lesser RP, Luders H, Morris HH, Dinner DS, Klem G, Hahn J, Harrison M. Electrical stimulation of Wernicke's area interferes with comprehension. *Neurology* 1986; 36: 658-63.

- Lieb JP, Engel J, Jr., Gevins A, Crandal PH. Surface and deep EEG correlates of surgical outcome in temporal lobe epilepsy. *Epilepsia* 1981; 22: 515-38.

- Luders H, Awad I, Burgess R, Wyllie E, Van Ness P. Subdural electrodes in the presurgical evaluation for surgery of epilepsy. *Epilepsy Res Suppl* 1992; 5: 147-56.

- Luders H, Hahn J, Lesser RP, Dinner DS, Morris HH, III, Wyllie E, *et al*. Basal temporal subdural electrodes in the evaluation of patients with intractable epilepsy. *Epilepsia* 1989; 30: 131-42.

- Lüders H, Lesser RP, Hahn J, Dinner DS, Morris H, Resor S, Harrison M. Basal temporal language area demonstrated by electrical stimulation. *Neurology* 1986; 36: 505-10.

- Luders H, Murphy D, Awad I, Wyllie E, Dinner DS, Morris HH, III, Rothner AD. Quantitative analysis of seizure frequency 1 week and 6, 12, and 24 months after surgery of epilepsy. *Epilepsia* 1994; 35: 1174-8.

- Lüders HO, Lesser RP, Morris HH. Negative motor responses elicited by stimulation of the human cortex. *Adv Epileptol* 1987; 16: 229-35.

- McBride MC, Binnie CD, Janota I, Polkey CE. Predictive value of intraoperative electrocorticograms in resective epilepsy surgery. *Ann Neurol* 1991; 30: 526-32.

- Morris HH, III, Luders H, Hahn JF, Lesser RP, Dinner DS, Estes ML. Neurophysiological techniques as an aid to surgical treatment of primary brain tumors. *Ann Neurol* 1986; 19: 559-67.

- Mosewich RK, So EL, O'Brien TJ, Cascino GD, Sharbrough FW, Marsh WR, et al. Factors predictive of the outcome of frontal lobe epilepsy surgery. *Epilepsia* 2000; 41: 843-9.

- Onal C, Otsubo H, Araki T, Chitoku S, Ochi A, Weiss S, et al. Complications of invasive subdural grid monitoring in children with epilepsy. *J Neurosurg* 2003; 98: 1017-26.

- Palmini A, Gambardella A, Andermann F, Dubeau F, Da Costa JC, Olivier A, et al. Intrinsic epileptogenicity of human dysplastic cortex as suggested by corticography and surgical results. *Ann Neurol* 1995; 37: 476-87.

- Paolicchi JM, Jayakar P, Dean P, Yaylali I, Morrison G, Prats A, et al. Predictors of outcome in pediatric epilepsy surgery. *Neurology* 2000; 54: 642-7.

- Ray A, Tao JX, Hawes-Ebersole SM, Ebersole JS. Localizing value of scalp EEG spikes: a simultaneous scalp and intracranial study. *Clin Neurophysiol* 2007; 118: 69-79.

- Rosenbaum TJ, Laxer KD, Vessely M, Smith WB. Subdural electrodes for seizure focus localization. *Neurosurgery* 1986; 19: 73-81.

- Rosenow F, Luders H. Presurgical evaluation of epilepsy. *Brain* 2001; 124: 1683-700.

- Rosenow F, Lüders HO. *Handbook of Clinical Neurophysiology: Presurgical assessment of the epilepsies with clinical neurophysiology and functional imaging.* Amsterdam: Elsevier, 2004.

- Rosenow F, Luders HO, Dinner DS, Prayson RA, Mascha E, Wolgamuth BR, et al. Histopathological correlates of epileptogenicity as expressed by electrocorticographic spiking and seizure frequency. *Epilepsia* 1998; 39: 850-6.

- Salanova V, Andermann F, Olivier A, Rasmussen T, Quesney LF. Occipital lobe epilepsy: electroclinical manifestations, electrocorticography, cortical stimulation and outcome in 42 patients treated between 1930 and 1991. Surgery of occipital lobe epilepsy. *Brain* 1992; 115 (Pt 6): 1655-80.

- Salanova V, Morris HH, III, Van Ness PC, Luders H, Dinner D, Wyllie E. Comparison of scalp electroencephalogram with subdural electrocorticogram recordings and functional mapping in frontal lobe epilepsy. *Arch Neurol* 1993; 50: 294-9.

- Schiller Y, Cascino GD, Busacker NE, Sharbrough FW. Characterization and comparison of local onset and remote propagated electrographic seizures recorded with intracranial electrodes. *Epilepsia* 1998; 39: 380-8.

- Schwartz TH, Bazil CW, Walczak TS, Chan S, Pedley TA, Goodman RR. The predictive value of intraoperative electrocorticography in resections for limbic epilepsy associated with mesial temporal sclerosis. *Neurosurgery* 1997; 40: 302-9.

- Semah F, Picot MC, Adam C, Broglin D, Arzimanoglou A, Bazin B, et al. Is the underlying cause of epilepsy a major prognostic factor for recurrence? *Neurology* 1998; 51: 1256-62.

- Spencer SS, Guimaraes P, Katz A, Kim J, Spencer D. Morphological patterns of seizures recorded intracranially. *Epilepsia* 1992; 33: 537-45.

- Stefan H, Hopfengartner R, Kreiselmeyer G, Weigel D, Rampp S, Kerling F, et al. Interictal triple ECoG characteristics of temporal lobe epilepsies: An intraoperative ECoG analysis correlated with surgical outcome. *Clin Neurophysiol* 2008; 119: 642-52.

- Tao JX, Ray A, Hawes-Ebersole S, Ebersole JS. Intracranial EEG substrates of scalp EEG interictal spikes. *Epilepsia* 2005; 46: 669-76.

- Uematsu S, Lesser R, Fisher RS, Gordon B, Hara K, Krauss GL, Vining EP, Webber RW. Motor and sensory cortex in humans: topography studied with chronic subdural stimulation. *Neurosurgery* 1992; 31: 59-71.

- Weinand ME, Wyler AR, Richey ET, Phillips BB, Somes GW. Long-term ictal monitoring with subdural strip electrodes: prognostic factors for selecting temporal lobectomy candidates. *J Neurosurg* 1992; 77: 20-8.
- Wennberg R, Quesney F, Olivier A, Rasmussen T. Electrocorticography and outcome in frontal lobe epilepsy. *Electroencephalogr Clin Neurophysiol* 1998; 106: 357-68.
- Wennberg R, Quesney LF, Lozano A, Olivier A, Rasmussen T. Role of electrocorticography at surgery for lesion-related frontal lobe epilepsy. *Can J Neurol Sci* 1999; 26: 33-9.
- Wetjen NM, Cohen-Gadol AA, Maher CO, Marsh WR, Meyer FB, Cascino GD. Frontal lobe epilepsy: diagnosis and surgical treatment. *Neurosurg Rev* 2002; 25: 119-38.
- Williamson PD, Boon PA, Thadani VM, Darcey TM, Spencer DD, Spencer SS, *et al*. Parietal lobe epilepsy: diagnostic considerations and results of surgery. *Ann Neurol* 1992a; 31: 193-201.
- Williamson PD, Spencer SS. Clinical and EEG features of complex partial seizures of extratemporal origin. *Epilepsia* 1986; 27 Suppl 2: S46-S63.
- Williamson PD, Thadani VM, Darcey TM, Spencer DD, Spencer SS, Mattson RH. Occipital lobe epilepsy: clinical characteristics, seizure spread patterns, and results of surgery. *Ann Neurol* 1992b; 31: 3-13.
- Wingkun EC, Awad IA, Luders H, Awad CA. Natural history of recurrent seizures after resective surgery for epilepsy. *Epilepsia* 1991; 32: 851-6.
- Wong CH, Birkett J, Byth K, Dexter M, Somerville E, Gill D, *et al*. Risk factors for complications during intracranial electrode recording in presurgical evaluation of drug-resistant partial epilepsy. *Acta Neurochir* (Wien) 2009; 151: 37-50.
- Wyler AR, Walker G, Somes G. The morbidity of long-term seizure monitoring using subdural strip electrodes. *J Neurosurg* 1991; 74: 734-7.
- Wyllie E, Comair YG, Kotagal P, Bulacio J, Bingaman W, Ruggieri P. Seizure outcome after epilepsy surgery in children and adolescents. *Ann Neurol* 1998; 44: 740-8.
- Wyllie E, Luders H, Morris HH, III, Lesser RP, Dinner DS, Rothner AD, *et al*. Subdural electrodes in the evaluation for epilepsy surgery in children and adults. *Neuropediatrics* 1988; 19: 80-6.

Depth-EEG recordings in extratemporal lobe epilepsies

Suela Dylgjeri, Mustapha Benmekhbi, Maysa Sarhan, Dominique Chaussemy, Maria Paola Valenti, Pierre Kehrli, Édouard Hirsch

University Hospitals, Strasbourg, France

"… in April 1939, Penfield performed trephination over both temporal regions and placed electrodes on the dura, intending to lateralize seizure origin in a patient with bitemporal epilepsy… the patient underwent surgery on April 21, revealing a meningocerebral scar in the posterior part of the left temporal lobe…brain stimulation and electrocorticography delineated the extent of resection, while preserving the speech area…"

■ SEEG as a methodology

Surgery is the treatment of choice for pharmacoresistant focal extratemporal lobe epilepsy (ETLE), but this condition remains a surgical challenge due to its complex underlying circuitry, etiology and long-term course associated with childhood onset. While technical advances have significantly improved the surgical management of focal ETLE, the outcomes achieved remain limited when compared to temporal lobe epilepsy surgery.

Invasive EEG plays a crucial role in the pre-surgical assessment of epileptic patients, recordings being routinely performed in most surgical centers for epilepsy, accounting for 25 to 50% of patients (Kahane & Francione, 2008). Commonly, depth-EEG recordings are used to determine the side of onset for temporal lobe epilepsies or to differentiate between frontal and temporal lobe seizures, using standardized intracerebral targets to avoid bias towards a specific exploration site (Engel & Crandall, 1986; Gloor, 1991; Olivier et al., 1983; Spencer, 1981). Rather than using standardized targets for electrodes placement, and relying on the interictal phases to determine abnormal brain activity, Talairach and Bancaud introduced a novel concept in the late sixties, based on recordings tailored to individual clinical presentations (Talairach & Bancaud, 1966). The authors developed stereo-electro-encephalography (SEEG), a method combining anatomo-electro-clinical correlations with the stereotactic placement of intracerebral electrodes in order to assess the origin and spread of ictal discharges prior to surgery. This method takes into account the dynamic and functional nature of seizures, considering their spatio-temporal organization within the brain, based on documented cortical and sub-cortical chronological topographies and temporal progress (Bancaud *et al.*, 1965; Talairach & Bancaud, 1973; Talairach *et al.*, 1974). SEEG is indicated when noninvasive anatomo-electroclinical data are conflicting, inconclusive or suggest the early involvement of highly functional, eloquent areas. The anatomo-functional presentation, comprising the anatomo-electro-clinical data previously obtained using noninvasive investigations, is used to define a working hypothesis with regards to the circuits involved according to which the subsequent intra-cerebral exploration is planned (Bancaud *et al.*, 1965; Bancaud *et al.*, 1973; Kahane & Francione, 2008; Kahane *et al.*, 2006; Munari & Bancaud, 1987; Munari *et al.*, 1986; Talairach & Bancaud, 1973; Talairach *et al.*, 1974). The electrodes are positioned in relation to the hypothesized epileptogenic network involved, keeping in mind that an erroneous implantation strategy will give misleading SEEG information and therefore entails the risk of a poor surgical outcome (Chauvel *et al.*, 1996).

■ Indications

Currently, indications for invasive presurgical monitoring like SEEG remain unclear, but a recent retrospective study showed that a large proportion of patients with no apparent lesions on MRI can still benefit from surgery following SEEG recordings (Cossu *et al.*, 2005).

While there are no defined criteria that can be routinely used to determine whether or not SEEG should be performed, it clearly appears more useful in ETLE rather than TLE, especially for cryptogenic cases. Taking into account its invasive nature, this investigation is rather used where there is evidence of wide extratemporal epileptogenic network engagement, frequent involvement of eloquent areas, specific etiologies or childhood onset epilepsies. These varied indications therefore make it more difficult to define standard exploration planning or resection techniques.

Considering the ictal clinical symptomatology as a seizure pattern using SEEG is particularly useful in ETLE, as this avoids the erroneous interpretation of isolated events or "signal-symptom" (Bancaud *et al.*, 1965) and this allows a better understanding and record of its common multilobar expression. The SEEG study is also particularly valuable in cases where extracerebral artifacts, such as hyperkinetic movements, render the fast seizure propagation over homologous contralateral regions difficult to account for using noninvasive EEG recordings.

Based on the current knowledge, SEEG appears much less needed for lesional epilepsies, including ETLE. It was shown that approximately half of patients suffering from different types of lesions underwent SEEG and the use of intracerebral recordings remains essential in the vast majority of cryptogenic cases, probably due to the high proportion of multilobar epilepsies in such patients (Kahane *et al.*, 1994; Munari *et al.*, 1995). Furthermore, the histological nature of a lesion, and/or its topography, may at least partially influence the decision.

Temporal plus epilepsies

Commonly, SEEG is performed in TLE when neocortical or extratemporal ictal onset is possible or when electro-clinical data suggest "temporal plus" seizures. The term "temporal plus epilepsies" was recently introduced and refers to bilobar or extratemporal seizure onset epilepsies that appear to further benefit from the joint resection of temporal and extra-temporal regions (Kahane et al., 2001; Ryvlin & Kahane, 2005).

In this context, and using SEEG recordings, the group of Kahane gave evidence of the involvement of temporo-polar regions (Kahane et al., 2002) as well as the insular (Isnard et al., 2000) and perisylvian cortex (Kahane et al., 2001) based on surgical case series.

The designation of extratemporal epileptogenic network has to include both temporal and extratemporal sites, for instance insulo-opercular, temporo-parieto-occipital junction, or anterior frontal cortex seizure spread patterns. The aim of a wide exploration planning is to identify potential extratemporal ictal onset regions to be included within the epilep-togenic zone, in addition to the temporal lobe. This methodology is necessary for the correct subsequent multilobar surgery that is individually tailored to optimize the surgical outcome.

Cases that require bilateral exploration remain rare, but when necessary, the side of dis-charges is first determined using noninvasive anatomo-electro-clinical data, and the implantation is usually asymmetric. Previously, these cases were erroneously considered as bitemporal epilepsies, with poor surgical outcomes, and these benefit from the use of SEEG to identify the additional epileptogenic regions that developed later during the course of the disease.

Frontal epilepsies

Frontal lobe epilepsy (FLE) surgery is the second most common resective surgery performed for pharmacoresistant epilepsy after temporal lobe resections, and patients with FLE dis-playing normal imaging are considered to be the most challenging when analyzing surgical outcomes (Jeha et al., 2007).

Currently, a defined "syndromic" classification of frontal lobe epilepsy is lacking, but it is commonly divided into central, premotor and prefrontal FLE with further medial and lateral subdivisions (Chauvel, 2003). Scalp EEG is often inadequate and limited, especially for the detection of mesial and basal foci, with an increased risk of misdiagnosis or "para-doxical lateralization" in addition to extra-cerebral artifacts with hyperkinetic seizures (Kellinghaus & Lüders, 2004).

Major advances in the understanding of the semiology of prefrontal seizures were achieved with the use of SEEG, demonstrating the complexity and individual variability characte-ristic of FLE (Chauvel, 2003; Jobst et al., 2000). Accordingly, clinical signs such as echo-lalia, singing and distal hand tapping with semi-purposeful movements, forms of "forced acting" or pseudo-compulsive behavior, were described as features of dorsolateral prefrontal seizures (Bancaud & Talairach, 1992; Bartolomei et al., 2007; Chauvel & Bancaud, 1994). On the other hand, prefrontal mesio-ventral cortical involvement is characterized by proximal purposeless and often violent movements (also called "hypermotor seizures") (Chauvel, 2003). Anterior cingulate region involvement is rather suggested when ictal emotional modifications are associated with stereotypical motor behaviors (Bancaud & Talairach, 1992) under the influence of known central pattern generators (Tassinari et *al.*, 2005). Other signs and symptoms justify the exclusion of defined areas from the abnormal neuronal firing region. For instance, the absence of language dysfunction during the ictal or post-ictal phases argues against an involvement of the dominant hemisphere and likewise retained consciousness during a seizure argues against the bilateral frontal or temporal lobe spread.

Based on this anatomo-functional understanding, it is important to accurately evaluate the extent of cortical involvement that generates recurrent seizures, as well as the extent of the region to be removed in order to yield a satisfactory decrease in the rate of these events, thereby emphasizing the essential role of pre-operative recording and mapping methods (Rasmussen, 1983). It clearly appears from the literature that invasive acute or chronic depth monitoring is usually indicated in FLE prior to surgery, as reported by several surgical centers (Quesney *et al.*, 1992; Schramm *et al.*, 2002).

The anatomical characteristics of the frontal lobe, such as the depth of its sulci and structures, combined with the presence of major eloquent and associative areas, and its multiple distant lobar connections, make the SEEG study essential, usually requiring a wide exploration, that is most often bilateral and almost always very asymmetric.

In 1989 Munari *et al.* reported the evaluation of SEEG in surgical cases, amongst which about a third of patients were investigated for FLE (Munari *et al.*, 1989). The stereotactic placement of electrodes allowed the simultaneous recording of electrical activity in both the mesial and lateral cortical areas, as well as extra-frontal, mainly temporal, sites in 75% of the cases. As a result, SEEG was shown to be effective in reducing the extent of the resection area, based on the analysis of the spatial patterns of the abnormal discharges.

In a recent multivariate analysis, the presence of a well-circumscribed lesion on the preoperative MRI was shown to be predictive of a good long-term surgical outcome (Elsharkawy *et al.*, 2008). This is consistent with the fact that a better rate of remission is noted in the presence of localized lesions, for instance in focal cortical dysplasia (FCD), in association with SEEG when this investigation is indicated (for lesions near or within eloquent areas), partly because it allows a more focused exploration (Colombo *et al.*, 2003; Francione *et al.*, 2003).

The involvement of a well-defined neural network such as the fronto-orbital, orbito-cingulate, mesial premotor or dorsolateral frontal cortex also allows a more efficient, targeted exploration. Hence, in cases of fronto-orbital epilepsies, the exploration will mainly be focused on the gyrus rectus, orbital cortex, frontal pole, lateral fronto-basal cortex, anterior cingulate gyrus and temporal pole. Similarly, seizures that are suspected to arise from the mesial wall of the premotor cortex are investigated within the supplementary motor area, pre-supplementary motor area, the cingulate motor area, cingulate gyrus and primary motor cortex. Using this systematic approach, very small epileptogenic regions can be identified, resulting in smaller surgical resections, some cases showing a good response to focal thermocoagulation (Chassagnon *et al.*, 2003; Schmitt *et al.*, 2006).

The clinical picture is very different in more complex cases, such as in "frontal multi-lobar cases" for which the ictal discharges often include central regions and still necessitate a particularly wide exploration planning as is the case with rapid quasi-simultaneous bilateral spreads (Talairach *et al.*, 1992). The anatomo-pathophysiological data are most important in cryptogenic cases, but unfortunately even combined with SEEG, the surgical outcomes remain mediocre for these epilepsies (*Case 1*).

Central region epilepsies

Central region exploration is indicated in cases where it is suspected to be involved as an epileptogenic zone. It also allows the "functionality" assessment of the ictal onset zone, particularly important in focal lesions like FCD, that are eligible for limited resections preventing further propagation to adjacent frontal and parietal structures. Using intracerebral electrodes it is possible to explore the depth of the rolandic fissure, as well as the descending motor and ascending sensory pathways. Nowadays the implantation procedure is automated, which facilitates oblique approaches and thus allows further exploration of the adjacent frontal and parietal areas with a reduced risk of post-operative functional deficits. The type of post-surgical deficits and the course of recovery are mainly dependent upon the anatomical location and extent of the cortical resection, as well as the disease-induced plasticity that occurred in the motor cortex and its projections. Ultimately, lower central cortical resection does not appear to cause significant long-term neurological deficits (Chassoux et al., 1999; Lehman et al., 1994).

As published literature emphasizes, the outcome of surgery is influenced by the pre-surgical evaluation method. Routine diagnostic methods allow approximately 40 to almost 60% of patients to remain practically seizure free in response to surgical resection in the long-term (Jeha et al., 2007; Rasmussen, 1991), but combined with SEEG mapping these results are increased to 70% and even 90% when considering lesion-related epilepsy such as FCD and dysembryoplastic neuroepithelial tumors (Trottier et al., 2008).

In patients suffering from disabling sleep related seizures with a frontal lobe origin, resective surgery following an accurate pre-surgical SEEG evaluation should also be considered, as it often provides excellent results for both seizures and epilepsy related sleep disturbances, particularly in Taylor-type FCD (Nobili et al., 2007).

Posterior

The literature reports fairly good surgical outcomes for posterior cortex epilepsy, preferably for occipital lobe resections rather than parietooccipital or parietal (Jehi et al., 2009), with better results in lesional-related epilepsies for both adults (Elsharkawy et al., 2009; Salanova et al., 1992) and children (Sinclair et al., 2005). Early surgery allows good seizure control and neuopsychological improvement, especially in children with FCD (Lortie et al., 2002).

The semiology of posterior epilepsy often reflects the propagation pattern of abnormal discharges, hence a misleading presentation in comparison to temporal lobe epilepsy. Also, the accuracy of scalp-EEG is dependent upon the type of intracerebral interictal distribution, particularly in medial and medio-lateral localizations and in non-lesional cases (Gavaret et al., 2009). The precise definition of the resection area using depth recording, electrocorticography (Salanova et al., 1992), subdural recording (Blume et al., 2005) and a presurgical protocol, plays a central role in favor of better surgical outcomes (Barba et al., 2005).

Commonly, the epileptogenic network involving the posterior cortex affects simultaneously the occipital, parietal and posterior temporal areas, sometimes combined with a multidirectional spread of discharges to the central, frontal, insulo-opercular and temporal regions. Considering the frequent involvement of the visual cortex and language areas in posterior epilepsy, be it due to the focal origin or the subsequent propagation, it is essential to investigate further using SEEG recordings to avoid as much as possible neurological deficits.

Exclusively posterior seizures, particularly with parietal onset, are mostly characterized by a subjective ictal semiology and are often followed by the expression of their propagation to central, frontal or temporo-mesial structures. In contrast, occipital onset is more frequently associated with mono or biocular nystagmus. Usually a large number of electrodes and complex arrangements are needed for the exploration, especially when the hypothetic ictal onset zone is in associative areas, such as the postero-medial aspect of the parietal lobe.

Also, a bilateral exploration is often required for cases presenting early and strong motor manifestations, leading to falls, and for patients where the scalp EEG suggests bi-occipital discharges with very rapid anterior spreading, or a bi-temporal propagation. Not surprisingly, the SEEG planning remains quite asymmetric in these cases, reflecting the hypothetical epileptogenic zone.

The classical targets in posterior SEEG planning are the peri-calcarin cortex, the inferior and superior parietal lobules, the posterior cingulate cortex, as well as junction territories such as the lingual lobule and fusiform gyrus, the angular and supra-marginal gyri, the precuneus, or the retrosplenial cortex.

Propagation from the occipital lobe to temporo-mesial structures and to the retrosplenial cortex are not rare and an exploration of both mesial and temporo-neocortical structures is essential (CASES).

Recently, a study reported a good surgical outcome for well defined lesional-related epilepsies with a pre-existent visual field defect, regardless of the pre-surgical evaluation type (Tandon et al., 2009). In these cases, the exploration planning can be kept within a restricted area, thereby avoiding subsequent visual deficits.

Multilobar discharges

Multilobar discharges are another important characteristic of ETLE and reflect the wide multi-lobar epileptogenic network involved in seizures, particularly evident when associative areas are affected. In this respect, the electro-clinical pattern is difficult to reproduce through stimulation protocols, thus challenging the accurate definition of the resection area (Kahane et al., 2001; Palmini et al., 1999; Quesney et al., 1992; Talairach et al., 1992) Posterior epilepsies are typically associated with multilobar discharges.

Munari and colleagues reported that for about 20% of patients studied by SEEG, the epileptogenic zone included distinct, but interconnected, regions in different lobes within one hemisphere, and when the epileptogenic zones were almost or completely removed, more than 80% of patients were cured, while when the removal was clearly incomplete, the percentage of seizure-free patients dropped to 10% (Munari et al., 1995).

SEEG exploration is especially useful in defining the epileptogenic zone in extratemporal and multilobar epilepsies, and it facilitates a tailored resection of extralesional cortex to obtain better surgical outcomes (Francione et al., 2003) (Case 2).

Multilobar discharges are particularly obvious in cases of extensive multilobar cortical dysplasia in infants, who commonly first present with devastating epilepsy that is a therapeutic challenge for seizure control, brain development, and psychosocial outcomes. There is limited experience in the context of surgical treatment for these lesions, with often not very encouraging results and a higher operative risk when compared to older children and adults. The introduction of disconnective techniques in the surgery for extensive multilobar cortical dysplasia in infants has made it possible to achieve excellent seizure control by maximizing the extent of surgical treatment to include the entire epileptogenic zone. These techniques decrease perioperative morbidity, and the long-term complications associated with large brain excisions, further maintaining the excellent short-term results obtained with resective surgery (Daniel *et al.*, 2007).

Multifocal discharges

Currently, depth recordings are rarely indicated to determine whether the epileptogenic zone is unifocal or multifocal. Patients with electro-clinical evidence of different epileptogenic foci are commonly excluded from surgery following noninvasive investigations. It is important to realize that different types of seizures are sometimes due to specific circuits or they can result from extensive abnormal areas that paradoxically are safe for resection. In specific cases, especially in the presence of lesions as in tuberous sclerosis complex, conducting a SEEG can help to establish the nature of the seizures, and although they may appear multifocal, in view of the SEEG results they can be reconsidered as surgical cases (Sivelle *et al.*, 1995). These cases illustrate to an extreme extent, the very complex and detailed analysis required when performing SEEG, from planning the investigation to the specific individually tailored surgery.

The use of SEEG prior to resective or disconnective surgery for intractable partial epilepsy in functional areas of the brain may provide excellent results on seizures and a moderate risk of permanent neurological deficits. The outcome certainly depends on the etiology of the epilepsy, with a seizure-free state achieved for 93% of Taylor-type FCD but only for 40% of cryptogenic epilepsies (Devaux *et al.*, 2008).

Consistent with these results, a better surgical outcome is achieved with limited exploration when SEEG is performed in the presence of lesions, for instance when abnormal areas are near or within eloquent cortex in cases of FCD.

■ Subjacent etiology

According to the literature, FCD appears to represent the major neuro-pathological abnormality present in more than a third of ETLE cases, following which developmental tumors are found in over a quarter of patients and encephalo-malacia is identified in another fifth. However, less than 20% of specimens showed pathological abnormalities even when surgery provided a good outcome for seizures. ETLE is commonly seen in children and usually results from congenital cortical malformations, this is in contrast to what is seen in adults, where the epilepsy usually results from tumors, injury or other acquired cortical abnormalities.

It is now well documented that the presence of a lesion in pharmacoresistant focal epilepsy is associated with good surgical outcomes, whereas cryptogenic cases, especially extratemporal epilepsies, still carry poor outcomes, reaching less than 50% seizure-free rates (Devaux et al., 2008; Tellez-Zenteno et al., 2010).

The clinical use of SEEG is much less valuable for lesional epilepsies, although about half of patients affected by lesion-related focal pharmacoresistant epilepsy still undergo SEEG studies in some Surgical Centres such as Grenoble and Milan (Kahane et al., 1994). It still remains a strong indication for specific lesional pharmacoresistant focal epilepsies such as extratemporal dysembryoplastic neuroepithelial tumors.

The major indication for SEEG is the presence of an unknown epileptic aetiology, for which the surgical outcomes are at least partly influenced by the hypothetical histological nature of a lesion and/or its topography.

In fact in SEEG terminology, the lesional zone refers to the brain area that presents an abnormal slow-wave activity or, in some cases, a major alteration of the background activity or even sometimes an electrical silence (Bancaud et al., 1973; Munari et al., 1986; Munari et al., 1983). This area is not necessarily associated with a noticeable lesion on the MRI, or with a lesion as assessed on pathological specimens (Bancaud et al. 1973; Bancaud, 1980; Munari et al., 1983, 1986), but it appears very important and needs to be taken into account for the final surgical decision.

Despite ongoing, rapid advances in MR techniques, a large proportion of all dysplasias remain undetected by magnetic resonance imaging, and it is acknowledged that even lesions visible on MRI may only be the "tip of the iceberg" (Luders & Schuele, 2006). Some studies report poor surgical prognosis for cortical developmental malformations in the absence of visible MRI abnormalities (Jeha et al., 2007), whereas SEEG studies yield excellent outcomes in such patients, as demonstrated by other authors (Nobili et al., 2007; Trottier et al., 2008).

Interestingly, FCD displays a characteristic SEEG pattern with epileptiform abnormalities including interictal and preictal rhythmic spike discharges and the occurrence of very fast ictal discharges within the same localized region, suggesting an underlying dysplastic lesion despite a normal MRI (Chassoux et al., 2000; Francione et al., 2003). The histological evaluation usually confirms a type IIB FCD (Taylor-type, with balloon cells) in the resected tissue. The epileptogenic zone is often larger than the lesion itself (Chassoux et al., 2000) and the SEEG is useful in assessing dysplastic lesions based on direct intra-lesional recordings, that can then combined with thermocoagulation often resulting in the complete control of seizures (Catenoix et al., 2008).

■ Children (last but not least)

The beneficial surgical outcome obtained in children argues in favor of early interventions, even when the seizure focus is outside of the temporal lobe (Adler et al., 1991). There is published evidence that the surgical outcome in FLE is better for children compared to adults, suggesting that cerebral plasticity may contribute to these results (Fauser et al., 2008) and this is particularly the case for tumor-associated epilepsy (Devaux et al., 2008).

Generally it is more complex to perform an SEEG in children than in adults and even more so in ETLE. Age-related peculiarities make localizing hypotheses more difficult to elaborate compared to adults, but the method remains feasible and safe even in children as young as 3 years of age (Kahane *et al.*, 2002; Kahane *et al.*, 1998).

■ New technologies

Recent technical advances have made oblique approaches more accessible, through robotized technology for intracranial electrodes implantation such as neuronavigaton. This allows a better exploration of both the lateral and mesial structures and the sulcus of Rolando despite its antero-posterior orientation, including motor and somato-sensory pathways. It also reduces the risks associated with implantation and often avoids other invasive assessments, such as cerebral arteriography. Exploration of the insula was recently described using these novel approaches as parasagittal electrodes, parallel to the insular cortex, were lowered with an entry point at the parieto-occipital junction (Robles *et al.*, 2009). This was entirely based on MRI scans and avoided passing through the opercula, with a reduced risk of injury to the perisylvian vessels. All these advantages are particularly important when SEEG is considered and performed in children.

■ Surgery... and conclusions

The concept of epileptogenic zone was developed by Talairach and Bancaud to emphasize the importance of planning surgical treatment based on abnormal neural activity recorded during seizures, rather than during the interictal phase. Later, Munari and Bancaud in 1987 (Munari *et al.*, 1989), further defined the epileptogenic zone as the site of beginning and primary organization of the epileptic seizures. More recently, Kahane and Francione in 2006 (Kahane *et al.*, 2006), suggested that the epileptogenic zone is only part of a wider entity, the epileptogenic network, referring to the multiple interconnected brain structures, including subcortical regions, involved in the initiation, propagation, and clinical expression of the epileptic seizures. The accurate assessment of the resection area should therefore be based on the thorough analysis of spontaneous seizures recordings within the context of the whole electro-clinical pattern. This includes analysis of the post-ictal phase and stimulation results, as well as the assessment of functional areas and technical aspects of the surgical approach.

There is clear evidence of improved surgical results for TLE, with or without the presence of a lesion on MRI, but the outcomes remain moderate for ETLE, especially for cryptogenic cases. In these cases, the complex epileptogenic networks, histological changes rather than MRI evidence of lesions, and early epilepsy onset associated with neuropsychological and behavioral implications, all make the SEEG investigation essential for an optimal management.

More than just a presurgical evaluation tool, SEEG is a comprehensive method based the analysis of the spatio-temporal dynamics of seizure discharges, known as the epileptogenic zone, rather than just focusing on their starting point, the ictal onset zone. Despite these recent improvements, this method still cannot unambiguously locate all the cortical areas to be removed for the complete, seizure-free, curative result.

Several novel analysis methods are being currently developed to interpret intracranial signals, usually as a joint effort with epileptologists. These tools are created in order to better identify the epileptogenic zone and hence understand the networks involved, with the ultimate ambition of improved surgical outcomes (Aubert *et al.*, 2009; Bartolomei *et al.*, 2008; Bragin *et al.*, 1999; Gardner *et al.*, 2007; Jacobs *et al.*, 2008; Schiff *et al.*, 2000; Schindler *et al.*, 2007; Wendling *et al.*, 2003; 2009).

The use of SEEG as a therapeutic option is currently regaining interest, as evidenced by thermocoagulation procedures that are now reintroduced, after being first developed in the sixties for epilepsy and psychosurgery. These techniques can be used in palliative care as demonstrated recently (Catenoix *et al.*, 2008; Guenot *et al.*, 2004). Thermocoagulation is safe, well-tolerated and almost free from permanent deficits. Its primary indication is when conventional respective surgery entails high risks or is contraindicated, bearing in mind that it does not exclude further surgery. Optimal results were obtained in the presence of well-defined lesional epilepsies like FCD, while further studies are still needed to improve technical aspects and to assess long-term outcomes.

■ Illustrative cases

Case I *(Figure I)*

We report the case of a 14 years old right-handed girl, with a background of familial consanguinity, no history of febrile convulsions and with a normal neuropsychological development until the age of 6 years old. The patient first presented with morpheic/nocturnal seizures, characterized by sudden awakening, fear, a hypertonic right arm and postictal dysphasia. The seizures were not adequately controlled, despite the use of several antiepileptic drugs (valproic acid, carbamazepine, topiramate, zonisamide and levetiracet). Neuropsychological assessments indicate an important and irreversible impairment first characterized by a continual deficit in attention, loss of inhibition and aggressive behavior. Later, the patient developed a deficit in verbal comprehension and fluency with a progression towards mutism, lack of initiative, perseveration and excessive inhibition. At 14 years old, a presurgical evaluation was performed that revealed a normal neurological examination. Video-EEG monitoring showed a symmetrical normal background activity, with normal bifrontal spikes, both synchronous and asynchronous, with a clear left predominance. Electroclinical seizures were recorded during sleep, clinically characterized by a sudden awakening, accompanied by fear. The patient usually looked around her then performed a bilateral "grimace" and bilateral hypertonic abduction of the arms with a right prevalence and a right and up oculo-cephalic deviation associated with verbigeration followed by aphasia during the postictal phase. The corresponding EEG showed a bilateral slowing of the background activity, a rhythmic bifrontal theta activity with left prevalence, followed by widespread biphasic spikes prior to the onset of a diffuse low voltage fast activity spreading over both hemispheres, with a left predominance. The brain MRI showed no visible anomalies *(Figure 1a)*. A very slight hypometabolism was noted in the left superior frontal gyrus on the FDG-PETSCAN analysis. Both the metabolic and genetic assessments were negative, in particular for ADNFLE, fragile X and ring chromosome 20. This anatomo-electro-clinical and functional presentation led us to offer an SEEG exploration to the patient, in order to define the epileptogenic zone in a cryptogenic frontal lobe epilepsy.

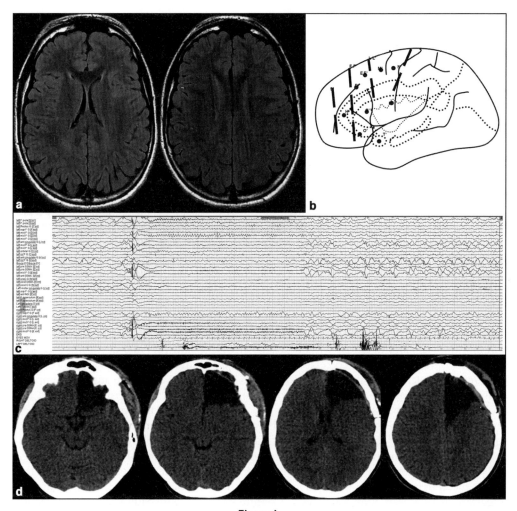

Figure 1.

The SEEG planning included a bifrontal exploration with an emphasis on the left side based on the prior hypothesis (*Figure 1b*). The spontaneous seizures recording and stimulation protocols were used to define the epileptogenic zone that included the left prefrontal area and anterior cingulate gyrus, bilateral pre-supplementary sensorimotor area (pre-SSMA) and SSMA, with a precedence and prevalence of the left side. In view of these results we proceeded to perform thermocoagulation in the left prefrontal and pre-SSMA (120 mA, 50 V, 20 sec) without significant results. Two months later, surgical resection was performed including the left prefrontal, pre-SSMA and SSMA areas and the left anterior cingulate gyrus. During the first 36-48 hours post-surgery, the patient was aphasic and presented a motor deficit of the right arm, with a subsequent complete spontaneous recovery. During the first week following surgery, the patient had one tonic-clonic generalized seizure. The histological specimen was negative. About 6 months post-surgery, the patient was seizure-free, with no behavioral disorder and a slight language improvement was noted.

Case 2 (Figure 2)

This is the case of a 13 years old, left-handed, girl without any significant family or personal history, who started having seizures at the age of 3 months old (spasms). At 6 months old, she also started having focal seizures characterized by clonic rightward eyes deviation associated with blinking. The EEG performed suggested a West syndrome and was treated with vigabatrin, further combined with benzodiazepines and stiripentol, to obtain an apparently seizure control for some years. Around the age of 7 years old, the seizures reappeared with an initial sensation of "vertigo" or right eye "jump" during which the patient was able to speak, followed by a hypertonic-dystonic posture of the arms. The postictal phase was short and without motor or language deficit. The seizures occurred in both diurnal and nocturnal clusters. At the age of 14, a pre-surgical evaluation was performed. MRI showed a thickened left occipito-temporal gyrus with a discrete hypersignal in FLAIR images, but no other MRI abnormalities were found (Figure 2a). The brain FDG-PETS-CAN showed hypometabolism over the left occipito-temporal regions. Video-EEG monitoring showed an asymmetric background activity characterized by a slow activity in the left posterior region, particularly occipito-temporal, with slow focal abnormalities and spikes over the left occipito-temporal region. Sleep increased the frequency of spikes and facilitated their propagation over the left occipito-temporo-parietal regions. Several electroclinical seizures were recorded during nocturnal sleep: the clinical pattern was characterized by an initial right ocular-cephalic deviation followed by a dystonic posture of the right hand, then a left cephalic deviation associated with a dystonic posture of the left arm and the legs, and eventually led to a further right oculo-cephalic deviation and stertorous respiration. The EEG correlation consisted in a flattening in T5-O1 followed by a rhythmic theta activity that further involved the left posterior and more anterior temporal regions and later spread over the controlateral regions, with a slow and depressed left occipito-temporo-parietal postictal phase. The neuropsychological evaluation revealed an impairment in cognitive functions, especially visuo-constructive and visuo-spatial, without behavioral disorders. The visual field assessment showed a homologous right infero-temporal partial quadrantanopsia. These anatomo-electro-clinical features led us to offer to the patient and her family a SEEG investigation, the main aim of which was to better define the epileptogenic zone and to avoid, if possible, an hemianopsia through a limited resection area without compromising the seizure outcome. The SEEG planning included the left occipito-temporo-parietal regions (Figure 2b). Several spontaneous seizures were recorded that, combined with the stimulation protocol, allowed to define the epileptogenic zone, which included the left calcarin cortex and temporo-mesial structures. Thermocoagulation was performed (120 mA, 50 V, 20 sec), including the anterior calcarin cortex, the inferior occipital gyrus and the posterior part of the lingual gyrus, resulting in an improvement in seizures frequency. One month later, surgical resection was performed with a posterior approach, including the left inferior occipital gyrus, the lingual and fusiform gyrus and the hippocampus. The histological specimens concluded in a non classified neuronal migration disorder. Although he visual field assessment revealed a larger deficit in the right temporal hemifield when compared to the pre-surgical state, the patient remains seizure-free around six months following surgery.

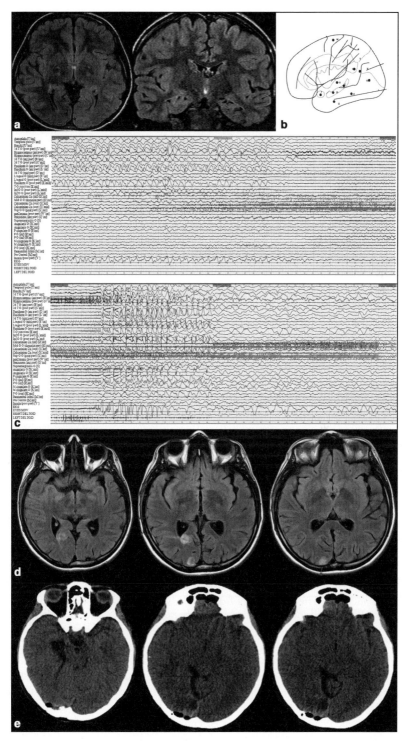

Figure 2.

References

- Adler J, Erba G, Winston KR, Welch K, Lombroso CT. Results of surgery for extratemporal partial epilepsy that began in childhood. *Arch Neurol* 1991; 48: 133-40.
- Aubert S, Wendling F, Regis J, McGonigal A, Figarella-Branger D, Peragut JC, *et al.* Local and remote epileptogenicity in focal cortical dysplasias and neurodevelopmental tumours. *Brain* 2009; 132: 3072-86.
- Bancaud J, Talairach J. Clinical semiology of frontal lobe seizures. *Adv Neurol* 1992; 57: 3-58.
- Bancaud J, Talairach J, Bonis A, *et al.* La stéréoencéphalographie dans l'épilepsie. Informations neuro-physio-pathologiques apportées par l'investigation fonctionnelle stéréotaxique. Paris: Masson, 1965.
- Bancaud J, Talairach J, Geier S, Scarabin JM. EEG et SEEG dans les tumeurs cérébrales et l'épilepsie. Paris: Edifor, 1973.
- Barba C, Doglietto F, De Luca L, Faraca G, Marra C, Meglio M, *et al.* Retrospective analysis of variables favouring good surgical outcome in posterior epilepsies. *J Neurol* 2005; 252: 465-72.
- Bartolomei F, Chauvel P, Wendling F. Epileptogenicity of brain structures in human temporal lobe epilepsy: a quantified study from intracerebral EEG. *Brain* 2008; 131: 1818-30.
- Bartolomei F, McGonigal A, Guye M, Guedj E, Chauvel P. Clinical and anatomic characteristics of humming and singing in partial seizures. Neurology 2007; 69: 490-2.
- Blume WT, Wiebe S, Tapsell LM. Occipital epilepsy: lateral versus mesial. *Brain* 2005; 128: 1209-25.
- Bragin A, Engel J Jr, Wilson CL, Fried I, Mathern GW. Hippocampal and entorhinal cortex high-frequency oscillations (100-500 Hz) in human epileptic brain and in kainic acid--treated rats with chronic seizures. *Epilepsia* 1999; 40: 127-37.
- Catenoix H, Mauguiere F, Guenot M, Ryvlin P, Bissery A, Sindou M, Isnard J. SEEG-guided thermocoagulations: a palliative treatment of nonoperable partiale epilepsies. *Neurology* 2008; 71: 1719-26.
- Chassagnon S, Minotti L, Kremer S, Verceuil L, Hoffmann D, Benabid AL, Kahane P. Restricted frontomesial epileptogenic focus generating dyskinetic behavior and laughter. *Epilepsia* 2003; 44: 859-63.
- Chassoux F, Devaux B, Landre E, Chodkiewicz JP, Talairach J, Chauvel P. Postoperative motor deficits and recovery after cortical resections. *Adv Neurol* 1999; 81: 189-99.
- Chassoux F, Devaux B, Landre E, Turak B, Nataf F, Varlet P, *et al.* Stereoelectroencephalography in focal cortical dysplasia: a 3D approach to delineating the dysplastic cortex. Brain 2000; 123 (Pt 8): 1733-51.
- Chauvel P. Can we classify frontal lobe epilepsy? In: Baumanoir A, Andermann F, Chauvel P, Mira LBZ, eds. *Frontal Lobe Epilepsies in Children.* London: John Libbey, 2003, pp. 59-64.
- Chauvel P, Bancaud J. The spectrum of frontal lobe seizures: with a note of frontal lobe syndromatology. In: Wolf P, ed. *Epileptic Seizures and Syndromes.* London: John Libbey and Company, 1994.
- Chauvel P, Vignal JP, Biraben A, Scarabin JM. Stereoelectroencephalography. In: Pawlik G, Stephan H, eds. *Focus Localization.* Berlin: Liga Verlag, 1996.
- Colombo N, Tassi L, Galli C, Citterio A, Lo Russo G, Scialfa G, Spreafico R. Focal cortical dysplasias: MR imaging, histopathologic, and clinical correlations in surgically treated patients with epilepsy. *AJNR Am J Neuroradiol* 2003; 24: 724-33.
- Cossu M, Cardinale F, Castana L, Citterio A, Francione S, Tassi L, *et al.* Stereoelectroencephalography in the presurgical evaluation of focal epilepsy: a retrospective analysis of 215 procedures. *Neurosurgery* 2005; 57: 706-18.

- Daniel RT, Meagher-Villemure K, Farmer JP, Andermann F, Villemure JG. Posterior quadrantic epilepsy surgery: technical variants, surgical anatomy, and case series. *Epilepsia* 2007; 48: 1429-37.

- Devaux B, Chassoux F, Landre E, Turak B, Abou-Salma Z, Mann M, *et al.* Surgical resections in functional areas: report of 89 cases. *Neurochirurgie* 2008; 54: 409-17.

- Elsharkawy AE, Alabbasi AH, Pannek H, Schulz R, Hoppe M, Pahs G, *et al.* Outcome of frontal lobe epilepsy surgery in adults. *Epilepsy Res* 2008; 81, 97-106.

- Elsharkawy AE, El-Ghandour NM, Oppel F, Pannek H, Schulz R, Hoppe M, *et al.* Long-term outcome of lesional posterior cortical epilepsy surgery in adults. *J Neurol Neurosurg Psychiatry* 2009; 80: 773-80.

- Engel JJ, Crandall PH. Intensive neurodiagnostic monitoring with intracranial electrodes. In: Gumnit R, ed. *Intensive Neurodiagnostic Monitoring.* New York: Raven Press, 1986, pp. 85-106.

- Fauser S, Bast T, Altenmuller DM, Schulte-Monting J, Strobl K, Steinhoff BJ, *et al.* Factors influencing surgical outcome in patients with focal cortical dysplasia. *J Neurol Neurosurg Psychiatry* 2008; 79 : 103-5.

- Francione S, Vigliano P, Tassi L, Cardinale F, Mai R, Lo Russo G, Munari C. Surgery for drug resistant partial epilepsy in children with focal cortical dysplasia: anatomical-clinical correlations and neurophysiological data in 10 patients. *J Neurol Neurosurg Psychiatry* 2003; 74: 1493-501.

- Gardner AB, Worrell GA, Marsh E, Dlugos D, Litt B. Human and automated detection of high-frequency oscillations in clinical intracranial EEG recordings. *Clin Neurophysiol* 2007; 118: 1134-43.

- Gavaret M, Trebuchon A, Bartolomei F, Marquis P, McGonigal A, Wendling F, *et al.* Source localization of scalp-EEG interictal spikes in posterior cortex epilepsies investigated by HR-EEG and SEEG. *Epilepsia* 2009; 50: 276-89.

- Gloor P. Preoperative electroencephalographic investigation in temporal lobe epilepsy: extracranial and intracranial recordings. *Can J Neurol Sci* 1991; 18: 554-8.

- Guenot M, Isnard J, Ryvlin P, Fischer C, Mauguiere F, Sindou M. SEEG-guided RF thermocoagulation of epileptic foci: feasibility, safety, and preliminary results. *Epilepsia* 2004; 45: 1368-74.

- Isnard J, Guenot M, Ostrowsky K, Sindou M, Mauguiere F. The role of the insular cortex in temporal lobe epilepsy. *Ann Neurol* 2000; 48: 614-23.

- Jacobs J, LeVan P, Chander R, Hall J, Dubeau F, Gotman J. Interictal high-frequency oscillations (80-500 Hz) are an indicator of seizure onset areas independent of spikes in the human epileptic brain. *Epilepsia* 2008; 49: 1893-907.

- Jeha LE, Najm I, Bingaman W, Dinner D, Widdess-Walsh P, Lüders H. Surgical outcome and prognostic factors of frontal lobe epilepsy surgery. *Brain* 2007; 130: 574-84.

- Jeha LE, O'Dwyer R, Najm I, Alexopoulos A, Bingaman W. A longitudinal study of surgical outcome and its determinants following posterior cortex epilepsy surgery. *Epilepsia* 2009; 50: 2040-52.

- Jobst BC, Siegel AM, Thadani VM, Roberts DW, Rhodes HC, Williamson PD. Intractable seizures of frontal lobe origin: clinical characteristics, localizing signs, and results of surgery. *Epilepsia* 2000; 41: 1139-52.

- Kahane P. Chabardes S, Minotti L, Hoffmann D, Benabid AL, Munari C. The role of the temporal pole in the genesis of temporal lobe seizures. *Epileptic Disord* 2002; 4 (Suppl 1): S51-8.

- Kahane P, Francione S. Stereoelectroencephalography. In: Lüders H, ed. *Textbook of Epilepsy Surgery.* Informa HealthCare, 2008.

- Kahane P, Francione S, Tassi L, Hoffmann D, Lo Russo GM, Benabid AL, Munari C. Results of epilepsy surgery: criteria for validation of presurgical investigations. *Boll Lega It Epil* 1994; 86/87: 405-19.

- Kahane P, Hoffmann D, Francione S, Tassi L, Di Leo M, Benabid A, Munari C. La stéréo-electro-encéphalographie chez l'enfant : outil diagnostique et préchirurgical. In: Bureau M, Kahane P, Munari C, eds. *Épilepsies partielles graves pharmaco-résistantes de l'enfant, Stratégies diagnostiques et traitements chirurgicaux.* Paris: John Libbey Eurotext, 1998, pp. 135-151.

- Kahane P, Huot J, Hoffmann D, *et al.* Perisylvian cortex involvement in seizures affecting the temporal lobe. In: Avanzini G, Beaumanoir A, Mira L, eds. *Limbic Seizures in Children.* London: John Libbey, 2001, pp. 115-127.

- Kahane P, Landre E, Minotti L, Francione S, Ryvlin P. The Bancaud and Talairach view on the epileptogenic zone: a working hypothesis. *Epileptic Disord* 2006; 8 (Suppl 2): S16-26.

- Kellinghaus C. Lüders HO. Frontal Lobe Epilepsy. *Epileptic Disord* 2004; 6: 223-39.

- Lehman R, Andermann F, Olivier A, Tandon PN, Quesney LF, Rasmussen TB. Seizures with onset in the sensorimotor face area: clinical patterns and results of surgical treatment in 20 patients. *Epilepsia* 1994; 35: 1117-24.

- Lortie A, Plouin P, Chiron C, Delalande O, Dulac O. Characteristics of epilepsy in focal cortical dysplasia in infancy. *Epilepsy Res* 2002; 51: 133-45.

- Lüders H, Schuele SU. Epilepsy surgery in patients with malformations of cortical development. *Curr Opin Neurol* 2006; 19: 169-74.

- Munari C, Bancaud J. The role of stereo-electro-encephalography (SEEG) in the evaluation of partial epileptic patients. In: Porter R, Morselli P, eds. *The Epilepsies.* London: Butterworths, 1987; pp. 267-306.

- Munari C, Francione S, Kahane P, Hoffmann D, Tassi L, Lo Russo G, Benabid AL. Multilobar resections for the control of epilepsy. In: Schmidek H, Sweet W, eds. *Operative Neurosurgical Technique.* Philadelphia: WB Saunders Company, 1995, pp. 1323-1339.

- Munari C, Giallonardo AT, Brunet P, Broglin D, Bancaud J. Stereotactic investigations in frontal lobe epilepsies. *Acta Neurochir Suppl* (Wien) 1989; 46: 9-12.

- Munari C, Musolini A, Blond S, *et al.* Stereo-EEG exploration in patients with intractable epilepsy: topographic relations between a lesion and epileptogenic areas. In: Schmidt D, Morselli P, eds. *Intractable Epilepsy: Experimental and Clinical Aspects.* New York: Raven Press, 1986; pp. 129-146.

- Munari C, Talairach J, Musolino A, *et al.* Stereotactic methodology of functional neurosurgery in tumoral epileptic patients. *Ital J Neurol Sci* 1983; (Suppl 2): 69-82.

- Nobili L, Francione S, Mai R, Cardinale F, Castana L, Tassi L, *et al.* Surgical treatment of drug-resistant nocturnal frontal lobe epilepsy. *Brain* 2007; 130: 561-73.

- Olivier A, Gloor P, Quesney LF, Andermann F. The indications for and the role of depth electrode recording in epilepsy. *Appl Neurophysiol* 1983; 46: 33-6.

- Palmini A, Andermann F., Dubeau F, da Costa JC, Calcagnotto ME, Gloor P, *et al.* Occipito-temporal relations: evidence for secondary epileptogenesis. *Adv Neurol* 1999; 81: 115-29.

- Quesney LF, Constain M, Rasmussen T, Stefan H, Olivier A. How large are frontal lobe epileptogenic zones? EEG, ECoG, and SEEG evidence. *Adv Neurol* 1992; 57: 311-23.

- Rasmussen T. Tailoring of cortical excisions for frontal lobe epilepsy. *Can J Neurol Sci* 1991; 18: 606-10.

- Rasmussen TB. Surgical treatment of complex partial seizures: results, lessons, and problems. *Epilepsia* 1983; 24 (Suppl 1): S65-76.

- Robles SG, Gelisse P, El Fertit H, Tancu C, Duffau H, Crespel A, Coubes P. Parasagittal transinsular electrodes for stereo-EEG in temporal and insular lobe epilepsies. *Stereotact Funct Neurosurg* 2009; 87: 368-78.

- Ryvlin P, Kahane P. The hidden causes of surgery-resistant temporal lobe epilepsy: extratemporal or temporal plus? Editorial review. *Curr Opin Neurol* 2005; 18: 125-7.

- Salanova V, Andermann F, Olivier A, Rasmussen T, Quesney LF. Occipital lobe epilepsy: electroclinical manifestations, electrocorticography, cortical stimulation and outcome in 42 patients treated between 1930 and 1991. Surgery of occipital lobe epilepsy. *Brain* 1992; 115 (Pt 6): 1655-80.
- Schiff SJ, Colella D, Jacyna GM, Hughes E, Creekmore JW, Marshall A, *et al.* Brain chirps: spectrographic signatures of epileptic seizures. *Clin Neurophysiol* 2000; 111: 953-8.
- Schindler K, Leung H, Elger CE, Lehnertz K. Assessing seizure dynamics by analysing the correlation structure of multichannel intracranial EEG. *Brain* 2007; 130: 65-77.
- Schmitt JJ, Janszky J, Woermann F, Tuxhorn I, Ebner A. Laughter and the mesial and lateral premotor cortex. *Epilepsy Behav* 2006; 8: 773-5.
- Schramm J, Kral T, Kurthen M, Blumcke I. Surgery to treat focal frontal lobe epilepsy in adults. *Neurosurgery* 2002; 51: 644-54.
- Sinclair DB, Wheatley M, Snyder T, Gross D, Ahmed N. Posterior resection for childhood epilepsy. *Pediatr Neurol* 2005; 32: 257-63.
- Sivelle G, Kahane P, De Saint Martin A, *et al.* La multilocalité des lésions dans la sclérose tubéreuse de Bourneville contreindique-t-elle une approche chirurgicale. *Epilepsies* 1995; 7: 451-64.
- Spencer SS. Depth electroencephalography in selection of refractory epilepsy for surgery. *Ann Neurol* 1981; 9: 207-14.
- Talairach J, Bancaud J. Lesion, "irritative" zone and epileptogenic focus. *Confin Neurol* 1966; 27: 91-4.
- Talairach J, Bancaud J. Stereotaxic approach to epilepsy. Methodology of anatomo-functional stereotaxic investigations. *Progr Neurol Surg* 1973; 5: 297-354.
- Talairach J, Bancaud J, Szikla G, Bonis A, Geier S. Approche nouvelle de la neurochirurgie de l'épilepsie. Méthodologie stéréotaxique et résultats thérapeutiques. *Neurochirurgie* 1974; 20 (Suppl 1): 1-240.
- Talairach J, Tournoux P, Musolino A, Missir O. Stereotaxic exploration in frontal epilepsy. *Adv Neurol* 1992; 57: 651-88.
- Tandon N, Alexopoulos AV, Warbel A, Najm IM, Bingaman WE. Occipital epilepsy: spatial categorization and surgical management. *J Neurosurg* 2009; 110: 306-18.
- Tassinari CA, Rubboli G, Gardella E, Cantalupo G, Calandra-Buonaura G, Vedovello M, *et al.* Central pattern generators for a common semiology in fronto-limbic seizures and in parasomnias. A neuroethologic approach. *Neurol Sci* 2005; 26 (Suppl 3): S225-232.
- Tellez-Zenteno JF, Hernandez Ronquillo L, Moien-Afshari F, Wiebe S. Surgical outcomes in lesional and non-lesional epilepsy: a systematic review and meta-analysis. *Epilepsy Res* 2010; 89: 310-8.
- Trottier S, Landre E, Biraben A, Chassoux F, Pasnicu A, Scarabin JM, *et al.* On the best strategies on the best results for surgery of frontal epilepsy. *Neurochirurgie* 2008; 54: 388-98.
- Wendling F, Bartolomei F, Bellanger JJ, Bourien J, Chauvel P. Epileptic fast intracerebral EEG activity: evidence for spatial decorrelation at seizure onset. *Brain* 2003; 126: 1449-59.
- Wendling F, Bartolomei F, Senhadji L. Spatial analysis of intracerebral electroencephalographic signals in the time and frequency domain: identification of epileptogenic networks in partiale epilepsy. *Philos Transact A Math Phys Eng Sci* 2009; 367: 297-316.

High frequency oscillations in extratemporal lobe epilepsy

Julia Jacobs[1], Jean Gotman[2]

[1] Department of Neuropediatrics, University of Freiburg, Germany
[2] Montreal Neurological Institute, Montreal, Quebec, Canada

In classical surface and intracranial EEG (iEEG), frequencies up to 50 Hz are commonly evaluated. Usually, the analysis of long-term EEG monitoring focuses on the identification of areas showing the first ictal activity (seizure onset zone – SOZ) as well as areas generating interictal epileptic spikes (irritative zone) (Rosenow & Luders, 2001). The identification of these areas in combination with neuroimaging, clinical and neuropsychological results often allows the planning of a surgical intervention in patients with medically intractable epilepsy. The majority of these patients have temporal lobe epilepsy (TLE) but a significant fraction has extra-TLE (ETLE) and this group is generally more difficult to treat. In some patients, the exact definition of one SOZ, the separation of ictal onset and propagation, as well as a complete delineation of epileptogenic areas are difficult. Postsurgical outcome may therefore be hard to predict or surgical planning may fail completely.

In recent years, analysis of EEG frequencies above 100 Hz has gained increased interest in the evaluation of epilepsy patients. Microelectrode EEG studies in patients with mesial temporal lobe epilepsy have shown a strong correlation between epileptogenic tissue and the occurrence of very short and distinct brain oscillations between 100 and 500 Hz (Bragin et al., 1999; Bragin et al., 2002). These oscillations, called high frequency oscillations (HFOs), have now also been recorded with macroelectrodes in mesial temporal and neocortical areas, and are therefore easier to record and on the verge of becoming useful in a clinical setting (Crepon et al., 2010; Jacobs et al., 2008).

■ Physiological and pathological HFOs

HFOs are divided into ripple (80-250 Hz) and fast ripple (250-500 Hz) oscillations depending on their frequency. Ripples were first detected in the mesial temporal structures in the freely moving rat (O'Keefe, 1990). Subsequently, these physiological oscillations were observed in the healthy hippocampus of rodents and cats as well as in the less epileptogenic hippocampus of patients with epilepsy (Bragin et al., 1999; Buzsaki et al., 1992; Chrobak & Buzsaki, 1996). In the human mesial temporal structures, ripples have been associated with memory consolidation processes (Axmacher *et al.*, 2008). Physiological ripples and fast ripples however are not limited to the mesial temporal structures but also occur in neocortical areas. Ripples occurred spontaneously in neocortical recordings of anesthetized cats (Grenier *et al.*, 2001). Physiological ripples, at least in the hippocampus, are believed to result from summated IPSPs from basket cells onto pyramidal cells. During the memory consolidation process, CA3 pyramidal cells fire during sharp waves and depolarize CA1 basket cells. This induces a ripple transported from the latter to CA1 pyramidal cell, in this way controlling pyramidal cell firing (Bragin *et al.*, 1999; Ylinen *et al.*, 1995).

Fast ripples have been recorded over the somatosensory cortex following vibrissae stimulation in rodents and median nerve stimulation in humans (Curio *et al.*, 1994; Jones & Barth, 1999). In humans, no spontaneous physiological fast ripples have been described, but it has to be kept in mind that all intracranial recordings have been limited to patients with epilepsy, for ethical reasons. Thus differentiation between spontaneous physiological and pathological oscillations is difficult and spontaneous HFOs in neocortical areas of seizure onset so far have been considered pathological, on the basis of correlation between epileptogenic areas and areas of HFO generation.

The relationship between HFOs and epileptogenic areas was first evaluated in detail using microwires in the limbic structures of rats and humans. These first studies suggested that ripples could be recorded with similar rates in the entorhinal cortex and in CA1-3 in both hippocampi in patients with temporal lobe epilepsy, while fast ripples were significantly more frequent on the more epileptic side. As ripples were known correlates of memory, first only fast ripples were considered pathological events (Bragin *et al.*, 1999; Bragin *et al.*, 2002; Staba *et al.*, 2004). Subsequent studies with macroelectrodes however found that ripple oscillations may be more frequent in epileptic hippocampus as well (Jacobs *et al.*, 2008; Jacobs *et al.*, 2009a), and that the relationship between HFOs recorded in microelectrodes and HFOs recorded in macroelectrodes is uncertain. In macroelectrode recordings, ripple and fast ripple oscillations have been clearly correlated with areas of seizure onset in extra temporal structures. As physiological HFOs are considered much less frequent in these areas, and particularly since most studies take place during slow wave sleep, it is likely that most HFOs that have been studied are pathological. Nevertheless, since ripples and fast ripples may also be physiological events, the term "pHFOs" (pathological HFOs) was introduced to describe ripples and fast ripples considered to be related to epileptogenesis (Engel, Jr. *et al.*, 2009).

pHFOs can most likely be generated in the same anatomical areas as physiological HFOs or in areas adjacent to them. Thus HFOs in humans with epilepsy may consist of a mixture of physiological and pathological HFOs. Physiological HFOs in the hippocampus show a correlation with CA3 sharp waves and it is hypothesized that they function to synchronize network in the hippocampal structures and allow memory consolidation. This function in memory consolidation suggests that they may be visible over large brain areas. In contrast, pHFOs are considered to be very locally restricted and to have small generators. It was shown that pathological fast ripples are generated in networks smaller than 1 mm^3 (Bragin *et al.*, 2002) and pathological ripples probably have similarly small generators.

To conclude, all oscillations described in the high frequency range so far are of low-amplitude and short duration. pHFOs additionally have very small generators which complicate their recording. The implications of these characteristics for the clinical use of pHFOs will be discussed below.

■ Evaluation pHFOs as makers of epilepsy

Several questions need to be answered to estimate the value of pHFOs for presurgical investigation. Are HFOs stable markers over time and in different conditions? Are they superior to known markers of epileptogenicity such as interictal spikes? And last but not least are they actually reflecting the epileptogenic potential of the underlying tissue?

Studies in the kianic acid rat model showed that areas generating fast ripples were stable over time for several weeks and remained well localized over this period (Bragin et al., 2003). In humans, similar observations were made over several nights during intracranial investigations (Zijlmans et al., 2009a). Medication and seizure frequency influenced the rate of HFOs but not their location nor the relative importance of different regions (Zijlmans et al., 2009a). Studies of wakefulness and different sleep stages found similar results: the rate of HFOs is highest in slow wave sleep and significantly lower in wakefulness and REM sleep (Bagshaw et al., 2009; Staba et al., 2004); the areas generating HFOs however remained the same. The same is true for the transitions from interictal, to preictal and ictal stages (Zijlmans et al., 2009b). Most studies have been performed on interictal data, which has the advantages of less artefact and longer periods compared to ictal data. But even at the beginning of seizures HFOs were most frequent in the SOZ and it was possible to distinguish between SOZ and propagating areas by analysing HFO rates (Jirsch et al., 2006). Thus HFOs appear to be stable events in regard to the localization during the period of intracranial investigation.

Intra-cranial investigations aim to identify the irritative zone and the SOZ. Interictal epileptic spikes are considered to reflect epileptic areas, even if experts disagree on the importance of removing the irritative zone to gain seizure freedom (Hufnagel et al., 2000). Studies have revealed a strong relationship between interictal spikes and HFOs, which is not completely understood (Urrestarazu et al., 2007). The analysis of isolated HFOs and HFOs co-occurring with spikes is complicated as spikes are invisible in the high-frequency filtered EEG that is needed to see HFOs. Three types of HFOs can be distinguished in regard to their relationship with spikes: they can occur independently of spikes, together with them and visible on the unfiltered spike (riding on the spike) or together with them and not visible on the unfiltered spike (Figure 1) (Urrestarazu et al., 2007). Thus it is also possible to distinguish between spikes with and without HFOs (Crepon et al., 2010; Jacobs et al., 2008). Despite this observed relationship in occurrence there is evidence that patho-physiological mechanisms of both types of events are different. Recurrent seizures during an intracranial investigation do not lead to a change in HFO activity (Zijlmans et al., 2009a), but result in an increase of spikes in the SOZ (Gotman, 1991; Spencer et al., 2008). In contrast, a reduction of antiepileptic medication results in an increase in HFOs (Zijlmans et al., 2009a), while spikes remain stable or decrease (Spencer et al., 2008). Thus HFOs behave differently from spikes and more similarly to seizures following medi-cation reduction. Moreover, HFOs show a different pattern during the transition from interictal to ictal periods than spikes. HFOs increase in the 10 seconds prior to the seizure, compared to the interictal period, and then even more during the first seconds of a seizure. Spikes in contrast showed a short preictal decrease prior to an increase in the seizure as well (Zijlmans et al., 2009b). Moreover, HFOs have proven to be more specific to the SOZ than spikes in general (Jacobs et al., 2008). Interestingly, spikes co-occurring with HFOs show a possibility to differentiate the SOZ nearly as well as HFOs alone. It is unclear how both types of events occur together and which circumstances within the tissue are needed to allow for this coupling, but the occurrence of HFOs seems to reflect more

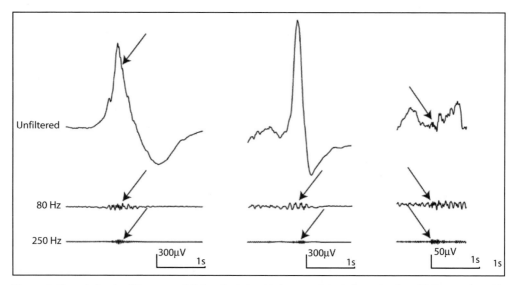

Figure 1. Example for the different possibilities of relationship between fast ripples and spikes. (A) Fast ripple visible in spike, "riding on the spike"; (B) Fast ripple not visible in spike; (C) Fast ripple visible, independently of a spike.

Top: non-filtered EEG; middle: EEG filtered with high-pass filter of 80 Hz; bottom: EEG filtered with high-pass filter of 250 Hz. The gain is identical in the three views.

Reprinted from Urrestarazu *et al.*, 2007, with permission of Elsevier.

epileptogenicity than the spikes alone. This was first underlined by studies linking the SOZ and predicting SOZ channels using rates of HFOs (Crepon *et al.*, 2010; Jacobs *et al.*, 2008; Jacobs *et al.*, 2009a). Similarly, a correlation was found between the occurrence of an epileptic response to electrical stimulation, namely seizures or after-discharges, and high rates of HFOs (Jacobs *et al.*, 2010b). Even stronger evidence has been found by establishing the correlation between the removal of HFO-generating areas and a good postsurgical outcome (Jacobs *et al.*, 2010a). The possibility to predict postsurgical outcome was better using HFOs than rates of spikes or the removal of the SOZ. Thus there is evidence from several perspectives that HFOs are providing additional information to that of established markers and that their rates may reflect epileptogenicity.

■ Specific features of neocortical HFOs

HFO studies that evaluated the differences in pHFO patterns depending on the brain area in which they are generated always focussed on contrasting mesial-temporal with neocortical HFOs. Thus the literature provides no information about the difference between neocortical temporal and extratemporal patterns of HFOs. This paragraph will therefore focus on diffe-rences between neocortical HFOs in general and mesial-temporal HFOs. Compared to HFOs generated in the mesial temporal lobe, neocortical HFOs have some specific characteristics. When comparing all HFOs, independently of whether or not they occur in the SOZ, the mean durations of neocortical ripples (77.5 ± 36.7ms) and fast ripples (28.3 ± 16.4ms) are significantly shorter than those of mesial temporal ripples (97.5 ± 44.2ms) and fast ripples (43.1 ± 28.9ms) (Jacobs *et al.*, 2008). Often, neocortical HFOs additionally have smaller amplitudes and therefore are less prominent than mesial temporal ones (*Figure 2*). Moreover, rates of neocortical HFOs (ripple: 4.3 ± 7.25/ min, fast ripples: 2.2 ± 4.5/ min) are significantly lower than those in mesial temporal structures (ripple: 21.9 ± 20.8/min, fast ripple: 19.8 ± 33.2/ min) (Jacobs *et al.*, 2008). The pathophysiological reasons for these differences remain unclear. High rates of mesial-temporal HFOs may on the one hand reflect the higher epileptogenic potential of these structures; on the other hand it may result from a larger number of spontaneous physiological HFOs interfering with the analysis of pHFOs in the mesial temporal structures. Nevertheless, comparisons between HFOs within mesial-temporal and neocortical areas still reveal significantly higher rates in the SOZ than outside (Jacobs *et al.*, 2009b). The different patterns of mesial temporal and neocortical HFOs have two practical implications for the analysis of HFOs.

First, in group studies of HFOs, for example for the predictability of the SOZ, patients with mesial temporal lobe epilepsy cannot be analysed in the same way as patients with neocortical epilepsies. Rates of HFOs in the mesial temporal structures may be higher outside the SOZ than neocortical rates inside the SOZ, while within the same structures rates of HFOs are always clearly higher in the SOZ than outside (Jacobs *et al.*, 2009b). Analysis becomes extremely hard to interpret in patients which are implanted in neocortical as well as mesial temporal structures. Second, automatic detection tools for HFOs, which will be discussed below, probably need adjustment for the different features of neocortical and mesial temporal HFOs.

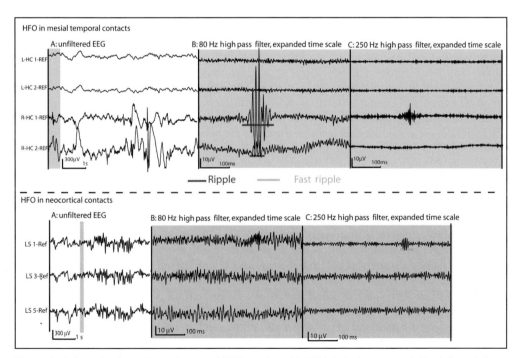

Figure 2. A) Example of typical mesial temporal HFOs in channel R-HC 1 (right hippocampus). The left panel shows the unfiltered EEG with a normal time scale; the middle shows the grey section from the left panel in extended time scale and high gain, and with a high pass filter of 80 Hz (ripple oscillation marked in blue); and the right the same section with a filter of 250 Hz (fast ripple oscillation marked in orange).
B) In contrast to A) the neocortical HFO recorded over LS 1-2 (left frontal region) is much shorter and of lower amplitude. The panels are the same as explained above.
Figures modified from Jacobs *et al.*, 2009a (part A) and Jacobs *et al.*, 2010b (Part B) with permission of Elsevier.

■ Technical challenges

Amplifier techniques allow more and more EEG systems to record with sampling rates above 1,000 Hz and thus theoretically enable to record HFOs. Nevertheless, the small generator size and a number of unknown features still pose many questions on the ability to identify HFOs before they can be used in clinical routine.

Methods of intracranial recording and contact sizes of intracranial electrodes vary greatly. In extratemporal epilepsies, different types of grid electrodes as well as depth electrodes are used. Epilepsy centres use contact sizes ranging from 0.8 mm^2 in custom made electrodes to 10 mm^2 in some of the commercially available electrodes. This difference most likely does not influence the visibility of events like interictal spikes, which are believed to result from synchronous firing of large cortical areas. It may interfere with the possibility to see HFOs generated in cortical surfaces as small as 1 mm^3. The signal to noise ratio may be reduced in large contacts, with the HFOs becoming invisible in the noise of surrounding neuronal activity. While initial data on HFOs were derived from microelectrodes, studies on custom made contacts with a size of 0.8 mm^2 in Montreal for the first time identified distinct epilepsy-related HFOs in a clinical standard recording (Jirsch et al., 2006). By now, HFOs have been seen in various types of standard grid recordings. Even recorded with sampling rates of only 1,024 Hz, HFOs below 300 Hz were shown to be more frequent in the SOZ (Crepon et al., 2010; Ochi et al., 2007; Worrell et al., 2008). Detailed studies have tried to compare simultaneous recording from larger and smaller contact sizes. One study comparing large macro electrodes (9.4 mm^2) with micro-contacts suggested that micro-contacts have better capabilities to record HFOs (Worrell et al., 2008). Another study used an arrangement of adjacent small (0.2 mm^2) and larger contacts (0.8 mm^2) recording 1 mm from each other (Chatillon et al., 2008). Surprisingly, despite the small size of HFO generators, no significant differences in rates of HFO could be found for the different contact sizes. It was hypothesised that the larger contacts may actually encompass several small generators at the same time and thus record HFOs adequately (Chatillon et al., 2008; 2010). The evidence however cannot be directly translated to even larger contact sizes as used in some commercial grids. HFO studies on such grids suggest that the ability to record HFOs may be good enough to detect the SOZ (Khosravani et al., 2009).

A second challenge in the use of HFO recordings is their actual detection. At the moment, automatic detection tools and visual detection have been used. For research questions, the latter is an interesting option. It allows evaluating different shapes of HFOs, analysing the HFO relationship with spikes and disregarding high frequency artefacts. Reviewer bias can be reduced by calculating an inter-rater agreement using Cohen's Kappa (Zelmann et al., 2009). It has been demonstrated that as few as five minutes of inter-ictal activity are enough to establish stable rates of HFOs (Zelmann et al., 2009). However, the data has to be marked on a very small EEG time scale, so the marking of one channel for 5 minutes of EEG can take up to one hour. Thus manual marking has the major disadvantage of being very time consuming (Jacobs et al., 2008; Urrestarazu et al., 2007).

Several automatic detection tools have been developed. They use techniques derived from frequency analysis and up to now no single detection methods has been used by the different work groups (Gardner et al., 2007; Staba et al., 2002). Most techniques combine a first automatic detection with a visual review of detected events (Crepon et al., 2010). Automatic detection methods have the advantage of being fast and independent of the reviewer's eye. All techniques however still face problems as the shape of the events may be strongly dependent on the brain region and baseline they are recorded from. It is only when combined with visual analysis that they provide information about the relationship between spikes and HFOs (Crepon *et al.*, 2010). Especially in neocortical epilepsy, users should keep in mind that detection thresholds as well as methods were established primarily in the mesial temporal structures. As HFOs in extratemporal epilepsy are smaller in amplitude and shorter, they may be harder to distinguish from the baseline.

■ Scalp-recorded high frequency activity

In regard to clinical use, an important question is whether it is possible to record HFOs with surface EEG. This would make the use of HFOs available for a larger group of patients as a non-invasive tool as well as partially overcome the spatial limitations of intracranial recordings. For stimulus-related high frequencies, recordings with magnetoencephalography (MEG) and surface EEG have been shown (Curio, 1999; Curio, 2000). The recording of spontaneous HFOs however poses two more challenges as their time of occurrence is unknown: first, differentiation from high frequency artefacts such as muscle is difficult; second, events cannot be averaged to increase the signal to noise ratio. Frequencies up to 150 Hz have already been correlated with some success with epilepsy (Kobayashi *et al.*, 2010). Kobayashi and co-workers found frequencies of 50 to 100 Hz to be present in infantile spasms (Kobayashi *et al.*, 2004) and Wu and co-workers could identify gamma activity correlating with the seizure onset in neocortical epilepsy in children (Wu *et al.*, 2008). It remains however unclear whether even higher frequencies could be detected and predictive. The assumed small size HFO generators may be reason for doubts that they are actually visible through the scalp.

■ Clinical applications of HFOs

Independently of a possibility to record HFOs with surface contacts, they could become a valuable marker of epileptogenicity in presurgical studies with intracranial electrodes.

In lesional neocortical epilepsy, investigators encounter several challenges, one of them being patients with larger lesions in whom parts of the lesion may involve functional areas (Boonyapisit *et al.*, 2003). The seizure onset may only be observed in parts of the lesion, but other areas may show interictal spiking or other evidence of epileptic potential such as hypometabolism on PET (Li *et al.*, 1997; Raymond *et al.*, 1995). It remains uncertain whether such lesions have to be removed partially or completely to achieve seizure freedom. Another challenge is seen in patients with several independent lesions such as tuberous sclerosis and nodular heterotopias (Barkovich & Kjos, 1992; Major *et al.*, 2009). Even after implanting electrodes into several lesion sites and finding one lesion to be predominantly involved in ictogenesis, the epileptogenic potential of the other lesions remains unclear and they may reduce the chances for a good postsurgical outcome (Rosenow & Luders, 2001). There is evidence that HFOs are not specific to pathological tissue changes in general but actually specific to areas of seizure generation (Jacobs *et al.*, 2009a). In patients in whom the SOZ only involved a small part of the lesion or was even outside the lesional areas, HFO rates were highest inside the SOZ and not in the remaining lesional areas (*Figure 3*). Thus HFOs may be an additional tool to identify those lesional areas that are part of the epileptogenic network and exclude those that will remain silent. Larger studies analysing different types of lesions are needed to further assess this approach. There has been some evidence that patients with focal cortical dysplasia in general may have extended areas with high rates of HFOs (Urrestarazu et al., 2007). In patients with mesial temporal sclerosis, the degree of cell loss correlates with the occurrence of fast ripples (Staba et al., 2007). Therefore, findings in one type of lesion may not be generalized for other types.

In non-lesional epilepsy, even implantation with a large coverage of grid electrodes sometimes results in problems to differentiate between areas of seizure onset and areas of propagation. Especially in patients with deep cortical generators, the first ictal activity on the grid may already result from fast propagation. HFOs may have the potential to differentiate between the generating tissue and propagated activity. Studies of ictal HFOs suggest that HFOs increased at the beginning of seizures in the contacts of the SOZ only in patients with a distinct focal seizure onset. Similar observations were not made for patients in whom the first recorded ictal activity was already widespread, suggestive of propagating activity (Jirsch et al., 2006).

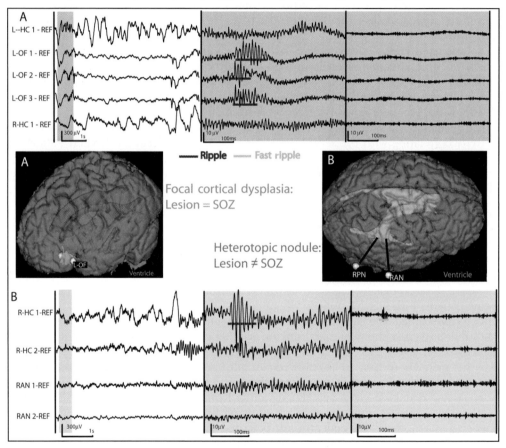

Figure 3. Relationship between the occurrence of HFOs and lesions. (A) example with a complete overlap of SOZ and lesion in a patient with a frontal focal cortical dysplasia (green). Ripples are displayed in the three contacts inside the lesion (L-OF 1-3). Panel explanations are the same as in *figure 2*. (B) example of a SOZ outside the lesional areas in a patient with nodular heterotopia (red) and a SOZ within both hippocampi. Ripples (blue) and fast ripples (orange) occur in the mesial temporal contacts (here contact R-HC1, right hippocampus) and not in the contacts within the nodular heterotopia (contact RAN1 & 2). Thus HFOs in these patients are specific to the SOZ not to the pathologically changed lesional areas.
Modified figure from Jacobs et al., 2009a, with permission of Elsevier.

Another clinical application would be the use of HFOs in a seizure prediction tool. If HFOs reflect epileptogenicity one could assume that their rates change prior to seizures. Two studies observed a change in HFO occurrence a few seconds (up to 10 sec.) prior to ictal activity (Khosravani *et al.*, 2005). (Zijlmans *et al.*, 2011). No systematic change however could be found during the 15, 5 or 1 minutes prior to ictal onset (Jacobs *et al.*, 2011). Better and more reliable automatic detection tools will be needed to perform valid studies on seizure prediction, evaluating HFO activity during several days of recordings.

A challenge for the use of HFOs is the inability to differentiate between physiological ripples and fast ripples and pHFOs. The interference is visible for mesial temporal areas and memory related ripples (Axmacher *et al.*, 2008), but the occurrence and interference of physiological HFOs, especially in the somatosensory areas, cannot be excluded for neocortical areas as well. Already, task-related gamma and high frequency increases are assumed to reflect cortical activation (Bauer *et al.*, 2006; Crone *et al.*, 1998). Rat models may suggest ways of differentiation between physiological and pathological HFOs as they allow to record from healthy cortex, which for ethical reasons is impossible in human (Engel, Jr. *et al.*, 2009). Validation studies may confirm findings in humans. A first study suggests that physiological ripples in the hippocampus can be increased in humans following a memory task (Axmacher *et al.*, 2008). Differentiation between pHFOs and physiological HFOs may therefore not only allow to use pHFOs for a clearer delineation of pathological areas, but the detection of physiological HFOs may help assess physiological function in the same areas.

Finally, HFOs may become an additional marker for the prediction of surgical outcome (Ochi *et al.*, 2007). One study evaluated the correlation between the removal of HFO-generating areas and postsurgical outcome in a mixed group of patients with neocortical and mesial-temporal epilepsy (Jacobs *et al.*, 2010a). In patients with a good postsurgical outcome (Engel classes 1 & 2), significantly more HFO-generating regions were removed than in those with a bad outcome (classes 3 & 4). In patients in whom a large part of HFO-generating tissue remained, a bad postsurgical outcome was observed. Some patients with a good removal of HFO-generating regions however still had a poor surgical outcome *(Figure 4)*. Therefore, a good outcome in this patient group could be predicted with less certainty. This is possibly arising from the limited electrode coverage of intracranial recordings, unable to record HFOs outside the range of electrodes. Prospective studies with more patients and different recording techniques will be necessary to conclude whether HFOs have a predictive value for postsurgical outcome. As inter-ictal studies only required recording of approximately 5 minutes, intra-operative ECoG recordings might also be tested for their ability to record HFOs. A recent study has demonstrated the ability of HFOs recorded with ECoG to predict post-surgical outcome (Wu *et al.*, 2010).

To conclude, evidence from different studies, centres and recording techniques suggest a close link between epileptogenicity and the occurrence of pHFOs. HFOs have been shown to provide additional information to the classical markers, namely the SOZ and interictal spikes. Recording techniques and results however still have to be assessed carefully and mechanisms behind HFO generation have not been completely understood. We suggested some possible clinical applications in extratemporal epilepsy, all of which still have to be validated further. Nevertheless, distinct HFOs may improve our understanding of epileptic tissue and most of the information can be acquired from a few minutes of interictal EEG.

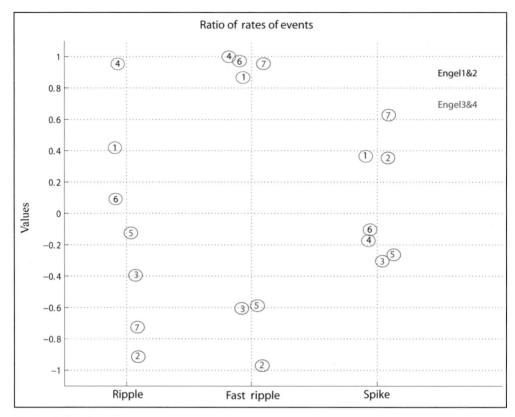

Figure 4. Correlation between the surgical removal of HFO generating areas and the postsurgical outcome in patients with extratemporal lobe epilepsy. Ratio of event rates in the removed areas to rates in the nonremoved areas for patients with good *versus* bad outcome regions generating high rates of ripples (R) and fast ripples (FRs) where more likely to have been removed in patients with good outcome. Patients with good outcome are in blue and patients with poor outcome in red circles. A number identifies each patient, so that it is possible to follow which marker (ripples on the left, fast ripples in the middle, spikes on the right) is indicative of the outcome in each patient. Values > 0 indicate that the majority of HFOs is removed and patients should therefore have a good outcome (blue circles). One patient (7) with a bad outcome had a good removal of fast ripple, but not of ripple oscillations. Bad outcome may be explained by remaining ripples or by fast ripples outside the recording reach of the electrodes. Modified figure from Jacobs et al., 2010a, with permission of Wiley Interscience.

References

- Axmacher N, Elger CE, Fell J. Ripples in the medial temporal lobe are relevant for human memory consolidation. *Brain* 2008; 131: 1806-17.
- Bagshaw AP, Jacobs J, LeVan P, Dubeau F, Gotman J. Effect of sleep stage on interictal high-frequency oscillations recorded from depth macroelectrodes in patients with focal epilepsy. *Epilepsia* 2009; 50: 617-28.
- Barkovich AJ, Kjos BO. Gray matter heterotopias: MR characteristics and correlation with developmental and neurologic manifestations. *Radiology* 1992; 182: 493-9.

- Bauer M, Oostenveld R, Peeters M, Fries P. Tactile spatial attention enhances gamma-band activity in somatosensory cortex and reduces low-frequency activity in parieto-occipital areas. *J Neurosci* 2006; 26: 490-501.

- Boonyapisit K, Najm I, Klem G, Ying Z, Burrier C, LaPresto E, *et al*. Epileptogenicity of focal malformations due to abnormal cortical development: direct electrocorticographic-histopathologic correlations. *Epilepsia* 2003; 44: 69-76.

- Bragin A, Engel J, Jr., Wilson CL, Fried I, Buzsaki G. High-frequency oscillations in human brain. *Hippocampus* 1999; 9: 137-42.

- Bragin A, Mody I, Wilson CL, Engel J, Jr. Local generation of fast ripples in epileptic brain. *J Neurosci* 2002; 22: 2012-21.

- Bragin A, Wilson CL, Engel J. Spatial stability over time of brain areas generating fast ripples in the epileptic rat. *Epilepsia* 2003; 44: 1233-7.

- Buzsaki G, Horvath Z, Urioste R, Hetke J, Wise K. High-frequency network oscillation in the hippocampus. *Science* 1992; 256: 1025-7.

- Chatillon CE, Zelmann R, Olivier A, Dubeau F, Gotman J. The effect of contact size on high frequency oscillations (HFOs) detection in human intracerebral EEG recordings. *Epilepsia* 2008; 49 (Suppl 7): 184.

- Chatillon CE, Zelmann R, Bortel A, Avoli M, Gotman J. Contact size does not affect high frequency oscillation detection in intracerebral EEG recordings in a rat epilepsy model. *Clin Neurophysiol* 2011 [Epub ahead of print].

- Chrobak JJ, Buzsaki G. High-frequency oscillations in the output networks of the hippocampal-entorhinal axis of the freely behaving rat. *J Neurosci* 1996; 16: 3056-66.

- Crepon B, Navarro V, Hasboun D, Clemenceau S, Martinerie J, Baulac M, *et al*. Mapping interictal oscillations greater than 200 Hz recorded with intracranial macroelectrodes in human epilepsy. *Brain* 2010; 133: 33-45.

- Crone NE, Miglioretti DL, Gordon B, Lesser RP. Functional mapping of human sensorimotor cortex with electrocorticographic spectral analysis. II. Event-related synchronization in the gamma band. *Brain* 1998; 121 (Pt 12): 2301-15.

- Curio G. High frequency (600 Hz) bursts of spike-like activities generated in the human cerebral somatosensory system. *Electroencephalogr Clin Neurophysiol* 1999 (Suppl); 49: 56-61.

- Curio G. Linking 600-Hz "spikelike" EEG/MEG wavelets ("sigma-bursts") to cellular substrates: concepts and caveats. *J Clin Neurophysiol* 2000; 17: 377-96.

- Curio G, Mackert BM, Burghoff M, Koetitz R, Abraham-Fuchs K, Harer W. Localization of evoked neuromagnetic 600 Hz activity in the cerebral somatosensory system. *Electroencephalogr Clin Neurophysiol* 1994; 91: 483-7.

- Engel J, Jr., Bragin A, Staba R, Mody I. High-frequency oscillations: what is normal and what is not? *Epilepsia* 2009; 50: 598-604.

- Gardner AB, Worrell GA, Marsh E, Dlugos D, Litt B. Human and automated detection of high-frequency oscillations in clinical intracranial EEG recordings. *Clin Neurophysiol* 2007; 118: 1134-43.

- Gotman J. Relationships between interictal spiking and seizures: human and experimental evidence. *Can J Neurol Sci* 1991; 18: 573-6.

- Grenier F, Timofeev I, Steriade M. Focal synchronization of ripples (80-200 Hz) in neocortex and their neuronal correlates. *J Neurophysiol* 2001; 86: 1884-98.

- Hufnagel A, Dumpelmann M, Zentner J, Schijns O, Elger CE. Clinical relevance of quantified intracranial interictal spike activity in presurgical evaluation of epilepsy. *Epilepsia* 2000; 41: 467-78.

- Jacobs J, LeVan P, Chander R, Hall J, Dubeau F, Gotman J. Interictal high-frequency oscillations (80-500 Hz) are an indicator of seizure onset areas independent of spikes in the human epileptic brain. *Epilepsia* 2008; 49: 1893-907.

- Jacobs J, LeVan P, Chatillon CE, Olivier A, Dubeau F, Gotman J. High frequency oscillations in intracranial EEGs mark epileptogenicity rather than lesion type. *Brain* 2009a; 132: 1022-37.
- Jacobs J, LeVan P, Dubeau F, Gotman J. Generation of High Frequency oscillations (80-500 Hz) in different anatomical structures and their relation to the Seizure onset zone. *Clinical neurophysiology* 2009b; 120: e29-e30.
- Jacobs J, Zelmann R, Jirsch J, Chander R, Dubeau CE, Gotman J. High frequency oscillations (80-500 Hz) in the preictal period in patients with focal seizures. *Epilepsia* 2009c; 50: 1780-92.
- Jacobs J, Zijlmans M, Zelmann R, Chatillon CE, Hall J, Olivier A, *et al*. High-frequency electroencephalographic oscillations correlate with outcome of epilepsy surgery. *Ann Neurol* 2010a; 67: 209-20.
- Jacobs J, Zijlmans M, Zelmann R, Olivier A, Hall J, Gotman J, *et al*. Value of electrical stimulation and high frequency oscillations (80-500 Hz) in identifying epileptogenic areas during intracranial EEG recordings. *Epilepsia* 2010b; 51: 573-82.
- Jirsch JD, Urrestarazu E, LeVan P, Olivier A, Dubeau F, Gotman J. High-frequency oscillations during human focal seizures. *Brain* 2006; 129: 1593-608.
- Jones MS, Barth DS. Spatiotemporal organization of fast (> 200 Hz) electrical oscillations in rat Vibrissa/Barrel cortex. *J Neurophysiol* 1999; 82: 1599-609.
- Khosravani H, Mehrotra N, Rigby M, Hader WJ, Pinnegar CR, Pillay N, *et al*. Spatial localization and time-dependant changes of electrographic high frequency oscillations in human temporal lobe epilepsy. *Epilepsia* 2009; 50: 605-16.
- Khosravani H, Pinnegar CR, Mitchell JR, Bardakjian BL, Federico P, Carlen PL. Increased high-frequency oscillations precede *in vitro* low-Mg seizures. *Epilepsia* 2005; 46: 1188-97.
- Kobayashi K, Oka M, Akiyama T, Inoue T, Abiru K, Ogino T, *et al*. Very fast rhythmic activity on scalp EEG associated with epileptic spasms. *Epilepsia* 2004; 45: 488-96.
- Kobayashi K, Watanabe Y, Inoue T, Oka M, Yoshinaga H, Ohtsuka Y. Scalp-recorded high-frequency oscillations in childhood sleep-induced electrical status epilepticus. *Epilepsia* 2010; 51: 2190-4.
- Li LM, Cendes F, Watson C, Andermann F, Fish DR, Dubeau F, *et al*. Surgical treatment of patients with single and dual pathology: relevance of lesion and of hippocampal atrophy to seizure outcome. *Neurology* 1997; 48: 437-44.
- Major P, Rakowski S, Simon MV, Cheng ML, Eskandar E, Baron J, *et al*. Are cortical tubers epileptogenic? Evidence from electrocorticography. *Epilepsia* 2009; 50: 147-54.
- O'Keefe J. A computational theory of the hippocampal cognitive map. *Prog Brain Res* 1990; 83: 301-12.
- Ochi A, Otsubo H, Donner EJ, Elliott I, Iwata R, Funaki T, *et al*. Dynamic changes of ictal high-frequency oscillations in neocortical epilepsy: using multiple band frequency analysis. *Epilepsia* 2007; 48: 286-96.
- Raymond AA, Fish DR, Sisodiya SM, Alsanjari N, Stevens JM, Shorvon SD. Abnormalities of gyration, heterotopias, tuberous sclerosis, focal cortical dysplasia, microdysgenesis, dysembryoplastic neuroepithelial tumour and dysgenesis of the archicortex in epilepsy. Clinical, EEG and neuroimaging features in 100 adult patients. *Brain* 1995; 118 (Pt 3): 629-60.
- Rosenow F, Luders H. Presurgical evaluation of epilepsy. *Brain* 2001; 124: 1683-700.
- Spencer SS, Goncharova II, Duckrow RB, Novotny EJ, Zaveri HP. Interictal spikes on intracranial recording: behavior, physiology, and implications. *Epilepsia* 2008; 49: 1881-92.
- Staba RJ, Frighetto L, Behnke EJ, Mathern GW, Fields T, Bragin A, *et al*. Increased fast ripple to ripple ratios correlate with reduced hippocampal volumes and neuron loss in temporal lobe epilepsy patients. *Epilepsia* 2007; 48: 2130-8.
- Staba RJ, Wilson CL, Bragin A, Fried I, Engel J, Jr. Quantitative analysis of high-frequency oscillations (80-500 Hz) recorded in human epileptic hippocampus and entorhinal cortex. *J Neurophysiol* 2002; 88: 1743-52.

- Staba RJ, Wilson CL, Bragin A, Jhung D, Fried I, Engel J, Jr. High-frequency oscillations recorded in human medial temporal lobe during sleep. *Ann Neurol* 2004; 56: 108-15.
- Urrestarazu E, Chander R, Dubeau F, Gotman J. Interictal high-frequency oscillations (100-500 Hz) in the intracerebral EEG of epileptic patients. *Brain* 2007; 130: 2354-66.
- Worrell GA, Gardner AB, Stead SM, Hu S, Goerss S, Cascino GJ, *et al.* High-frequency oscillations in human temporal lobe: simultaneous microwire and clinical macroelectrode recordings. *Brain* 2008; 131: 928-37.
- Wu JY, Koh S, Sankar R, Mathern GW. Paroxysmal fast activity: an interictal scalp EEG marker of epileptogenesis in children. *Epilepsy Res* 2008; 82: 99-106.
- Wu JY, Sankar R, Lerner JT, Matsumoto JH, Vinters HV, Mathern GW. Removing interictal fast ripples on electrocorticography linked with seizure freedom in children. *Neurology* 2010; 75: 1686-94.
- Ylinen A, Bragin A, Nadasdy Z, Jando G, Szabo I, Sik A, *et al.* Sharp wave-associated high-frequency oscillation (200 Hz) in the intact hippocampus: network and intracellular mechanisms. *J Neurosci* 1995; 15: 30-46.
- Zelmann R, Zijlmans M, Jacobs J, Chatillon CE, Gotman J. Improving the identification of High Frequency Oscillations. *Clin Neurophysiol* 2009; 120: 1457-64.
- Zijlmans M, Jacobs J, Khan YU, Zelmann R, Dubeau F, Gotman J. Relationship between ictal and interictal high frequency oscillations in patients with focal epilepsy. *Clin Neurophysiol* 2011; 122: 664-71.
- Zijlmans M, Jacobs J, Zelmann R, Dubeau F, Gotman J. High-frequency oscillations mirror disease activity in patients with epilepsy. *Neurology* 2009a; 72: 979-86.

Seizure detection and epileptic focus stimulation in extratemporal lobe epilepsy

Gregory K. Bergey, Christophe C. Jouny

Johns Hopkins Epilepsy Center, Department of Neurology, Johns Hopkins University School of Medicine, Baltimore, USA

■ Seizure detection in the context of therapy

Intracranial monitoring is most commonly performed for the presurgical evaluation of patients with intractable epilepsy who cannot have their seizures adequately lateralized or localized with ictal scalp monitoring. Often these patients are patients with unremarkable imaging. Neocortical epilepsy, whether temporal or extratemporal, can present challenges because of the rapid and broad regional propagation that occurs. The clinical evaluation of these patients appropriately is aimed at defining the seizure onset zone to better direct surgical therapy and hopefully improve outcome. The other chapters in this section discuss this evaluation in detail. This chapter will discuss the concept of seizure detection from intracranial leads in the context of non-surgical therapy, specifically closed-loop responsive neurostimulation (RNS) (Bergey 2008; 2009). This therapy, currently under review by the FDA, is typically reserved for patients who are not optimal surgical candidates or who have failed to have their seizures controlled by surgery, patients with multifocal epilepsy, and those with bilateral epileptogenic regions. Many of these potential candidates for RNS therapy have neocortical and extratemporal lobe epilepsy (ETLE).

■ Types of neurostimulation

Therapeutic neurostimulation can be divided into two basic subgroups, programmed or chronic stimulation and responsive stimulation. Chronic or programmed stimulation delivers recurrent therapy to a site (*e.g.* vagus nerve, anterior thalamus) thought to potentially modulate seizure activity. Responsive neurostimulation is designed to respond to the seizure activity and to deliver electrical therapy in response to this activity (Bergey, 2009). As such, in contrast to programmed stimulation, such therapy requires detection of ictal activity and it is thought that detection and stimulation at or near the seizure focus is optimal. The principles of this therapy will be discussed further below.

Advantages shared by all types of neurostimulation are mechanisms of action thought distinct from antiepileptic drug actions, and the lack of drug related side effects on cognition or other functions. There is no risk of hypersensitivity reactions, no hepatic or hematologic toxicity and no risk for teratogenicity. Both the anterior thalamic stimulator and responsive neurostimulation require placement of intracranial leads; the vagus nerve stimulator (VNS) stimulates extracranial structures (Ben-Menachem, 2001). Stimulation of intracranial structures, in contrast to stimulation of the vagus nerve, however, produces no sensation or discomfort for the patient. All types of neurostimulation require periodic "battery changes" typically after several years (depending upon stimulation parameters) during which time the entire device is replaced. While this is same day surgery, general anesthesia is required.

With chronic or programmed stimulation the stimulation site may be remote from the seizure onset zone; seizure detection is not required for application of this therapy (open-loop). The VNS, the only FDA approved chronic stimulation therapy for epilepsy, was approved in 1997 following 5 controlled trials with 454 patients (Morris & Mueller, 1999). VNS is approved for patients with partial seizures, although it has been used in patients with intractable primary generalized epilepsy. In the pivotal trials, about 26% of patients had a 50% reduction in their seizures at 3 months, but this increased to 43% of patients after 2 years (Morris & Mueller, 1999). Only a small percentage of patients with VNS became seizure free (less than 3%). There is no evidence or expectation that VNS would be more or less effective in patients with ETLE. VNS would be appropriate therapy in medically intractable patients who are not candidates for surgery and who are expected to experience an improvement in quality of life with seizure reduction, but not seizure freedom.

Anterior thalamic stimulation is another chronic stimulation paradigm. Pivotal blinded studies (SANTÉ, Medtronics) have recently been completed (Fisher et al., 2010). These studies in patients with intractable partial seizures have demonstrated a 38% reduction in seizures during the blinded evaluation period that increased to 60% over the next year of unblinded therapy. Whether this improved efficacy with longer term follow-up after completion of the blinded protocol reflects additional medication adjustments or some other factor is not known. In many of the neurostimulation trials, efficacy improves with time, suggesting some type of neuromodulation. Because the anterior thalamus has much more extensive influence on temporal lobe structures (Bertram 2001; 2008) it is thought that anterior thalamic stimulation will be more effective for temporal lobe onset partial seizures than for seizures of extratemporal lobe onset. Programmed stimulation with the anterior thalamic stimulation was approved for use in the European Union in 2010, but the FDA is requesting additional information before granting approval in the United States.

■ Principles of responsive neurostimulation

The concept of responsive neurostimulation is that, in contrast to chronic, programmed stimulation, a closed-loop device will detect seizure activity early and deliver therapy that will disrupt or terminate the seizure. The goal is not to prevent seizures since the principle of RNS relies on seizure detection. The goal is to prevent a partial seizure from evolving from a simple partial (e.g. an aura or sensory phenomena) or electrical seizure into a disabling seizure (e.g. one with alteration of consciousness). While extratemporal neocortical partial seizures propagate more rapidly than do mesial temporal onset seizures, there is still time for intervention with responsive therapy. There is considerable controversy over what constitutes a seizure and this will not be resolved in this chapter. Suffice it to say that 10-20 seconds of clear ictal activity in one brain region (*e.g.* mesial temporal) might produce clinical symptoms, whereas similar activity in another brain region (*e.g.* frontopolar) might not. The authors here would consider both seizures, independent of the clinical manifestations.

Seizure detection in the context of closed-loop therapy is therefore much different than seizure detection in an epilepsy monitoring unit (EMU). In the EMU, detection software can utilize the entire record for detection and can therefore more readily sort out interictal epileptiform activity from ictal events. In fact retrospective review is even acceptable since the goal is to detect seizures for visual inspection and presurgical planning. With intracranial electrode arrays confounding artifacts are much less common. When, however, as in the case of responsive neurostimulation, seizure detection is required online within seconds of seizure onset so that therapy can be triggered, then the challenges for the detection software are considerably greater even with intracranial electrodes (Jouny *et al.*, 2010a).

Partial seizures are self-limited events. In a study of intracranial recordings, mesial temporal lobe onset partial seizures lasted a median of 106 seconds, significantly longer than extratemporal neocortical partial seizures where the median duration was 78 seconds (Afra *et al.*, 2008). In many patients the seizure duration of partial seizures without secondary generalization are remarkably similar, suggesting an intrinsic dynamic of the epileptic network. While the number of partial seizures often increases with antiepileptic drug (AED) withdrawal, and the number of secondarily generalized seizures increases, it is not established that the duration of the complex partial seizures changes with AED withdrawal.

The hypothesis underlying responsive neurostimulation is that stimulation can change the dynamics of the seizure to result in early seizure termination. The analogies to defibrillation some authors have made are not appropriate; RNS therapy delivers very low intensity currents (12 mA maximum) designed to alter seizure evolution, not to repolarize tissue as in cardiac stimulation. Early proof of principle studies demonstrated that these small currents could terminate afterdischarges produced during cortical stimulation of humans (Lesser *et al.*, 1999). Neuronal network models have shown that stimulation can terminate repetitive bursting and that in fact inhibitory connections are not a requirement, *i.e.* that excitatory currents can disrupt seizure dynamics (Franaszczuk *et al.*, 2003).

Current concepts of closed-loop responsive stimulation rely on very early seizure detection, not detection of a preictal period or seizure prediction. Early detection is much more reliable and computationally less demanding than prediction at present. Although stimulation remote from the seizure onset zone could conceivably produce seizure termination, since seizures are network phenomena, it is felt that having the stimulating electrodes near the seizure onset zone is desirable because the goal of therapy is early seizure detection so that therapy can be delivered before the partial seizures propagate to produce disabling symptoms. While closed-loop intervention after seizure propagation might still produce earlier seizure termination than would normally happen without therapy, it is less likely to have a significant impact if alteration of consciousness has already occurred. The currently employed seizure detection algorithms in the Neuropace RNS® employ simple concepts (either alone or in combination) of line-length, area under the curve, and half wave, in part because they are computationally efficient for use in low-power implantable devices. Most epileptic seizures with rapid, repetitive, increased synchronous activity will have increases in one or more of these parameters.

■ Characteristics of early partial seizure onset

Identification of seizure onset from intracranial EEG recordings in the EMU during presurgical evaluations is traditionally done by visual inspection. Seizure onset can be characterized by various patterns of activity. Periodic or quasi periodic spiking, rhythmic non-spiking activity, and low voltage fast activity are examples of types of seizure onset. An accompanying chapter by Jacobs and Gotman in this volume discusses the importance of low voltage fast activity as an early feature of neocortical onset seizures. This activity will result in increases in line length and area under the curve due to the rhythmic activity. As computational capabilities increase, it is hoped that more sophisticated early seizure detection can be developed that will result in increased sensitivity and specificity. The following discussion of complexity changes early in seizure onset is designed to provide insights into seizure dynamics. These complexity measures are not yet online tools, but may be in the future. Others (Meier *et al.*, 2008; Osorio *et al.*, 2002) have developed wavelet-based parameters for detection of seizures from intracranial recordings.

One can analyze the ictal signal in various ways. Because partial seizures are rapidly evolving events, such common analytic tools such a FFT are not ideal. Similarly, methods that rely on quasi-stationary periods or assume linear characteristics of the signal may misrepresent the signal. One of the most appropriate methods for signal analysis of seizure activity is the matching pursuit (MP) method (Mallat and Zhang, 1993) which is a method for time-frequency analysis that provides detailed decomposition of any signal, even rapidly changing ones. The MP method makes no assumptions about linearity or nonlinearity of the signal. The MP method decomposes a signal into simpler signals called atoms. The most commonly used atoms are those based on the Gabor function which is a Gaussian modulated oscillation.

A common feature seen at the onset of most partial seizures is an increase in signal complexity (Jouny *et al.*, 2005; 2010). This is seen whether the ictal onset clearly contains mixed frequencies or if the signal is dominated by a predominant monotonic frequency. This increase in complexity occurs whether the activity is low voltage fast activity or higher voltage lower frequency activity. Jouny *et al.* have developed a way of quantifying signal complexity, the Gabor atom density (GAD) method (Jouny *et al.*, 2003). This method quantifies the number of atoms necessary to represent the signal as derived from the MP decomposition. *Figure 1* illustrates an example of a brief frontal neocortical onset seizure. As is common for these types of partial seizures, the early seizure onset is characterized by an electrodecremental change in the signal associated with the development of prominent low voltage fast activity. The time-frequency decomposition reveals both the increased contributions of the higher frequency components and the increased number of atoms necessary to represent the signal. The GAD plot (dark line) quantifies this signal complexity change. At time 20 seconds, after the conclusion of the seizure, the signal is also of low amplitude, but in this postictal window the complexity is actually lower than baseline. These changes in frequency and complexity associated with seizure onset and evolution are often difficult to appreciate with mere visual assessment of the intracranial EEG (ICEEG) signal.

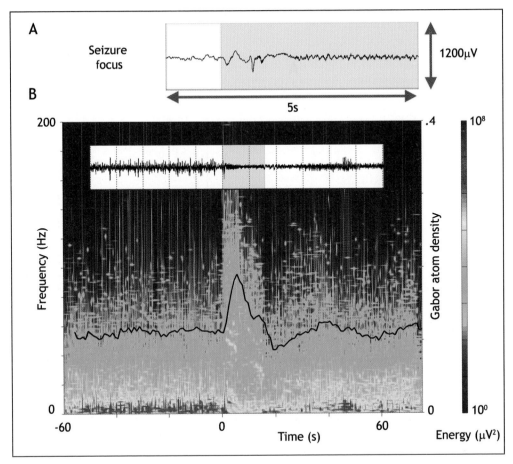

Figure 1. Intracranial EEG recordings of a partial seizure onset with neocortical localization over a 5 second window **(A)** and time-frequency decomposition of the entire seizure with one minute before and after the seizure **(B)**. Onset of a neocortical onset seizure may often be short in duration and only presents subtle changes that cannot be identified solely based on the amplitude of the signal. The frequency shift at onset is better assessed by the matching pursuit decomposition and a derived measure the Gabor atom density (black trace).

Early seizure detection is facilitated by the fact that seizures originating from a given focus in a given patient have very similar dynamics, particularly early in the seizure. This can be shown using the GAD complexity measure *(Figure 2)*. Examination of the corresponding time-frequency decompositions (not shown) would also reflect this similarity. This similarity of seizure onset allows for tuning of any early detection method, particularly one using intracranial recordings, to the specific patient, improving specificity of detection (Qu *et al.*, 1997; Shoeb *et al.*, 2004).

Figure 3 illustrates this similarity of early seizure dynamics from recurrent frontal neocortical seizures. This figure demonstrates that propagation patterns for seizures originating from the same focus can be similar whether examining the raw ICEEG data or GAD propagation maps which plot the changing GAD measure of complexity. This representation highlights the fact that signal complexity changes parallel seizure propagation. Also shown is the dramatic drop in signal complexity in the post-ictal period. Note the abrupt

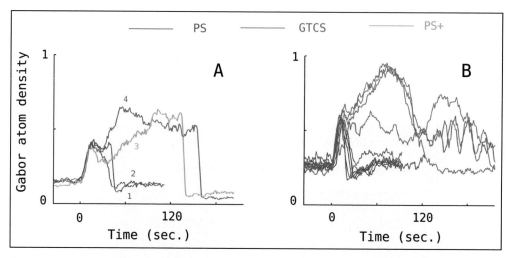

Figure 2. Gabor atom density plots of stereotypical onset of partial onset seizures in two patients (A and B) with neocortical onset epilepsy. Despite the various types of seizures, the dynamic of each onset, as characterized by the Gabor atom density, remains extremely similar within each patient. The dynamic of the early stage of the seizure is similar regardless of the later evolution of the seizures into a partial seizure (blue), a partial seizure with secondary focus (green) or a generalized tonic-clonic seizure (red). Similarity of seizure onset dynamic is the basis of current early seizure onset detection techniques (Jouny et al., 2007).

seizure termination, particularly in the second seizure of *figure 3*. This abrupt, spontaneous termination in all channels is the predominant termination pattern (Afra, Bergey and Jouny, unpublished data) for the majority of both temporal and extratemporal partial seizures. This spontaneous termination follows changes in seizure dynamics as organized rhythmic seizure activity becomes more intermittent prior to termination. This pattern of spontaneous terminiation was a factor in developing the hypothesis that external stimulation could potentially lead to earlier seizure termination.

■ Responsive neurostimulation for partial seizures: current status

The Neuropace RNS® device is implanted into a recess in the skull where a titanium ferrule is inserted and secured *(Figure 4)*. The device itself contains a microprocessor that can be programmed for both seizure detection parameters and closed-loop stimulation parameters. Programming and downloading of data can be done via a transcranial wireless communication device placed over the implant location. Two electrode arrays, either depths or strips can be connected. The electrodes are placed in brain regions thought to be near the seizure onset zone based on previous ictal recordings, either scalp or intracranial. Multiple contacts can be stimulated as either anode or cathode and up to five therapies are delivered after each detection. Typical pulse durations are in the range of 160 μs with stimulus durations of 100-200 ms. While various stimulus frequencies can be employed, 100-200 Hz is the most commonly used range. The device records the time and number of detections and closed-loop therapy. A limited number of electrocorticographic events (ECoGs) can be stored in the device, but these can be readily downloaded to a remote server and reviewed. As mentioned previously, the Neuropace RNS® utilizes relatively simple detection algorithms. The detection parameters can be revised and tuned for the given seizure morphology and new parameters can be tested on previously recorded seizures to determine if these modifications produce earlier or more reliable seizure detection.

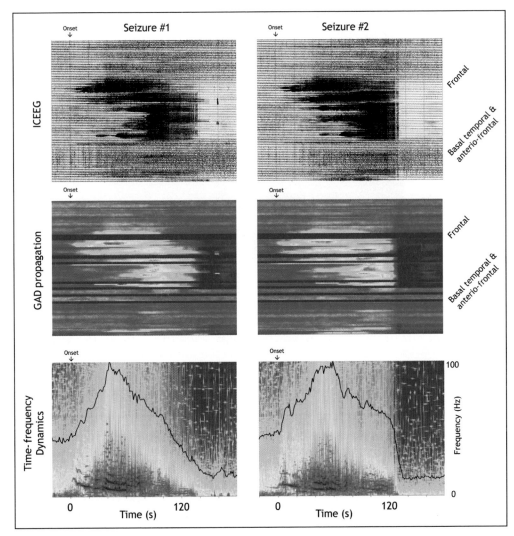

Figure 3. Similarity of dynamic propagation of two neocortical onset partial seizures in the same patient recorded days apart. Top panels show the ICEEG traces for the seizures with frontal electrodes at the top and the basal temporal and anterio-frontal electrodes at the bottom. Middle panels show the GAD propagation maps which quantify the propagation of epileptiform activity. Electrodes order is similar to that of the ICEEG above. Lower panels show the time-frequency and GAD plot for the electrode closest to the focus. Time 0 is the time of the onset. For detection of seizure done a posteriori, similarity of the evolution of the seizure can be used to improved seizure identification.

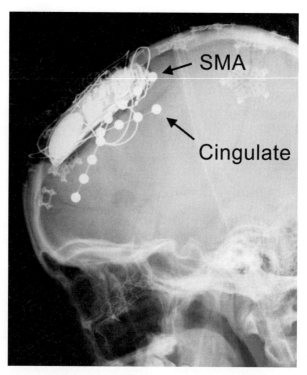

Figure 4. Skull film of patient with Neuropace® responsive neurostimulator. Patient has intractable complex partial seizures with frontal lobe onset (documented by previous invasive video-EEG monitoring). The two connected subdural strips are in the region of the left interhemispheric SMA and left cingulated gyrus. An additional strip is not connected to the device.

The responsive neurostimulation using the Neuropace RNS® system has been demonstrated to be effective for patients with refractory partial onset seizures (Morrell, 2011). Recruitment of 191 patients was done at 32 sites. Because intracranial stimulation is not perceived by the patient (in contrast to VNS therapy) the trial could be conducted in a blinded fashion. Patients represented a mix of those with intractable partial epilepsy from various brain regions. The pivotal trials were completed in 2009; the results of these trials have not yet been published in peer reviewed journals, but have been reported at national meetings (Morrell et al., 2008; 2009). Preliminary case reports and reviews have been published (Bergey 2008; Sun et al., 2008; Fountas et al., 2005; Anderson et al., 2008). A significant 29% reduction in seizures occurred over the 12 week blinded evaluation period. With long-term therapy during the period following the blinded protocol period these responder rates improved (46% had a 50% or greater reduction in their seizures). This suggests the possibility that neuromodulation such as seen with other types of neurostimulation may play a role, but since this occurred during the unblinded period, other factors may also be involved. It is not known whether subgroups of patients such as mesial temporal onset or extratemporal lobe neocortical onset responded more favorably than others, but patients with extratemporal onset seizures did benefit from the responsive stimulation. The Neuropace RNS® was well tolerated with only rare self-limited treatment related adverse events. Therapies can be delivered for years; good electrode impedances were maintained (platinum electrodes). *Figure 5* illustrates an example of a downloaded detection and therapy in a patient with frontal lobe neocortical partial seizures. This illustration shows very early seizure detections despite an onset pattern that is low voltage fast activity. Two trains of therapy were delivered but this did not prevent continued seizure evolution. In this patient it was thought (from later more extensive intracranial recordings) that the seizure onset zone was somewhat removed from the stimulating electrode.

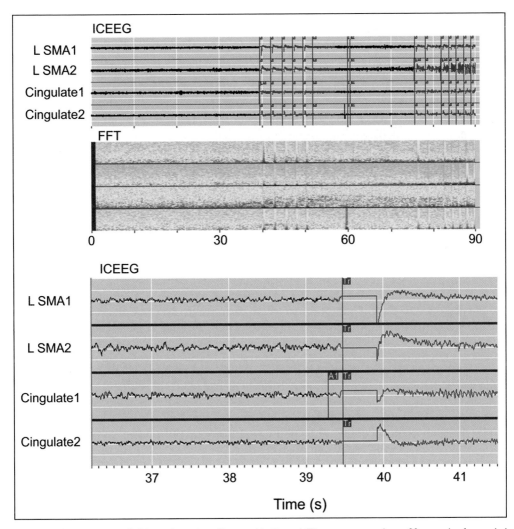

Figure 5. A seizure recorded from the patient illustrated in *figure 4*. The upper trace shows 90 seconds of recorded activity including the seizure and illustrates the detections (blue) and multiple delivered therapies. The middle trace is the FFT of the epoch showing the increased high frequency activity. The lower trace illustrates the time from 36 to 42 seconds, illustrating the low voltage high frequency activity that triggered the closed-loop responsive therapy (stimulus artifact). In this instance and in the top panel the closed-loop therapy did not terminate the seizure, probably because the stimulating electrode was not over the seizure onset zone. This data is data recorded from the Neuropace® device and downloaded by the patient to the remote server.

With the current detection algorithms used with the closed-loop Neuropace RNS® system, the system can be tuned to be very sensitive, *i.e.* not to miss any epileptiform activity lasting 2 seconds or more. This sensitivity, however, results in detections and therapy that often number over 500 per day. While the total amount of closed-loop stimulation delivered is still quite brief, clearly not all of these events are destined to become partial seizures, even with the most liberal definition of a seizure. These are not false positive detections *per se* because they are detecting abnormal epileptiform activity. Responsive closed-loop therapy is, however, delivered following all detected events. Whether this additional stimulation provides added benefit is not known.

Evaluation of the efficacy of neurostimulation is much different than the assessment of efficacy of a new AED. In AED trials a range of doses can usually be determined based on tolerability and projected efficacy. This is much more difficult with trials of neurostimulation. The optimal stimulation parameters have not been established for chronic programmed or responsive closed-loop stimulation and these parameters may be different for different patients depending upon the dynamics of their seizures. The blinded treatment period in the Neuropace RNS® trial is relatively short (12 weeks) and could well occur before determination of optimal stimulation parameters. Failure to respond optimally to RNS therapy therefore can be due to a variety of factors. In some patients the exact seizure onset zone may be difficult to determine, particularly if previous intracranial monitoring was not done (this was not required for the trial). Therefore stimulation may be remote from the seizure onset zone. Multifocal seizure onsets can further confound therapy.

The goal of responsive neurostimulation is to detect partial seizures early with high sensitivity and to provide therapy that will result in early seizure termination prior to evolution to disabling seizures. The fact that responsive neurostimulation has been demonstrated to produce significant reduction of disabling partial seizure in patients with medically intractable partial seizures represents a gratifying first step in the application of this novel therapy. There are many reasons to hope that further refinement of patient selection and therapeutic parameters will improve upon these early results. Neurostimulation with approved devices as treatment for epilepsy in patients with intractable partial seizures who are not optimal candidates for seizure surgery (and this includes many patients with ETLE) represents a reasonable alternative to additional AED trials. Closed-loop responsive therapy is the most technologically advanced neurostimulation therapy and as such potentially holds the greatest future promise. Studies of stimulus parameters using neural network models may assist in determination of the optimal stimulation parameters (Anderson et al., 2007; 2009). Closed-loop responsive therapy could also employ other treatment modalities such as focal cooling or focal drug application (Burton et al., 2005; Fujii et al., 2010; Stein et al., 2000). While current RNS therapy relies on early seizure detection, the potential exists for applications of RNS to preictal periods if reliable, computationally efficient prediction algorithms could be developed and implemented.

References

- Afra P, Jouny CC, Bergey GK. Duration of complex partial seizures: An intracranial electrode study. *Epilepsia* 2008; 49: 677-84.
- Anderson WS, Kudela P, Cho RJ, Bergey GK, Franaszczuk PJ. Studies of stimulus parameters for seizure disruption using neural network simulations. *Biol Cybern* 2007; 97: 173-94.

- Anderson WS, Kossoff EH, Bergey GK, Jallo GI. Implantation of a responsive neurostimulator device in patients with refractory epilepsy. *Neurosurg Focus* 2008; 25: E12.

- Anderson WS, Weinberg S, Kudela P, Bergey GK, Franaszczuk PJ. Phase dependent stimulation effects on bursing activity in a neural network cortical simulation. *Epilepsy Res* 2009; 84: 42-55.

- Ben-Menachem E. Vagus nerve stimulation, side effects, and long-term study. *J Clin Neurophysiol* 2001; 18: 415-8.

- Bergey GK. Responsive neurostimulation for the treatment of epileptic seizures. In: Schelter B, Timmer J, Schulze-Bonhage, A, eds. *Seizure Predicition in Epilepsy – From Basic Mechanisms to Clinical Applications*. Weinheim: Wiley-VCH, 2008, pp. 299-306.

- Bergey GK. Brain Stimulation. In: Shorvon S, Engel, J, Perucca E, eds. *Treatment of Epilepsy*, 3rd edition. Hoboken: Wiley, 2009 pp 1025-1034.

- Bertram EH, Williamson JM, Scott C, Mangan PS, Zhang DX. The midline thalamus: alterations and a potential role in limbic epilepsy. *Epilepsia* 2001; 42: 967-78.

- Bertram EH, Zhang DX, Williamson JM. Multiple roles of midline dorsal thalamic nuclei in induction and spread of limbic seizures. *Epilepsia* 2008; 49: 256-68.

- Burton JM, Peebles GA, Binder DK, Rothman SM, Smyth MD. Transcortical cooling inhibits hippocampal-kindled seizures in the rat. *Epilepsia* 2005; 46: 1881-7.

- Fisher RS, Salanova V, Witt T, *et al*. Electrical stimulation of the anterior nucleus of thalamus for treatment of refractory epilepsy. *Epilepsia* 2010; 5: 899-908.

- Fountas KN, Smith JR, Murro AM, *et al*. Implantation of a closed-loop stimulation in the management of medically refractory focal epilepsy: a technical note. *Stereotact Funct Neurosurg* 2005; 83: 153-8.

- Franaszczuk PJ, Kudela P Bergey GK. External excitatory stimulation can terminate repetitive bursting in neural network models. *Epilepsy Res* 2003; 53: 65-80.

- Fujii M, Fujioka H, Oku T, Tanaka N, Imoto H, Maruta Y, Nomura S, Kajiwara K, Saito T, Yamakawa T, Yamakawa T, Suzuki M. Application of focal cerebral cooling for the treatment of intractable epilepsy. *Neurol Med Chir (Tokyo)* 2010; 50: 839-44.

- Jouny, C, Franaszczuk PJ, Bergey GK. Characterization of epileptic seizure dynamics using the Gabor atom density. *Clin Neurophysiol* 2003; 114: 426-37.

- Jouny CC, Franaszczuk PJ, Bergey GK. Signal complexity and synchrony of epileptic seizures: is there an identifiable preictal period? *Clin Neurophysiol* 2005; 116: 552-8.

- Jouny CC, Adamolekun B, Franaszczuk PJ, Bergey GK. Dynamics at the seizure focus: differential effects of secondary generalization revealed by complexity measures. *Epilepsia* 2007; 48: 297-304.

- Jouny CC, Franaszczuk PJ, Bergey GK. Early seizure detection: considerations and applications. In: Rho, JM, Sankar R, Cavazos JE, eds. *Epilepsy: Scientific Foundations of Clinical Management*, 2nd Edition. New York: Marcel Dekker Inc, 2010a, pp 567-582.

- Jouny CC, Bergey GK, Franaszczuk PJ. Partial seizures are associated with early increases in signal complexity. *Clin Neurophysiol* 2010; 121: 7-13.

- Lesser RP, Kim SH, Beyderman L, *et al*. Brief bursts of pulse stimulation terminate afterdischarges caused by cortical stimulation. *Neurology*1999; 53: 2073-81.

- Mallat SG, Zhang ZF. Matching pursuits with time-frequency dictionaries. *IEEE Trans Sig Proc* 1993. 41(12): 3397-415.

- Meier R, Dittrich H, Schulze-Bonhage A, Aertsen A. Detecting epileptic seizures in longterm human EEG: A new approach to automatic online and real-time detection and classification of polymorphic seizure patterns. *J Clin Neurophysiol* 2008; 25: 119-31.

- Morrell MJ, Hirsch LJ, Bergey G, *et al*. Long-term safety and efficacy of the RNS™ system in adults with medically intractable partial onset seizures. *Epilepsia* 2008; 49: 481-2.

- Morrell MJ, and the RNS System Pivotal Investigators. *Results of a multicenter double blinded randomized controlled pivotal investigation of the RNS™ system for treatment of intractable partial epilepsy in adults.* American Epilepsy Society, 2009, Abstr 1.102.
- Morrell MJ, RNS System in Epilepsy Study Group. Responsive cortical stimulation for the treatment of medically intractable partial epilepsy. *Neurology* 2011; in press.
- Morris GL 3rd, Mueller WM. Long-term treatment with vagus nerve stimulation in patients with refractory epilepsy. The Vagus Nerve Stimulation Study Group E01-E05. *Neurology* 1999; 53: 1731-5.
- Osorio I, Frei MG, Giftakis J, *et al.* Performance reassessment of a real-time seizure detection algorithm on long ECoG series. *Epilepsia* 2002; 43: 1522-35.
- Qu H, Gotman J. A patient-specific algorithm for the detection of seizure onset in longterm EEG monitoring: Possible use as a warning device. *IEEE Trans Biomed Eng* 1997; 44: 115-22.
- Shoeb A, Edwards H, Connolly J, Bourgeois B, Treves T, Guttag J. Patient-specific seizure onset detection. *Epilepsy Behav* 2004, 5 (4): 483-98.
- Stein AG, Eder HG, Blum DE, Drachev A, Fisher RS. An automated drug delivery system for focal epilepsie. *Epilepsy Res* 2000; 39: 103-14.
- Sun FT, Morrell MJ, Wharen RE, Jr. Responsive cortical stimulation for the treatment of epilepsy. *Neurotherapeutics* 2008; 5: 68-74.

Electrical stimulation of invasive electrodes in extratemporal lobe epilepsy

Caspar Stephani[1], Hans O. Lüders[2]

[1] Department of Clinical Neurophysiology, University of Göttingen, Göttingen, Germany

[2] The Neurological Institute, Department of Neurology, University Hospitals Case Medical Center, Cleveland, Ohio, USA

■ Technical aspects of brain stimulation

The object of electrocortical stimulation

The nervous system uses electrical currents to process information. Neurons, axons and dendrites are the elements of the nervous system that provide the neuroanatomical basis for the transmission of currents. 10% of a unit volume of the cerebral cortex is composed of neurons. 30% are filled by axons and 30% by dendrites, 10% by glia cells and around 12% by spines. The remaining 8% space contains extracellular matrix and blood vessels (Braitenberg & Schütz, 1998). The density of neurons within the cerebral cortex is estimated to be $10^5/mm^3$ (Schütz & Palm, 1989). And the total number of neurons in the cerebral cortex of man has been calculated to be approximately $1\text{-}2 \times 10^{10}$ neurons (Braendgaard et al., 1990). Pyramidal cells, stellate cells and Martinotti cells are the three main classes of neurons in the cerebral cortex according to a recent classification based on morphological characteristics (Braitenberg & Schütz, 1998). Up to 85% of all neurons are pyramidal cells.

Estimations from light- and electronmicroscopical cortical sections postulate a total length of axons within a volume of 1 mm^3 of 2-4 km whereas the total length of dendrites per mm^3 is estimated to be around 450 m. This ratio of nearly 10 to 1 between the length of axonal and dendritic elements in the cerebral cortex is due to the greater thickness of the latter. However, there are approximately 10 times more synapses per dendrite compared to axon (Braitenberg & Schütz, 1998). The large majority of these axons is thought to be of intracortical origin. Even in the primary sensory areas receiving prominent afferents from brainstem nuclei and the diencephalon only about 20% of synapses are of extracortical origin (White, 1986).

Synapses link these basic elements to each other. The size of a synapse in mouse cortex is between 320 and 380 nm and the number of synapses per mm^3 is approximately 7.2×10^8 per mm^3. This figure was found to be roughly the same in different areas of the cortex and also in different cortical layers. Therefore the ratio of synapses to neuron depends mainly on the local neuronal density and size of the neurons and differs considerably between cortical areas and species. For the primary motor cortex it has been estimated that this ratio is of 13,000 and 60,000 in mice and men respectively whereas the number of synapses per neuron in the visual cortex was 7,000 and 5,600 respectively (Cragg, 1967). Based on morphological criteria in electron micrographs 89% of all synapses are classified as type I synapses whereas the remaining 11% are classified as type II synapses (Gray, 1959). It has been suggested that these two morphological entities represent excitatory (type I) and inhibitory (type II) synapses respectively (Uchizono, 1965). In general, pyramidal cells are the presynaptic element of type I synapses and stellate cells are the presynaptic element of type II synapses. Spines are the postsynaptic element in 75% of all synapses and synapses on spines are thought to be almost exclusively type I synapses. The distribution of synapses on an axon collateral does not appear to follow a recognizable pattern and may in fact follow a random distribution (Braitenberg & Schütz, 1998).

The medium of electrocortical stimulation

There are two main categories in which techniques to stimulate the brain electrically are classified Electrical stimulation of the brain can be performed with invasive electrodes or non-invasively. Invasive stimulation techniques include intracranial implantation of subdural, epidural or depth electrodes. Non-invasive techniques of brain stimulation include transcranial magnetic stimulation (TMS) and transcranial direct current stimulation (tDCS). Non-invasive stimulation methods have come to greater attention in the past 25 years. This review, however, will only refer to invasive stimulation.

Parameters of stimulation

Invasive electrical stimulation represents a non-physiological activation of the central nervous system. It does not mimic the elaborate physiological mechanisms that lead to selective excitation and inhibition of specific neurons in the central nervous system. Still, it may mimic some of basic effects mediated by a given neuronal circuit.

The following technical parameters influence the effectiveness of invasive electrical stimulation: i) polarity of the stimulus, ii) current intensity, iii) pulse width, iv) frequency, v) waveform, vi) phase, vii) train duration, viii) electrode configuration, ix) size of the electrode. Understanding the contributions of these factors to the effects of electrocortical stimulation is important. The constellation of parameters described here affects not only thresholds of stimulation to elicit a certain response but may change the quality of response. Therefore, it is essential to select the appropriate stimulus parameters for specific purposes.

Polarity: The term "polarity" in electrical stimulation may refer to the arrangement of the two electrodes being "monopolar" or "bipolar". This will be discussed below in the section "electrode configuration". In this paragraph the term polarity refers to the direction of the stimulating current, *i.e.* if the stimulating electrode is the anode or the cathode. Previous studies consistently have shown that "monopolar" cathodal pulses are significantly more effective as compared to "monopolar" anodal stimulation for eliciting action potentials in the central nervous system with intracerebral stimulation. Varying ratios of cathodal to anodal threshold currents between 3 and 12 for single pyramidal tract cells in the motor-sensory cortex of the cat (Stoney et al., 1968) and 3.19 and 7.7 for surface stimulation of the dorsal column of cats (BeMent & Ranck, 1969) were reported. Besides, the stimulation threshold for "negative pulses" were consistently less than those for "positive pulses" in cortical and subcortical stimulation of monkeys (Mihailovic & Delgado, 1956). Increasing the intensity of a cathodal stimulus to several times the threshold current a paradoxical blocking of an action potential may occur. While the outward current in direct proximity to the stimulating cathode depolarizes the nerve fiber an inward current in the more distant parts of the fiber will hyperpolarize these parts accordingly. Therefore, strong stimulation can lead to a complete block of the action potential on either side of the axon abolishing stimulation *(Figure 1)*. This effect has been named "anodal surround" referring to the anodal-like effect in the periphery of cathodal stimulation (Ranck, 1975). As a consequence the fibers closest to the stimulating cathode may not necessarily be stimulated most effectively. In fact, no excitation takes place in a core around the electrode tip while comparable fibers in a surrounding shell are stimulated. The same may be true in a reverse pattern for anodal stimulation.

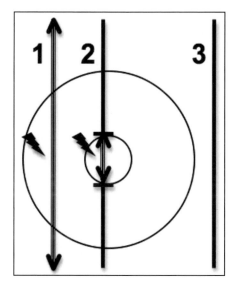

Figure 1. The "anodal surround" effect. Vertical lines represent nerve fibers. The circles are centered around a hypothetical cathodal current source. Fiber 1 will be stimulated. Cathodal current strength reaches stimulation threshold, while anodal inward current does not. Fiber 2 will be depolarized being closest to the current source. But the action potential will be blocked by a strong hyperpolarizing current as indicated by the inner circle. Fiber 3 will not be depolized being to far away from the current source.

By analyzing latencies of evoked responses it could be shown that when using threshold currents with anodal surface stimulation of the baboon's motor cortex, the axon hillock of pyramidal tract cells would be excited directly while cathodal surface stimulation with the same stimulation threshold activates pyramidal tract cells via presynaptic elements (Hern et al., 1962). The same study could demonstrate that the minimal threshold for direct excitation of pyramidal tract cells is smaller with anodal surface stimulation as compared to cathodal surface stimulation *(Figure 2)*. Interestingly, there was a systematic spatial differences between the effectiveness of anodal and cathodal stimulation with the latter being more effective in more precentral areas compared to anodal stimulation. Others, when stimulating the motor cortex of the cat found that anodal surface stimulation was more effective in exciting Betz cells than cathodal stimulation (Phillips, 1956). It is also interesting that the stimulation threshold for eliciting a clinical response by surface cathodal stimulation of the somatosensory cortex was smaller than for surface anodal stimulation and that the ratio of both was found to be between 0.6 and 0.9 while such a difference could not be found with cortical surface stimulation of the precentral gyrus (Libet et al., 1964).

Current intensity: This is the single most important parameter of electrical stimulation. The current intensity required to elicit a clinical response or to excite a nerve fiber or neuron depends on the cerebral region and the cerebral structure stimulated. When comparing stimulation of motor and sensory cortex the threshold current intensity for eliciting either a movement from the precentral gyrus or a sensation from stimulation of the postcentral gyrus appears to be similar using comparable parameters of stimulation (Penfield & Boldrey, 1937; Libet, 1964). However, producing *motor responses* with electrical stimulation of the postcentral gyrus requires much higher threshold currents than in the precentral gyrus (Vogt & Vogt, 1919; Foerster, 1936). Also, the electrode type is of importance and intracerebral microelectrodes and depth electrodes generally require lower or much lower stimulating currents to elicit a certain response as compared to cortical surface stimulation (Stoney et al., 1968). The minimum stimulation threshold for direct activation of axons can be as low as 0.1 μA when stimulating interneurons of the ventral horn of the spinal cord of cats (Jankowska & Roberts, 1972). It can be calculated that this value corresponds to an electrode tip 30 μm distance from an axon. A minimum stimulation threshold of 1 μA at a distance of 45 μm was also proposed (Stoney et al., 1968). These values are important since they represent the slope of threshold-distance relationships which often shows a parabolic correlation between threshold current and distance from a given element to be excited. In *figure 4* this relationship is depicted on a double-logarithmic table given a fixed set of conditions according to Ranck (1975). Additionally, studies in monkeys have shown that the stimulation threshold also depends on the physiological state of the animal under investigation (Delgado, 1981). Namely, the stimulation threshold for inducing saccades by electrical stimulation of the frontal eye field (FEF), the dorsomedial frontal cortex (DMFC) or the primary visual cortex (V1) depends on the state of preactivation of the visual system. Free-viewing or active fixation, location of the fixation and concurrent existence or non-existence of reward are such important factors (Tehovnik & Slocum, 2004).

Pulse width: The pulse width or pulse duration has major effect on the stimulation intensity required to elicit a response. In order to minimize the charge needed for electrical stimulation, a pulse width of 100 μs or less has been recommended (Barry et al., 1973). Others observed a significant decrease in stimulation threshold when increasing pulse width to 0.5 msec and suggested an optimal pulse width in the vicinity of 0.5 msec (Libet, 1973). Therefore, a pulse width between 100-500 μs may be regarded as most effective (Mihailovic & Delgado, 1956). Due to different time constants of different structural parts of the nervous system it may be possible to selectively stimulate certain neuronal elements. A brief pulse width would preferentially stimulate axons or axon hillocks (Ranck, 1975; Nowak & Bullier, 1998). It is important to remember, that using longer pulse widths does not facilitate the response anymore but may be more likely to induce repetitive discharges.

Frequency: Stimulation frequencies from 30 to 250 Hz are associated with the lowest stimulation intensities for eliciting motor or autonomic responses with cerebral stimulation when other stimulation parameters are left constant (Mihailovic & Delgado, 1956). In the motor cortex a qualitative change in response to electrical stimulation can be observed when changing the stimulation frequency. Single contractions follow a stimulus rate up to 30 Hz, smooth movements will be induced with frequencies between 60 and 500 Hz and jerky, sudden onset movements with frequencies between 1,000 and 5,000 Hz (Lilly et al., 1952; Mihailovic & Delgado, 1956). It could be shown that electrical stimulation of the motor cortex with a stimulation frequency of 50 Hz induces clonus of 4-8 Hz repetition rate. When decreasing the stimulation frequency to 20 Hz the frequency of the clonus decreases as well. Stimulation frequencies below 20 Hz does not induce stable clonus (Hamer et al., 2002). Therefore, temporal summation of pulses may be a relevant mechanism in the generation of clonus. In accordance with these findings, subdural electrode recordings during tonic-clonic seizures show a polyspike-wave pattern time-locked to the clonic movements as revealed by muscle action potential recordings (Hamer et al., 2003). Temporal summation of subthreshold potentials has been suggested as one possible explanation of the good effectiveness of higher frequency stimulation regarding the stimulation threshold (Ranck, 1981). In order to induce temporal summation or facilitation the interstimulus interval needs to be sufficiently small and may not exceed a few time constants of the membrane. Studies in simple monosynaptic models could show that increasing presynaptic stimulation rates up to frequencies of 500 Hz can facilitate the postsynaptic potential (Curtis & Eccles, 1960). Beyond stimulation frequencies of 500 Hz the stimulating current threshold will not be reduced and may in fact begin to increase (Mihailovic & Delgado, 1956; Libet, 1964). Livingston (1950) reported that changing the stimulation-frequency even may reverse effects from excitation to inhibition. While high-frequency stimulation (30-60 Hz) of the frontal eye-field resulted in eye-version to the contralateral side, stimulation of a same point in the frontal eye-field at frequencies between 1 to 12 Hz could produce ipsilateral eye-version. However, this finding from electrocortical stimulation in macaque monkeys has not been substantiated by other studies. Contrasting to this report and in accordance with own observations, there were generally no significant changes of the quality of a somatosensory response after electrical stimulation of the postcentral gyrus when stimulation frequencies were modified from 15 to 120 Hz (Libet, 1973). Still, a considerable importance of the stimulus frequency for stimulation of the somatosensory cortex has been established when 250 stimuli were applied to the ventral posterior lateral nucleus of the thalamus by depth electrodes. None of these stimuli did elicit a conscious sensory response with a frequency of 1.8 Hz of suprathreshold currents up to 20 times the threshold current for eliciting conscious sensory responses by stimulus pulses to the skin. In contrast, stimulation with 60 Hz of the threshold current intensity for producing a sensation by stimulation of the skin was able to elicit paresthesias (Libet et al., 1967).

Waveform: Waveforms generated are either sinusoidal, square-waves or exponential-decay-waves. Few data are available concerning the actual effect of single waveforms for intracranial stimulation. Still, the significance of the waveform itself is regarded as low for the response of the nerve-cell population stimulated (Delgado, 1981).

Phase: A single stimulus cycle can be either mono- or biphasic regardless of the waveform. Mihailovic and Delgado (1956) did not find a significant difference of "monophasic" cathodal compared to biphasic pulses regarding the stimulation thresholds for producing motor responses. On the other hand the risk of tissue injury with application of monophasic current has been highlighted (Lilly et al., 1952) whereas prolonged stimulation with biphasic stimulation was found to be well-tolerated (Lilly et al., 1955). In a rat model 5 minutes of continuous monophasic stimulation with depth electrodes induced cerebral lesions that further increased with duration and intensity of stimulation while biphasic stimulation at the same intensity did not produce such lesions (Piallat et al., 2009). This difference between monophasic and biphasic stimulation has been attributed to the balanced current flow reducing accumulation of charges at the electrode contacts. Such lesions may not occur when the duration of stimulation is sufficiently brief.

Train duration : The appropriate train duration depends on the purpose of stimulation. Cerebral tissue can be stimulated electrically by a brief single pulse of a few microseconds duration evoking single action potentials. On the other extreme continuous brain stimulation for several months and longer has been used for therapeutic indications (Delgado, 1981). For locating motor representations by intra- or extraoperative electrocorticography a train duration of 1-3 seconds often is sufficient and prolonging stimulation will only increase the risk of inducing an epileptic seizure. The chance opf inducing an epileptic seizure is particularly high in the motor cortex even in patients not suffering from epilepsy (Libet, 1973). As already discussed above, the response to stimulation of the motor cortex may be influenced by the stimulation frequency. But the train duration also has a significant influence on the clinical response as well. Whereas myoclonic movements will be typical following single electrical stimuli or brief train durations of less than 0.5 sec, increasing the train duration will more likely produce tonic or even combined clonic-tonic or sequential movements. At the same time the minimum train duration for eliciting a somatosensory sensation by electrical stimulation of the somatosensory cortex (pulse width 0.5 msec, frequency 30/s or 60/s) is 0.4-1.0 sec. This value was found to be considerably stable over a range of different pulse widths, varying polarity and electrode configuration and electrode sizes. Still, Libet *et al.* (1967) reported that sensory evoked responses may be recorded by subdural electrodes after skin stimuli despite the lack of any conscious sensory experience. Neither the threshold current nor the quality of the response will change with prolonging stimulation whereas reducing the train duration affects both (Libet, 1964). Interestingly, the superficial cortical application of γ-amino-butyric-acid (GABA) does not change the stimulation threshold or type of sensory experience reported with electrocortical stimulation of the somatosensory cortex. This indicates that the mechanisms that are most important for the mediation of a conscious sensory response are centered in deeper cortical layers and that "postsynaptic responses of apical dendrites and other neuronal elements in the superficial cortical layers of sensory cortex (including the neuropil of the molecular layer) are not necessary for the production of a subjective sensory experience" (Libet, 1973). This is consistent with the observation of Clark *et al.* (1969) that somatosensory evoked potentials could be markedly reduced and almost vanished after inhalation of cyclopropane whereas the reported sensation did not change.

In contrast, depths electrodes implanted for therapeutic indication in movement disorders can be stimulated continuously while the risk for epileptic seizures remains relatively very low.

Another tissue-depending factor related to train duration is the fatigability of the tissue stimulated. Brain tissue depending of its fatigability has been subdivided into three categories: 1) quickly (within seconds) fatigable parts of the brain (motor cortex), 2) slowly (within minutes) fatigable parts of the brain (caudate nucleus), 3) parts of the brain with no evidence of fatigability (lateral hypothalamus) (Delgado, 1981). On the other hand, in some brain tissue fatigability may decrease when stimulation-free intervals are interspersed with more prolonged continuous electrical stimulation (Delgado *et al.*, 1976). For different cortical areas the time-interval after which the electrical properties of excitability and fatigability are restituted varies. For example, an interval between two trains of stimulation of 30 seconds and more has been recognized as being adequate for preventing post-stimulus facilitation after stimulating motor or sensory cortex (Libet *et al.*, 1964).

Electrode configuration : It is also important to chose between bipolar and monopolar electrode configuration for cortical stimulation. In fact, any stimulation is always bipolar. Nevertheless, monopolar stimulation refers to a set of two electrodes where one electrode, the reference, is distant from the other electrode, which we expect to produce the desired effect as a cathode or anode. Bipolar stimulation refers to a set of two electrodes in close proximity in which each of the two electrodes can produce a cortical response. However, the field of excitation depends more on parameters like pulse width and stimulus intensity than on the electrode configuration (Gallistel, 1981). The effect of stimulation usually is very focal at one electrode contact even in the case of bipolar stimulation. Since the size of the electrical field is not necessarily determined by the electrode configuration, the disadvantage of the bipolar configuration is that it frequently is difficult to assign a clinical response to one of the two electrodes which have been stimulated. In the case of a bipolar electrode configuration it is important to consider the arrangement of the electrodes with respect to the direction of the elements excited as it has been shown that it is the electrical field along a nerve fiber which determines the effectiveness of a stimulation. Brain structures parallel to the electric field are much easier to excite as compared to brain structures with a perpendicular orientation (Ranck, 1975).

This has been studied in the dorsal columns of cats where it could be shown that the stimulating current for bipolar electrode configurations perpendicular to the nerve fibers required threshold currents exceeding those for stimulation of the same elements with an arrangement parallel to the fibers by a factor of 4-5 (Rudin & Eisenman, 1954). Since polarizing effects of brain stimulation depend on the amount of current applied to the tissue, generally constant current stimulation is preferred over constant voltage stimulation as the latter will depend much more on the resistance of the stimulated tissue.

Size of the electrode : This problem has not been studied in detail. Studies with surface electrodes have shown that the total threshold current needed to elicit a conscious sensory response would increase twofold when using a 2 mm electrode instead of a 1 mm electrode and fourfold when using a 10 mm electrode compared to a 1 mm electrode. Since a tenfold increase in diameter equals a 100 fold increase in surface area the threshold current per mm^2 is reduced to 4% of the values obtained with a 1 mm electrode (Libet et al., 1964). In this report no differences in the clinical responses were found between stimulating the 1 mm electrode *vs* stimulating the 10 mm electrode at 4 times higher stimulus intensity. Mechanisms of spatial facilitation were suggested as possible explanation for the reduction in current density threshold.

In order to minimize the current delivered to the nervous system by electrical stimulation pulse durations of approximately 0.1 msec, a stimulation frequency of 100 Hz and only brief train durations of cathodal pulses are suggested (Gallistel, 1981). Besides, to avoid accumulation of charges at one electrode biphasic stimulation can be used.

The effect of electrocortical stimulation

For electrical cortical stimulation to be effective the stimulating current must initiate an action potential either in a neuron, axon or dendrite. In order to produce an action potential the resting membrane potential has to be depolarized. The resting membrane potential (V_m) is the difference between the voltage inside the cell (V_i) and the voltage outside the cell (V_e).

$$V_m = V_i - V_e \quad (1)$$

To change the membrane potential the voltage of either or both sides of the membrane has to be changed. Current flow is restricted by resistances and neuronal membranes have significant resistances to current flow. In the case of extracellular electrical stimulation, the current outside the neuron flows freely while, due to the resistance of membrane and cytosol, it has difficulty to cross the membrane and to flow inside the neurons. Hence, voltage changes inside and outside a neuronal structure differ with a significantly greater change at the outer side of the membrane in the case of extracellular electrical stimulation. Thus, neuronal membranes usually are depolarized in the direct vicinity of a cathode and hyperpolarized in the direct vicinity of an anode. This makes cathodal current more effective than anodal current for direct excitation concerning intracerebral stimulation. At the same time cathodal stimulation on the cortical surface will induce depolarization in the neuronal dendrites being generally closer to the surface whereas a hyperpolarization takes place in cell-body and axon (*Figure 2*). In case of cortical surface anodal stimulation the opposite effect is elicited, namely hyperpolarization at the cortical surface and depolarization in the cell body and axon (Nair *et al.*, 2008).

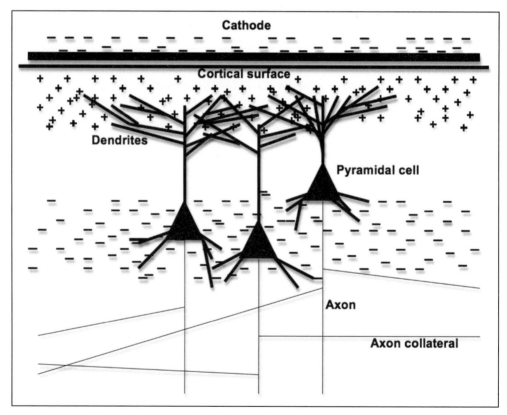

Figure 2. llustration of the effect of electrical stimulation of the cortical surface.
Cathodal surface stimulation will depolarize more superficial parts of the cortex. At the same time, the parts of pyramidal cells being more susceptible to electrical stimulation (axon initial segment, axons) will be hyperpolarized. Opposite effects will follow anodal surface stimulation (referring to Nair *et al.*, 2008).

Due to the relatively low threshold of axonal elements to electrical stimulation, it can be expected that surface anodal stimulation should be more likely to induce action potentials compared to surface cathodal stimulation (Asanuma & Sakata, 1967). However, experimental results are not always consistent with these theoretical conclusions.

There are two questions we need to resolve to permit a better understanding of the physiological effects produced by electrical cortical stimulation:

1) Which neuronal elements are excited by electrical stimulation?

2) How far does the effect of electrical stimulation reach?

For both questions it is important to specify the neural elements that are being stimulated as well as the parameters of the electrical stimulation. Therefore it is essentially imposible to derive generally applicable answers to these questions.

1) Extracellular stimulation does change the membrane potential of all structures close to the stimulating electrodes. Nevertheless, different parts of the nervous system show different degrees of excitability. Two tissue-specific parameters reflect excitability of a specific system or structure. The rheobase I_r is the minimum current necessary to induce a response in a system. The chronaxie C refers to the minimum pulse duration for eliciting a certain response at a current strength twice that of the rheobase. The following equation is the function of the strength-duration

$$I = I_r (1 + C/t) \quad (2)$$

where I is the current, I_r the rheobase current, C the chronaxie and t the pulse duration. Therefore this formula describes the dependence between threshold current and pulse duration. Pulse-duration curves for extracellular electric stimulation have an asymptotic course if one plots the duration of a stimulus on the abscisse and the intensity of the stimulus on the ordinate *(Figure 3)*. It represents a correlate of excitability and shows characteristic values for different elements of the CNS.

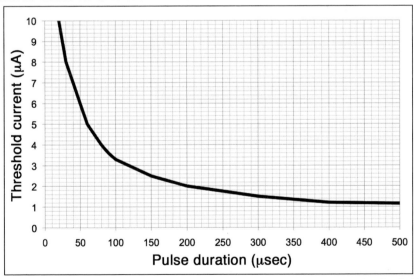

Figure 3. Strength-duration relation for stimulation of nerve fibers. This graph indicates the threshold current necessary to produce an action potential in a nerve fiber at a given pulse width. The rheobase is the threshold current when the pulse duration is infinite. The chronaxie is the pulse duration at twice the rheobase current. Values in this graph are approximations only (referring to Nowak & Bullier, 1998).

Studies established the lower chronaxies of axons and axon initial segments as compared to cell bodies or dendrites (Nowak & Bullier, 1998). This difference is most likely due to the higher density of sodium current channels in axons and axon hillocks compared to cell bodies and neurons. The densities of these channels in the axon is greater by a magnitude of 1 to 3 as compared to a cell body. Another factor which may be responsible for this difference is the higher resistivity of the membrane at the cell body compared to lower resistivities in the axon and especially at the nodes of Ranvier.

Stimulation of myelinated fibers or white matter repeatedly has been shown to have chronaxies of less than 200 µs (Ranck et al., 1975). Such short chronaxies most probably reflect the chronaxie of the nodes of Ranvier which most likely are the central nervous system elements with the shortest chronaxie. On the other hand the chronaxie of cell bodies largely exceeds that of axons by a factor of up to 40 (Nowak & Bullier, 1998). The consequence of this relationship is that at a given stimulus intensity and pulse duration the myelinated fibers will be the first activated elements in the CNS. It also suggests that excitation may be induced selectively at a specific CNS structure when its chronaxie is known.

Additionally, several factors of fiber anatomy influence the efficacy of electrical stimulation. About 70% of the fibers of the pyramidal tract are myelinated (Weil & Lassek, 1929). The diameter of a myelinated axon correlates directly with the internodal distance (ratio of 1 by 120) (Hess & Young, 1949), the conduction velocity (1 µm of axon diameter per 6 m/second of conduction velocity) (Hursh, 1939) and negatively with the chronaxie (BeMent & Ranck, 1969; Nowak & Bullier, 1998). Similar principles apply to the peripheral nerves. Studies investigating the threshold currents for eliciting an action potential along the course of an axon found periodic low thresholds every 500 to 1,125 µm with peak to valley threshold current ratios of 1.25 to 2.42 (BeMent & Ranck, 1969) most likely corresponding to the periodicity of the nodes of Ranvier. As already mentioned above, these are the structures of central myelinated fibers which are stimulated first by intracerebral stimulation whereas the high resistance and low capacitance of the myelinated fiber parts makes them more refractory to electrical stimulation.

Still, in case of extracellular electrical stimulation by depth or subdural electrodes current strength and pulse duration often exceed threshold values of several neuronal elements and, therefore, there is no selectivity of stimulation.

2) Concerning the distribution of the electrical field of an extracellular stimulation the voltage V at any point in a volume conductor is:

$$V = Is/4\pi r \quad (3)$$

with V being directly proportional to the the current I and the specific resistivity of the tissue s but inversely proportional to the distance from the pole r (Asanuma and Sakata 1967). The current density at a given point around a monopolar electrode can be calculated by the following equation:

$$J = I/4\pi r^2 \quad (4)$$

where J is the current density, I the current intensity of the electrode and r the distance of the given point from the electrode. Therefore, current density decreases with the square of the distance from the stimulating electrode (Nathan et al., 1993).

Experiments have shown that stimulation of the motor cortex with cortical surface electrodes just above the threshold for eliciting a movement activates Betz cells at a distance of up to 4 mm (Phillips, 1956). It has been shown also that direct excitation of pyramidal cells with microelectrodes is restricted to the "immediate vicinity of the stimulating microelectrode" (Stoney et al., 1968). Also the amplitude of an action potential evoked by intracortical microstimulation in pyramidal cells is inverse to the square distance from the stimulating electrode.

Current distance relations have been reported by Ranck (1975) who reviewed the relevant literature at that time and calculated a diagram of current distance relations for intracortical electrical stimulation with pulse durations of 200 μs. A simplified form with approximate values of this diagram is shown by *figure 4*. These values allow to approximate the maximal distance at which a intracortical stimulation may be effective.

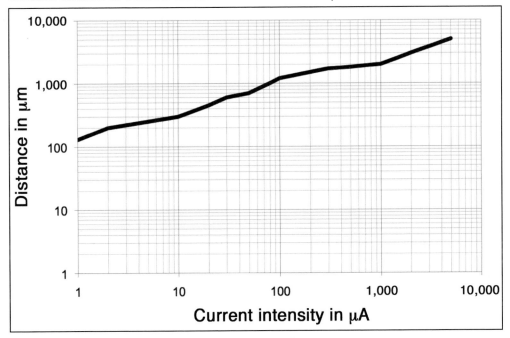

Figure 4. Current-distance relation of myelinated fibers. Double-logarithmic diagram representing a 100-fold range of distance and a 10,000-fold range of current. Monopolar cathodal depth electrode, pulse-width 200 μs. Electrical stimulation at a given current intensity will affect myelinated fibers up to the distance indicated by the graph (reffering to Ranck, 1975).

Variability of responses to invasive electrical stimulation

Early on, instability of responses to electrical stimulation of the cortex has been reported (Leyton & Sherrington, 1917). While maintaining all stimulation parameters constant the stimulation of the same cortical site may evoke responses differing in quality, quantity or topical distribution. This property has been found to depend on two main factors. On the one hand, the general context in which the stimulation is performed may influence the results. Stimulation of the central gray in monkeys may produce offensive or defensive behavior depending on the company of a submissive or dominant partner, respectively (Delgado, 1981). On the other hand, some parameters of stimulation including polarity, electrode diameter, stimulation frequency may influence the results obtained from stimulation of a single cortical point as discussed above. Besides, the response of a certain point in the Rolandic cortex may be either facilitated or inhibited by prior stimulation of the same or an adjacent cortical point (Leyton & Sherrington, 1917; Libet, 1973). In addition, the stimulus threshold just varies over time. The mechanisms of this variation are not known.

Safety of invasive electrical stimulation

Implantation of intracranial electrodes for diagnostic purposes is a potential harmful procedure that may only be justified after careful interdisciplinary assessment of the benefit-risk ratio. Still the general perioperative risk of this method is small compared to its invasiveness. The major concerns are related to the risk of brain surgery necessary for implantation of invasive electrodes and include primarily hemorrhages and infection. Less frequent complications of intracranial electrode placement are due to material defects or possible hazardous effects of the stimulation. The most common complication of placement of intracranial electrodes is that of inctracerebral hemorrhage. Among 50 consecutive patients with intracranial electrodes Ross et al., (1996) reported one case with a small subdural bleeding. But in a series of 198 patients who had invasive electrodes implanted, between 1,980 and 1,997 complications occurred in 52 monitoring sessions with infection and transient neurologic deficits occurring in approximately 10% of the cases. Additionally, increased intracranial pressure, epidural hematoma and infarction were reported in 1.5-2.5% of the patients. The death of one patient during grid implantation was also reported. The complication rate was directly correlated with the duration of the monitoring and the number of implanted electrodes. Notably, there was a significant tendency for decrease in complication rate over the time-course under investigation (Hamer et al., 2002). Similar rates of epidural or subdural bleedings of 1-2% were reported in another more recent study on 185 patients while the infection rate was reported to be as low as 1% (Fountas & Smith, 2007).

A second hazard arises from the electrical stimulation itself and two major concerns are related to the risk of tissue damage by the procedure of electrical stimulation. On the one hand the electrode itself carries a risk for potentially hazardous effects on the nervous system. This effect mainly depends on the metal used for the electrode contact. Investigations on the tolerability of several materials implanted chronically into the cerebral cortex (no electrical stimulation was applied) classified the contact material into non-reactive material (aluminum, gold, platinum, tungsten, silicon), reactive material (tantalum, nichrome, molybdenum, titanium dioxide) and toxic materials (copper, silver, iron, cobalt) (Fischer et al., 1957; Stensaas & Stensaas, 1978). Even though stainless steel has been used frequently as a material for electrical stimulation of the brain, studies have shown that tissue damage can occur with this material with mono- or biphasic stimulation. Under comparable conditions this was not observed with electrodes made of platinum or platinum-iridium (Wetzel et al., 1969; Harnack et al., 2004). On the other hand, the general risk of tissue injury by electrical stimulation of the cortex depends mainly on the total amount of coulombs passed onto the tissue (MacIntyre et al., 1959). With increasing train duration, pulse width or stimulation frequency the total amount of electrical charges passed increases. Therefore, more extensive tissue damage can be produced with any type of electrode depending on these parameters. This is the principle of thermocoagulation which is used in experiments with animal models to mark the location of electrode contacts within the nervous system. For example direct current "application of 3 mA for 30 sec through an electrode 0.12 mm in diameter with a 1 mm exposed tip produces a destruction of 1 to 2 mm in diameter" (Delgado, 1981). Therapeutically, thermocoagulation with depth electrodes has been used in the 1960s to treat behavioral disorders and more recently focal epilepsy (Catenoix *et al.*, 2008). On the other hand, post-mortem analysis in patients with chronic deep brain stimulation for different indications has shown very little substantial tissue damage favouring good tolerability of chronic electrical stimulation with suitable parameters (Pilitsis *et al.*, 2009). Still, it has been reported that repeated daily stimulation of amygdala and hippocampus may induce persistent changes in these brain structures and can cause focal epilepsy (Delgado, 1981). On the other hand, the same technique of electrical stimulation may diminish excitability and act anticonvulsive when applied to deep brain structures like the anterior thalamus, the subthalamic nucleus or the hypothalamus. These phenomena of kindling and "negative kindling" respectively highlight the risks of brain stimulation and the importance of defining parameters and conditions of stimulation. In order to minimize tissue damage, stimulation parameters producing the least total amount of current flow should be chosen.

Electrical stimulation of the central nervous system excites various neuronal elements in the vicinity of the stimulating electrodes. Susceptibility to stimulation differs between neuronal elements being highest in axons and initial axon segments. Stimulation acts focal at the stimulating electrodes independ if monopolar or bipolar stimulation is used. Selecting appropriate stimulus parameters may minimize the risk of tissue damage by electrical stimulation.

■ Functional aspects of brain stimulation

The most important application of electrocortical stimulation is for mapping of eloquent or indispensable cortex prior to resective brain surgery including:
- Broca's and Wernicke's language areas in the posterior inferior frontal lobe and a region around the inferior anterior parietal lobe respectively;
- The primary motor area (Brodmann's area 4);
- The primary visual area (Brodmann's area 17);
- The primary sensory area (Brodmann's areas 3, 1 and 2).

The degree of restoration of function after removal or loss of eloquent cortex varies depending on the amount of removed tissue and the type of eloquent cortex that has been damaged or removed.

Even though functional neuroanatomy is not bound to sulcal or gyral borders (Zilles & Amunts, 2010) we will summarize some results of electrocortical stimulation of extratemporal lobe areas on the basis of the fundamental division of the cortical surface into the cerebral lobes. Besides we will introduce the cytoarchitectonic divisions of each lobe considering John Hughlings-Jackson's statement that "differentiation of function implies differentiation of structure and differentiation of structure means differentiation of function" (Foerster, 1936).

Frontal lobe

Macroscopical anatomy

The frontal lobe is the part of the brain anterior to the central sulcus. Basolaterally the lateral sulcus separates it from the temporal lobe whereas on the mesial surface an auxiliary line between the end of the mesial part of the central sulcus and the cingulate sulcus represents the border between frontal and parietal lobe. The anterior cingulate gyrus may or may not be counted as part of the frontal lobe since it has also been considered as one part of the limbic lobe (Nieuwenhuys *et al.*, 2008). Still, one third of the entire cortical surface belongs to the frontal lobe and it is the largest cerebral lobe by surface and volume. A structure that further macroscopically subdivides the frontal lobe is the precentral sulcus, the anterior border of the precentral gyrus. This sulcus is nearly parallel to the central sulcus. The superior and inferior frontal sulci run in a caudo-rostral direction from the precentral sulcus to the frontal pole and, therefore, parcel the lateral surface of the frontal lobe into a superior, middle and inferior frontal gyrus. The inferior frontal gyrus between the inferior frontal sulcus and the lateral sulcus can be divided into three further sections. Ascending sulci from the lateral sulcus allow to differentiate a caudal pars opercularis or the frontal operculum that covers the anterior insula, a pars triangularis adjacent to the frontal operculum and a pars orbitalis in the rostral part of the inferior frontal gyrus. The frontal operculum and the triangular part of the inferior frontal gyrus are thought to be the macroscopical correlates of Broca's area in the dominant cerebral hemisphere. The orbitofrontal cortex is synonymous with the basal surface of the frontal lobe overlying the orbital bone. Its most prominent structures are the olfactory sulcus where the olfactory tract carries the olfactory fibers originating in the olfactory bulb. Medial to the olfactory sulcus and lateral to the longitudinal cerebral fissure is the rectal gyrus. The orbital cortex lateral to the olfactory sulcus macroscopically can be divided into 4 further gyri: the posterior, anterior, lateral and medial orbitofrontal gyrus.

Microscopical anatomy:

Brodmann (1909) established 15 cytoarchitectonically different areas within the frontal lobe. These are areas 4, 6, 8, 9, 10, 11 each extending over the lateral and mesial surface of the frontal lobe, the adjacent area 12 that is restricted to the mesial and orbitofrontal surface of the frontal lobe, and areas 44, 45, 46 and 47 that cover the middle and inferior areas of the lateral frontal lobe. Areas 24, 25, 32 and 33 are on the mesial hemisphere and mainly correspond to the anterior cingulate gyrus and contiguous structures (*Figures 5 and 6*).

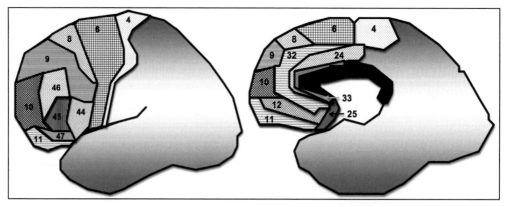

Figures 5 and 6. Lateral and medial aspect of the brain. The schematic areas of the frontal lobe are shown according to the cytoarchitectonic studies of Brodmann (1909). Areal numbers refer to Brodmann (1909).

In this classification area 4 is the most caudal part of the frontal lobe. It includes the anterior wall of the central sulcus and in the high caudal part of the cerebral convexity extends to the posterior wall of the precentral gyrus. Histologically it is the typical type of agranular cortex. This type of cortex shows large pyramidal cell layers III and V whereas the granule cell layers II and IV are poorly developed. In the classification of fundamental cortical architectures by von Economo and Koskinas (1925), the agranular cortex was labeled as heterotypical cortex of type I in contrast to the heterotypical cortex of type V which shows incomplete pyramidal cell layers III and V and prominent granular cell layers and is characteristic of the primary sensory cortex. Area 4, as a special case of agranular cortex, is characterized by the presence of the largest neurons of the cerebral cortex, the giant Betz pyramidal cells in the lamina V of the cortex (*area gigantopyramidalis*). The axons of these neurons constitute the corticospinal tract. The length of their axons as well as the size of their cell bodies decreases successively from the paracentral lobule to the foot of the lateral hemisphere. Oskar and Cécile Vogt (1919) divided this cortex into 3 subareas namely from dorsal to ventral areas 4a, 4b and 4c. Receptor architectonical studies on the other hand have lead to the subdivision of the primary motor cortex (area 4 of Brodmann) into an anterior and a posterior part based on different in densities of muscarinergic M2 receptors (Geyer *et al.*, 1996). The cortex of area 4 belongs to the broadest cortical areas reaching a thickness of up to 5 mm. The amount of myelin is high in area 4 especially in the supra- and infrastriatal layers whereas the lines of Baillarger (white fibers in layer V and IV, respectively outer and inner line) are less developed. If the presence of the giant Betz cells is taken as the fundamental criterion in defining the limits of area 4, this area mainly includes the anterior wall of the precentral gyrus and does run on its crown only in the dorsal parts of the precentral gyrus in humans. Though, the degree to which area 4 extend onto the precentral gyrus is variable (Foerster, 1936).

The precentral gyrus corresponds mainly to area 6 showing the characteristics of agranular cortex but lacking Betz' giant pyramidal cells. It also is characterized by the reappearance of a stripe of Baillarger hence its alternative latin name *area agranularis frontalis unistriata*. Area 6 occupies the crown of the precentral gyrus extending into the precentral sulcus in the superior and middle frontal gyrus. Subdivisions within this large cortical area have been introduced based on studies on the old world monkey (Cécile & Oskar Vogt, 1919). These authors named the caudal part of area 6 covering the anterior parts of the precentral gyrus as area 6aα. The adjacent rostral part of Brodmann's area 6 including dorsal parts of Brodmann's area 8 was termed area 6aβ. The foot of area 6 of Brodmann adjacent to the lateral fissure and including the frontal operculum was delineated as area 6b by the Vogts.

Area 8 of Brodmann, which is anterior to area 6, is usually classified as dysgranular cortex and shows incompletely developed granular layers. In contrast to area 4 and area 6 both lines of Baillarger are present in this area. Again, this area does only partially coincide between the maps of Brodmann (1909) and Oskar and Cécile Vogt (1919). As mentioned, the dorsal part of Brodmann's area 8 is part of area 6aβ of the map of the Vogts' (1919). Additionally, the latter authors divided their area 8 into a dorsal area 8αβδ and a ventral area 8γ anterior to area 6. Their area 8γ includes caudal parts of Brodmann's area 9 and 44. However, the Vogts delineated these areas in non-human primates only.

Areas 9, 10 and 11 as well as area 12 on the medial surface of the frontal lobe cover the frontal pole. These areas show characteristics of granular cortex. The remaining areas of the lateral frontal surface are areas 46 on the anterior middle and inferior frontal gyri, area 44 approximately corresponding to the pars opercularis of the inferior frontal gyrus, area 45 nearly corresponding to the pars triangularis and area 47 which corresponds to the basal part of the inferior frontal gyrus. Areas 46 and 9 together are often designated as dorsolateral prefrontal cortex. On the medial surface 4 agranular areas numbered area 24, 25, 32 and 33 together form the anterior cingulate gyrus which shows cytoarchitectonically an agranular structure.

Recent studies in rhesus monkeys led to a newer classification of cortical areas in the motor cortex by Matelli et al (1991). Compared to the classical cytoarchiteconic maps of Brodmann (1909) and the Vogts (1919), this new classification takes into account histological, neurochemical and functional data (Figures 7 and 8). Even though derived from studies in animals, it has been shown that this revised classification may also apply to the human cerebral cortex (Fink et al., 1997). The terminology of this new parcellation of cortical areas in the frontal lobe designates distinct frontal areas by the letter F together with classifying numbers. Area F1 in that classification is nearly identical with area 4 by Brodmann and is located in the most caudal part of the frontal lobe. Analogue areas to area 4 of Brodmann have been delineated in all comprehensive cytoarchitectonic studies. Even though defined by different investigators and different methods terms like area 4, F1 or MI are often used synonymously in the literature to designate the primary motor area. This is due to the good agreement on the histological demarcation of this area and its reproducible structure-function correlation (Nieuwenhuys et al., 2008). Area 6, rostral to area 4, is divided into several separate areas according to this new classification. Area F4 is situated in the most ventral part of Brodmann's area 6 with a separate area F5 in the most rostroventral part of area 6. Topographically these areas may correspond to Broca's area. In the dorsal part of area 6 on the lateral surface of the hemisphere there are two areas, namely area F2 and rostral to F2 area F7. On the mesial hemisphere just frontal to area F1 resides area F3 with a more rostral area F6 adjacent to it. Areas F2 and F3 as well as areas F6 and F7 most closely correspond to the areas 6aα and 6aβ respectively as defined by Cécile and Oskar Vogt (1919). It has been worked out by Matelli et al. (1991) that these areas may best be summarized in two functionally different groups. Areas F1 to F5 are closely related to the corticospinal system by either giving rise to direct corticofugal fibers or by internally connecting predominantly to area F1. Additionally, these areas receive their main afferents from the parietal cortex. In contrast, the rostral areas F6 and F7 project to brainstem nuclei and receive afferents that preferentially originate from the prefrontal cortex. An important distinctive feature of this new classification is its histological distinction between premotor areas on the mesial and lateral surface in contrast to the Vogts (1919) or Bailey and von Bonin (1951) who did not report such a difference. Based on electrocortical stimulation studies in humans and animals the existence of a complete motor representation restricted to the mesial surface of the hemisphere – named the supplementary motor area (SMA) – was postulated already in the 1950s (Penfield & Welch, 1951; Woolsey et al., 1952). Therefore, the histological and neurochemical findings by Matelli et al. (1991) may confirm the existence of this functionally distinct area. Moreover, within the mesial surface the more caudal area F3 was proposed to be the supplementary motor area proper (SMA proper) and the more rostral area F6 on the mesial surface was functionally associated with the pre-SMA (Figure 8). Concerning connectivity, area F3 is strongly connected to area F1. In contrast, area F6 does not project to the primary motor cortex whereas there are rich connections with premotor area F5 (Luppino et al., 1993). Regarding other parts of the mesial frontal surface the anterior cingulate gyrus i.e. area 24 of Brodmann has also been separated into two areas, the rostral cingulate motor area (CMAr) and the caudal cingulate motor area (CMAc) respectively. Both give rise to direct corticospinal fibers while they receive prominent afferents from the prefrontal cortex and limbic structures (Morecraft & van Hoesen, 1998).

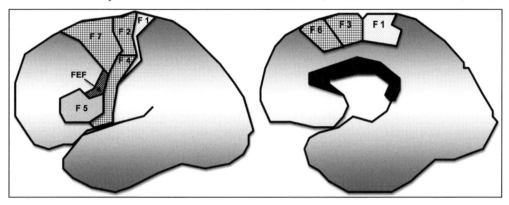

Figures 7 and 8. Lateral and medial aspect of the brain. The schematic areas of the frontal lobe represent areas of the motor and premotor cortex based on histological, neurochemical and functional data according to Matelli *et al.* (1991) and Nieuwenhuys *et al.* (2008). Areal numbers increase from caudal to rostral. F: Frontal, FEF: Frontal eye field.

The control of eye movements occupies specialized cortical areas in each hemisphere. Functional studies have located the frontal eye field (FEF) within the rostral area 6 or dorsal area 8 of Brodmann who did not define a cytoarchitectonically distinct area as opposed to the Vogts whose area 8αβδ as a subfield of area 8 does correspond to the functionally defined frontal eye field *(Figure 7)*. The existence of such a distinct subfield is supported also by histochemical studies of Rosano *et al.* (2003).

Areas 44 and 45 on the lateral surface are anterior to the ventral part of area 6. Area 44 is classified as dysgranular cortex and resides in a transitional zone between the agranular premotor and the granular prefrontal cortex *(Figure 5)*. Its cytoarchitectonical attributes are large pyramidal cells in layers III and V and an incompletely developed inner granular layer IV. Area 45 in contrast shows a more granular pattern with a clearly recognizable layer IV (Amunts *et al.*, 1999). Both areas are thought to constitute the anatomical correlate of Broca's speech area in the ventral inferior frontal gyrus. In contrast to area 45 which shows no definite interhemispheric differences, area 44 is considerably more extensive on the left hemisphere and may reveal a neuroanatomical core element of language lateralization (Amunts *et al.*, 1999). Concerning connectivity, it is well known that Broca's area is strongly interconnected with Wernicke's speech area by the arcuate fasciculus. The main afferents of Broca's area reach inferior parts of the primary motor cortex. However, this schematic view on mechanisms of language perception and production has been modified substantially by findings of functional neuroimaging, lesional studies and electrocortical stimulation (Nieuwenhuys *et al.*, 2008).

The prefrontal cortex occupies 29% of the cerebral cortex in humans. It comprises 17% of the Chimpanzee's cerebral cortex being the closest primate relative of humans, 7% of the macaque's cortex and around 3% of the rabbit's cerebral cortex (Brodmann, 1909). Generally the laminar pattern of the prefrontal areas is granular or dysgranular. Concerning the prefrontal cortex the numbering scheme of Brodmann (1909) is still in use but has been modified by Walker (1940) based on studies in the macaque monkey.

Modifications concern the extension of areas 9 and 46 as well as areas 12 and 25 (*Figures 5 and 6*). The lateral prefrontal cortex is a crucial area for sensorimotor integration. It receives dominant afferents especially from the temporoparietal association areas while maintaining feed-back connections to these areas. Brodmann subdivided the orbitofrontal cortex in areas 11 and 47. Whereas Walker (1940) generally used the classification of Brodmann and redefined some areal borders he introduced two new areas on the orbitofrontal surface namely areas 13 and 14. These numbers had not been used in Brodmann's map of the human cerebral cortex but originally correspond to insular areas in non-human primates (Brodmann, 1909). More recent work confirms these contributions to the cytoarchitecture of the frontal lobe (Petrides & Pandya, 1999). Öngür *et al.* (2003) introduced additional subfields to the 4 areas 11, 47/12, 13 and 14 (*Figure 9*). Their detailed map may serve as a modern basis for functional characterization of the orbitofrontal cortex. The general cytoarchitectonic pattern of the orbitofrontal cortex shows a caudorostral increase in granularity resembling the general organization of the prefrontal cortex (Nieuwenhuys *et al.*, 2008). In contrast to the lateral prefrontal cortex the mesial frontal and orbitofrontal areas are highly interconnected to limbic and paralimbic structures. A high degree of interconnectivity is a further characteristic of the mesial frontal and orbitofrontal areas.

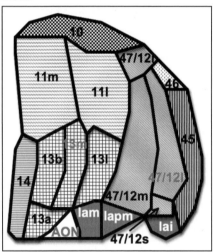

Figure 9. Basal aspect of the frontal lobe/orbitofrontal cortex. Distribution of cortical fields according to Öngür *et al.* (2003) and Nieuwenhuys *et al.* (2008). Areal numbers are partially based on the numbering scheme of Brodmann (1909) but are refined by specifying letters (m: medial, l: lateral).
AON: anterior olfactory nucleus, Iam: medial agranular insula, Iapm: posteromedial agranular insula, Iai: intermediate agranular insula. Parts of areas 10, 11, 12, 45, 46, 47 can be found on the lateral or medial aspect of the frontal lobe.

Functional anatomy

Motor areas

Area 4: Clinical observation has been the foundation of neurological reasoning. Theories of functional specialization and localization were based on correlating clinical symptoms with histopathological examinations. Prominent historic examples are the studies of Paul Broca on the neuroanatomical basis of aphasia (1865) and the works of John Hughlings-Jackson (1880) on the cortical origin of phenomena observed with epileptic seizures. The introduction of cortical stimulation with electrical current in the second half of the XIXth century complemented the pioneering clinical work of Broca, Jackson and others.

Today, the frontal lobe is still classified into motor and premotor cortex reflecting differences in response to electrocortical stimulation. The literature on electrocortical stimulation of the motor and premotor cortex is abundant and includes studies on humans, non-human primates and other vertebrates. Indeed, the recognition of a distinct specialized area of the cortex producing motor responses after electrocortical stimulation was an influential neuroscientific discovery of the XIXth century (Fritsch & Hitzig 1870). In 1870 Fritsch and Hitzig demonstrated that movements were most reliably elicited after electrical stimulation of a region directly anterior to the central sulcus. Shortly after these first experiments in dogs, the first electrical stimulation of human cerebral cortex was reported by Bartholow (1874). Bartholow, an American neurologist from Ohio, directly stimulated the cerebral cortex underneath a destructing skull lesion. The motor effects of electrical stimulation were then intensively studied in different non-human primates. Very influential results came from Leyton and Sherrington (1917). In 3 non-human primate species they recognized a primary motor area on the precentral gyrus and described the somatotopic distribution of motor responses closely comparable to the results later obtained from electrical stimulation studies in humans. Leyton and Sherrington (1917) observed a temporal instability of responses despite "a well-fixed topographical scheme". This temporal instability was attributed to different physiological states of the cortical points stimulated depending on the pattern of connectivity and temporally shifting intracortical influences. Infrequently they also found motor responses after stimulation of the postcentral gyrus "under certain circumstances". They concluded that the primary motor cortex was a "synthetic organ for compounding and re-compounding" motion based on fractional movements, 400 of which they elicited. Cécile and Oskar Vogt (1919, 1954) were able to correlate the results of their electrical stimulation with a myeloarchitectonic map of the cortex of non-human primates. They provided evidence for the relation of function and cytoarchitectonic structure in the cerebral cortex. Like Leyton and Sherrington (1917) they regarded motor responses after stimulation of the postcentral gyrus as secondary to neuronal spreading of the stimulus to the M1 area and presented experimental evidence by proving extinction of motor phenomena upon stimulation of the postcentral gyrus after disruption of intergyral association fibers. These experiments exclude volume conduction of the stimulus as an explanation for motor responses obtained by stimulation of the postcentral gyrus. Other lines of evidence helped to refine the motor cortex to the precentral gyrus instead of the complete perirolandic cortex. First, ablation of the precentral gyrus abolished motor effects of electrocortical stimulation of the postcentral gyrus. This observation held true even for focal ablations which extinguished motor effects with stimulation of corresponding regions in the postcentral gyrus. Second, marked degeneration of corticospinal tract fibers in the spinal cord was observed after excision in the prefrontal gyrus while excision of the postcentral gyrus did produce only subtle degeneration of the pyramidal tract. Third, it had been described repeatedly that the threshold for producing movements with electrocortical stimulation was lowest in the precentral gyrus and that movements after stimulation of the postcentral gyrus occurred only with much higher stimulation intensities (Leyton & Sherrington, 1917; Vogt & Vogt, 1919). Fourth, destruction of the precentral gyrus invariably was found to be associated with paresis of the contralateral hemibody whereas destruction of the postcentral gyrus was not.

With the advances obtained by electrocortical stimulation for localizing motor areas in animals the usefulness of electrical stimulation for localizing brain function during neurosurgical operations in humans had been recognized. The technique was introduced in neurosurgical centers of that time, very notably by Victor Horsley in London and later Harvey Cushing in Boston. An early comprehensive text on results of electrocortical stimulation was published by Fedor Krause (1931) who practiced in Berlin for most of his lifetime. He published a topographic map of the precentral gyrus that already included much of the findings on the topography of the motor cortex later published by Foerster (1936) and Penfield and Boldrey (1937). This map was based on intraoperative faradic stimulation of 142 patients who underwent brain surgery for the treatment of epilepsy. For the scientific analysis of his results Krause excluded patients with macroscopical lesions or abnormalities of the rolandic cortex and with unreliable responses to stimulation. Additionally, stimulation was usually repeated three times. While this technique provided outlasting scientific findings the indication for its application was to identify the area of the cortex that was believed to be the seizure onset zone. At that time, this technique therefore was primarily applied to patients with "Jacksonian-seizures" or with an early involvement of the motor system. The motor area as defined by Krause resides on the whole precentral gyrus corresponding to the cytoarchitectonic areas 4 and the caudal part of area 6 of Brodmann. Importantly, the cytoarchitectonically caudal border of area 4 is sharp often corresponding to the bottom of the central sulcus whereas the anterior border tends to fade into area 6 (Krause, 1931). Krause also quotes the subjective impressions of the patients during stimulation who mainly reported the perception of an involuntary movement lacking sensory phenomena.

Otfried Foerster (1936) published a further important monograph on motor areas. He claimed a good agreement between the physiological results of his stimulation and cytoarchitectonic results from the Vogts (1919). He summarized experiences with electrocortical stimulation of about 300 patients. Compared to Krause (1931) Foerster's map is more detailed. For the sake of completeness we will repeat the sequence of motor representations on the precentral gyrus especially since there is a loss of information within the available pictograms representing the organization of the motor cortex *(Figure 10)*. Beginning at the foot of the paracentral lobule there is a representation for the bladder and rectum. Dorsally the representation of the toes follows and extends slightly onto the edge of the hemisphere. Stimulation there does produce joint movements of all toes and occasionally of the hallux alone. Foot movements are located rostral to the former on the paracentral lobule and the most dorsal part of the precentral gyrus on the lateral hemisphere. Again more rostral and more dorsal is the focus for movements of the leg with an adjacent focus of the thigh which has its main representation on the lateral precentral gyrus. Therefore, the representation of the lower extremity is not arranged parallel to the central sulcus but directed oblique in a caudo-rostral manner. Additionally, it is important to bear in mind that the cortical field for the motor representation of the lower extremity extends over the mesial as well as over dorsal parts of the lateral hemisphere and is not restricted to the one or the other *(Figure 10)*. Foerster mentions that statistically foci for knee-extension are more prevalent than those for knee-flexion whereas hip-flexion is more often seen with electrocortical stimulation than hip-extension. The sequence of the adjacent representation of the trunk begins with abdominal muscles, lumbal muscles of the spine, followed by the representation of the chest and thoracal muscles of the spine. Foerster stated that singultus will most often be produced with stimulation of the anterior part of the motor area of the trunk. Consecutively from dorsal to ventral shoulder, upper arm, forearm, hand, small finger, fourth finger, middle finger, index finger and thumb form the field of the upper extremity. It is specified that in general extension of any joint of the upper extremity tends to be more frontal compared to the representation of flexor movements of arm, hand or fingers. This principle is concordant with results from Krause (1911; 1931). Moreover, Foerster (1936) delineated that the foci for pronation and supination of the hand are localized more dorsal as compared to those foci representing flexion and extension of the hand. Then the following cortex includes representation of neck muscles including the musculus sternocleidomastoideus and the platysm. Foerster (1936) described that the ipsilateral musculus sternocleidomastoideus will be activated with stimulation of the neck field producing a contralateral version of the face. The representation of face muscles then begins with the upper facial muscles for forehead and eyelids followed by the lower facial muscles of the upper lip, the lower lip, corner of the mouth, chin. Then, the motor representation of the tongue can be found with electrocortical stimulation producing a contralateral deviation of the tongue. Jaw-movements will be the consequence of stimulation of areas ventral to the representation of the tongue and include mouth-opening, -closure and -shift. Again Foerster (1936) mentions activation of an ipsilateral chewing muscle namely the musculus pterygoideus lateralis. The remaining area of the precentral gyrus is responsible for innervation of the velum palatinum, the pharyngeal muscles and the laryngeal muscles. Characteristically, these structures have bilateral cortical representations in each hemisphere and electrocortical stimulation produces symmetrical movements of these intracavital muscles. The same is true for the jaw muscles as well as the upper facial muscles responsible for eyeclosure and raised eyebrows. Bilateral movements after electrocortical stimulation are largely due to bilateral projection of the pyramidal tract rather than callossal spread as supported by preserved bilateral effects of electrical stimulation after callosotomy (Foerster, 1936). The existence of a highly topographic organization of the motor cortex therefore was further substantiated by these results. Foerster (1936) did not distinguish between the results produced by stimulation of area 4 and those that followed stimulation of the posterior part of area 6aα. Moreover, it is not entirely clear how frequently he was able to stimulate the anterior wall of the precentral gyrus which includes a substantial part of area 4. Still, he reported clear differences in excitability when stimulating area 4 and 6. With the method of unipolar galvanic stimulation the threshold current for eliciting movements from area 4 was reported to be 0.3-0.5 mA and the threshold current for producing the same movement from area 6 (Brodmann, 1909) or 6aα (Vogt & Vogt, 1919) was 1.5-2.0 mA. It may be stated that this author despite the minute description of localization in the motor cortex was aware of the variable responses that follow repeated stimulation of the same cortical focus and the probabilistic character of a cortical map as had been described before (Leyton & Sherrington, 1917). The relative temporal dynamics and gradual differences in the motor cortex have been highlighted in more recent reports (Sanes & Donoghue, 1997). It was also interesting to notice that when isolating a small focus of the motor cortex from its surrounding structures the movements elicited by electrocortical stimulation were very fractionated and no complex movements were elicited. This supports the theory that intracortical spread of stimulating current and secondary physiological activation are essential neurophysiological features explaining the variability of responses to electrocortical stimulation (Vogt & Vogt, 1919). Additionally, it is important to bear in mind that the corticospinal tract accounts not for the major part of efferent fibers arising from the motor cortex. It was suggested that as few as 15% of the corticonuclear and corticospinal fibers arise from the primary motor cortex (Creutzfeldt, 1983). Besides, Tower (1940) reported that dissection of the pyramidal tract on a cervical level abolishes most distal movements while those of the proximal joints are much less affected.

Penfield and colleagues (1937; 1950) confirmed the previous reported results from Krause (1911; 1931) and Foerster (1936). Moreover, Penfield and his colleagues were the first to present a synthesis of their information on perirolandic electrocortical stimulation in the figurines of the homunculus, being an essence of the electrophysiological studies on the motor cortex. Again, the results of Krause, Foerster and Penfield were very similar to the studies in primates (Leyton & Sherrington, 1917; Vogt & Vogt, 1919) confirming their validity. Later, studies with other species further confirmed the existence of a fine somatotopical organization in the motor cortex (Asanuma & Sakata, 1967).

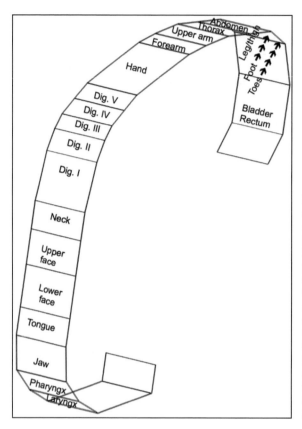

Figure 10. Scheme of the sequence of representations of bodyparts in the primary motor cortex (referring to Foerster, 1936; and Penfield & Rasmussen, 1950). The representation of the lower extremity extends over the medial and partially over the lateral hemisphere as indicated by arrows. In the filed for trunk representation the muscles of the corresponding segment of the spine are included. Within the representation of the upper extremity electrocortical stimulation produces more often flexion than extension. The latter is represented more anterior compared to the former. The muscles of jaw and more so pharynx and laryngx have a bilateral representation. This figure is schematized and does not take into account the gyral and sulcal anatomy.

Premotor cortex: In analogy to the qualification of sensory areas as SI or SII, there is a common terminology for motor areas using the term MI for the primary motor area including cytoarchitectonic areas 4 and caudal parts of area 6 and using the term MII for secondary motor areas commonly named premotor areas with the localization in Brodmann's rostral area 6 and caudal area 8 or area 6aβ of the Vogt's (Woolsey *et al.*, 1952). Early experiments by the Vogts (1919), Foerster (1936), Kleist and others showed that electrical stimulation of area 6 produces either contralateral version of the head, the eyes and the trunk or synergistic movements of the contralateral extremities *i.e.* elevation of the arm, flexion of the forearm, pronation of the hand and flexion of the fingers. Hand opposite extensor movements and synergisms affecting the contralateral lower extremity with combined flexion or extension in the major joints have also been reported. The Vogts (1919) and Foerster (1936) concluded that the area therefore was involved in adversion of the hemibody to the contralateral side. Foerster denied a somatotopic organization of the premotor area while Kleist (1934), based on lesion studies, proposed an organization with a fronto-ventral representation of the head and a more caudo-dorsal representation of the extremities. Penfield, however, concluded from his studies that the results obtained by the Vogts, Foerster and others were in great part the result of volume conduction of the stimulus to the SMA (Penfield & Rasmussen, 1950). The results from early experiments were obtained using very high stimulation intensities suggesting that they could have elicited afterdischarges or actually epileptic seizures. Penfield and

Rasmussen (1950) and Macpherson *et al.* (1982), however, reported that characteristically predominantly proximal movements were obtained when stimulating the premotor area and fine finger movements did not occur.

Supplementary motor area (SMA): As mentioned above, Foerster (1936) already described a premotor area on the upper lateral surface and the mesial surface anterior to the primary motor area which induced predominantly contraversive movements upon electrocortical stimulation. In contrast, Penfield and colleagues however concluded that complex movements with a contralateral version were seen only with electrocortical stimulation in the medial wall of the frontal cortex anterior to the precentral sulcus (Penfield & Welch, 1951). This area not only has been recognized by many studies of electrocortical stimulation but has also been somatotopically defined with the representation of the head being most rostral and that of the lower extremities most caudal (Fried *et al.*, 1991). A corresponding cytoarchitectonical area in the mesial wall of the frontal lobe has been recognized in non-human primates as well as in humans (Matelli *et al.*, 1991; Zilles *et al.*, 1995). This area corresponds to the area F3 as defined in cytoarchitectonic studies of the motor cortex of the macaque and was labeled SMA-proper in humans *(Figure 11)*. The SMA-proper includes a complete body map. More recently, the idea of a more extensive SMA including mostly mesial but occasionally also lateral premotor areas has reappeared (Dinner & Lüders, 2008). Characteristically, movements elicited by electrocortical stimulation of the SMA are more proximal, can be bilateral and are tonic as compared to primary motor responses which typically are clonic, contralateral and preferentially distal (Lim *et al.*, 1994). Other types of responses to stimulation of the SMA were described including vocalization, speech arrest, paresthesia, inhibition of movement, and autonomic changes (Dinner & Lüders, 2008). The existence of such non-motor responses in the SMA is a main reason for its other denomination as supplementary sensorimotor area (SSMA) *(Figure 11)* (Lim *et al.*, 1994). The supplementary frontal eye field which is discussed in the following paragraph of this text probably is part of the SMA or the pre-SMA. Also, the supplementary negative motor area most likely corresponds to the pre-SMA anterior to the SMA.

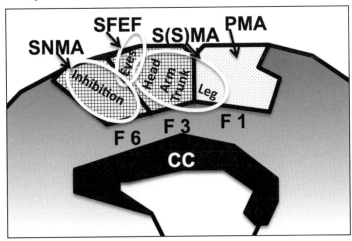

Figure 11. Medial aspect of the frontal lobe. Functional organization of the medial premotor cortex as revealed by electrocortical stimulation. PMA: primary motor cortex, S(S)MA: supplementary (sensory)motor area, SFEF: supplementary frontal eye field, SNMA: supplementary negative motor area, CC: corpus callosum. The S(S)MA corresponds well with the cytoarchitectonical field F3 and extends into ventral parts of medial F1. The SNMA is located in cytoarchitectonic area F6.

Frontal eye field (FEF): All previously mentioned authors or groups identified a special area within the premotor cortex concerned with eye movements. This area functionally is often referred to as frontal eye field *(Figure 7)*. In Brodmann's map of the cortical areas the frontal eye field is part of area 8 and not delineated separately. Oskar and Cécile Vogt (1919) were able to find a myeloarchitectonic distinct area corresponding to the premotor area that produced eye-movements to the contralateral side in the old world monkey which they named area $8\alpha\beta\delta$. It is located rostral to the prefrontal gyrus in the caudal part of the middle frontal gyrus. Foerster (1936) describes that the version lasts as long as the stimulus inducing it and sometimes includes a slight upward, infrequently a downward component while changes of the size of the pupils are absent. A pure upward or downward gaze as well as an isolated eye movement can not be induced by electrocortical stimulation of area $8\alpha\beta\delta$ according to Foerster (1936). Confirmatory, out of 19 patients studied who had electrocortical stimulation of subdural grids, 15 presented purely contralateral and conjugate horizontal eye-version, whereas 4 showed an additional upward component. The majority of these eye-movements was qualified as saccadic type (Godoy et al., 1990). Most likely, the preponderance of horizontal eye-movements after electrocortical stimulation reflects the predominance of abductive or adductive effects of the eye muscles (Livingston, 1950). Two cases have been described recently in which stimulation of the caudal part of the middle frontal gyrus as well as an epileptic seizure with seizure activity in the frontal lobe produced disconjugate eye-movements with the amount of ipsilateral adduction exceeding the amount of contralateral abduction. This uneven conjugation was interpreted as co-activation of version and vergence of the contralateral eye and favours a hypothesis of "control of all voluntary eye movements" by the cortical eye fields (Thurtell et al., 2009). Foerster (1936) found that intraoperative stimulation of the frontal eye field induced eye-movement alone without a head movement. Nevertheless, in more recent studies of stimulation of this area conjugated, contralateral eye version followed by head version were noticed in more than 50% of the patients (Godoy et al., 1990; Penfield & Rasmussen, 1950). No visual or other sensory phenomena are associated with stimulation of this area and Foerster (1936) indicates that the lack of a visual aura with early eye-movements in epileptic seizures arising from this area is a semiologically localizing characteristic. Penfield and Rasmussen (1950) did however report on occasional eye-sensations with stimulation of this area. Since the primary motor area does not have an own representation for eye movements its destruction does not affect the gaze-control confirming the independent system of efferents of the frontal eye field. This field is not only functionally distinct compared to its surrounding areas but is attributed with a comparably low stimulation threshold between 3 and 6 mA of galvanic current. This is considerably lower than the threshold current of the adjacent premotor area $6a\beta$ according to Foerster (1936). Again, these results may have been contaminated by the occurrence of afterdischarges, epileptic seizures or volume conduction.

Penfield and Rasmussen (1950) described observations of eye movements in a wider precentral area. In two thirds the rostral part of the precentral gyrus and the caudal parts of the adjacent frontal gyri more closely corresponding to the aforementioned area recognized by the Vogts (1919) and Foerster (1936) were the sites which produced eye movements after electrical stimulation. Another third of eye-movements occurred with stimulation of the caudal part of the precentral gyrus corresponding to the primary motor cortex. Whereas stimulation of the former area was mainly followed by contralateral eye-version stimulation of the latter produced variable responses including ipsilateral version, upward rotation and convergence. It has to be qualified that these responses often were associated with additional phenomena like head version, eyelid movements, movements of facial muscles and jaw muscles. Therefore the question whether the variability of these results is partially due to epiphenomena of the electrocortical stimulation may be addressed. Similarly, contralateral head movements were produced with stimulation of the anterior precentral gyrus or the adjacent frontal convolutions and less frequently as well as more variable in nature after stimulation of the motor cortex. Therefore two thirds of the versive movements in the studies of Penfield and Rasmussen (1950) are comparable to the results obtained by Foerster (1936) indicating a premotor area on the lateral surface relevant for conjugate eye movements.

A minute description of effects of stimulation of the frontal eye field has been published by Livingston (1950) who could attribute lateralization of a version to the stimulation-frequency used. Low stimulation frequencies between 1 and 10 Hz did produce ipsilateral version whereas the more common stimulation-frequencies between 30 and 60 Hz did induce contralateral movements. It is the opinion of the same author that the frontal eye-field is relevant for voluntary eye-movements compared to the occipital eye-field which is involved in the subconscious gaze-control. The existence of a distinct cytoarchitectonic zone in the caudal part of the middle frontal gyrus on the side of the precentral sulcus recently was re-established (Rosano et al., 2003).

Another distinct supplementary eye-field in the dorsomedial prefrontal cortex has been described and may correspond to the adversive eye-movements Foerster (1936) observed with stimulation of the medial cerebral surface (Figure 11). It is located anterior to the representation of the head of the SMA. Its first detailed description was carried out by electrical microstimulation in monkeys (Schlag & Schlag-Rey, 1987). Contralateral vesion of the eyes and sometimes subsequent contralateral head-version is seen when this region is stimulated as has been confirmed in humans (Lim et al., 1994). Interestingly, this area was found to be involved in learning-processes of eye-movements (Tehovnik et al., 2000).

Field for mastication: Vogt and Vogt (1919) recognized an additional cortical field in the foot of the precentral gyrus just superior to the lateral fissure. This area 6b is considerably small but has been recognized as an area associated with the action of mastication. Electrocortical stimulation of this area produces movements of chewing and swallowing (Foerster, 1936). This area is distinct from the adjacent primary motor area as its stimulation can induce rhythmic and coordinated movements associated with mastication. This includes rhythmic movements of the jaw as well as licking movements. Also voalizations are described. Penfield and Rasmussen (1950) found a different representation of mastication including the ventral part of the postcentral rolandic areas. They proposed a consecutive representation of the alimentary motor system in the foot of the perirolandic cortex with representations of the tongue (1), the throat (2), salivation (3) and mastication (4). It should be qualified here, that there is sparse support for this subfield in the more recent literature.

Negative motor area (NMA): In front of area 6b as well as the ventral parts of area 6aα resides area 8γ in the classification of the Vogts (1919). Stimulation of this area does not produce movements when electrically stimulated. Therefore a more detailed discussion of its function is not available in the early literature on electrocortical stimulation. Nevertheless, the Vogts (1919) reported that the clinical effects of stimulation of area 6b i.e. complex oral movements did immediately rest when area 8γ was stimulated at the same time and reappeared when stimulation of area 8? was stopped. This special effect lead to a nomination of this area as "suppressor area" (Figure 12). Foerster was not able to reproduce these effects but described that he had repeatedly observed disruption of sustained oral automatisms induced by electrocortical stimulation of area 6b when area 8γ was immediately stimulated thereafter. For long this effect was not further investigated. Then, in the last decades there were several reports of "negative motor responses" following stimulation of the inferior frontal gyrus immediately anterior to the precentral gyrus (Lüders et al., 1988). Lüders et al. (1985) presented a case of a patient undergoing invasive presurgical epilepsy monitoring who when stimulated at an electrode contact on the inferior frontal gyrus felt paralyzed in the left arm and face and was unable to perform movements of the left upper hemibody and tongue leading to a speech arrest. A definition of a negative motor response as "an inability to perform a certain voluntary movement or to sustain a voluntary muscle contraction at a stimulation intensity that did not produce any symptoms or signs" has been proposed (Lüders et al., 1988). Movements of the tongue, the eyes, the hands, the feet were affected in decreasing frequency by stimulation. Therefore, this inferior lateral frontal area most closely corresponding to area 8γ of the Vogts (1919) was termed negative motor area.

Negative motor effects have been observed with stimulation of other areas as well, especially on the mesial frontal surface anterior to the supplementary motor area (*Figure 11*). This area anatomically most closely corresponds to the pre-SMA, rostral to the face representation of the supplementary motor area and is regarded as supplementary negative motor area (Smyth 2008). Reports on akinetic epileptic seizures also provide evidence for the existence of such negative motor areas (Noachtar & Lüders, 1999; Villani et al., 2006). Still, there are very few reports presenting evidence from electrocorticography or electrocortical stimulation for the confirmation of the localization of these areas. And Mikuni et al. (2006) observed that negative motor phenomena after electrocortical stimulation were much wider distributed than previously thought reporting on such phenomena along the precentral perirolandic area of the complete lateral hemisphere.

The electrophysiological significance of this effect is not well understood. One main hypothesis explains the negative effect of stimulation of these premotor areas with a disruption of preparatory executive processes for performance of movements.

A useful screening procedure in practical terms to test for negative motor areas during electrocortical stimulation is reading. If hesitation, slowing or disruption of reading occur other motor functions like different types of tongue movements, eye movements, and movements of the extremities should be tested. Corresponding to the execution of the reading task the patient should be instructed to initiate these movements briefly before the onset of stimulation (Smyth, 2008).

Speech areas

Broca's area: The production of speech is one of the most elaborated functions of the human brain. It is widely known that this process relies on an unimpaired interaction of the various language areas. In traditional concepts, the executive organs of speech reside in the frontal lobe whereas the receptive aspects of speech are located in temporal and parietal areas (*Figure 12*). Penfield and Roberts (1959) reported on the first large series of patients in whom language function during electrocortical stimulation was systematically studied. Indeed, these authors preferred to use the term electrical interference instead of stimulation. Penfield and Roberts (1959) argued that "stimulation" of any part of the cortex is in nature an interference with cortical function whether its effect may be positive or negative. They recognized several effects on speech produced by their methods of interference namely: Total arrest of speech/inability to vocalize spontaneously (1), hesitation and slurring of speech (2), distortion of words and syllables (3), repetition of words and syllables (4), inability to name with retained ability to speak (5), misnaming with evidence of perseveration (6), misnaming (7). This different types of speech interference, however, do not have differential cortical representations. It rather appears that these responses represent the pattern of lingual abnormalities which can occur with electrical interference of any point of the cortical network of speech areas representing symptoms of transient failures of the speech system. Therefore, whereas vocalization as the positive effect of stimulation in speech areas can be evoked solely in regions of the frontal lobe – the primary and the supplementary motor area (Foerster, 1936; Penfield & Rasmussen, 1949; Lim et al., 1994) – the negative effects will occur at much wider distribution predominantly around the Sylvian fissure of the dominant hemisphere. However, the authors confirmed that alteration of the right hemisphere by electrical interference or cortical tissue affects speech very infrequently.

Penfield and Roberts (1959) ranked the speech areas due to the occurrence of sustained postoperative deficits and regarded the temporoparietal speech area as indispensable, the inferior frontal speech area as partially "dispensable in some patients at least" and the supplementary motor area as generally dispensable with transient loss of speech but a more eminent importance when other speech areas are disturbed for any reason. It may be annotated that the supplementary speech area at the supplementary motor area as described by Penfield and Roberts (1959) may coincide with the supplementary negative motor area in the mesial frontal lobe as described by Lüders et al. (1988). A more recently described speech area in the basal temporal lobe most likely is also not associated with persistent aphasia after resection of its anterior part (Lüders et al., 1991). There is some evidence that resection of the posterior part of the basal; temporal language area may produce alexia without agraphia.

In order to detect any negative response it is necessary to instruct the patient properly. There is a common set of tasks used to test for interference with speech. Basic exercises during electrical interference are reading sentences, object naming, auditory comprehension, spontaneous speech. Additional test include reading words aloud, verb generation from pictures, verb generation from nouns, repetition of spoken words/phrases, auditory naming or word stem completion (Tandon, 2008).

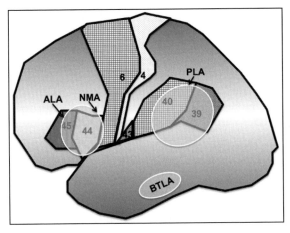

Figure 12. Lateral aspect of the frontal lobe. Speech areas as revealed by electrocortical stimulation. Stimulation of these areas produces "negative" phenomena i.e. interference with speech perception and production. ALA: anterior language area (Broca's area), PLA: posterior language area (Wernicke's area), BTLA: basal temporal language area, NMA: negative motor area. Numbers indicate cytoarchitectonic areas of Brodmann. These language areas are present in the dominant hemisphere only. The NMA corresponds to the location of the ALA in the dominant hemisphere.

Prefrontal cortex: Typically, stimulation of the prefrontal cortex including the frontal pole, the dorsolateral prefrontal cortex and the orbitofrontal cortex does not produce any recognizable clinical response.

Summary: The frontal lobe covers one third of the brain and includes the main effector organ of the brain, the motor cortex. Its minute description in the past has been largely advanced by electrocortical stimulation. Besides giving rise to the main part of the pyramidal tract in the primary motor area many frontal areas participate in the preperation of movements including those for the production of speech. The frontal eye field and the negative motor area on the lateral hemisphere as well as the supplemtary sensorymotor area, the supplementary frontal eye field and the supplementary negative motor area on the medial hemisphere are other distinct areas of the frontal lobe which have been discovered by the application of electrocortical stimulation.

Parietal lobe

Macroscopical anatomy

The parietal lobe is the part of the cortex that lies in between the frontal and the occipital lobe and is adjacent to the temporal and insular lobes in its ventral part. It is the only cerebral lobe that is macroscopically directly connected to the four other lobes of the cerebral cortex. This is the reason it has been regarded as an intermediate cortex in large parts. Even though the primary sensory cortex occupies the rostral part of the parietal lobe most of its surface is often classified as association cortex. This view on the parietal lobe is justified also by phylogenetic aspects since the association areas of the brain within the neocortex grow overproportionally compared to those areas concerned with primary afferent and efferent functions. The parietal lobe is separated from the frontal lobe by the central sulcus which is extended by a vertical line connecting to the cingulate sulcus on the medial surface of a hemisphere. The caudal border of the parietal lobe is the parietooccipital sulcus and the subparietal sulcus on the medial surface. The demarcation between the parietal lobe and the insular lobe is the circuminsular sulcus. And an arbitrary horizontal line extending the posterior ramus of the lateral sulcus separates the temporal from the parietal lobe.

Additionally to these neuroanatomical borders a separation of the parietal lobe into four functionally different areas has been proposed (Nieuwenhuys et al., 2008). First, the primary sensory cortex covering only a narrow strip in the posterior central sulcus and postcentral gyrus in the anterior or rostral part of the parietal lobe. Second, the superior parietal lobule in between the superior postcentral gyrus and the superior parieto-occipital sulcus. It is divided from the third functional area, the inferior parietal lobule, by the intraparietal sulcus. Important structures within the inferior parietal lobule are the supramarginal gyrus and the angular gyrus which surround parts of the posterior end of the temporal lobe. The parietal operculum may be regarded as a fourth functionally separate unit of the parietal lobe. It covers the posterior part of the insula and connects the insula anatomically to the postcentral gyrus and the supramarginal gyrus.

Microscopical anatomy

Brodmann distinguished 10 different cortical areas within the parietal lobe (*Figures 13 and 14*). The postcentral gyrus can be further divided into 3 different areas which are from rostral to caudal area 3, area 1 and area 2. Area 3 is further subdivided into area 3b and area 3a. Area 3a represents a transitional cortical stripe between the primary motor and the primary sensory cortex in the bottom of the central sulcus. These parietal areas are narrow cortical areas nearly parallel to the central sulcus and each other and extend over the postcentral gyrus including the anterior wall of the postcentral sulcus. Their characteristics are the prominent and fully developed granular layers II and IV as well as the presence of both lines of Baillarger. The afferents of areas 3b, 1 and 2 stem from the sensory nuclei of the thalamus. These areas therefore are the primary cortical representation of these sensory qualities. Each of the primary sensory areas 3, 1 and 2 includes a complete somatotopically arranged cortical map. These primary sensory areas are heavily interconnected between each other and connect to various parts of the superior parietal lobule.

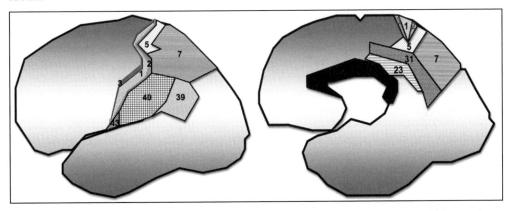

Figures 13 and 14. Lateral and medial aspect of the brain. The schematic areas of the parietal lobe are shown according to the cytoarchitectonic studies of Brodmann (1909). Areal numbers refer to Brodmann (1909).

According to Brodmann (1909) the superior parietal lobule includes area 5 adjacent to area 2 (*Figures 13 and 14*). It is homologue with area 5a of the Vogts. Brodmann's area 5 is a narrow area that covers the most caudal part of the paracentral lobule and the caudal wall of the postcentral sulcus in the dorsal part of the lateral hemisphere corresponding to the superior parietal lobule. Compared with areas 3, 1 and 2 the presence of large pyramidal cells in layer V is characteristic for area 5. This area is regarded as unimodal somatosensory association cortex. It receives afferents mainly from the primary somatosensory cortex. The main part of the superior parietal lobule is occupied by area 7 of Brodmann. It covers the superior parietal cortex between area 5 and the parietooccipital sulcus. It is homologue with area 5b in the nomenclature of Cécile and Oskar Vogt (1919). This area extends to the parieto-occipital sulcus caudally and the parietal sulcus ventrally. Compared to area 5 or 5a respectively the pyramidal cells in layer III and V are rather small and a subdivision of layer IV into two sublayers is typical of this area. The polymodal association area 7 receives processed visual information from the occipital lobe via the dorsal processing stream, sensory information via intracortical afferents from the adjacent sensory areas and is connected to the frontal cortex. Connections to the dorsal part of the prefrontal cortex, to the dorsal part of area 8 and to the supplementary motor area (SMA) are of main-importance in this area.

The intraparietal sulcus even though currently not further differentiated by human cytoarchitectonical maps presents special cytoarchitectonics and distinct patterns of connectivity in macaques which are further supported by data from functional imaging in humans

(Grefkes & Fink, 2005). 5 different areas within the intraparietal sulcus were differentiated. These areas were named from rostral to caudal the anterior intraparietal area (AIP), the ventral intraparietal area (VIP), the medial intraparietal area (MIP), the lateral intraparietal area (LIP) and the caudal intraparietal area (CIP). These different areas within the intraparietal sulcus have strong feed-forward and feed-back connections with special areas of the frontal lobe and may be regarded as "interface between perceptive and motor systems." (Nieuwenhuys et al., 2008).

The inferior parietal lobule has been subdivided into area 40 and area 39 by Brodmann (1909). Area 40 roughly includes the supramarginal gyrus whereas area 39 includes the angular gyrus. Here the maps of Brodmann (1909) and the Vogts' (1919) who subdivided this part of the parietal lobe into an anterior area 7b and a posterior area 7a vary considerably. Both areas each show a completely developed laminar pattern with small pyramidal cells. The two most relevant structures within the inferior parietal lobule are the aforementioned angular gyrus and supramarginal gyrus. The angular gyrus is connected to visual areas by the dorsal and ventral processing stream, with the intraparietal sulcus, with the superior temporal gyrus, the posterior cingulate, as well as different areas of the frontal lobe e.g. the anterior part of the dorsal premotor cortex, area 8 and prefrontal areas. The supramarginal gyrus has strong connections to the primary and secondary sensory areas, to the superior parietal association areas and to several areas of the frontal lobe including the anterior cingulate cortex, the supplementary motor area, Area 44, 45 and 46 (Gregoriou et al., 2006).

The parietal operculum has been further divided into area 43 and parts of area 40 (*Figure 13*). Nevertheless, more recent subdivisions differentiate 4 cortical areas within the parietal operculum (*Figure 15*). Two caudal opercular areas termed OP1 and OP2 correspond to the opercular part of area 40 as described by Brodmann (1909) and two more ventral areas termed OP3 and OP4 most closely correspond to Brodmann's area 43 (Eickhoff et al., 2006). A former functional classification of areas within the parietal operculum also distinguished a parietal ventral area and a second somatosensory area also labeled SII. The parietal ventral area was found to be interconnected with area 3b, the parietal association areas, the medial auditory field and the frontal eye field. SII is densely connected to the primary sensory cortex, the inferior parietal lobule and the parietal ventral area in studies of the cerebral cortex of the macaque monkey (Disbrow et al., 2003). Regarding the new cytoarchitectonic subdivisions within the parietal operculum the parietal ventral area may correspond to area OP4 or Brodmann's area 43 and SII may be analogue to area OP1 or the parietal opercular part of Brodmann's area 40.

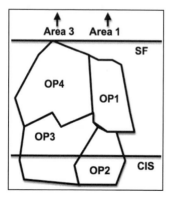

Figure 15. Lateral aspect of the hypothetically unfolded parietal operculum. Four cytoarchitectonicaly different areas have been delineated recently (referring to Eickhoff et al., 2006). Few data on electrical stimulation of the parietal operculum are available. Evoked potential studies in non-human primates and functional neuroimaging data indicate distinct secondary somatotopically organized somatosensory representations concordant with this cytoarchitectonic organization. OP: parietal operculum, SF: Sylvian fissure, CIS: circuminsular sulcus.

Receptor architectonics of the parietal lobe revealed a exceptionally high density of M2 receptors in area 3b. The glutamatergic AMPA-receptor is more concentrated in the areas 3a and 2 of Brodmann. Generally, the differences in receptor distribution appear to be most prominent when differences in cytoarchitecture are prominent. The receptor pattern therefore probably is less specific in the parietal association areas (Zilles & Palomero-Gallagher, 2001).

Functional anatomy

Primary sensory area: Primary cortical somatosensation is represented in the postcentral gyrus including the posterior bank of the central sulcus. Knowledge on the function of the postcentral gyrus was based on findings of postmortal pathological examinations of the brain that were correlated with reported sensory loss or when such sensory loss occurred after a defined surgical resection of parts of the cerebral cortex (Krause, 1931). Sensory effects of electrocortical stimulation in the cerebral cortex can not be assessed in non-human mammals. Therefore, knowledge about the detailed functional organization of somatosensory areas developed much later than that on motor areas depending on the results of intra- or interoperative electrocortical stimulation in humans. One of the first reports on intraoperative electrical stimulation of the postcentral gyrus in humans was published by Harvey Cushing (1909). He elicited sensory phenomena by stimulation of the postcentral gyrus in two patients which lend support to the theory of a primary sensory representation in the postcentral gyrus, a disputed topic at that time. Despite their numerous findings on motor effects with intraoperative electrocortical stimulation, Krause and Schum (1931) could not present satisfying data regarding somatosensory effects induced by this technique. The first detailed description of the responses of the postcentral gyrus to electrocortical stimulation was presented by Otfried Foerster (1936) who had performed intraoperative cerebral stimulation for several decades. In contrast to the application of galvanic current as preferred by Krause (1931) he found that faradic current was effective in eliciting sensory phenomena while stimulating the postcentral gyrus. He was the first to establish the somatotopic arrangement of the primary sensory cortex and proved it was similar to the somatotopic organization of the primary motor cortex. He was also able to stimulate the medial surface of the hemispheres especially the paracentral lobule. The posterior part of the paracentral lobule represents the anterior part of the medial parietal lobe and shows a sensory representation of genital organs including the bladder and rectum. Sensations of urinary urge and rectal tenesms were induced by stimulation of this area. Foerster (1936) pointed out that there were no sexual sensations produced by stimulation of the paracentral lobule. The same opinion was shared by Penfield and Rasmussen (1950). The adjacent most dorsal part of the paracentral lobule will produce sensations in the digits of the contralateral foot upon electrocortical stimulation. This sequence may reflect partially a segmental order of the cortical sensory representation beginning with sacral segments in the most ventral part of the paracentral lobule. Nevertheless, the cortical representation of sensation does not strictly follow the order of dermatoms in its further course. The following area of the postcentral gyrus on the lateral surface then includes the known sequence of sensory representations which is: foot, leg, thigh, abdomen, chest, shoulder, arm, hand, small finger, ring finger, middle finger, index finger, thumb, collum, back of the head, face (forehead, middle face, lips, chin), intraoral cavity. Also, pharyngeal and laryngeal sensations were produced at the most ventral portion of the postcentral gyrus.

Some annotations concerning this pattern have to be added. When bilateral sensations were described it was with stimulation of the face-area and more so the intraoral cavity, the pharynx and the larynx. This bilateral pattern of sensations in the ventral parts of the lateral surface has been reproduced by studies of electrocortical stimulation in non-human primates and humans (Penfield & Rasmussen, 1950). More recently, bilateral responses to sensory stimulation of the lips and the intraoral cavity in humans were recorded by a magnetoencephalography (MEG) (Disbrow et al., 2003). Primarily ipsilateral sensations were not described by Foerster (1936) as opposed to others who occasionally found ipsilateral sensations after stimulation of the most ventral portion of the postcentral gyrus (Penfield & Rasmussen, 1950). Qualities of sensations produced upon stimulation of the postcentral gyrus were heterogeneous and would often be described as tingling or pins and needles, buzzing, vibrating, tickling, itching, cold. This variability of qualities reported may not only be expression of the patients' individual perceptions but may represent the stimulation of different somatosensory areas as defined by cytoarchitectonic methods. As introduced in the previous paragraph, Brodmann (1909) initially described 4 separate cytoarchitectonic patterns in the postcentral gyrus namely, from rostral to caudal, areas 3a, 3b, 1 and 2. Area 3a at the bottom of the central sulcus predominantly receives afferents from muscle spindles. Its main projections are to the primary motor area indicating that it is a sensory-motor relay cortex. The majority of afferents from the ventroposterior thalamus terminate in area 3b. This area represents the core somatosensory area as supposed by studies on connectivity and functional activation in the fMRI (Grefkes & Fink, 2006). Its macroanatomical correlate is the posterior bank of the central sulcus. The adjacent area 1 on the anterior crown of the postcentral gyrus also receives thalamic afferents transmitting light touch and vibration and it is possible that it was primarily this area that was stimulated when patients reported a sensation of vibration with electrocortical stimulation. Area 2 receives afferents from joint-receptors as well as corticocortical fibers from the adjacent areas 1 and 3b. Occasionally, as Foerster mentioned (1936), patients described the feeling of a movement without objective evidence of a real movement. Whether a sense of buzzing or the aforementioned sense of a movement without the evidence for motion results from stimulation of area 2 is speculative as well. Nonetheless, all primary sensory areas were shown to include a complete somatotopic map of the body and therefore may serve as separate somatosensory representations (Nieuwenhuys et al., 2008).

Foerster (1936) pointed out that painful sensations were exceptionally rare when stimulating the postcentral gyrus. The observation of other investigators supports this observation suggesting a separate central representation of the afferents arising from the dorsal column and those coming from the spinothalamic tract. Foerster and also other authors stated that a complete anesthesia is unlikely to be of cortical origin (Krause & Blum, 1931). Therefore, probably not the whole spectrum of sensation is represented in the postcentral gyrus.

Concerning sensory qualities elicited with cortical stimulation of the parietal lobe Foerster (1936) mentioned cases where stimulation of the ventral part of the postcentral gyrus especially at the representation of tongue, intraoral cavity and pharynx produced unpleasant sour or putrefacient taste phenomena. In his discussion of these findings he refers to cortical lesions including the most ventral portion of the postcentral gyrus that were associated with anesthesia of the face, the inner cheek and the tongue which did not affect gustation. With this contradictions and quoting other researchers of that time he put his findings into question by leaving the location of the cortical representation of gustation open. Penfield and Rasmussen did not report any gustatory sensation when stimulating the primary sensory cortex (1950).

The results of Foerster (1936) contributed significantly to the understanding of the central sensory system. However, the most comprehensive data on somatosensory responses to intraoperative stimulation were published in the monographs of Penfield and colleagues (e.g. Penfield & Rasmussen, 1950). In 1950 Penfield and Rasmussen reported on a collected series of about 1,000 sensory responses elicited in the rolandic cortex. 75% of the sensory responses they produced with galvanic stimulation were of postcentral origin whereas 25% were produced by stimulation of the precentral gyrus. Besides, in 15 cases they were able to stimulate the anterior or posterior bank of the central sulcus after excision of the postcentral or precentral gyrus respectively. The same as Foerster (1936) they reported sensations of "numbness, tingling, or a feeling of electricity" as typical responses to electrocortical stimulation of the posterior bank of the central sulcus. They also refer to a sense of movement without objective evidence for a real movement as distinct type of response as Foerster (1936) did. This is accordant with our own observations of electrical stimulation of subdural and depth electrodes close to or within the rolandic cortex which occasionally produced this sense of a movement upon stimulation.

Despite the fact that not infrequently they observed sensory phenomena produced with stimulation of the precentral gyrus, Penfield and Rasmussen (1950) concluded that "the major cortical representation of somatic sensation (proprioceptive and discriminatory) is in the postcentral gyrus." This conclusion was supported by the observation that ablation of the precentral gyrus in contrast to ablation of the postcentral gyrus "does not seem to interfere with sensory perception."

The maps that have been generated by the work of Foerster (1936) and Penfield and colleagues (1950) resemble each other closely confirming their reliability. However, there are minor discrepancies. The representation of the neck and the back of the head were found to be extensions of the trunk and shoulder region dorsal to the representation of arm and hand by Penfield and Rasmussen (1950) whereas Foerster (1936) reported evidence for a representation of the neck and the back of the head between the representation of the fingers and that of the face therefore being more comparable to the sequence of representations in the primary motor cortex. Even though Penfield and Rasmussen decided to draw the representation of neck and posterior head between that of the shoulder and the upper extremity their original data were more heterogeneous. They described that about two thirds of the corresponding responses were at the position described above whereas the other third of sensations in the neck and the back of the head occurred after stimulation of the area between hand and face representation of even more ventrally thus corresponding with the descriptions of Foerster (1936).This point does not appear to be finally solved. Penfield and colleagues not only introduced the motor-homunculus as mentioned above but also a sensory homunculus as a figurine presenting the relative distortions of functional cortical representations compared to the bodies anatomy shortly after Foerster's report (Penfield & Boldrey, 1937). The analogue figurine of the primary motor representation depicts the differences in the central representation of sensation and primary movements. Whereas the motor representations of the hand and wrist are larger in the primary motor area, the lower face and especially the lips are overrepresented in the sensory cortex compared to the primary motor cortex.

In addition there is a sensory representation of the genital region in the ventral part of the paracentral lobule whereas such a representation can not be found in the primary motor area.

Secondary somatosensory areas: Interest in the secondary somatosensory areas was stimulated by studies of electrographically recorded evoked potentials in animals that provided evidence for additional areas responsive to sensory stimulation (Adrian, 1943). Sensory responses of the forelimbs and the hindlimbs were recorded in the most ventral portion of the postcentral gyrus (ventral to the primary somatosensory area of the face and the intraoral cavity as defined by Foerster [1936] in humans). Interestingly, Penfield also reported having noticed such responses when stimulating around the postcentral gyrus at the junction with the Sylvian fissure but initially interpreted them as "escape of current to the internal capsule". Later Penfield and Rasmussen (1950) reported reliably reproducible sensory phenomena of the upper and lower extremities with electrocortical stimulation of that area. At that time they were unable to define a clear somatotopic map from the results of electrocortical stimulation. They called this area as the second somatosensory area. The exact location and extend of this (these) area(s) is still a matter of discussion.

Besides, the concept of a second somatosensory system has been expanded. More recently new cytoarchitectonic maps as well as studies with functional imaging and evoked potentials provided new evidence for several secondary somatosensory areas (Eickhoff *et al.*, 2007; Coq *et al.*, 2004). Four different somatosensory maps in the parietal operculum and the adjacent insula were delineated and may each contain complete body maps. Still, removal or ablation of these secondary sensory areas did not lead to any noticeable sensory loss in the studies of Penfield and Rasmussen (1950). This cortex therefore was declared as "dispensable" and secondary compared to the primary sensory area. Electrocortical stimulation of depths electrodes introduced perpendicular to the lateral surface of the hemisphere and penetrating the parietal operculum were shown to elicit illusions of rotation, translations and feeling of body motion. These findings were assessed as support for a representation of vestibular function in the peri-Sylvian cortex including the parietal operculum (Kahane *et al.*, 2003). But electrical stimulation of the parietal is performed particularly infrequent and further reports on parietal opercular function based on this technique are sparse.

Sensory phenomena can be found with stimulation of other parts of the parietal lobe. Stimulation of the superior parietal lobe *i.e.* area 5a and 5b in the nomenclature of Vogt and Vogt (1919) or areas 5 and 7 by Brodmann can elicit sensory phenomena contralateral to the stimulated hemisphere. Foerster (1936) reported that often these sensations affect the whole hemibody and that stimulation of sufficient duration can involve the ipsilateral hemibody as well (Foerster, 1936). As mentioned above, unfortunately we do not know if these more prolonged stimulations may have induced afterdischarges or actual epileptic seizures. Foerster (1936) also operated on patients whose rolandic cortex had been severely injured secondary to a trauma. Electrocortical stimulation of the superior parietal lobule in these patients produced the characteristic sensations as mentioned above whereas stimulation of the residual postcentral gyus or the structures around the central sulcus was not able to induce somatosensation. This evidence suggests the presence of a somatosensory representation in the superior parietal lobule that is independent of the postcentral gyrus (Foerster, 1936). Foerster (1936) reported also patients with lesional epilepsy of the superior paracentral lobule who presented with epileptic seizures starting with somatosensory auras affecting the whole contralateral hemibody. Nevertheless, these clinico-pathological observations were not validated by electrographic recordings a technique that had just been introduced at that time. No somatotopic distribution of sensory responses has been established in this area. The sensations induced by stimulation of the superior parietal lobule were reported as being similar to those that followed stimulation of the postcentral gyrus even though painful sensations were more frequently encountered with stimulation of the superior parietal lobule. The existence of an independent somatosensory representation in the superior parietal lobe has not been documented by other authors.

No somatosensory phenomena were produced by electrocortical stimulation of the inferior parietal lobule *i.e.* area 7a and 7b of the Vogts (1922) or area 39 and 40 of Brodmann (1909). In accordance cortical lesions of the inferior parietal lobule do not produce somatosensory deficits unless they penetrate the afferents to the postcentral gyrus in the white matter underneath the cortex. Unfortunately, we do not find reported corresponding evidence of stimulation of these areas from studies of Penfield and colleagues concerning effects on somatosensation (1937; 1950).

Electrical stimulation of the superior and inferior parietal lobule usually does not produce neglect or apraxia, neurological deficits frequently observed in patients with lesions in these areas. This may be due to inadequate clinical testing during electrical stimulation of these areas. Kleinman *et al.* (2007) observed that electrical stimulation of the inferior parietal lobe interfered with the ability to recognize gaps in circles and to correctly divide a line into equal halves. The authors also reported that electrical stimulation results correctly predicted a postoperative deficit after resection of epileptogenic tissue in the inferior parietal lobule in one patient and therefore may be a valid tool to more precisely estimate consequences of cortical resections in the parietal lobe (Kleinman *et al.*, 2007). Nevertheless, a highly cooperative patient is required. Wellmer and colleagues (2009) stressed the necessity for a structured testing procedure during electrocortical stimulation especially for testing of complex functions as speech.

It is important to stress that the occurrence of sensory phenomena by electrical stimulation is not restricted to electrocortical stimulation of the parietal lobe. We already quoted the findings of Penfield and Rasmussen (1950) whose sensory responses of the perirolandic cortex were precentral in 25%. Similarly, secondary sensory phenomena in the perisylvian region have been described after stimulation of post- and precentral cortex. Stimulation at the parieto-occipital junction of the right hemisphere was found to be able to disrupt visuospatial functions (Fried *et al.*, 1982). As introduced in the previous part of this chapter the polymodal association cortex of the parietal lobe has strong connections with the frontal lobe. It is likely, therefore, that that part of the cortex participates in planning and awareness of movements. Indeed, in a study using intraoperative electrocoritcal stimulation of the right inferior parietal region Desmurget *et al.* (2009) reported that patients felt the desire to move the contralateral hand, arm and foot. Stimulation of the left inferior parietal region on the other hand produced the intention to move the lips and to talk. This feeling was even intensified when increasing stimulation intensity. It is important, however, to remember that electrical stimulation of the postcentral gyrus can produce motor responses in a significant proportion of patients (Penfield & Jasper, 1954). Electrical stimulation at near motor threshold frequently produces subclinical muscle contraction in selected muscles that the patient may perceive as "intention to move".

Speech areas: Stimulation of posterior and inferior parts of the parietal lobe often can remain clinically asymptomatic. The most relevant exception to this rule is the stimulation of the parietotemporal junction *(Figure 12)*. Electrocortical stimulation of the dominant lobe posterior inferior parietal area and the temporoparietal junction elicits aphasias. These areas, which are not clearly defined neuroanatomically, are also know as Wernicke's speech region and for a long time have been associated with perception and processing of speech. Lesions of this area in the dominant hemisphere are associated with receptive aphasia. As already discussed in the previous paragraphs on speech function in the frontal lobe, electrical stimulation of Wernicke's area does not induce positive phenomena like induction of words, phrases, or thoughts but interferes globally with speech comprehension and production. Foerster (1936) did not report on stimulation-induced aphasia. Penfield and colleagues (1950; 1959), however, observed a variety of aphasic symptoms after electrocortical interference in Wernicke's areas.

Motor effects: It has to be mentioned that the postcentral gyrus has also been associated with rudimentary motor function. This theory arose secondary to electrocortical stimulation of the postcentral gyrus which occasional produced restricted movements. Nonetheless, Cecile and Oskar Vogt (1919) demonstrated that this phenomenon could be extinguished after either disrupting the corticospinal fibers arising from the precentral gyrus or after discontinuation of the U-fibers that intracortically connect the pre- and postcentral gyrus. Based on these observations motor-phenomena after stimulation of the postcentral gyrus have been attributed to spread of excitation rather than as evidence for a motor representation in the postcentral gyrus. The threshold for eliciting movements tends to be higher than in the primary motor cortex. There is an isosomatotopic arrangement of the results of stimulation of the postcentral gyrus compared to the primary motor cortex.

Foerster (1936) observed that stimulation of the postcentral gyrus produced complex adversive movements comparable to those that occurred after stimulation of area 6aα and 6aβ and that were independent of the functional integrity of the primary motor area. No somatotopy regarding these synergistic movements was noticed and Foerster suggested that this effect is mediated by direct efferents of the postcentral gyrus. Foerster (1936) describes flexor-synergisms with stimulation of area 5a (Vogt & Vogt 1919). Contralateral flexion in hip, knee, foot, elbow and hand were most frequently the result of stimulation of area 5a. An early ipsilateral involvement after electrocortical stimulation was described as characteristic for this area. The adjacent area 5b on the other hand was shown to elicit a forced version of the head and the eyes to the contralateral side during stimulation. Areas 5a and 5b (area 7 of Brodmann) both were thought to induce their effect via an own efferent system since ablation of the perirolandic cortex did not extinguish the versive movements described above. Both areas did exhibit high thresholds of stimulation for motor responses. Threshold for induction of their sensory effects as qualified was much lower. This also refers to areas 3, 1 and 2 which exhibit their motor effects at thresholds exceeding those for inducing sensory phenomena. Foerster claims that area 22 can produce movements upon stimulation as well and describes its effect as complex contralateral versive movements as with stimulation of the postcentral areas mentioned before. All these complexes motor phenomena induced by parietal lobe stimulation by Foester (1936) have not been reproduced by other authors. The high intensity of stimulation used by Foerster (1936) clearly suggests that the results were induced by spreading of the stimulus into classical frontal lobe motor areas or the induction of epileptic seizures.

The parietal lobe is the main receptor organ of the brain for somatosensory information. Small parts in its anterior part receive direct peripheral information the arrangement of which parallels the configuration of the primary motor area as discovered by electrocortical stimulation. With exception of this and the posterior speech area stimulation of most

parts of the parietal lobe does not produce measurable clinical effects in a routine extraoperative stimulation setting. These silent areas represent multimodal interfaces for orientation and motion in three-dimensional space.

Occipital lobe

Macroscopical anatomy

The occipital lobe is the most caudal part of the telencephalon. Its anterior border on the
lateral surface usually is defined by the occipital sulcus and the superior end of the parieto-
occipital sulcus. On the medial surface the parieto-occipital sulcus separates the parietal
and the occipital lobe whereas no clear landmark divides the temporal and the occipital
lobe. Therefore an occipitotemporal line in continuation of the parieto-occipital sulcus
commonly defines the rostral basomedial border of the occipital lobe. The occipital lobe
centers around the calcarine sulcus that divides the medial surface of the occipital lobe
in a superior and inferior part. The occipital lobe is as far as it is known exclusively
concerned with processing of visual information. Nevertheless, the visual system exceeds
the aforementioned borders of the occipital lobe including parts of the temporal, parietal
and even frontal lobes. No evidence exists for visual processing in the insular lobe. It is
estimated that about one third of the cerebral cortex in humans and up to 50% of the
cerebral cortex in macaques is concerned with the processing of visual information emphasizing its relative importance and complexity in the cerebral processing of information
(Gulyás, 1998).

Microscopical anatomy

Cytoarchitectonically the occipital lobe is divided into several hierarchically organized
areas *(Figures 15-18)*. The occipital pole with the primary visual cortex area 17 of Brodmann receives the main visual afferents. This area is easily identified by a dense layer of
myelinated fibers that is even recognizable macroscopically in sections through area 17.
This layer is called stria of Gennari after Francesco Gennari who described its characteristic structure in 1782. The division of the occipital lobe into striate primary and extrastriate secondary occipital cortex was primarily derived from the existence of this stripe in
the primary visual cortex as well. The borders between the primary *i.e.* striate and its
surrounding secondary *i.e.* extrastriate cortices were repeatedly found to be very sharp.
Nevertheless, whereas the extent of Brodman's area 17 is well-defined the demarcation
and functional characterization of many extrastriate areas is less precise. According to
Brodmann there are 3 major cytoarchitectonic areas in the occiptal lobe centering around
the calcarine sulcus and the occipital pole. These areas are from caudal to rostral area 17,
area 18 and area 19 *(Figures 16 and 17)*. Area 18 and area 19 represent the extrastriate
visual cortex in that classification. Areas 18 and 19 rely mainly on the afferent input from
the primary visual cortex. Nevertheless, it is well-known that the lateral geniculate body
of the thalamus not only projects to the primary visual cortex but also to visual association
cortex since visual responsiveness is partially retained even after total ablation of both
primary visual cortices (Bullier *et al.*, 1994).

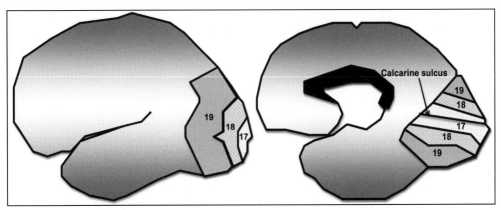

Figures 16 and 17. Lateral and medial aspect of the brain. The schematic areas of the occipital lobe are shown according to the cytoarchitectonic studies of Brodmann (1909). Areal numbers refer to Brodmann (1909).

Recent studies of visual physiology have led to new subdivisions of the visual system of non-human primates. This terminology assigns the capital letter "V" followed by a subsequent figure increasing from caudal to rostrally to every cortical area involved in visual processing. Therefore the primary visual cortex *i.e.* Brodmann's area 17 is named V1 whereas subsequent areas in the processing stream of visual information are named V2, V3, V4, etc. (*Figures 18 and 19*). Between 25 and 30 different areas have been described in the extrastriate occipital cortex of non-human primates. Key properties of the organization of these areas are the functional separation of the visual cortex and its hierarchical structure. Thus it is thought that already starting at the primary visual cortex visual processing uses separated areas for decoding the different functional aspects of visual objects like motion, form and color. For example, area V4 has been associated with colour-representation repeatedly (Zeki, 1980). One concern of these maps certainly is the degree of comparability to humans. Still, there has been a good amount of overlap in the comparative neuroanatomy of these maps in different non-human species thus supporting generally the validity of this map (Gulyás, 1998). And 8-10 of the visual areas described in non-human primates have been recognized in humans so far (*Figures 18 and 19*) (Nieuwenhuys *et al.*, 2008).

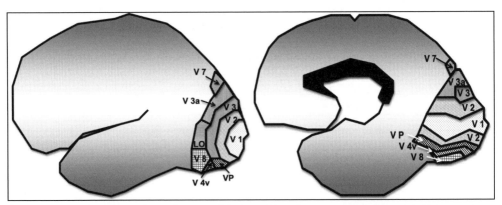

Figures 18 and 19. Lateral and medial aspect of the brain. The schematic areas of the occipital lobe are shown according to histological and functional data referring to Nieuwenhuys *et al.* (2008). Area V1 represents the striate cortex. Successive numbers refer to refined extrastriate areas. VP: ventral posterior area of V3, LO: lateral occipital area.

Receptor architectonical studies have also shown that the densities of several groups of receptors, including the gamma-Amino-butyric-acid A (GABA-A)-receptor, glutamatergic receptors, muscarinergic M1 and M2 as well as nicotinergic acetylcholine receptors, serotonergic 5-HT1a and 5 HT2a receptors and noradrenergic receptors are highest in area V1 of the visual system. Moreover, changes in densities of these receptors between area 17 and area 18 coincide with established cytoarchitectonical borders in most cases (Zilles & Amunts, 2009). Nevertheless, supporting the theory of structure-function relation on the one hand these findings may be due to the overall higher neuronal density in the primary visual cortex.

Functional anatomy

Character of visual sensations: The first reports on electrical stimulation of the occipital lobe have been published by Fedor Krause (1911) and Otfried Foerster (1929). Both reported the occurrence of visual sensations in the central or visual hemifield after stimulation of the contralalateral occipital lobes. Foerster (1929) showed that stimulation of the anterior calcarine sulcus would lead to phosphenes that moved from the periphery towards the center of vision and stimulation of the occipital pole lead to phosphenes in the central visual field that remained steady. Stimulation of the upper bank of the calcarine fissure lead to moving stimuli in the contralateral lower visual quadrant and stimulation of the lower bank of the calcarine fissure to moving phosphenes in the upper quadrant of the contralateral visual field. These sensations usually were colourless (Foerster, 1929). Penfield and Rasmussen (1950) reported that with very few exceptions elementary visual sensations resulted exclusively from stimulation of the occipital lobe. The visual sensations produced by intraoperative stimulation of primary or secondary visual cortices were reported as very elementary and simple sensations like "a brilliant ball, a star, a streak, a wheel, a spot or a flash, a shadow, a light." These responses should be classified as phosphenes *i.e.* simple visual sensations that are not produced by the influx of light through the eye. The fact that scotomes are not infrequently described in epileptic seizures arising from the occipital lobe indicates that the scotome Krause (1911) reported in one patient during electrical stimulation of the occipital lobe may have been due to afterdischarges or induction of an epileptic seizure.

Even though forms may sometimes become more complex it generally holds true that these responses to occipital electrocortical stimulation "bore little resemblance to things a man sees in his environment." (Penfield & Rasmussen, 1950). Interestingly, Salanova *et al.* (1992) state that more complex hallucinations can occur as visual auras in 15-20% of the patients with occipital lobe epilepsy and stimulation of basal temporo-occipital areas did produce complex and colored visual perceptions (Lee *et al.*, 2000). Still, electrocortical stimulation is probably incapable of producing more complex figures without spread of activity to different regions of the brain.

Penfield's and Rasmussen's results are in line with subsequent studies of cortical stimulation of the occipital lobe and Brindley 1982 confirmed that phosphenes are solely generated by stimulation of the occipital cortex. Besides, there is evidence that electrocortical stimulation of the occipital cortex elicits almost exclusively visual phenomena. Although reports of induction of eye-movements or frontal headache exist these phenomena are thought to be secondary to the induced visual perceptions in the visual field and the stimulation of meningeal pain fibres respectively (Brindley, 1982).

The effects of occipital stimulation can also be induced in blind persons. This is one of the sources for research in "prosthesis for the blind" *i.e.* induction of visual phenomena by cortical stimulation that may be able to produce rudimentary visual impressions of the outer world (Brindley & Lewin, 1968). These authors studied the effects of chronically implanted cortical electrodes in selected blind patients. In these patients, stimulation of areas 17 and 18 which were variably covered with electrodes did not show definite differences in appearance. Most induced phosphenes were described as being of "point-like" appearance with some being elliptical or linear therefore resembling what Penfield and Rasmussen (1950) had described before. They were "always of light, not darkness". Also the phosphenes did not cease within a stimulation, but lasted as long as the stimulus was applied to the cortex and in some cases did overlast a strong stimulation for several minutes. We have only seen this in patients in whom the electrical stimulation elicited afterdischarges in the occipital pole. In those cases, the visual hallucinations disappeared as soon as the afterdischarge stopped. Failures of inducing phosphenes in these two areas were felt to be related to technical or anatomical constraints rather than being correlate of functional variation (Brindley, 1982). Additionally, induction of pairs of phosphenes generally was stable in repeated testing over the course of 3 years. Also the internal consistency of maps was shown to be high.

Bak *et al.* (1990) investigated the effects of cortical stimulation and intracortical microstimulation within the occipital pole in 3 patients undergoing surgery for the treatment of epilepsy. They found that the stimulation threshold for inducing phosphenes is 10-100 times lower with intracortical electrodes compared to direct cortical stimulation. In absolute figures the lowest threshold for inducing phosphenes recorded in their procedure was at $20 \, \mu A$ for intracortical electrodes in a depth of 2-3 mm. In contrast, the corresponding threshold on the cortical surface were between 1 and 2 mA. The nature of the induced phosphenes was in the opinion of these authors similar between those two modalities of stimulation. However, whereas cortical stimulation tended to induce flickering phosphenes, intracortical stimulation induced steady phosphenes synchronized with on- and offset of the stimulation. Moreover, it was reported that phosphenes induced with low stimulation thresholds tended to be colored and somewhat larger compared to stronger stimuli.

There is evidence for the presence of color-specific areas in the more rostral parts of the occipital lobe. In recent years several reports using functional imaging techniques have identified areas V4 and V8 as possible central representation of color perception (Hadjikhani *et al.*, 1998; Brewer *et al.*, 2005).

Retinotopy of visual sensations: The results of cortical stimulation have contributed to the elucidation of the retinotopic distribution within the visual cortex. Still, first important insights into the central representation of vision have been derived from visual field defects of patients with circumscribed lesions of the occipital lobe. Although this technique carries imprecision it allowed for topical differentiation of central and peripheral vision in the occipital pole and medial occipital surface respectively (Holmes, 1918). It has been confirmed by electrocortical stimulation that the occipital pole of one hemisphere harbors the representation of the central fovea and thus represents central vision (Dobelle *et al.*, 1979). The classical neuroanatomical view of cerebral visual representation is further supported by reports from Brindley (1982) who stated that "there is a clear tendency for high electrodes to produce low phosphenes and vice versa" and that "there is probably a slight tendency for rostral electrodes to produce peripheral phosphenes and caudal electrodes to produce phosphenes near the point of fixation" *(Figures 20 and 21)*. Still, even though nearness of electrodes indicated nearness of phosphenes exceptions to this rule were found to be not infrequent. This is on the one hand certainly an effect of the incompleteness of coverage of cortical surface especially within the sulci of the occipital lobe. On the other hand it may be due to multiple retinotopic maps within occipital cortex.

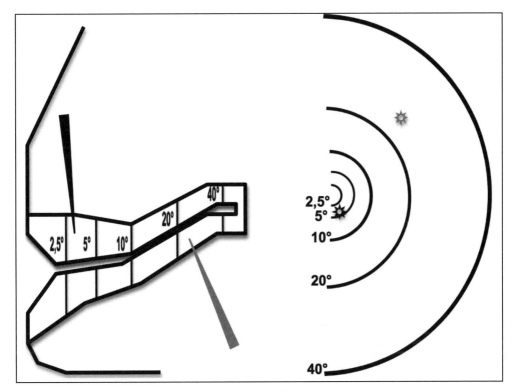

Figures 20 and 21. Medial aspect of the left occipital pole. The primary visual cortex surrounding the calcarine fissure is delineated. The vertical lines indicate the approximate representation of the annotated angle of the right visual field as shown on the right. Asterisks in the right visual hemifield show the presumed location of a phosphene induced by electrical stimulation of the primary visual cortex as indicated by colour-concordant electrodes on the left. The upper quadrant of the visual hemifield is represented in the lower wall of the contralateral calcarine fissure and vice versa. In analogy to other primary cortical areas peripheral-central distortion discloses information content.

No final consensus exists regarding the question of foveal representation. Evidence exists supporting the so-called "split-fovea" theory which says that the central vision is represented bilaterally (Lavidor & Walsh, 2004). Holmes (1918) investigated patients with occipital lesions and concluded that "the macular region has not a bilateral representation." This conclusion is generally accepted. There is only few other evidence in the literature supporting Foerster's (1929) report of a bilateral foveal representation based on his electrocortical stimulation studies and observations on patients with lesions of the occipital lobe. Still, occasionally responses to electrocortical stimulation of the occipital lobe in the studies of Penfield and Rasmussen (1950) were reported to having occurred in the ipsilateral hemifield.

The occipital lobe is exclusively concerned with the processing of visual information. The classical cytoarchitectonic tripartition of the occipital lobe has been advances in the recent past. However, the distinct topic arrangement of the visual field and its location in the primary visual or striate cortex remains the core structure of the occipital lobe. Electrortical stimulation most often produces phophenes with stimulation of the primary visual but also the secondary visual areas. Therefore this technique has not been capable of producing clinical responses that reliably distinguish primary and secondary visual cortex.

Insular lobe

Macroscopical anatomy

Even though there is full continuity of cortex between the insula and its neighboring cortical areas the hidden position of this structure explains its name. It may be justified to refer to the insula as the fifth lobe of the brain since its central position does not allow a definite allocation to one of the surrounding cerebral lobes. This cortical area was first described by Johann Christian Reil in 1809 (Reil, 1809). The insula is overlapped by the frontal, the temporal and the parietal operculum. It has a triangular shape. Macroscopically it is characterized by an anterior part with three short gyri divided by 2 short sulci and a posterior part with two gyri subdivided by a single long gyrus. Anterior and posterior insula are separated by the central sulcus of the insula. The sulcus which lies between the insula and the surrounding cerebral cortex is called circuminsular sulcus.

Microscopical anatomy

Microscopically the insula shows some interesting characteristics. In early cytoarchitectonic studies, Brodmann found evidence for at least two different areas in the insula: the granular part in the posterior insula and the agranular part in the anterior part (Brodmann, 1909). And even though Brodmann generally used numbers to label cortical areas that showed re-identifiable characteristics the insular cortex was not included into that system. Still in the cytoarchitectonic studies in monkeys he divided the insular cortex into 4 different areas labeled area 13 – 16. Three cytoarchitectonically different areas have been described in studies of the insular cortex of the old world monkey by Mesulam and Mufson (1982) *(Figure 22)*. The anterior and ventral part of the anterior insula is an agranular cortex without identifiable granular layers. Therefore this part of the insula resembles the three-layered allocortex. The overall myelin content was found to be low in this part of the cortex. Posterior to the agranular cortex there is a dysgranular sector with five to six cortical layers. There, the layer II is incompletely developed and is not clearly separated from layer III which lacks a typical organization. More dorsally this layer shows a developing columnar arrangement. On the other hand the prominent hyperchromic neurons of layer V decrease from more anterior to more posterior parts of the insula. The myelin content of this area is low again and it has been stated that "the lines of Baillarger are almost totally absent" (Mesulam & Mufson, 1982). The granular sector of the insula shows a fully developed isocortical pattern with prominent layers II and IV. The inner and outer lines of Baillarger are present and the whole sector has the highest myelin concentration within the insula. In the most recent description of the insular cytoarchitecture based on standardized observer-independent methods the posterior insular cortex has been refined into two different granular areas. Additionally the dysgranular insular cortex has been subdivided into three different areas as well *(Figure 22)*. Given the variety of symptoms induced by electrocortical stimulation of the insula those subdivisions may well correspond to functional differences (Kurth *et al.*, 2010).

Chemoarchitectonically there is not much information available regarding specific patterns of the insular lobe. Still the density of acetylcholinesterase (AchE) in the insula has been investigated by Mesulam and Mufson (1982). They found peak concentrations in the anterior insula and a gradual decline in direction to the posterior insula which shows the lowest density of AchE within the insula.

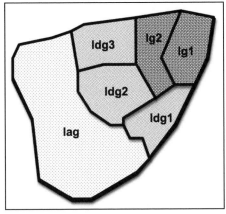

Figure 22. Lateral aspect of the insula lobe. A marked reduction in granularity from caudal to more rostral parts is typical of the insula cortex. A tripartition of the insula into a granular, dysgranular and agranular area (Mesulam & Mufson, 1982) has partially been refined more recently (Kurth *et al.*, 2010). Ig: granular insula, Idg: dysgraular insula, Iag: agranular insula.

Regarding comparative neuroanatomy these authors found similar patterns of cyto- and myeloarchitecture in the insula, the orbitofrontal cortex and the temporal polar cortex. In their concept these cortical areas center around the prepiriform cortex from which on a radial evolution from agranular over a transitional dysgranular to a granular cortex can be demonstrated. This is of importance since it reflects the pattern of connectivity of the insula which most likely influence its functional properties. Hence, one of the characteristics of connectivity at least in the insula is that its cortical areas tend to connect to those cortical areas which show similar cytoarchitectural properties. Therefore the anterior agranular insula is strongly interconnected with orbitofrontal, entorhinal and other limbic cortices with agranular cytoarchitecture. These connections moreover are often reciprocal. The posterior granular insula on the other hand mainly receives afferents from the thalamus, the amygdala and different sensory cortices with exception of the visual cortex (Mufson & Mesulam, 1982).

Functional anatomy

The inaccessible anatomy of the insula has been the reason for the fact that its functional role was and partially still is not decoded. Even exposure of a whole hemisphere after a craniotomy would under normal circumstance not allow to gain access to the insula *e.g.* for electrocortical stimulation. Nevertheless, it is mainly the progress in the diagnosis and treatment of epilepsy from the middle of the XXth century onwards that resulted in a few but valuable studies performing electrocortical stimulation of the insula. The reported evidence has contributed to the understanding of the insula function. The most persistent findings in these studies will be briefly discussed now. Penfield and Faulk (1955) published first results on intraoperative insular stimulation secondary to the introduction of temporal lobectomies for patients with temporal lobe epilepsies. In these patients the part of the insula underneath the temporal operculum was exposed so that intraoperative recordings on their epileptogenicity and electrocortical stimulation could be performed in selected cases. Much of what was proposed then still represents a valid frame for insula function based on electrocortical stimulation. The authors reported on a series of 36 patients. Eighty two points on the insula cortex were stimulated and gave electroclinical responses. Two main groups of clinical responses were obtained almost in equal numbers.

Viscerosensation and -motion: The first type of response related to visceral sensations. Responses did not prevail in a certain area of the insular cortex and no clear viscerotopic distribution could be established. Viscerosensory phenomena were most often located to the "xiphoid process, the epigastrium, or the umbilicus". The character of these abdominal sensations was described as "something funny to the abdomen, also "gurgling", "rolling", "pain", "nausea", "scratching". In 6 cases gastrographic recordings were obtained from patients and showed marked variation from the baseline gastric motility *i.e.* either inhibition or activation in 4 patients. This reveals evidence for the assumption that some of the viscerosensory phenomena primarily represent perception of a visceromotor activity a thought that has been clearly expressed by Penfield and Faulk (1955). Also they found that after unilateral complete removal of one insular lobe there was marked alteration in gastric motility in one case. Corresponding evidence for visceromotor representation in the insula exists from animal studies. Electrical stimulation of the insula leads to decrease in gastric tone and motility as well as a decrease in blood pressure and heart frequency in monkeys. It is important to mention that although these effects could also be obtained from stimulation of the orbitofrontal cortex and the temporopolar cortex stimulation of the lateral cortical surface did not produce a similar pattern of clinical responses. This renders an unspecific autonomic reaction of the cerebral cortex to electrocortical stimulation unlikely. The reported effects on gastric motility in this study could be extinguished by sectioning of the vagal nerve supporting the theory of a vagal nerve representation in the insula (Hoffman & Rasmussen, 1953). Babkin and Speakman (1950) also reported inhibition but not increase of gastric motility from stimulation of the insular-orbitofrontal and anterior cingulate cortex of the dog. Therefore it may not be easy to explain the divergent sympathetic and parasympathetic effects of insular stimulation. On the other hand recordings of neuronal responses to visceral sensory stimuli in rats showed that within different regions of the insular cortex there were responses to gastric mechanoreceptor input, taste stimuli, cardiovascular baroreceptor stimulation and arterial chemoreceptors (Cechetto & Saper, 1987). Therefore, the evidence from electrocortical stimulation supports that beside the viscerosensory and -motor system other autonomic function has a representation in the insula. Stimulation of the right insula cortex of rats has been shown to decrease blood pressure and heart rate whereas the opposite was demonstrated for stimulation of the left insular cortex (Oppenheimer & Cechetto, 1990). Nevertheless, a reverse pattern of lateralization was demonstrated for the human insulae concerning effects of electrocortical stimulation on blood pressure (Oppenheimer *et al.*, 1992). More recently the proposed insular involvement in autonomic regulation has supported statistical associations that were found to exist between an increased risk for cardiac arrhythmias and death following strokes involving the insula (Abboud *et al.*, 2006). Nevertheless, criticism has been raised by stating that this association is a confounder of infarct size (Borsody *et al.*, 2009). Regarding viscerosensory or -motor effects of electrocortical stimulation of the human insula other available studies are those of Ostrowsky (2000) and Isnard (2004). These authors stimulated stereotactically implanted depths electrodes in patients with drug-resistant epilepsy. They elicited sensations of "abdominal heaviness, thoracic constriction, unpleasant ascending epigastric and retrosternal sensation, sudden flush, or nausea" and rarely abdominal pain (Isnard et al., 2004). These responses were not restricted to a certain part of the insula even though predominance in the anterior and middle insula can be derived from their schemes. Like in the study of Penfield and Faulk (1955) visceral phenomena were among the most common responses to stimulation representing 22% of all evoked clinical responses in the insula (Isnard et al., 2004). The most recent reports on this topic confirmed these results stating that 12% of clinical responses after stimulation of insular depth electrodes were associated to visceral sensations (Nguyen et al., 2009). The locations of electrode contacts that produced viscerosensitive symptoms in this study also predominated in the more anterior and middle part of the insula (Figure 23).

Results of stimulation of the insula and adjacent cortex were the basis for the hypothesis of a alimentary or feeding pattern represented in the insula and periinsular region. Based on results from Babkin and van Buren (1951) who found such a sequence in the cortex of the dog the proximity of representation of chewing, swallowing, salivation at the foot of the lateral rolandic surface, the intraoral sensations and taste represented in the superior opercular and insular cortex and the viscersosensory and -motor representation in the anterior and middle insular cortex in humans are in agreement with this term.

Somatosensation: Penfield and Faulk (1955), after having induced a variety of symptoms by stimulation of the insula stated that "among all the types of response, only two seemed to be statistically important (a) the visceral (sensory and motor) and (b) the somatic (sensory)." Indeed, somatosensory responses are the second large group of symptoms that are induced by stimulation of the insula cortex (Figure 23). Penfield and Faulk (1950) stated that the somatosensory responses were variously described by the patients as "tingling", "warmth", "numbness", "tightness", "vibration", "shock", and simply as "sensation" in different parts of the body. Sensations reportedly were occasionally ipsilateral to the stimulated insula or even bilateral. Similar experiences were described by Isnard et al. (2004). In their group of 50 patients with insular depth electrodes 43% of all responses were somatosensory "neutral or unpleasant nonpainful paresthesias, such as pins and needles or slight electric current". As much as 62% of all responses in 36 insular sites were interpreted as somatosensation in the reports of Nguyen et al. (2009). Both studies confirmed that stimulation of the insula occasionally produces ipsilateral or bilateral sensations.

Nociception and thermosensation: One special quality of somatosensory phenomena needs to be discussed additionally. The special sensory responses of warmth and pain were produced in all larger reports on human insular stimulation. Even though not separately discussed in some studies (Penfield & Faulk, 1955; Nguyen et al., 2009). However, Isnard et al. (2004) made inferences on these special qualities stating that among the 58 somatosensory responses they recorded 10 were warmth sensations and 9 painful or violent. The part of the insula representing pain was more closely defined to the two posterior thirds on the insular cortex (Mazzola et al., 2009). Also these authors found a somatotopic distribution of the 49 painful responses they had collected. Painful sensations of the face were found to be more rostrally located compared with those of the limbs. And the representation of painful sensations of the upper limbs was found to be above those of the lower limbs. The reports on sensations of warmth and painful sensations are of more general interest since those responses usually can not be obtained from electrocortical stimulation of the primary sensory cortex. The cortical representation of this quality therefore is less well-established with the posterior insula being one of the possible locations for a primary cortex of afferents processing pain and warmth (Figure 23).

Gustation: Another rather small subgroup of gustatory sensations may be worth to be discussed for the same reason. This quality has been reported to occur after stimulation of the insula in all the aforementioned reports. This quality was subsummated within the group of viscerosensitive responses by Penfield and Faulk (1955) as well as among the 12% viscerosensitive responses of the study from Nguyen *et al.* (2009). And olfactogustatory responses were separately reported by Isnard *et al.* (2004) representing only 2% of their responses. Still, gustation as a sensation induced by electrical stimulation may be regarded as a separate quality of responses within the insula *(Figure 23)*. Additionally, dysgeusia or ageusia *i.e.* disturbance or loss of taste will normally not be found after lesions of the area of the postcentral gyrus representing the face and the intraoral cavity (Foerster, 1936). One reason for this may be the anatomical complexity of afferents involved in taste discrimination coming from the VIIth, the VIIIth and the Xth cranial nerve.

Other responses: Other clinical responses that have been evoked by insular cortical stimulation are auditory sensations in the posterior insula close to the gyrus of Heschl, dysarthric speech, sensation of unreality, vestibular responses and psychical illusions. Even though these responses were partially reproduced in independent studies their low frequency does not allow clear conclusions regarding their cortical representation. This is also due to the fact that all results on insular stimulation in humans stem from presurgical or intraoperative management of patients with epilepsy. Additionally, not all studies could exclude the occurrence of afterdischarges during stimulation. Subsequently, a subgroup of the reported clinical responses of insular stimulation may indeed represent activation of physiological or pathological neuronal networks or even distant cortical sites.

Nevertheless, in general the results of different groups obtained with different techniques of cortical stimulation can be regarded as comparably solid. However, despite the various functional representations in the insula as demonstrated by electrocortical stimulation results from the few reports of insular lobectomy or partial insula excision report that patients post-surgically do not necessarily exhibit clear neurological deficits (Penfield & Faulk, 1955; von Lehe *et al.*, 2009). On the one hand, very specialized testing may be required to detect deficits occurring after insular resections. A lack of postsurgical dysfunctions may on the other hand argue for secondary or tertiary processing in the insula and a mainly integrative function of that cortex.

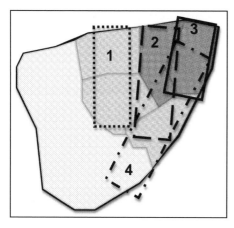

Figure 23. Lateral aspect of the insula lobe. The approximate locations of four different functional zones in the posterior and middle insular areas are indicated by four numbered rectangular fields displayed on a scheme of the insula. 1: gustation, 2: viscerosensation, 3: thermosensation and nociception, 4: somatosensation. Referring to Isnard *et al.* (2004), Mazzola *et al.* (2009) and own results.

The insula is almost solely accessible for electrocortical stimulation with depth electrodes. Due to the complexity of its anatomy and the implantation of such electrodes the data on insula function based on electrical stimulation are scarce. The majority of symptoms obtained by electrocortical stimulation of the insula can either be classified as somatosensory or viscerosensory responses. Special sensations as warmth and pain or taste are evoked less frequently but constantly and may have a primary representation in the insula.

References

- Abboud H, Berroir S, Labreuche J, Orjuela K, Amarenco P. Insular involvement in brain infarction increases risk for cardiac arrhythmia and death. *Ann Neurol* 2006; 59: 691-9.
- Adrian ED. Afferent areas in the brain of ungulates. *Brain* 1943; 66: 89-103.
- Amunts K, Schleicher A, Bürgel U, Mohlberg H, Uylings HBM, Zilles K. Broca's region revisited: Cytoarchitecture and intersubject variability. *J Comp Neurol* 1999; 412: 319-41.
- Asanuma H, Sakata H. Functional organization of a cortical efferent system examined with focal depth stimulation in cats. *J Neurophysiol* 1967; 30: 35-54.
- Babkin BP, Speakman TJ. Cortical inhibition of gastric motility. *J Neurophysiol* 1950; 13 (1): 55-63.
- Babkin BP, Van Buren JM. Mechanism and cortical representation of the feeding pattern. *Arch Neurol Psychiat* 1951; 66: 1-19.
- Bailey P, von Bonin G. *The isocortex of man*. Urbana: University of Illinois Press, 1951, 301 p.
- Bak M, Girvin JP, Hambrecht FT, Kufta CV, Loeb GE, Schmidt EM. Visual sensations produced by intracortical microstimulation of the human occipital cortex. *Med Biol Eng Comput* 1990; 28: 257-9.
- Bartholow R. Experimental investigations into the functions of the human brain. *Am J Med Sci* 1874; 67: 305-13.
- Barry FE, Walter MS, Gallistel CR. On the optimal pulse duration in electrical stimulation of the brain. *Physiol Behav* 1973; 12: 749-54.
- BeMent SL, Ranck JB. A quantitative study of electrical stimulation of central myelinated fibers. *Exp Neurol* 1969; 24: 147-70.
- Borsody M, Gargano JW, Reeves M, Jacobs B. Infarction involving the insula and risk of mortality after stroke. *Cerebrovasc Dis* 2009; 27: 564-71.
- Braendgaard H, Evans SM, Howard CV, Gundersen HJ. The total number of neurons in the human neocortex unbiasedly estimated using optical dissectors. *J Microsc* 1990; 157: 285-304.
- Braitenberg V, Schütz A. *Cortex: Statistics and geometry of neuronal connectivity*. Berlin/Heidelberg: Springer, 1998, 249 p.
- Brewer AA, Liu J, Wade AR, Wandell BA. Visual field maps and stimulus selectivity in human ventral occipital cortex. *Nature Neurosci* 2005; 8 (8): 1102-9.
- Brindley GS. Effects of electrical stimulation of the visual cortex. *Hum Neurobiol* 1982; 1: 281-3.
- Brindley GS, Lewin WS. The sensations produced by electrical stimulation of the visual cortex. *J Physiol* 1968; 196: 479-93.
- Broca P. Sur le siège de la faculté du langage articulé. *Bull Soc d'Antrophol Paris* 1865; 6: 377-93.
- Brodmann K. *Vergleichende Lokalisationslehre der Großhirnrinde des Menschen*. Leipzig: Barth JA, 1909, 324 p.
- Bullier J, Gerard P, Salin P-A. The role of area 17 in the transfer of information to extrastriate visual cortex. In: Peters A, Rockland KS, eds. *Cerebral Cortex – Volume 10 – Primary visual cortex in primates*. New York: Plenum Press, 1994: 301-30.

- Catenoix H, Mauguière F, Guénot M, Ryvlin P, Bissery A, Sindou M, Isnard J. SEEG-guided thermocoagulations – A palliative treatment of nonoperable partial epilepsies. *Neurology* 2008; 71: 1719-26.

- Cechetto DF, Saper CB. Evidence for a viscerotopic sensory representation in the cortex and thalamus in the rat. *J Comp Neurol* 1987; 262: 27-45.

- Clark DL, Butler RA, Rosner BS. Dissociation of sensation and evoked responses by a general anesthetic in man. *J Comp Physiol Psychol* 1969; 68: 315-9.

- Coq J-O, Qi H, Collins CE, Kaas JH. Anatomical and functional organization of somatosensory areas of the lateral fissure of the new world Titi monkey *(callicebus moloch)*. *J Comp Neurol* 2004; 476: 363-87.

- Cragg BG. The density of synapses and neurons in the motor and visual areas of the cerebral cortex. *J Anat* 1967; 101: 639-54.

- Creutzfeldt OD. *Cortex Cerebri*. Berlin; Heidelberg; New York; Tokyo: Springer-Verlag, 1983, 484 p.

- Curtis DR, Eccles JC. Synaptic action during and after repetitive stimulation. *J Physiol* 1960; 150: 374-98.

- Cushing H. A note upon the faradic stimulation of the postcentral gyrus in conscious patients. *Brain* 1909; 32: 44-53.

- Delgado JMR. Depth stimulation of the brain. In: Patterson MM, Kesner RP, eds. *Electrical stimulation research techniques*. London: Academic Press, 1981: 105-40.

- Delgado JMR, Degado-Garcia JM, Conde M, Robles SS. Fatigability of caudate nucleus stimulation in cats. *Neuropsychologia* 1976; 14: 11-21.

- Desmurget M, Reilly KT, Richard N, Szqthmari A, Mottolese C, Sirigu A. Movement intention after parietal cortex stimulation in humans. *Science* 2009; 324: 811-3.

- Dinner DS, Lüders HO. Cortical mapping by electrical stimulation of subdural electrodes: supplementary sensorimotor area in humans. In: Lüders HO, ed. *Epilepsy surgery*. London: Informa healthcare, 2008: 991-1000.

- Disbrow EA, Litinas E, Recanzone GH, Padberg J, Krubitzer L. Cortical connections of the second somatosensroy area and the parietal ventral area in macaque monkeys. *J Comp Neurol* 2003; 462: 382-99.

- Disbrow EA, Hinkley LBN, Roberts TPL. Ipsilateral representation of oral structures in human anterior parietal somatosensory cortex and integration of inputs across the midline. *J Comp Neurol* 2003; 467: 487-95.

- Dobelle WH, Turkel J, Henderson DC, Evans JR. Mapping the representation of the visual field by electrical stimulation of humans visual cortex. *Am J Ophthalmol* 1979; 88 (4): 727-35.

- Eickhoff SB, Schleicher A, Zilles K, Amunts K. The human parietal operculum. I. Cytoarchitectonic mapping of subdivisions. *Cereb Cortex* 2006; 16: 254-67.

- Eickhoff SB, Grefkes C, Zilles K, Fink G. The somatotopic organization of cytoarchitectonic areas on the human parietal operculum. *Cereb Cortex* 2007; 17: 1800-11.

- Fink GR, Frackowiak RS, Pietrzyk U, Passingham RE. Multiple nonprimary motor areas in the human cortex. *J Neurophysiol* 1997; 77: 2164-74.

- Fischer G, Sayre GP, Bickford RG. Histologic changes in the cat's brain after introduction of metallic or plastic coated wire used in electroencephalography. *Mayo Clinic Proc* 1957; 32: 14-22.

- Foerster O. Beiträge zur Pathophysiologie der Sehbahn und der Sehsphäre. *J Psychol Neurol* 1929; 39: 463-85.

- Foerster O. Motorische Felder und Bahnen. In: Bumke O, Foerster O, eds. *Handbuch der Neurologie*. Berlin: Springer, 1936: 1-440.

- Fountas KN, Smith JR. Subdural electrode-associated complications: A 20-year experience. *Stereotact Funct Neurosurg* 2007; 85: 264-72.

- Fried I, Katz A, McCarthy G, Sass KJ, Williamson P, Spencer S, Spencer DD. Functional organization of human supplementary motor cortex studied by electrical stimulation. *J Neurosci* 1991; 11 (11): 3656-66.
- Fried I, Mateer C, Ojemann G, Wohns R, Fedio P. Organization of visuospatial functions in human cortex – evidence from electrical stimulation. *Brain* 1982; 105: 349-71.
- Fritsch G, Hitzig E. Über die elektrische Erregbnarkeit des Grosshirns. *Arch Anat Physiol Wiss Med* 1870; 30: 300-32.
- Gallistel CR. Subcortical stimulation for motivation and reinforcement. In: Patterson MM, Kesner RP, eds. *Electrical stimulation research techniques*. London: Academic Press, 1981: 141-71.
- Geyer S, Ledberg A, Schleicher A, Kinomura S, Schormann T, Bürgel U, Klingberg T, Larsson J, Zilles K, Roland PE. Two different areas within the primary motor cortex of man. *Nature* 1996; 382: 805-7.
- Godoy J, Lüders H, Dinner DS, Morris HH, Wyllie E. Versive eye movements elicited by cortical stimulation of the humane brain. *Neurology* 1990; 40: 296-9.
- Gray EG. Electron microscopy of synaptic contacts on dendrite spines of the cerebral cortex. *Nature* 1959; 183: 1592-3.
- Grefkes C, Fink GR. The functional organization of the intraparietal sulcus in humans and monkeys. *J Anatomy* 2005; 207: 3-17.
- Grefkes C, Fink GR. Somatosensorisches System. In: Schneider F, Fink GR, eds. *Funktionelle MRT in Psychiatrie und Neurologie*. Berlin: Springer, 2006: 280-96.
- Gregoriou GA, Borra E, Matelli M, Luppino G. Architectonic organization of the inferior parietal convexity of the macaque monkey. *J Comp Neurol* 2006; 496: 422-51.
- Gulyás B. Functional organization of human visual cortical areas. In: Rockland KS, Kaas JH, Peters A, eds. *Cerebral Cortex – Volume 12 – Extrastriate cortex in primates*. New York: Plenum Press, 1998: 743-75.
- Hadjikhani N, Liu AK, Dale AM, Cavanagh P, Tootell RBH. Retinotopy and color sensitivity in human visual cortical areas V8. *Nature Neurosci* 1998; 1 (3): 235-41.
- Hamer HM, Lüders HO, Knake S, Fritsch B, Oertel WH, Rosenow F. Electrophysiology of focal clonic seizured in humans: a study using subdural and depth electrodes. *Brain* 2003; 126: 547-55.
- Hamer HM, Lüders HO, Rosenow F, Najm I. Focal clonus elicited by electrical stimulation of the motor cortex in humans. *Epilepsy Res* 2002; 51: 155-66.
- Hamer HM, Morris HH, Mascha EJ, Karafa MT, Bingaman WE, Bej MD, Burgess RC, Dinner DS, Foldvary NR, Hahn JF, Kotagal P, Najm I, Wyllie E, Lüders HO. Complications of invasive video-EEG monitoring with subdural grid electrodes. *Neurology* 2002; 58: 97-103.
- Harnack D, Winter C, Meissner W, Reum T, Kupsch A, Morgenstern R. The effects of electrode material, charge density and stimulation duration on the safety of high-frequency stimulation of the subthalamic nucleus in rats. *J Neurosci Methods* 2004; 138: 207-16.
- Hern JEC, Landgren S, Phillips CG, Porter R. Selective excitation of corticofugal neurons by surface-anodal stimulation of the baboon's motor cortex. *J Physiol* 1962; 161: 73-90.
- Hess A, Young JZ. Correlation of intermodal length and fibre diameter in the central nervous system. *Nature* 1949; 164: 490-1.
- Hoffman BL, Rasmussen T. Stimulation studies of insular cortex of *Macaca Mulatta*. *J Neurophysiol* 1953; 15: 343-51.
- Holmes G. Disturbances of vision by cerebral lesions. *Br J Ophthal* 1918; 2: 353-84.
- Hughlings-Jackson J. On right or left-sided spasm at the onset of epileptic paroxysms, and on crude sensation warnings, and elaborate mental states. *Brain* 1880; 3 (2): 192-206.
- Hursh JB. Conduction velocity and diameter of nerve fibers. *Am J Physiol* 1939; 127: 131-9.
- Isnard J, Guénot M, Sindou M, Mauguière F. Clinical manifestations of insular lobe seizures-a stereo-electroencephalography study. *Epilepsia* 2004; 45: 1079-90.

- Jankowska E, Roberts WJ. An electrophysiological demonstration of the axonal projections of single spinal interneurones in the cat. *J Physiol* 1972; 222: 597-622.
- Kahane P, Hoffmann D, Minotti L, Berthoz A. Reappraisal of the human vestibular cortex by cortical electrical stimulation study. *Ann Neurol* 2003; 54: 616-24.
- Kleinman JT, Sepkuty JP, Hillis AE, Lenz FA, Heidler-Gary J, Gingis L, Crone NE. Spatial neglect during electrocortical stimulation mapping in the right hemisphere. *Epilepsia* 2007; 48 (12): 2365-58.
- Kleist K. *Gehirnpathologie: vornehmlich auf Grund der Kriegserfahrungen*. Leipzig: Barth, 1934: 344-1408.
- Krause F. *Chirurgie des Gehirns und Rückenmarks nach eigenen Erfahrungen, vol 11, Band 2*. Berlin: Urban und Schwarzenberg, 1911: 178-828.
- Krause F, Schum H. Die epileptischen Erkrankungen, ihre anatomische und physiologische Unterlagen sowie ihre chirurgische Behandlung. In: *Die spezielle Chirurgie der Gehirnkrankheiten: 3 Bände/II. Band*. Stuttgart: Enke, 1931: 427-91.
- Kurth F, Eickhoff SB, Schleicher A, Hoemke L, Zilles K, Amunts K. Cytoarchitecture and probabilistic maps of the human posterior insular cortex. *Cereb Cortex* 2010; 20: 1448-61.
- Lavidor M, Walsh V. The nature of foveal representation. *Nature Rev Neurosci* 2004; 5: 729-35.
- Lee HW, Hong SB, Seo DW, Tae WS, Hong SC. Mapping of functional organization in human visual cortex: Electrical cortical stimulation. *Neurology* 2000; 54 (4): 849-54.
- Leyton ASF, Sherrington CS. Observations on the excitable cortex of the chimpanzee, orang-utan, and gorilla. *Q J Exp Physiol* 1917; 11: 135-222.
- Von Lehe M, Wellmer J, Urbach H, Schramm J, Elger CE, Clusmann H. Insular lesionectomy for refractory epilepsy: management and outcome. *Brain* 2009; 132: 1048-56.
- Libet B. Electrical stimulation of cortex in human subjects, and conscious sensory aspects. In: Iggo A, ed. *Handbook of sensory physiology Vol. II. Somatosensory system*. Berlin-Heidelberg: Springer, 1973: 744-90.
- Libet B, Alberts WW, Wright EW, Delattre LD, Levin G, Feinstein B. Production of threshold levels of conscious sensation by electrical stimulation of human somatosensory cortex. *J Neurophysiol* 1964; 27: 546-78.
- Libet B, Alberts WW, Wright EW, Feinstein B. Responses of human somatosensory cortex to stimuli below threshold for conscious sensation. *Science* 1967; 158: 1597-600.
- Lilly JC, Austin GM, Chambers WW. Threshold movements produced by excitation of cerebral cortex and efferent fibers with some parametric regions of rectangular current pulses (cats and monkeys). *J Neurophysiol* 1952; 15: 319-41.
- Lilly JC, Hughes JR, Alvord EC, Galkin TW. Brief, noninjurious electric waveform for stimulation of the brain. *Science* 1955; 121: 468-9.
- Lim SH, Dinner DS, Pillay PK, Lüders H, Morris HH, Klem G, et al. Functional anatomy of the human supplementary sensorimotor area: results of extraoperative electrical stimulation. *Electroencephal Clin Neurophysiol* 1994; 91: 179-93.
- Livingston RB. Ispilaterale und kontralaterale Augenbewegungen nach elektrischer Reizung des frontalen oculomotischen Gebietes des Affen. *Arch Psych Ztschr Neurol* 1950; 185: 690-700.
- Lüders H, Lesser RP, Dinner DS, Hahn JF, Salanga V, Morris HH. The second sensory area in humans: evoked potential and electrical stimulation studies. *Ann Neurol* 1985; 17 (2): 177-84.
- Lüders H, Lesser RP, Dinner DS, Morris HH, Wyllie E, Godoy J. Localization of cortical function: New information from extraoperative monitoring of patients with epilepsy. *Epilepsia* 1988; 29 (S2): 56-65.
- Lüders H, Lesser RP, Hahn J, Dinner DS, Morris HH, Wyllie E, Godoy J. Basal temporal language area. *Brain* 1991; 114: 743-54.

- Luppino G, Matelli M, Camarda R, Rizzolatti G. Corticocortical connections of area F3 (SMA-Proper) and areas F6 (Pre-SMA) in the macaque monkey. *J Comp Neurol* 1993; 338: 114-40.
- MacIntyre WJ, Bidder TG, Rowland V. The production of brain lesions with electric currents. *Proc Nat Biophys Conf.* 1st 1957 (published 1959): 723-32.
- Macpherson JM, Marangoz C, Miles TS, Wiesendanger M. Microstimulation of the supplementary motor area (SMA) in the awake monkey. *Exp Brain Res* 1982; 45: 410-6.
- Matelli M, Luppino G, Rizzolatti G. Architecture of superior and mesial area 6 and the adjacent cingulate cortex in the macaque monkey. *J Comp Neurol* 1991; 311: 445-62.
- Mazzola L, Isnard J, Peyron R, Guénot M, Mauguière F. Somatotopic organization of pain responses to direct electrical stimulation of the human insular cortex. *Pain* 2009; 146: 99-104.
- Mesulam MM and Mufson EJ. Insula of the old world monkey. I: Architectonics in the insulo-orbito-temporal component of the paralimbic brain. *J Comp Neurology* 1982; 212: 1-22.
- Mihailovic L, Delgado JMR. Electrical stimulation of monkey brain with various frequencies and pulse durations. *J Neurophysiol* 1956; 19 (1): 21-36.
- Mikuni N, Ohara S, Ikeda A, Hayashi N, Nishida N, Taki J, Enatsu R, Matsumoto R, Shibasaki H, Hashimoto N. Evidence for a wide distribution of negative motor areas in the perirolandic cortex. *Clin Neurophysiol* 2006; 117: 33-40.
- Morecraft RJ, Van Hoesen GW. Convergence of limbic input to the cingulate motor cortex in the rhesus monkey. *Brain Res Bull* 1998; 45 (2): 209-32.
- Mufson EJ and Mesulam MM. Insula of the old world monkey. II. Afferents cortical input and comments on the claustrum. *J Comp Neurol* 1982; 212: 23-37.
- Nair DR, Burgess R, McIntyre CC, Lüders H. Chronic subdural electrodes in the management of epilepsy. *Clin Neurophyiol* 2008; 119: 11-28.
- Nathan SS, Sinha SR, Gordon B, Lesser RP, Thakor NV. Determination of current density distributions generated by electrical stimulation of the human cerebral cortex. *Electroenceph Clin Neurophysiol* 1993; 86: 183-92.
- Nguyen DK, Nguyen DB, Malak R, Leroux JM, Carmant L, Saint-Hilaire JM, Giard N, Cossette P, Bouthillier A. Revisiting the role of the insula in refractory partial epilepsy. *Epilepsia* 2009; 50 (3): 510-20.
- Nieuwenhuys R, Voogd J, van Huijzen C. Synopsis of main neocortical regions. In: Nieuwenhuys R, Voogd J, van Huijzen C, eds. *The human central nervous system, 4th edition.* Berlin, Heidelberg: Springer, 2008: 592-649.
- Noachtar S, Lüders HO. Focal akinetic seizures as documented by electroencephalography and video recordings. *Neurology* 1999; 53 (2): 427-9.
- Nowak LG, Bullier J. Axons, but not cell bodies are activated by electrical stimulation in cortical gray matter. I. Evidence from chronaxie measurements. *Exp Brain Res* 1998; 118: 477-88.
- Öngür D, Ferry AR, Price JL. Architectonic subdivision of the human orbital and medial prefrontal cortex. *J Comp Neurol* 2003; 460: 425-49.
- Oppenheimer SM, Cechetto DF. Cardiac chronotropic organization of the rat insular cortex. *Brain Res* 1990; 533: 66-72.
- Oppenheimer SM, Gelb A, Girvin JP, Hachinski VC. Cardiovascular effects of human insular cortex stimulation. *Neurology* 1992; 42 (9): 1727-32.
- Ostrowsky K, Isnard J, Ryvlin P, Guénot M, Fischer C, Mauguière F. Functional mapping of the insular cortex: Clinical implications in temporal lobe epilepsy. *Epilepsia* 2000; 41 (6): 681-6.
- Penfield W, Boldrey E. Somatic motor and sensory representation in the cerebral cortex of man as studied by electrical stimulation. *Brain* 1937; 60 (4): 389-443.
- Penfield W, Faulk ME. The insula-further observations on its function. *Brain* 1955; 78: 445-70.
- Penfield W, Rasmussen T. Vocalization and arrest of speech. *Arch Neurol Psychiatry* 1949; 61: 21-7.

- Penfield W, Rasmussen T. *The cerebral cortex of man: a clinical study of localization of function.* New York: MacMilian, 1950, 248 p.
- Penfield W, Roberts L. *Speech and Brain Mechanisms.* Princeton, New Jersey: Princeton University Press, 1959, 286 p.
- Penfield W, Welch K. The supplementary motor area of the cerebral cortex. *Arch Neurol Psychiatry* 1951; 66: 289-317.
- Petrides M, Pandya DN. Dorsolateral prefrontal cortex: comparative cytoarchitectonic analysis in the human and the macaque brain and corticocortical connection patterns. *Eur J Neurosci* 1999; 11: 1011-36.
- Phillips CG. Cortical motor threshold and the thresholds and distribution of excited Betz cells in the cat. *Quart J Exp Physiol* 1956; 41: 70-84.
- Piallat B, Chabardès S, Devergnas A, Allain M, Barrat E, Bernabid AL. Monophaisc but not biphasic pulses induce brian tissue damage during monopolar high-frequency deep brain stimulation. *Neurosurg* 2009; 64: 156-63.
- Pilitsis JG, Chu Y, Kordower J, Bergen DC, Cochran EJ, Bakay RAE. Postmortem study of deep brain stimulation of the anterior thalamus: case report. *Neurosurg* 2008; 62: 530-2.
- Ranck JB. Which elements are excited in electrical stimulation of mammalian central nervous system: A review. *Brain Res* 1975; 98: 417-40.
- Ranck JB. Extracellular stimulation. In: Patterson MM, Kesner RP, eds. *Electrical Stimulation Research Techniques.* London: Academic Press, 1981: 1-36.
- Reil JC. Die sylvische Grube. *Arch Physiol* (Halle) 1809; 9: 195-208.
- Rosano C, Sweeney JA, Melchitzky DS, Lewis DA. The human precentral sulcus: Chemoarchitecture of a region corresponding to the frontal eye fields. *Brain Res* 2003; 972: 16-30.
- Ross DA, Brunberg JA, Drury I, Henry TR. Intracerebral depth electrode monitoring in partial epilepsy: the morbidity and efficacy of placement using magnetic resonance image-guided stereotactic surgery. *Neurosurg* 1996; 39 (2): 327-33.
- Rudin DO, Eisenman G. The action potential of spinal axons *in vitro. J Gen Physiol* 1954; 37: 505-38.
- Salanova V, Andermann F, Olivier A, Rasmussen T, Quesney LF. Occipital lobe epilepsy: electroclinical manifestations, electrocorticography, cortical stimulation and outcome in 42 patients treated between 1930 and 1991. *Brain* 1992; 115: 1655-80.
- Sanes JN, Donoghue JP. Static and dynamic organization of motor cortex. *Adv Neurol* 1997; 73: 277-96.
- Schlag J, Schlag-Rey M. Evidence for a supplementary eye field. *J Neurophysiol* 1987; 57 (1): 179-200.
- Schütz A, Palm G. Density of neurons in the cerebral cortex of the mouse. *J Comp Neurol* 1989; 286: 442-55.
- Smyth P. Cortical mapping by electrical stimulation of sudural electrodes: negative motor areas. In: Lüders HO, ed. *Epilepsy Surgery.* London: Informa healthcare, 2008: 983-90.
- Stensaas SS, Stensaas LJ. Histopathological evaluation of materials implanted in the cerebral cortex. *Acta Neuropath* 1978; 41: 145-55.
- Stoney SD, Thompson WD, Asanuma H. Excitation of pyramidal tract cells by intracortical microstimulation: effective extent of stimulating current. *J Neurophysiol* 1968; 31: 659-69.
- Tandon N. Cortical mapping by electrical stimulation of subdural electrodes: language areas. In: Lüders HO, ed. *Epilepsy Surgery.* London: Informa healthcare, 2008: 1001-15.
- Tehovnik EJ, Sommer MA, Chou I-H, Slocum WM, Schiller PH. Eye fields in the frontal lobes of primates. *Brain Res Rev* 2000; 32: 413-48.
- Tehovnik EJ, Slocum WM. Behavioural state affects saccades elicited electrically from neocortex. *Neurosci Biobehav Rev* 2004; 28: 13-25.

- Thurtell MJ, Mohamed A, Lüders HO, Leigh RJ. Evidence for three-dimensional cortical control of gaze from epileptic patients. *J Neurol Neurosurg Psychiat* 2009; 80: 683-5.
- Tower SS. Pyramidal lesion in the monkey. *Brain* 1940; 63: 36-90.
- Von Economo C, Koskinas GN. *Die Cytoarchitektonik der Hirnrinde des erwachsenen Menschen*. Berlin: Springer, 1925, 810 p.
- Uchizono J. Characteristics of excitatory and inhibitory synapses in the central nervous system of the cat. *Nature* 1965; 207: 642-3.
- Villani F, D'Amico D, Pincherle A, Tullo V, Chiapparini L, Bussone G. Prolonged focal negative motor seizures: A video-EEG study. *Epilepsia* 2006; 47 (11): 1949-52.
- Vogt C, Vogt O. Die physiologische Bedeutung der architektonischen Rindenfelderung auf Grund neuer Rindenreizungen. *J Psychol Neurol* 1919; 25: 399-461.
- Vogt C, Vogt O. Gestaltung der topistischen Hirnforschung und ihre Förderung durch den Hirnbau und seine Anomalien. *J Hirnforschung* 1954; 1: 1-46.
- Walker EA. A cytoarchitectural study of the prefrontal area of the macaque monkey. *J Comp Neurol* 1940; 73: 59-86.
- Weil A, Lassek A. The quantitative distribution of the pyramidal tract in man. *Arch Neurol Psychiat* 1929; 22: 495-510.
- Wellmer J, Weber C, Mende M, von der Groeben F, Urbach H, Clusmann H, Elger CE, Helmstaedter C. Multitask electrical stimulation for cortical language mapping: Hints for necessity and economic mode of application. *Epilepsia* 2009; 50 (10): 2267-75.
- Wetzel MC, Howell LG, Bearie KJ. Experimental performance of steel and platinum electrodes with chronic monophasic stimulation of the brain. *J Neurosurg* 1969; 31: 658-69.
- White EL. Terminations of thalamic afferents. In: Jones EG, Peters A, eds. *Cerebral cortex, vol. 5. Sensory-motor areas and aspects of cortical connectivity*. New York: Plenum, 1986: 271-89.
- Woolsey CN, Settlage PH, Meyer DR, Sencer W, Pinot Hamuy T, Travis AM. Patterns of localization in precentral and "supplementary" motor areas and their relation to the concept o a premotor area. *Res Publ Assoc Nerv Ment Dis* 1952; 30: 238-64.
- Zeki S. The representation of colours in the cerebral cortex. *Nature* 1980; 284: 412-8.
- Zilles K, Amunts K. Receptor mapping: architecture of the human cerebral cortex. *Curr Op Neurol* 2009; 2: 331-9.
- Zilles K, Amunts K. Centenary of Brodmann's map – conception and fate. *Nature Rev Neurosci* 2010; 11 (2): 139-45.
- Zilles K, Palomero-Gallagher N. Cyto-, myelo-, and receptor architectonics of the human parietal cortex. *Neuroimage* 2001; 14 S8-S20.
- Zilles K, Schlaug G, Matelli M, Luppino G, Schleicher A, Qü M, Dabringhaus A, Seitz R, Roland PE. Mapping of human and macaque sensorimotor areas by integrating architectonic, transmitter receptor, MRI and PET data. *J Anat* 1995; 187: 515-37.

Cortico-cortical evoked potentials in extratemporal lobe epilepsy

Mohamad Koubeissi, Michael Zell

The Neurological Institute, Department of Neurology,
University Hospital Case Medical Center, Cleveland, USA

■ Introduction

Determining candidacy for extratemporal lobe epilepsy (ETLE) surgery is often challenging, and identification of the seizure focus and eloquent cortex frequently necessitates intracranial monitoring. Disclosing pathways of seizure propagation, largely part of the symptomatogenic zone, is crucial for understanding seizure semiology. The distinction between seizure onset and seizure propagation regions can lead to limited resection of the seizure onset zone rather than seizure propagation regions. Such distinction can be facilitated by studying brain connectivity.

Understanding brain connectivity in ETLE surgery is also important in terms of identifying eloquent cortical areas. Higher cortical processing of certain functions, such as language, takes place in noncontiguous cortical regions. For methodologic reasons, three types of connectivity among spatially segregated regions of the brain have been investigated. These are anatomical, functional, and effective connectivity. A proper understanding of each type and its associated limitations is essential for a obtaining a better understanding of brain connectivity.

Anatomical connectivity refers to actual anatomical links between two areas of the brain. This can be studied using tract-tracing methods post-mortem, or by diffusion tensor imaging (DTI) studies, a common method for exploring anatomical connectivity *in vivo*. DTI can reveal similarly-oriented fibers without reliable identification of the effective connections between two brain areas (Catani *et al.*, 2002). Because many neuroscientific investigations are more concerned with the brain's response to stimuli than with the physical characteristics of neurons, anatomical connections provide limited insight on their own, although they may implicate function (Lee *et al.*, 2003).

A better understanding of the relationships between brain regions can be gained by studying functional connectivity, defined as "the temporal correlations between spatially remote neurophysiological events" (Friston, 1993), and effective connectivity, defined as "the influence that one neural system exerts over another either directly or indirectly" (Friston *et al.*, 1993). While functional connectivity identifies areas that demonstrate similar behavior or statistical interdependence and refers to patterns observed in neural activity, effective connectivity offers insight into a possible explanation of their origins. Effective connectivity characterizes brain activity in relation to a causal or acausal model; that is, whether noncontiguous brain regions affect a change in each other or not (Lee *et al.*, 2003). This model, constrained by a combination of neuroanatomical, neurophysiological, and functional neuroimaging data, represents the most recent iteration of a general trend from merely describing what the brain does to a theory of how it does it.

Effective connectivity is studied through two general approaches. The first, based on the principle of temporal precedence, infers that two areas, A and B, may share an effective connection if an activity in A occurs consistently and reliably before activity in B. The second method relies on perturbing the system and observing the resulting activity. This method affords two primary advantages over studying temporal precedence in that it allows manipulation and subsequent observation to be conducted under explicit experimental control, and that it allows for the stimulation of a relatively small focus of the brain, allowing the assessment of the interaction between a specific area and other unperturbed areas.

Recording cortico-cortical evoked potentials (CCEPs) studies fall into effective connectivity research. Combining the observations from CCEP study with brain imaging obtained through PET and fMRI can provide a better understanding of functional integration of the brain. CCEP investigations can have results that are far-reaching, but in particular can help shed light on the mechanism and processing of complex neurological activity, identify functional areas that have reorganized outside of their expected locations, inform surgical decisions in epilepsy patients with secondary epileptic foci, and possibly aid in predicting postoperative outcomes following resective surgery (Koubeissi *et al.*, in submission).

■ Technical aspects of CCEPs

In order to separate an evoked response from the normal background activity at an electrode, a large number of stimulus trials are typically averaged using specialized computer software. The exact number of trials necessary to minimize background activity has fluctuated in various papers, but it is generally agreed that the number of trials should be sufficient to reduce the background activity to as close to zero potential as possible. This is based on a central understanding of EEG recordings that over enough time, the average electrical potential at a given point will be zero. That is, it is equally likely to observe a positive deflection as a negative one, and given a high enough sample, the average activity will reduce to zero.

In studying CCEPs, most investigators have solely relied on visual analysis to identify and describe evoke potential signals. Methods for visual evaluation have been largely standardized to ensure a consistent methodology across studies, but this approach necessarily restricts the results and introduces a certain level of subjectivity to the analysis. In particular, given the vast number of potential inter-areal connections in the human brain, a visual approach limits the breadth of analysis by the time and availability of properly trained investigators. Additionally, by necessitating visual evaluation, this method relies on an element of human error that, given the immensity of the data set, exposes the analysis to a not insignificant degree of error. Until a better and more reliable approach is implemented, however, the standardized visual method will continue to be used that, although limited, has produced meaningful results.

Under the current methodology, the response is visually examined for each connection, and any responses are evaluated individually. The latency of each response is measured from the stimulation artifact to the first peak of the first identifiable deflection. Viewing the response with both a bipolar and a referential montage can increase accuracy and reduce potential interference nearby electrodes. Some studies have been successful using a reference to the average of electrodes in the same strip or bundle to reduce artifact (Lacruz et al., 2007). The amplitude of the initial deflection is measured by first drawing a line connecting the onset to the offset of the peak. The amplitude is then equal to the height of a vertical line from the crest of the waveform to the intersection with the above-described line. Subsequent deflections, when present, are measured from the peak to the preceding trough (Matsumoto et al., 2004).

A recent paper identified a response as significant if the amplitude was at least twice the amplitude of the preceding 400 ms of background activity (Lacruz et al., 2007). Although this approach has proven effective where it has been applied, we do not believe it is statistically robust and merits further consideration. In particular, when a large number of stimulus samples are averaged, the preceding background activity is likely to be at or near zero potential. Consequently, activity that is twice this background activity is likely still an extremely small voltage and therefore may not be statistically significant. Instead, we propose that the standard for inclusion be voltages that lie beyond two standard deviations from the mean background activity. Not only does this represent a more statistically based criterion, but also will produce more accurate results.

Recent studies have analyzed the presence of evoked responses using two similar, but functionally different, statistical methods. One such approach is Fischer's exact test, a statistical approach that is used to compare two categorical variables that result in classifying data in one of two different ways where sample sizes are small. The test is used to examine the significance of the association between the two kinds of classification. In this case, Fischer's exact test is used to compare the presence of responses to stimulation between epileptogenic and non-epileptogenic hemispheres (Lacruz et al., 2007). The method is similar to the chi-square test, though better suited for small sample sizes. Another statistical analysis that has been utilized in recent studies is the paired student's t-test, a two-sample test of the null hypothesis involving both a categorical and a quantitative variable (Koubeissi et al., in submission). In practical terms, this test determines the statistical significance of a signal observed at a given point occurring due to a real phenomenon as opposed to a normal and unremarkable result. In this application, the student's t-test is used to determine whether the latency and amplitude of an observed response is statistically different from what would be expected even in the absence of connectivity.

As our ability to study and measure different aspects of brain activity expands, there is an increasing demand for innovate methods of studying the resulting data. In particular, recent research has focused on ways to develop robust models for explaining the dynamic nature of the brain and the underlying neural connectivity. This approach marks a shift from simply using statistical analysis to describe observations of neural activity to developing models that help predict and explain these observations. These methods model the brain as a set of complex causal functions, the behavior of which is determined by a variety of physiologic parameters or external perturbations (Lee et al., 2003).

Broadly termed "dynamic causal modeling", new research has yielded methodologies such as structural equation modeling (Buechel and Friston, 1997), multivariate autoregressive models, and the Volterra approach (Friston, 2001). In general, these approaches attempt to reduce the highly nonlinear behavior of the brain to a predictable linear problem of estimating outcomes given a set of experimental inputs and measured responses. These methodologies have their shortcomings, however, and tend to be useful when limited to investigating only the outputs that vary with a particular experimental procedure and not from the natural state of the brain. Additionally, this type of analysis is not relevant to a system with noncontrollable dynamic elements that have their own intrinsic activity, such as epileptic foci (Lee *et al.*, 2003).

A current focus of analytical technique centers on the use of time-series. This approach comprises methods of analyzing time series data – a sequence of data points measured at successive, uniform time intervals – in order to extract meaningful statistics and characteristics from an event. Some of these approaches are already in use with EEG/MEG and LFP recordings and are gaining traction in fMRI and PET data analysis. Several techniques within this category are presently being explored. One such approach involves independent component analysis (ICA), a method for separating a single time series from a complex background. This technique identifies the individual activity with the maximum independence from the background activity. Another approach, called hierarchical decomposition, characterizes a "fingerprint" of the underlying activity that is associated with or even may contribute to certain types of seizures. This method involves decomposing the brain activity from a population of seizures across many different patients in order to identify a common signal (Lee *et al.*, 2003).

These types of mathematical approaches to understanding brain activity come with caveats, however. At their core, the methods in this line of study rely on understanding phenomena through a process of reducing the whole to its constituent parts and subsequently building up a mechanistic understanding of each step. This approach ignores the principles of synergy that emerge from self-organizing systems, however. In other words, the dynamic complexity of the human brain may not be explained as simply the sum of its parts; there may be a holistic understanding that differs greatly from a reductionist one (Lee *et al.*, 2003).

Safety

As in any medical research, patient safety in CCEP is of the utmost importance. Consistently and without exception, however, CCEP methodology has been effectively used without compromising patient safety or care. Research has demonstrated that with attention to certain details, CCEP can be a safe procedure to study effective connectivity between regions of the brain in neurosurgery candidates (Brugge *et al.*, 2003).

The most relevant safety concerns center around controlling charge density to avoid damage to the cortical tissue during stimulation. The most direct way to reduce charge density to non-damaging levels is by limiting the amplitude and frequency of the stimulus. Most CCEP studies tie the choice of stimulus intensity to the current safely used during functional mapping. Functional mapping is typically performed at 50 Hz at an intensity that does not produce afterdischarges or clinical signs. Since CCEP is only performed at 1 Hz, exposing the cortical tissue to significantly less charge density over time, it is generally agreed the current intensity used for functional mapping represents a suitable upper limit for safety. Some researchers have selected a CCEP stimulus intensity at 80% of the current used in functional mapping, setting an upper limit at 10-12 mA if no clinical signs or afterdischarges were present at 15 mA standard cortical stimulation for mapping (Matsumoto *et al.*, 2007).

The second way to reduce charge density in cortical tissue is by controlling the way the current is applied. Previous research has typically applied electrical stimulation in a bipolar fashion across a pair of adjacent electrodes. This methodology provides three primary advantages with positive influence on patient safety. First, it reduces stimulus artifact by focusing the stimulation on a narrow focus of tissue as the electrodes are typically less than 1 cm apart (Lacruz *et al.*, 2007). Second, it avoids the buildup of electrical charge that could potentially be harmful to the patient and potentially trigger a seizure by removing the charge quickly with the opposite polarity of the bipolar wave. Finally, this approach minimizes the polarization of the electrodes themselves that could potentially decrease the efficacy over time (Matsumoto *et al.*, 2007). Research has demonstrated that when these considerations are heeded, the safety of patients undergoing CCEP is not a troublesome issue.

Feasibility

Although CCEP investigation is limited to patients undergoing presurgical evaluation for epilepsy surgery and is necessarily restricted by the availability of these patients, the procedure itself has low feasibility requirements. During the recording of CCEPs, the subjects can remain either sitting or lying in a bed, and testing does not require cessation of personal activity such as talking or eating (Matsumoto *et al.*, 2007). Since electrodes and EEG recording are typically already in use for these patients, CCEP testing requires only the addition of a current source. In general, assuming the availability of suitable patients, CCEP testing is a relatively simple procedure to perform.

■ CCEPs and seizure propagation pathways

Identification of the epileptogenic zone, based solely on seizure semiology and non-invasive EEG monitoring, is not straightforward, especially in non-lesional patients. Seizures with identical semiology may originate in different areas of the brain, for they may start in clinically silent cortical regions and secondarily propagate to other areas producing clinical and electrographic manifestations. For example, seizures that originate in the posterior cingulate region may appear identical to temporal lobe seizures semiologically and electrographically (Koubeissi *et al.*, 2009). Similarly, the initial ictal symptoms of non-lesional parietal lobe epilepsy often reflect areas of seizure propagation rather than seizure origin (Cascino *et al.*, 1993), possibly accounting, at least in part, for the surgical failures in non-lesional epilepsy. Extensive implantation of intracranial electrodes is frequently done in patients with discordant or inconclusive findings on non-invasive testing facilitating recording CCEPs (Koubeissi *et al.*, 2010). CCEPs may help reveal the effective connections between brain regions and allow for a better understanding of potential pathways for propagation.

Case study I

A 52 year-old woman began having seizures nine years after a head trauma. MRI showed a region of gliosis and cystic encephalomalacia in the inferior aspect of the right frontal lobe and anterior insula. Video-EEG monitoring with scalp electrodes, however, captured three seizures that were both semiologically and electrographically suggestive of mesial temporal lobe epilepsy. After implantation of depth electrodes, subsequent monitoring revealed three seizures arising from the right orbital frontal lobe with secondary propagation to the mesial temporal structures, and later, to the insula. The patient underwent 1-Hz electrical stimulation of the depth electrodes in the frontal, insular, and temporal regions, and the electrocorticograms (ECoG) was averaged time-locked to the electrical stimuli. CCEPs demonstrated connectivity between her orbitofrontal seizure onset zone and the insula, and between the insula and the anterior hippocampus (*Figure 1A*). No CCEPs were seen in the hippocampus upon stimulating the orbitofrontal seizure onset zone. Resective surgery was performed on the right orbital frontal seizure onset zone, while the mesial temporal structures were left unaltered. The patient remains seizure free one year after the surgery (Karanec *et al.*, 2011).

The difference between the sequence of seizure propagation as seen on the ECoG and connectivity as suggested by CCEPs suggests the possibility that seizure propagation from the orbitofrontal region to the hippocampus occurred via the insula. While the insular ictal discharge on the ECoG was initially too subtle to be recognized, it became clearly discernible after involvement of the hippocampus, possibly a more irritative zone than the insula. A tentative conclusion is that brain regions may serve as stepping stones for seizure propagation before synchronization of their electrical activity results in clear ictal discharges.

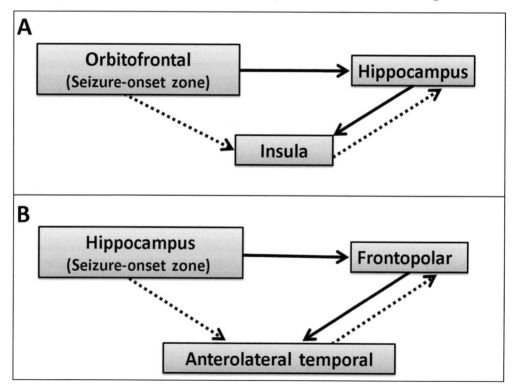

Case study 2

A 24-year-old man has history of meningoencephalitis at age 7 and onset of epilepsy at age 12 with a brain MRI showing left hippocampal atrophy. Video-EEG monitoring with scalp electrodes captured four seizures arising in the left frontopolar region with secondary spread to the left anterior temporal region. Both the EEG findings and the ictal semiology suggested frontopolar epilepsy. After implantation of depth electrodes, his seizure onset zone proved to be the left hippocampal body and head, with secondary spread to the frontopolar region. Concomitant scalp electrode monitoring missed the hippocampal discharge, and showed ictal changes only after propagation to the frontal pole. Similar to Case #1, this patient also underwent 1-Hz stimulation. His CCEPs demonstrated connectivity between the hippocampus and anterolateral temporal cortex, and between the Anterolateral temporal cortex and the frontal pole, but not between the hippocampus and the frontal pole (*Figure 1B*). The patient underwent left temporal lobectomy and remained seizure free at his three-month follow up (Karanec *et al.*, 2011).

In this patient the lateral temporal cortex played a similar role to that played by the insula in Case #1 in that, while it had direct connectivity with the seizure onset zone (by CCEPs), it showed the ictal discharge at a later stage than the, presumably only-indirectly connected, frontal pole. Such conclusions and their clinical value need to be assessed in more patients. Thorough analyses of latencies, morphology, and voltages of CCEPs in light of spontaneous seizure discharges are ongoing to infer better understanding of seizure dynamics.

■ CCEPs and eloquent brain function

Understanding connectivity within eloquent cortical regions may be important to minimize functional deficits in planning resective surgery for intractable ETLE. Both electrophysiologic methods, such as EEG and magnetoencephalography (Bowyer *et al.*, 2005, Crone *et al.*, 1998, Crone *et al.*, 1998, Crone *et al.*, 2001), and functional neuroimaging techniques, such as PET and fMRI (Buchel *et al.*, 1998, Sharp *et al.*, 2004), have shown that language and motor functions invoke neural processes in a number of several spatially separate brain regions. These studies, however, do not explain how these regions are connected. Few studies using CCEPs have helped elucidate these connections and draw inferences regarding the significance and consequence of inter-areal connectivity.

CCEPs in the language system

Matsumoto *et al.* studied connectivity within the language system with CCEPs in eight patients with medically intractable partial epilepsy (Matsumoto *et al.*, 2004). After standard electrocortical mapping of language, the authors stimulated electrodes in language regions by a square wave pulse of 0.3 ms duration at a frequency of 1 Hz and a current 80% of that used for mapping or that caused afterdischarges (Matsumoto *et al.*, 2004). Stimulation at electrodes located within the anterior language area elicited two distinct fields of CCEPs: one at the posterior language area, and another at the frontal operculum. CCEPs consisted of two primary negative potentials, N1 and N2, in 7 of 8 subjects. CCEPs were also observed between the perisylvian and extrasylvian language areas, specifically the basal temporal areas (Matsumoto *et al.*, 2004). Thus, this study recorded inter-areal connections in the human language system using CCEPs, revealing cortico-cortical connections within the perisylvian language area and between the perisylvian and extrasylvian language areas. The investigators postulated that these connections are made through long and short association fibers or through cortico-subcortico-cortical pathways. The connectivity demonstrated by the findings support the contemporary concepts of language organization and processing. Importantly, these findings most likely are consistent within the general human population and represent normal brain function, as the epileptogenic focus in each subject was outside of the perisylvian language area (Matsumoto et al., 2004).

Another CCEP study of the language system aimed at investigating connectivity between the perisylvian cortex and both basal temporal regions. Previous electrocortical stimulation mapping studies have demonstrated that electrical stimulation of the basal temporal language area (BTLA) results in language deficits, ranging from complete expressive, receptive, and repetition deficits at high stimulation frequencies to aphasic symptoms at lower ones (Lüders et al., 1986, Lüders et al., 1991). Research findings have suggested that the role of the BTLA is to match a conceptual entity to its phonographical representation (Lüders et al., 1991, Usui et al., 2003, Usui et al., 2005) and it has been posited that such functionality is bilaterally distributed (Lüders et al., 1991). Although bilateral representation of BTLA functionality has been observed through event-related potentials (Nobre et al., 1994) and functional neuroimaging (Sharp et al., 2004), this study aimed to investigate in vivo connectivity between the perisylvian and bilateral basal temporal areas.

Using a CCEP protocol similar to that of the previously discussed study, patients implanted with subdural electrodes as part of the presurgical evaluation of medically intractable epilepsy underwent CCEP testing to demonstrate connectivity between the posterior language area and ipsilateral basal temporal cortex. Additionally, CCEPs were used to demonstrate connectivity between the left posterior superior temporal gyrus, considered to be a receptive language area, and bilateral basal temporal areas. Like the previous study, stimulation was applied at a rate of 1 Hz, but the intensity was set at a starting current of 2.5 mA and increased in 1 mA increments to a maximum current of 8.5 mA (Koubeissi et al., in submission). Similar to the Matsumoto et al. study (2004), single-pulse electrical stimulation of electrodes located in the posterior language area resulted in a CCEP field in the anterior language area, and one in the ipsilateral basal temporal cortex. As compared to the anterior language area, the CCEPs in the basal temporal cortex were of a longer latency, but of similar morphology and voltage. In both areas, the CCEPs were captured focally over one or two electrodes with a voltage drop of over 50% in neighboring electrodes, suggesting the presence of a real, and not artifactual, response (Koubeissi et al., in submission). CCEPs were also recorded between the left posterior superior temporal gyrus and bilateral basal temporal areas. Single-pulse stimulation of the left posterior superior temporal gyrus produced CCEPs in both basal temporal cortices in three of the four patients and CCEPs in the left posterior inferior frontal gyrus in two of four patients. The CCEPs observed over both basal temporal regions displayed similar morphology in the same subject and were recorded focally over a single electrode. Importantly, the response in the basal temporal region was observed only focally over the fusiform gyrus (Koubeissi et al., in submission).

The results of this study provided direct support for a link between higher order visual and auditory areas through substantial connectivity between the basal temporal cortex and the posterior language area. Additionally, the study provides evidence for two-way connectivity between the left perisylvian area and bilateral basal temporal cortices, supporting the view that the role of the basal temporal cortex in linking visual semantic knowledge with phonological representation is bilaterally represented (Koubeissi *et al.*, in submission).

CCEPs in the motor system

The motor system is another functional network that has been investigated by CCEPs. Like in the language system, CCEP studies of the motor system have aimed to connect the observations from neuroimaging and functional output to better understand the connections between the spatially separate regions involved in motor function. A better understanding of connectivity has far-reaching implications, but there exists a clear application to the study of epilepsy by shedding valuable light on the pathophysiology of seizure motor semiology and the tendency for the rapid spread of epileptic discharges throughout the motor region. Practically, it is thought that a better understanding of how discharges spread throughout motor areas could play a role in improving the relatively poor outcomes associated with epilepsy surgery in patients with frontal lobe epilepsy.

In a recent study, seven patients with implanted subdural electrodes for the presurgical evaluation of epilepsy were tested with CCEPs to investigate the *in vivo* effective connectivity between the lateral motor cortex and the medial motor cortex (Matsumoto *et al.*, 2007). The CCEP protocol was consistent with the aforementioned studies with the current set at 80-100% of the intensity that produced either clinical signs or afterdischarges during electrocortical stimulation mapping at 50 Hz. If no clinical signs or afterdischarges were observed at 15 mA during functional mapping, then the intensity was set at 10-12 mA for the CCEP analysis (Matsumoto *et al.*, 2007). To study connectivity between the lateral and medial motor cortices, each of the two locations served as both stimulation and observation sites. Subsequent to testing at both locations, the electrodes in the lateral cortex that showed the highest amplitude response from stimulation of the medial cortex were themselves stimulated in order to test for reciprocal connections (Matsumoto *et al.*, 2007).

The results supported evidence for interconnectivity between the medial and lateral motor cortices. Across all subjects, stimulation of the medial motor cortex resulted in a lateral motor cortex CCEPs. Similar results were observed from stimulation of the lateral motor cortex, where CCEPs in the medial motor cortex were also observed in all of the patients tested. Importantly, there was an observed shift in the CCEP distribution as the site of stimulation moved along the rostral-caudal axis. Regression analysis revealed a positive correlation between the sites of stimulation and maximum CCEP response for both stimulation sites, suggesting that along the rostral-caudal axis, anatomically homologous areas of the lateral and medial motor cortices are connected with each other (Matsumoto *et al.*, 2007). The results were interpreted in terms of their functional implications by comparing the sites where CCEPs were elicited with the cortical function of those sites based on earlier functional mapping. In 12 out of the 17 stimulation sites in the medial cortex, the elicited CCEP in the lateral cortex occurred in somatotopically similar locations. In lateral cortex stimulation, 18 out of 22 stimulation sites elicited CCEP fields encompassing homologous motor function in the medial motor cortex. These findings suggest a high degree of functional correlation tied to the location of a stimulus and the resulting evoked potential (Matsumoto *et al.*, 2007).

This study also investigated the reciprocity of CCEPs by evaluating whether stimulating the area of maximum CCEP response projected back to the original site of stimulation. With the medial motor cortex as the site of initial stimulation, reciprocal connections were observed in 17 out of 18 (94%) of the stimulus sites, with the maximum response of the second CCEP located exactly at the location of the initial stimulation in 9 sites (50%). When the site of initial stimulation was in the lateral motor cortex, reciprocal connections were observed in 25 out of the 32 (78%) stimulus sites, with the maximum second CCEP exactly at the site of initial stimulation in 8 sites (25%). These results suggest a high degree of reciprocity between foci in the medial and lateral motor cortices (Matsumoto et al., 2007).

CCEPs in other networks

In this section, we present preliminary data regarding connectivity between the posterior cingulate gyrus (PCG) and mesial temporal structures and connectivity of the insula. We conducted these studies in patients with non-lesional TLE who underwent implantation of depth electrodes in the mesial temporal lobe as well as in other areas know to be connected to the mesial temporal structures, such as the insula and the PCG, among others, in order to rule out ETLE with secondary propagation to the temporal lobe.

We first present a case that illustrates the clinical importance of connectivity between PCG and the medial temporal lobe.

Case Study 3

A 22-year-old right handed man presented with intractable automotor seizures with alteration of awareness (Koubeissi et al., 2009). His video-EEG monitoring showed an ictal EEG pattern consisting of a rhythmic buildup of 2 to 5 Hz activity in the right temporal region evolving into 8 to 9 Hz. Interictally, the EEG showed spikes and spike-wave complexes in the right anterior to mid-temporal regions, observed primarily during sleep. His brain MRI revealed a $1 \times 0.9 \times 0.7$ cm cortical mass on the right PCG. Despite the clear EEG findings pointing to the temporal lobe, the presence of the known cingulate lesion prompted depth electrode implantation in the right PCG and the mesial temporal structures. The recorded seizures began with a burst in the right cingulate followed by a low-voltage, 40 Hz activity that secondarily spread to the mesial temporal depth electrodes after 20-30 seconds. Interictally, epileptiform discharges were seen in the right amygdala and hippocampus, with and without synchronous epileptiform activity in the PCG. The patient underwent resection of the PCG lesion and became seizure free at 2 years of follow-up (Koubeissi et al., 2009).

This case and similar cases have prompted studying the posterior cingulate gyrus by depth electrode recordings in patients with normal MRIs, but with scalp EEG recordings suggesting TLE. Four women (ages 23 to 58 years) with intractable nonlesional temporal lobe epilepsy underwent implantation of depth electrodes for seizure-focus localization. Implanted areas included anterior, middle, and posterior hippocampi; amygdalae; and PCG. Single pulse stimulation (1 Hz, pulse width 0.3 msec, at 2-10 mA) was applied to implanted structures. Cerebro-cerebral evoked potentials (CCEPs) with early and late components were recorded bidirectionally between PCG and ipsilateral hippocampus (n = 3). Stimulation of PCG elicited responses throughout the hippocampus, with maximal amplitude posteriorly (n = 2). Stimulation of the anterior, middle, and posterior hippocampal electrodes elicited CCEPs in the PCG region, with maximum amplitude upon stimulation of the posterior hippocampus (n = 2), and anterior hippocampus (n = 1). The location of the PC electrodes in the patient with no MTL CCEPs was different from PC electrode locations in the others.

This results constitute *in vivo* demonstration of connectivity between the PCG and the hippocampus, and confirm connectivity within the default mode network of the brain. This network is an anatomically defined system that is active during undisturbed thinking. Two of its subsystems, the medial temporal lobe, involved in memory retrieval, and the medial prefrontal subsystem, involved in construction of mental simulations, converge on the PCG. Neuroimaging has demonstrated functional connectivity among these structures, and CCEPs corroborated this connectivity neurophysiologically. In addition, the PCG may represent a link between sensory and limbic systems, as it receives input from auditory, visual, and somatosensory association cortices (Koubeissi *et al.*, 2010).

CCEPs and insular connectivity

We also used CCEPs to explore the connectivity of the insular cortex. The functions of this brain region include such functions as emotional processing, homeostasis, perception, self-awareness, and cognitive function. These activities, inasmuch as they require involvement of multiple brain regions, suggest robust connectivity between the insula and other areas of the brain. Functional neuroimaging has identified potential connectivity between the insula and the cingulate gyrus, and tract tracing in animals has provided evidence of reciprocal projections between the insula and the central nucleus of the amygdala, among other regions. Because many of the higher functions associated with the insula are thought to be unique to humans, even robust results from animal models do not ensure similar outcomes in humans. This following results disclosed some evidence of insular connectivity using neurophysiological methods *in vivo*.

The subjects consisted of five women, ages ranging from 23 to 58 years old, who underwent implantation of depth electrodes for the presurgical evaluation of intractable epilepsy. Implantation targets included the anterior, middle, and posterior insulae, posterior cingulate, and mesial temporal structures. Stimulation was delivered to the implanted electrodes through a single pulse, 1 Hz current with a pulse width of 0.3 msec and an intensity of 2-10 mA. The stimulation revealed CCEPs with early and late components recorded in the insula upon stimulating the hippocampus, lateral temporal neocortex, parahippocampus, amygdala, and posterior cingulate gyrus. Stimulation of the insula elicited CCEPs in the amygdala, hippocampus, and parahippocampus, but not in the cingulate or temporal neocortex. These results suggest bidirectional connectivity between the insula and the amgydala, hippocampus and parahippocampus, but only unidirectional connectivity with the cingulate and temporal neocortex. Additionaly, one patient had three depth electrodes implanted in each insula, and bidirectional interinsular CCEPs were seen with latencies ranging from 39 to 50 msec.

This study represents a novel *in vivo* demonstration of insular connectivity to mesial temporal structures, lateral temporal neocortex, posterior cingulate and contralateral insula. This observed connectivity is consistent with the role of the insula in emotional processing and other higher functions that require processing over different brain regions. Additionally, the results may shed light on potential seizure propagation pathways.

■ Limitations

Despite the successes and knowledge that have been achieved through CCEP research, there are several important limitations to note. Some of the limitations are a function of CCEP representing a relatively nascent field of study, and these issues will hopefully be resolved through further research and insight. Chief among these is the present difficulty in mathematically and objectively describing and characterizing evoked potentials. Other factors, on the other hand, represent fundamental limitations of CCEP research that will be difficult to overcome.

One of the fundamental limitations of CCEP research is that it is only applicable in conjunction with patients receiving a presurgical evaluation of medically intractable epilepsy. This poses several problems. First, this restricts potential subjects to a relatively limited population, making it difficult to be discriminating and to perform studies on large sample sizes. Additionally, it is difficult to guarantee that a particular cortex has not been damaged or been subject to reorganization as part of the pathology of the disease (Koubeissi et al., in submission). Thus, it raises the question of whether or not effective connectivity determined in this population is translatable to the general human population. Recent CCEP research has showed, however, that no significant differences have been observed between epileptogenic and non-epileptogenic hemispheres. This suggests that effective connectivity between regions of the brain is broadly preserved in patients with epilepsy. This is not a surprising conclusion, in fact, because the effective connectivity being studied is a factor of axonal pathways, while epilepsy is primarily a cortical disorder. Nevertheless, since it has been asserted that epilepsy can effect a substantial rewiring of brain connections, differences between epileptic and non-epileptic patients must be considered when generalizing any finding to the general population (Lacruz et al., 2007).

Another fundamental limitation of CCEP research is that decisions regarding the number, position, and distribution of implanted depth electrodes are made solely based on clinical considerations to evaluate patients as pre-surgical candidates. These decisions can lead to insufficient coverage of a particular region by electrodes, potentially creating false-negative CCEP results. It should be considered, then, that any observations and conclusions about connectivity resulting from CCEP analysis represent a "lower limit" of the true effective inter-areal connectivity. This is because while the presence of an evoked potential identifies an effective connection between two regions, the absence of one does not imply the opposite. Instead, a negative result could be a result of several factors, including, but not limited to, the null hypothesis that there exists no connectivity between two regions. For instance, there could be insufficient coverage of a region by electrodes or the dispersion of neural impulses throughout neighboring tissue could render an EEG recording of a particular site unremarkable (Lacruz et al., 2007). The inability to choose implantation sites for depth electrodes based on research requirements also restricts the ability to study anatomically homologous regions across multiple patients. Nevertheless, with a sufficiently large number of patients in a study and the relatively limited number of electrode implantation protocols, a significant number of electrodes are assumed to be within broadly similar areas. As a result, although there is considerable individual variation in responses, broad patterns tend to emerge from a patient population (Lacruz et al., 2007).

Finally, patient comfort and safety is always a chief concern when performing any sort of medical research, and these considerations have important implications in CCEP studies. For example, some patients may find it uncomfortable to undergo functional mapping of a particular cortex, inherently limiting the conclusions that can be inferred from any observed results (Koubeissi *et al.*, in submission). Due to the proven safety of CCEP protocols, concerns regarding patient safety are not often met, but still merit mentioning when discussing potential limitations.

References

- Bowyer SM, Fleming T, Greenwald ML, Moran JE, Mason KM, Weiland BJ, *et al.* Magnetoencephalographic localization of the basal temporal language area. *Epilepsy Behav* 2005; 6: 229-34.
- Brugge JF, Volkov IO, Garell PC, Reale RA, Howard MA, 3rd. Functional connections between auditory cortex on Heschl's gyrus and on the lateral superior temporal gyrus in humans. *J Neurophysiol* 2003; 90: 3750-63.
- Buchel C, Price C, Friston K. A multimodal language region in the ventral visual pathway. *Nature* 1998; 394: 274-7.
- Cascino GD, Hulihan JF, Sharbrough FW, Kelly PJ. Parietal lobe lesional epilepsy: electroclinical correlation and operative outcome. *Epilepsia* 1993; 34: 522-7.
- Catani M, Howard RJ, Pajevic S, Jones DK. Virtual *in vivo* interactive dissection of white matter fasciculi in the human brain. *Neuroimage* 2002; 17: 77-94.
- Crone NE, Miglioretti DL, Gordon B, Lesser RP. Functional mapping of human sensorimotor cortex with electrocorticographic spectral analysis. II. Event-related synchronization in the gamma band. *Brain* 1998; 121 (Pt 12): 2301-15.
- Crone NE, Miglioretti DL, Gordon B, Sieracki JM, Wilson MT, Uematsu S, *et al.* Functional mapping of human sensorimotor cortex with electrocorticographic spectral analysis. I. Alpha and beta event-related desynchronization. *Brain* 1998; 121 (Pt 12): 2271-99.
- Crone NE, Hao L, Hart J, Jr., Boatman D, Lesser RP, Irizarry R, *et al.* Electrocorticographic gamma activity during word production in spoken and sign language. *Neurology* 2001; 57: 2045-53.
- Friston KJ, Frith CD, Liddle PF, Frackowiak RS. Functional connectivity: the principal-component analysis of large (PET) data sets. *J Cereb Blood Flow Metab* 1993; 13: 5-14.
- Friston KJ, Frith CD, Frackowiak RSJ. Time-dependent changes in effective connectivity measured with PET. *Human Brain Mapping* 1993; 11.
- Karanec K, Maciunas R, Miller J, Nehamkin S, Lüders H, Koubeissi MZ. Studying seizure propagation pathways with cortical-cortical evoked potentials. *Neurology* 2011.
- Koubeissi MZ, Jouny CC, Blakeley JO, Bergey GK. Analysis of dynamics and propagation of parietal cingulate seizures with secondary mesial temporal involvement. *Epilepsy Behav* 2009; 14: 108-12.
- Koubeissi MZ, Maciunas R, Miller J, Smith K, Nehamkin S, Lüders H. Connectivity between the posterior cingulate and mesial temporal structures. *Epilepsia* 2010; 51.
- Koubeissi MZ, Sinai A, Franaszczuk P, Lesser RP, Crone NE. Connectivity between perisylvian and bilateral basal temporal cortices. *Cerebral Cortex*, in submission *[please update if possible]*.
- Lacruz ME, Garcia Seoane JJ, Valentin A, Selway R, Alarcon G. Frontal and temporal functional connections of the living human brain. *Eur J Neurosci* 2007; 26: 1357-70.
- Lee L, Harrison LM, Mechelli A. A report of the functional connectivity workshop, Dusseldorf 2002. *Neuroimage* 2003; 19: 457-65.
- Lüders H, Lesser RP, Hahn J, Dinner DS, Morris H, Resor S, *et al.* Basal temporal language area demonstrated by electrical stimulation. *Neurology* 1986; 36: 505-10.

- Lüders H, Lesser RP, Hahn J, Dinner DS, Morris HH, Wyllie E, *et al.* Basal temporal language area. *Brain* 1991; 114 (Pt 2): 743-54.
- Matsumoto R, Nair DR, LaPresto E, Najm I, Bingaman W, Shibasaki H, *et al.* Functional connectivity in the human language system: a cortico-cortical evoked potential study. *Brain* 2004; 127: 2316-30.
- Matsumoto R, Nair DR, Lapresto E, Bingaman W, Shibasaki H, Luders HO. Functional connectivity in human cortical motor system: a cortico-cortical evoked potential study. *Brain* 2007; 130: 181-97.
- Nobre AC, Allison T, McCarthy G. Word recognition in the human inferior temporal lobe. *Nature* 1994; 372: 260-3.
- Sharp DJ, Scott SK, Wise RJ. Retrieving meaning after temporal lobe infarction: the role of the basal language area. *Ann Neurol* 2004; 56: 836-46.
- Usui K, Ikeda A, Takayama M, Matsuhashi M, Yamamoto J, Satoh T, *et al.* Conversion of semantic information into phonological representation: a function in left posterior basal temporal area. *Brain* 2003; 126: 632-41.
- Usui K, Ikeda A, Takayama M, Matsuhashi M, Satow T, Begum T, *et al.* Processing of Japanese morphogram and syllabogram in the left basal temporal area: electrical cortical stimulation studies. *Brain Res Cogn Brain Res* 2005; 24: 274-83.

Section V:
Surgery and outcome
of extratemporal lobe epilepsies

Implantation of depth electrodes – stereo-electro-encephalography (SEEG) – in extratemporal lobe epilepsy

**Massimo Cossu, Francesco Cardinale,
Laura Castana, Laura Tassi, Stefano Francione, Roberto Mai,
Ivana Sartori, Lino Nobili, Francesca Gozzo, Marco Schiariti,
Giorgio Lo Russo**

*"C. Munari" Epilepsy Surgery Centre, Ospedale Niguarda Ca' Granda,
Milano, Italy*

■ Introduction

While temporal lobectomy accounts for the highest proportion of resective procedures performed in patients with drug-resistant symptomatic focal epilepsies, largest series (Schramm, 2008), as well as the personal experience (*Table I*), indicate that extratemporal cases correspond to approximately 30% of resective surgery for epilepsy. Extratemporal epilepsy represents a special challenge, owing to the specific features of the epileptic networks involved in seizure generation. Furthermore, the epileptogenic zone (EZ) may include critical cortical and subcortical areas, as those involved in sensory-motor, linguistic and visual functions. Also for these reasons, surgery for extratemporal epilepsy provides less satisfactory results if compared to temporal lobe resections (Tellez-Zenteno, 2005); additionally, patients with extratemporal epilepsy require invasive EEG monitoring more often than those with temporal lobe epilepsy (Roper, 2009), as demonstrated also by our own experience.

In recent years the increasing interest in epilepsy surgery has been largely dependent on the development of refined brain imaging techniques that contribute to the appropriate selection of patients. In particular, last generation Magnetic Resonance Imaging (MRI) provides crucial information for the identification of the EZ, that is the cortical area of origin and of primary organization of the ictal discharge (Kahane, 2006), enabling to disclose even subtle brain lesions, such as small foci of cortical dysplasia.

Table I. Type of resection (extratemporal or including temporal lobe) in 944 cases of epilepsy surgery operated on at "C. Munari" Epilepsy Surgery Centre, Niguarda Hospital, Milan, Italy

Type of resection	Operated on patients	
	n.	%
Extratemporal	302	32
Temporal unilobar ML + Temporal	642	68
Total	944	100

n.: number of cases; ML: multilobar.

Nevertheless, the identification of the EZ and, consequently, the formulation of a surgical strategy, does not depend only on the recognition of a possible etiological factor of the epilepsy (the so-called epileptogenic lesion), but relies on the accurate evaluation of electro-clinical data and on their consistency, as to localization, with the anatomical findings.

In a considerable proportion of patients this work up relies exclusively on non-invasive presurgical investigations. This proportion, which is highly dependent on the team's experience, available technical supports and attitudes in patients' selection, is represented approximately by 70% of the cases operated on in our Centre, and includes most of surgically treated temporal lobe epilepsies. In the remaining patients, a large amount of whom is represented by extratemporal cases, the non-invasive presurgical evaluation is not sufficient to clearly identify the EZ, and therefore intracranial EEG monitoring is required.

In this Chapter, indications, technical aspects, results and complications of stereotactic implantation of intracerebral electrodes are discussed, with particular attention to extratemporal epilepsies.

■ Historical perspective

stereo-electro-encephalography(SEEG) was developed in the Neurosurgical Unit of the Sainte-Anne Hospital in Paris (Talairach, 1974), where stereotactic investigations of epileptic patients with intracerebral electrodes were inspired to a newly elaborated concept: epileptic seizures were regarded to as a dynamic process, with a spatial-temporal, often multidirectional, organization, which is best defined referring to a 3-dimensional arrangement (Bancaud, 1965). The site of origin and of primary organization of this dynamic process in focal epilepsies, whose surgical removal results in control of seizures, was defined as the EZ.

With these premises, the Saint Anne group developed the methodology of SEEG which enabled to address the complex requirements of defining in the 3D space and time the organization of the ictal discharges by tailored "explorations" (arrangements of intracerebral electrodes). These were aimed to the verification of a previously formulated coherent hypothesis as to localization of the EZ, based upon available anatomo-electro-clinical findings peculiar of each single case. For these purposes, several needs should be satisfied: the electro-clinical definition of epilepsies must rely on the recording of spontaneous seizures, and not be limited to recording of static interictal electrical abnormalities; the structures presumed to be involved in the ictal electrical onset and in the primary and secondary organization of the ictal discharge should be previously defined, included in the plan of exploration and surgically reached with the precision of the stereotactic technique; unlike the early studies with intracerebral electrodes (Spiegel, 1950), a primary role was assigned to the exploration of cortical structures, since the dynamic organization of the ictal discharges was presumed to follow cortical trajectories. For this latter purpose, owing to the inter-individual variability of cortical anatomy, the stereotactic localization of different cortical areas required an approach based on a statistically built up proportional reference system which used the intercommissural line, as identified by contrast ventriculography, as the baseline landmark. This approach enabled to incorporate the anatomy of each single patient into a flexible anamorphotic reference system (Talairach, 1988). Furthermore, stereotactic and stereoscopic tele-angiography provided excellent definition of the gyral and sulcal anatomy of the brain, and allowed to plan avascular trajectories for electrode placement through a double grid mounted on the custom-made Talairach's frame (Talairach, 1980).

Since the pioneering experience of the Paris group, the development of modern neuroradiology and of image-fusion techniques has progressively increased the safety of the methodology and the accuracy of stereotactic targeting of intracerebral structures (Heyman, 1997). Nevertheless, the baseline concepts of a single "stereotactic environment", where electrophysiological, morphological and functional information may be imported and entered in a dynamic process of correlation to define the 3-dimensional organization of an epileptic discharge, are still topical in the current era of SEEG and they have been relevant for the development of modern epilepsy surgery and stereotactic neurosurgery (Chauvel, 2001).

■ Indications

As a consequence of the growing experience of the teams dedicated to the selection of patients and of the refinement of available diagnostic tools, mainly in the field of neuroimaging, the indications to invasive diagnostic procedures are now reduced. Nevertheless, a considerable proportion of cases require a SEEG investigation. More than half of the patients who will receive an extratemporal resection have a SEEG exploration, as compared to one forth of cases submitted to temporal unilobar or multilobar plus temporal resections (Table II).

From a general point of view, invasive recordings are indicated whenever the non-invasive investigations fail to correctly localize the EZ. This is the result of a varying degree of incoherence among anatomical, electrical and clinical findings, which is peculiar for every given patient. Although this means that indications to a SEEG exploration are usually

Table II. Proportion of patients who underwent a SEEG exploration before an extratemporal resection and, respectively, a resection including the temporal lobe

Type of resection	SEEG/resections (%)
Extratemporal	169/302 (56)
Temporal unilobar ML + Temporal	160/642 (25)

SEEG: Stereo-Electro-Encephalo-Graphy; ML: multilobar.

customized to the requirements of single cases, a retrospective analysis of our experience allows to group the indications into different patterns of anatomo-electro-clinical incoherence that configure the need for invasive monitoring (Cossu, 2005), which can be schematically summarized as follows:

1) With no definite anatomical abnormality seen on MRI, scalp ictal/interictal EEG findings are partially or fully discordant with ictal clinical semiology;

2) With a well-documented focal abnormality seen on MRI, scalp ictal/interictal EEG findings and/or ictal clinical semiology suggest a wide involvement also of extralesional areas;

3) Irrespective of MRI evidence, ictal clinical semiology is discordant with an apparently localizing ictal scalp EEG pattern;

4) Either MRI, scalp ictal EEG, or ictal clinical semiology suggest an early involvement of highly eloquent areas, when their relationships with the epileptogenic zone has to be established and functional mapping is needed, so that both the prognosis for resection regarding seizures and the associated surgical risks can be defined;

5) Large focal, hemispheric, multifocal, or bilateral abnormalities are seen on MRI, with ictal scalp EEG and clinical evidence of more localized/lateralized ictal onset.

■ Planning of SEEG explorations

General principles

The available non-invasive anatomo-electro-clinical data are reviewed to formulate a coherent hypothesis of localization of the EZ and to plan a consistent tailored strategy of exploration. This decisional process requires a good experience in the interpretation of electro-clinical patterns of focal seizures, as well as a detailed knowledge of the functional anatomy of the brain, including that of both intra- and inter-hemispheric connections. Furthermore, one has to take into account the intrinsic peculiarities of multilead intracerebral electrodes, which, despite a limited coverage of the cortical surface compared to subdural strips or grids, enable an accurate sampling of the structures encountered along its trajectory, from the entry site to the final impact point. In this way, the investigation may include lateral and mesial surface of the different lobes, fissural and deep-seated cortices, as well as different kinds of lesions.

The implantation strategy should be addressed to record from the regions considered the most likely origin of the discharge (including the lesion, if present) as well as from all the structures possibly involved in the organization of the discharge through the more common pathways of propagation, as suggested by available electro-clinical findings. Furthermore, one should arrange the exploration taking into consideration also possible alternative hypothesis of localization, with number and sites of additional electrodes consistent with the likelihood of these hypotheses. The aim to obtain all the possible information from the SEEG exploration should not be pursued at the expense of an excessive number of electrodes. The possible involvement of eloquent regions in the ictal discharge requires their judicious coverage, with the twofold goal to assess their role in the seizure organization and to define the boundaries of a safe surgical resection.

Patterns of exploration

The SEEG methodology emphasizes a tailored strategy of exploration, which results from the anatomo-electro-clinical features of every case, therefore rejecting a standardized arrangement of electrodes. Nevertheless, when retrospectively considering our SEEG experience, a number of typical patterns of coverage are clearly recognizable, and some illustrative examples of the more frequent of them will be herein detailed.

Cases of temporal lobe epilepsy with consistent anatomo-electro-clinical findings are usually operated on after non-invasive investigations. SEEG recordings may be required in patients in whom the supposed epileptogenic area, though probably involving the temporal lobe, is suspected to extend also to extratemporal areas (Ryvlin, 2005). In these cases, the main implantation patterns point to disclose a preferential spread of the discharge to the insulo-opercular complex, to the temporo-parieto-occipital junction, or to the anterior frontal cortex. Sampling of extratemporal areas must be wide enough to provide information also to identify a possible extratemporal origin of the seizures that could not have been anticipated with certainty according to scalp EEG and clinical findings.

Owing to the large volume of the frontal lobe, one can expect that a high number of electrodes is required for an adequate coverage of this region. In most patients, however, taking into account ictal clinical data and the related surface EEG expression, such a very large sampling can be avoided, and the exploration is focused on (but not restricted to) a more limited portion of the frontal lobe. The suspicion of an orbito-frontal epilepsy, for instance, often requires to investigate both the gyrus rectus and the orbital cortex (using oblique electrodes that also evaluate the frontal pole), the lateral fronto-basal cortex, the anterior cingulate gyrus (including Brodmann areas 32 and 24), and the anterior portion of the temporal lobe. In the same way, seizures that are thought to arise from the mesial wall of the premotor cortex are evaluated by targeting at least the rostral and caudal part of the supplementary motor area (SMA), the pre-SMA, different portions of the cingulate gyrus, as well as the primary motor cortex, mainly for functional mapping purposes. Proceeding this way, hypothesis-based sampling often allows localization of the seizure onset zone in the frontal lobe, and in some cases may allow identifying very small epileptogenic regions (Chassagnon, 2003). Occasionally, frontal lobe explorations may be bilateral, but almost always very asymmetric, because the question of the "affected side" is usually addressed to before placement of electrodes.

Rolandic electrodes are placed when MRI shows anatomical abnormalities within or close to this region and/or when its involvement in the EZ may be suspected, with the aim to evaluate the rolandic participation to the ictal discharge and to obtain a functional mapping by intracerebral electrical stimulations. This is not infrequently required when seizures are suspected to start in the frontal or parietal lobes and to propagate subsequently to the perirolandic areas. In the central region, intracerebral electrodes are particularly helpful to sample the depth of the rolandic fissure, as well as the descending motor and ascending sensory pathways.

In the posterior quadrant of the hemisphere, placement of electrodes limited to a single lobe is extremely uncommon, due to the frequent simultaneous involvement of several occipital, parietal and posterior temporal structures, as well as to the possible multidirectional spread of the discharges to supra and infra-sylvian regions. However, though multidirectional, posterior discharges often show a preferential spreading pattern that has to be adequately assessed by employing implantation strategies which mainly focus on parietal, occipital and temporal areas.

■ Technical aspects

Stereotactic neuroradiology

The correct positioning of intracerebral electrodes must fulfill two essential conditions:
- accurate targeting of desired intracerebral structures;
- minimal risk of vessel injury and of iatrogenic intracranial hemorrhage.

The first requirement is addressed employing adequate datasets of structural and, if needed, functional neuroimaging. These should therefore include:
- all the appropriate sequences demonstrating the presumed epileptogenic lesion(s), if present. T2-weighted fluid attenuation inversion recovery (FLAIR) sequences, for instance, are particularly helpful to detect subtle cortical malformations, and T1-weighted Inversion Recovery (IR) sequences provide an excellent definition of the grey-white matter interface and of the gyro-sulcal cortical arrangement;
- if required, areas of activation at functional MRI (fMRI) may be included, as well as Diffusion tensor imaging for fibre-tracking (DTI-FT) if functionally critical structures deserve special attention in the exploration strategy;
- a volumetric dataset (usually FFE T1-weighted sequence in the axial plane, voxel 0.46 × 0.46 × 1 mm, no gap, reconstruction matrix 560 × 560), which usually represents the reference dataset for subsequent co-registration of other images.

Furthermore, to minimize the risk of vascular damage, brain angiography (via selective intra-arterial injection of radio-opaque contrast medium) of the pertinent vessels is obtained. Usually, both a frameless 3D rotational acquisition and traditional 2D projective angiograms in stereotactic conditions (Talairach frame) are acquired. For 2D images, two series of angiograms are obtained by both an orthogonal and a slightly oblique incidence (+/- 6 degrees) of the X-ray beam. The coupled vision of corresponding phases of the two series enables a stereoscopic (pseudo-3D) effect, which is particularly helpful to discern vascular structures laying in different anatomical planes.

Once the image datasets are acquired, they are co-registered to the reference dataset (the T1-3D sequence) and imported into the planning software (Voxim, IVS, Chemnitz, Germany), and the exploration may be prepared according to the defined strategy, planning avascular trajectories which reach the desired targets with the accuracy of the stereotactic technique (*Figure 1*).

The work-flow of the imaging acquisition and post-processing is constantly updated in our Centre, with the following aims:
- to concentrate the invasive maneuvers in a single procedure, by acquiring the neuroimages without referential devices fixed to the skull;
- to develop fully automatic procedures for coregistrations of all volumetric datasets and for segmentation of both brain tissue and vessels;
- to increase the signal/noise ratio in all images;
- to plan the trajectories in a 3D environment, with multiplanar recostructions and 3D renderings (volume and/or surface renderings) of the brain surface, vessels, lesions, areas of cortical activations, and tracts of white matter;

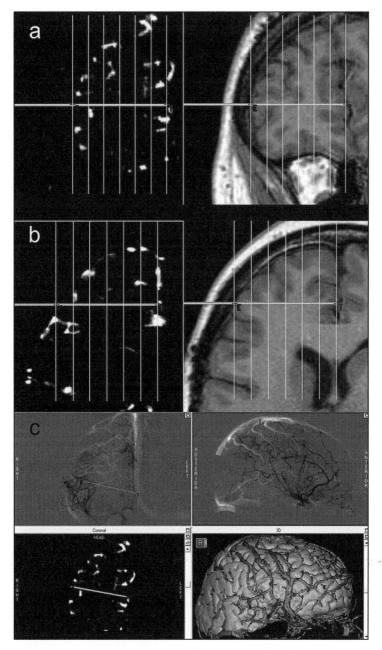

Figure 1. Screen snapshots from the module of trajectory planning (Voxim, IVS, Chemnitz, Germany). The trajectory plan of an electrode intended to sample the anterior part of the cingulate gyrus, with an entry point in the anterior lateral frontal cortex of the right hemisphere is shown.

a) The plan is detailed with respect to the 3D angiography (left box) and the MRI in the coronal plane.

b) Same as in a), in the transverse plane.

c) The trajectory plane is represented in the lateral and frontal views of a "combo" digital 2D angiogram (upper boxes) and in a different plane of the 3D angiography (left lower box), as well as in the reconstructed 3D cortical surface and vessels (right lower box).

– to reduce the sources of error in the trajectory plans and in the surgical implantation (for instance eliminating the slight but unavoidable error in frame repositioning, see below);
– to normalize inter-subjects datasets in a probabilistic atlas with non-linear registrations, in order to collect population data for research purposes;
– to make all useful information available for neuronavigation at the time of resective surgery.

With these main goals in mind, we are integrating the traditional methodology with the use of several open source medical softwares.

Placement of electrodes

Implantation of intracerebral electrodes is performed usually in a separate frame-based procedure (in order to dedicate all the required time to the accurate planning of trajectories), under general anesthesia.

Commercially available, platinum-iridium, semiflexible multilead intracerebral electrodes (diameter 0.8 mm; 5 to 18 contacts of 1.5 mm length, 2 mm apart) are employed, the number of electrodes per patient averaging approximately 12 electrodes. The exploration is unilateral in most cases; bilateral (only occasionally symmetrical) explorations account for less than 20% of the procedures.

Antibiotics (cephamezine, in a single bolus, 1-2 gr i.v. depending on patient's weight) are routinely administered at anesthesia induction.

The trajectories of the electrodes are planned in order to impact as many desired structures as possible. Targeting of deep-seated or mesial structures such as the *amygdala, hippocampus*, cingulated gyrus, gyrus rectus, mesial convolutions of the frontal, parietal and occipital lobes is feasible, as well as excellent sampling of the insular cortex by electrodes inserted through the supra- or infra-sylvian opercula or by a retro-insular trajectory with a dorso-lateral entry point. Intracerebral electrodes allow also an excellent coverage of deep-seated cortical malformations, like periventricular or subcortical heterotopic clusters of gray matter.

As far as the coverage of specific brain areas is concerned, out of the 427 patients investigated by SEEG so far in our Centre, 306 (72%) received at least one electrode into the frontal lobe, 320 (75%) into the temporal lobe, 333 (78%) into the central lobe, 296 (69%) into the parietal lobe, 194 (45%) into the occipital lobe and 154 (36%) into the insula. Of course, patients subsequently operated on by an extratemporal resection had a prevailing extratemporal electrode coverage. Nevertheless, placement of temporal electrodes also in these cases was not uncommon, as the chances of an early spread to the temporal lobe of an ictal discharge originated had to be investigated, as well as the possibility that a presumed extratemporal discharge could actually originate within the temporal lobe with atypical EEG and clinical features.

For the implantation of each electrode, a skull percutaneous trephination is performed with a 2.1 mm twist drill, guided through a computer-assisted passive robot (NeuroMate, Renishaw Mayfield SA, Nyon, Switzerland) with a tool holder attached to a five-degrees of freedom arm which enables placement of electrodes along practically infinite trajectories. The dura is perforated by low-current monopolar coagulation. Minor leakage of cerebro-spinal fluid is often observed at this stage, but it does not require particular attention.

Titanium hollow pegs (external diameter 2.45 mm), for the insertion and the fixation of the electrodes, are then screwed to the skull. A rigid stylet (diameter 0.8 mm) is then advanced through the peg as far as the established target under fluoroscopic control, in order to trace the intracerebral track of the electrode. After removal of the stylet, the electrode is inserted and advanced to the target. A plastic cap fixes the electrode to the peg and prevents possible CSF leakage. EEG signal provided by all implanted electrodes is checked in the operating room, enabling replacement of malfunctioning electrodes, which is however an uncommon occurrence. The cables are sutured to the skin and a sterile medication is applied. Skull 3D volumetric CT scan with implanted electrodes is then obtained and co-registered with the 3D-T1 MRI. Using appropriate windows, a blended image is obtained, which includes single contacts of electrodes visualized within the 3D MRI (*Figure 2*), enabling to correlate the recorded electrical activities with the generating cerebral structure. The patient is then awakened from anesthesia and moved to the recovery room.

Intensive Video-EEG monitoring usually starts the day following implantation, with the purpose of recording patient's habitual ictal manifestations. After an adequate number of seizures is obtained, the patients undergo the sessions of intracerebral electrical stimulations (see below). Mean duration of Video-SEEG monitoring approximates 10 days.

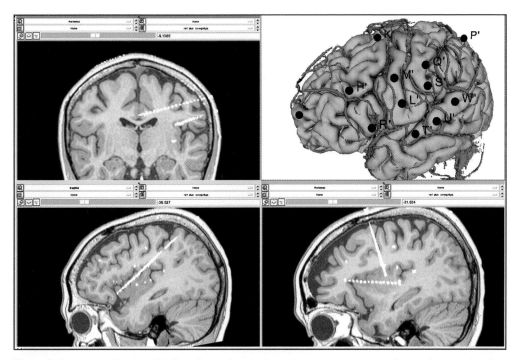

Figure 2. Screen snapshot from 3D Slicer (www.slicer.org), representing in the upper right box the cortical surface reconstructed from the 3D MRI and the cortical impact points of each intracerebral electrode, indicated with upper case letters. In the other boxes the multiplanar reconstructions include the 3D MRI and the intracerebral electrodes extracted from a co-registered volumetric CT scan. Single contacts of each electrode and their intracerebral locations are easily recognizable. Note the two electrodes sampling, with most contacts, the insular cortex and placed along trajectories with a post-central and, respectively, a fronto-polar entry points, as well as an electrode with its inner contacts placed into the cingulated cortex.

Removal of electrodes

Once monitoring is completed, electrodes are withdrawn. In most patients local anesthesia is employed, though sedation may be required in less cooperative patients and children. The plastic caps are removed, and then each electrode is gently withdrawn and accurately inspected in order to check its integrity. Once all the hollow pegs have been unscrewed, a skin suture is applied to each electrode entry site and a sterile medication applied. The patient is usually discharged the day after.

■ SEEG-guided functional mapping

High- and low-frequency intracerebral electrical stimulations, delivered to pairs of contiguous contacts, have the two-fold goal to induce habitual ictal manifestations and to provide a functional map of the implanted regions (Kahane, 1993; Munari, 1993).

Intracerebral electrical stimulations performed for functional purposes enable the identification of regions related to different critical functions: primary somatomotor and somatosensory, visual, acoustic and speech. Positive responses consist of either objective clinical events (e.g.: clonic jerks of circumscribed body districts, errors in naming or reading, tachyphemia) or subjective manifestations (dysesthesic sensations, positive or negative visual and acoustic phenomena) concurrent with electrical stimulations. For primary sensory-motor functions low-frequency stimulations (frequency 1 Hz, duration of single stimulus 2-3 msec, current intensity 0.4-3 mA) are preferred. In most cases, positive responses may be obtained from stimulations both in grey and white matter, thus allowing mapping critical pathways extensively. For this latter purpose, planning of electrode trajectories may be supported by DTI-FT imaging. Speech and visual areas are mapped using a combination of low and high-frequency (frequency 50 Hz, duration of single stimulus 1 msec, current intensity 1-3 mA) stimulations. Low-frequency stimulations are usually adequate in inducing subjective acoustic changes, the effect of high frequencies resulting often unpleasant for the patient.

Chronic intracerebral seizure monitoring coupled with functional mapping is crucial in distinguishing between patients with early ictal involvement of highly eloquent regions, for whom the impact of postoperative permanent deficits must be balanced against the severity of epilepsy, and those with later spread of the discharge to these structures, who can be operated on with limited surgical risks and with predictable benefit on seizures. Functional mapping allows anticipating potentially acceptable postoperative deficits, such as visual field defects in posterior temporal, occipital and parietal resections, as well as to evaluate the risk-to-benefit ratio of excisions close to more critical regions, such as sensory-motor and language areas. Though similar functional information can be obtained also from acute intraoperative electrical cortical stimulation, the following points must be stressed. First, chronic SEEG intracerebral electrical stimulations makes mapping of both cortex and fibres feasible, allowing to plan safer resections also in potentially critical subcortical areas. Second, availability of functional information before and not during surgery allows the patient to participate in the discussion of the risk-to-benefit balance in a relaxing and comfortable setting. Third, intraoperative electrocorticography only exceptionally results in spontaneous seizures recording, which is essential in evaluating the actual ictal involvement of eloquent areas.

■ Contribution of SEEG to resective extratemporal epilepsy surgery

The contribution of SEEG in addressing the decision whether to operate or not, the choice of an adequate surgical strategy, and the results of SEEG-guided resections may vary among different epilepsy surgery teams.

Out of the 329 patients operated on in our Centre following a SEEG investigation since 1996, 169 (51.3%) received a purely extratemporal resection, with frontal lobe resections prevailing over other sites of surgery (*Table III*). The results on seizures indicate that 57% of these cases are in Engel's Class I (patients free of disabling seizures), with frontal lobe resection providing slightly better results than other localizations (*Table III*).

There is general agreement that results of surgery performed after invasive EEG monitoring are not as satisfying as those obtained in patients submitted only to non-invasive presurgical investigations (Janszky, 2000). Furthermore, extratemporal epilepsies may represent puzzling cases for several reasons, including the often-confounding ictal semiology, difficulty of scalp EEG interpretation, complexity of epileptic network organization, involvement of functionally critical structures in the epileptogenic zone. Therefore, results on seizures after SEEG-based extratemporal resections, although not as gratifying as those obtained in temporal lobe epilepsies, should be regarded to as excellent, considering the high degree of complexity of these cases.

Table III. Sites of surgery and results on seizures (FU > 12 months) in the 169 patients who received a SEEG-based extratemporal resection

Site of extratemporal resection	n. (%)	Engel's Class I (%)
Frontal	103 (61%)	60%
Frontal "plus"	21 (12%)	50%
Posterior	33 (20%)	50%
Including rolandic	12 (7%)	58%
Total	169 (100%)	57%

Sites were divided in: frontal, frontal "plus" (additional opercular or insular corticectomy), posterior (occipital and parietal unilobar or bilobar resections), including rolandic (frontal or parietal resections extended to the primary sensory-motor areas). Seizure outcome was assessed by the Engel's classification.

■ Complications

As far as indications to SEEG monitoring are concerned, the potential risks, implied by the violation of anatomical structures for purely diagnostic purposes, should be taken into consideration.

Severe intracerebral haemorrhage is the most feared complication of intracerebral electrode placement (Sperling, 2001). In a series of 560 SEEG cases, three (0.5%) were operated on for removal of intracerebral hematomas developed after electrode implantation (Talairach, 1973). It is not clear whether these authors observed other cases with intracranial bleeding which did not require surgical treatment, but it is unlikely that such cases were diagnosed by the neuroradiological techniques available in the pre-CT scan or MRI era, even if mild neurological impairment was evident following implantation of intracerebral electrodes. The Montreal group experienced 1 subdural bleed out of 170 cases (0.6%) investigated with intracerebral electrodes (Espinosa, 1994). Mortality has also been associated to such complication, with 2 deaths (1.4%) from intracerebral haemorrhage reported in a series of 140 patients (Engel, 1983). In a series of 100 SEEG cases one death secondary to an intracerebral clot (1%) has been reported in a patient under anticoagulant treatment for deep vein thrombosis (Guenot, 2001).

Our group has recently reported the morbidity associated to the SEEG technique described in the present chapter (Cossu, 2005). Out of 215 procedures in 211 patients, complications of different nature occurred in 12 SEEG procedures, for an overall incidence of morbidity as high as 5.6%. There were 3 acute symptomatic intracerebral haemorrhages which required emergency surgical evacuation, 5 asymptomatic intracranial bleedings detected at post-implantation MRI, 1 obstructive hydrocephalus due to a clot in the aqueduct in a patient with a platelet disorder, 1 symptomatic brain abscess, 1 focal cortical oedema and 1 retained broken electrode. In two cases (0.9%) a permanent motor deficit resulted from massive intracerebral bleeding.

■ SEEG: only a diagnostic tool?

Though SEEG is merely a diagnostic tool, the employment of this technique for possible therapeutic purposes has been suggested (Catenoix, 2008). Following a complete SEEG monitoring, intracerebral electrodes may be used to generate focal lesions in the SEEG-defined EZ. A thermocoagulation with a diameter of 5-7 mm may be produced by a radio-frequency generator connected to adjacent electrode contacts. By these means, a variable number of lesions may be placed in the cortical areas selected according to the SEEG data, with no relevant morbidity. This technique, though deserving further evaluation in order to assess its feasibility, safety and efficacy, has been proposed as a possible option in cases with a limited and well confined EZ, or when resective surgery is contraindicated for functional reasons as in several cases of extratemporal epilepsies that should be excluded from resective surgery (*Figure 3*).

■ Conclusions

Results of SEEG-based resective surgery in focal symptomatic, drug-resistant extratemporal epilepsies indicate that electro-clinical evaluation with stereotactically implanted intracerebral electrodes enables to offer an effective treatment to a substantial number of difficult cases. Nevertheless, this gratifying picture is dependent on the accurate selection of patients and on the rigorous scrutiny of their anatomo-electro-clinical data, with the aim to formulate a working hypothesis as to the presumed localization of the epileptogenic zone, which will be verified by SEEG with a consistent strategy of exploration. This means that, considering the potential risks linked to an invasive diagnostic procedure, SEEG evaluation should be reserved to a highly selected sub-population of epileptic patients.

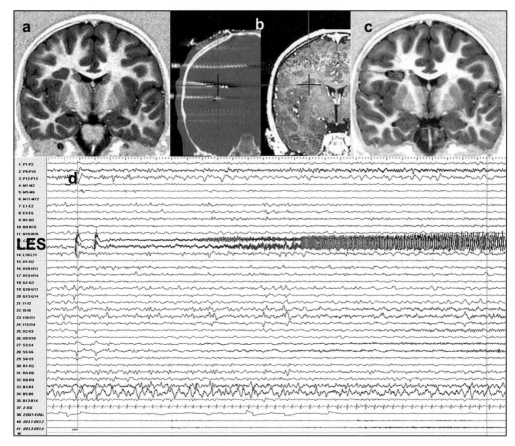

Figure 3. a) The Inversion Recovery coronal MRI shows a nodular heterotopy within the centrum semiovale of the right hemisphere of a 8-year-old boy with focal drug-resistant seizures. **b)** Post-implantation CT scan and co-registered MRI showing the electrode contacts sampling the lesion (black crosses). **c)** Coronal Inversion Recovery MRI after selective radio-frequency thermo-coagulation of the electrodes recording from the heterotopic nodule. **d)** Intrecerebral EEG. LES indicates the traces recording from the nodule. Electrical ictal activity involving exclusively the lesion is clearly shown.

References

- Bancaud J, Talairach J, Bonis A, Schaub C, Szikla G, Morel P, Bordas-Ferrer M. La *stéréo-électro-encéphalographie dans l'épilepsie*. Paris: Masson: 1965, 321 p.

- Catenoix H, Mauguiere F, Guenot M, Ryvlin P, Bissery A, Sindou M, Isnard J. SEEG-guided thermocoagulations. A palliative treatment of nonoperable partial seizures. *Neurology* 2008; 71: 1719-26.

- Chassagnon S, Minotti L, Krémer S, Verceuil L, Hoffmann D, Benabid AL, Kahane P. Restricted frontomesial epileptogenic focus generating dyskinetic behaviour and laughter. *Epilepsia* 2003; 44: 859-63.

- Chauvel P. Contribution of Jean Talairach and Jean Bancaud to epilepsy surgery. In: Lüders HO, Comair YG, eds. *Epilepsy Surgery 2nd edition*. Philadelphia: Lippincott Williams & Wilkins, 2001: 35-41.

- Cossu M, Cardinale F, Castana L, Citterio A, Francione S, Tassi L, *et al.* Stereo-EEG in the presurgical evaluation of focal epilepsy: a retrospective analysis of 215 procedures. *Neurosurgery* 2005; 57: 706-18.

- Engel JJ, Crandall PH, Rausch R. The partial epilepsies. In: Rosenberg R N, Grossman RG, eds. *The Clinical Neurosciences.* New York: Churchill Livingstone, 1983: 1349-80.

- Espinosa J, Olivier A, Andermann F, Quesney F, Dubeau F, Savard G. Morbidity of chronic recording with intracranial depth electrodes in 170 patients. *Stereotact Funct Neurosurg* 1994; 63: 63-5.

- Guenot M, Isnard J, Ryvlin P, Fischer C, Ostrowsky K, Mauguiere F, Sindou M. Neurophysiological monitoring for epilepsy surgery: the Talairach SEEG method. *Stererotact Funct Neurosurg* 2001; 77: 29-32.

- Heyman D, Menegalli-Boggelli D, Lajat Y. Adaptation of the Talairach technique to the evolution of medical imaging. *Stereotact Funct Neurosurg* 1997; 68: 59-63.

- Janszky J, Jokeit H, Schulz R, Hoppe M, Hebner A. EEG predicts surgical outcome in lesional frontal lobe epilepsy. *Neurology* 2000; 54: 1470-6.

- Kahane P, Tassi L, Francione S, Hoffmann D, Lo Russo G, Munari C. Manifestations électrocliniques induites par la stimulation électrique intracérébrale par "chocs" dans les épilepsies temporales. *Neurophysiol Clin* 1993 ; 22: 305-26.

- Kahane P, Landrè E, Minotti L, Francione S, Ryvlin P. The Bancaud and Talairach view on the epileptogenic zone: a working hypothesis. *Epileptic Disord* 2006 ; 8 (Suppl 2): S-16-S26.

- Munari C, Kahane P, Tassi L, Francione, S, Hoffmann D, Lo Russo G, Benabid AL. Intracerebral low frequency electrical stimulation: a new tool for the definition of the "epileptogenic area"? *Acta Neurochir* 1993; Suppl. 58: 181-5.

- Roper SN. Surgical treatment of the extratemporal épilepsies. *Epilepsia* 2009 ; 50 (Suppl. 8): 69-74.

- Ryvlin P, Kahane P. The hidden causes of surgery-resistant temporal lobe epilepsy: extratemporal or temporal plus? *Curr Opin Neurol* 2005; 18: 125-27.

- Schramm J, Clusmann H. The surgery of epilepsy. *Neurosurgery* 2008; 62 (SHC Suppl 2): SHC463-SHC481.

- Sperling MR. Depth electrodes. In: Lüders HO, Comair YG, eds. *Epilepsy Surgery 2nd edition.* Philadelphia: Lippincott Williams & Wilkins, 2001: 597-611.

- Spiegel EA, Wycis HT. Thalamic recordings in man with special reference to seizure discharges. *Electroencephalogr Clin Neurophysiol* (1950) 2: 23-39.

- Talairach J, Bancaud J. Stereotaxic approach to epilepsy. Methodology of anatomo-functional stereotaxic investigations. *Progr Neurol Surg* 1973; 5: 297-354.

- Talairach J, Szikla G. Application of stereotactic concepts to the surgery of epilepsy. *Acta Neurochir* 1980; Suppl. 30: 35-54.

- Talairach J., Tournoux P. *Co-planar Stereotaxic Atlas of the Human Brain: 3-Dimensional Proportional System: An Approach to Cerebral Imaging.* New York-Stuttgard: Georg Thieme Verlag, 1988, 122 p.

- Talairach J, Bancaud J, Szikla G, Bonis A, Geier S, Vedrenne C. Approche nouvelle de la neurochirurgie de l'épilepsie. Méthodologie stérérotaxique et résultats thérapeutiques. *Neurochirurgie* 1974; 20 (Suppl. 1): 1-240.

- Tellez-Zenteno JF, Dhar R, Wiebe S. Long-term seizure outcomes following epilepsy surgery: a systematic review and meta-analysis. *Brain* 2005; 128: 1188-98.

Electrocorticography

Warren T. Blume, Giannina M. Holloway

London Health Sciences Centre, University Campus, Epilepsy Unit;
Professor, University of Western Ontario, London, ON, Canada

■ Introduction

Current health care economic pressures commonly influence the selection of patients for this procedure and its operating room duration. These restrictions place a premium on pre-operative evaluation and surgical planning. Fortunately, advances in: i) clinical analysis; ii) invasive EEG (subdural or depth recording); and iii) more precise imaging by MRI all have contributed to more accurate pre-operative localization of epileptogenesis. This reduces or eliminates intraoperative decisions, often obviating the need for electrocorticography (ECoG). However, several situations remain where ECoG can further refine the locus of intractable epilepsy thus increasing the effectiveness of resective surgery. This chapter describes these circumstances; some procedural and analytical data that we have found beneficial are also included.

■ Indications: type of lesion

Whether or not an ECoG will be required hinges upon congruity of data localising epileptogenesis (seizure semiology, EEG, MRI), and the complexity of pathophysiology associated with a given epileptogenetic lesion.

For example, seizures from a cavernous angioma arise from its immediate periphery. Therefore, in most cases ECoG would add little to intra-operative assessment.

Among patients with temporal lobe epilepsy, seizures originate in the mesial temporal region in about 90% (So, 1991; Blume *et al.*, 2001). The most common histological finding in patients with mesial temporal originating seizures is mesial temporal sclerosis (MTS). The association between MTS and prolonged febrile seizures of infancy has been established, but the *nature* of any causal relationship has remained elusive. Moreover, MTS may occur with, and may be consequent to, another lesion ("dual pathology"), *e.g.* cortical dysplasia (CD). Neuroimaging may not always detect this second lesion. That lesion may create its own epileptic pathophysiology with a complex interaction with MTS. Such lesions are usually located in the temporal lobe, but occipital lesions may also create epileptogenic input to the mesial temporal area (Blume *et al.* 2005). If non-invasive and invasive EEG does not clarify the nature of any interactive neurophysiology, ECoG may be required.

CD lesions are highly epileptogenic: ECoG may display recurrent focal seizures, high frequency spikes or continuous epileptiform discharges (CEDs) (Palmini, 2010; Gambardella *et al.*, 1996) *(Figure 1)*. Moreover, unlike some other epilepsy etiologies, these EEG and ECoG patterns reliably delimit the area of epileptogenesis. However, multifocal spikes and bisynchronous spikes occur in about 70% of CD patients, suggesting a complex interactive epileptogenesis (Jiang *et al.*, 2010).

Tuberous sclerosis complex (TSC) is frequently associated with medically intractable epilepsy due to single or multiple cortical lesions, usually apparent on imaging. Tubers consist of dysmorphic neurons, giant cells and an excess number of astrocytes. The common multifocality of TSC epilepsy demands considerable pre-operative semiological, EEG and single photon emission computed tomography (SPECT) investigation. Subdural recordings, involving multiple lobes, may also be needed. Adding to the complexity is emerging evidence of subtle structural abnormalities of the brain, distinct from tubers (Crino, 2010).

Arteriovenous malformations (AVMs) are associated with epilepsy in about 40% of cases and may be the presenting symptom in about 20% (Paterson & McKissock, 1956). However, AVMs are currently treated by material such as balloons inserted intravascularly into the AVM from a peripheral artery approach. Any approach that reduces or obliterates the AVM will abolish or significantly reduce a related seizure tendency without cortical resection, obviating the need for ECoG. Management of large, complex AVMs with focal epilepsy may require ECoG if subdural EEG is deemed impractical or risky.

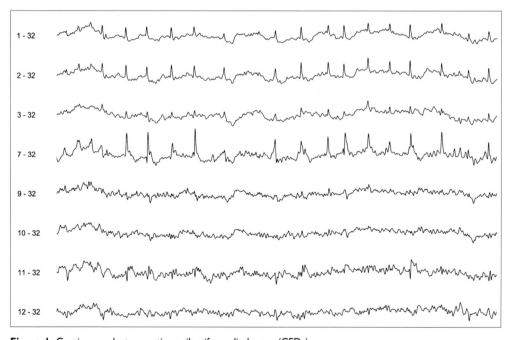

Figure 1. Continuous electronegative epileptiform discharges (CEDs).
Principally at positions 7 (right inferior frontal), and 2, 1 (right superior temporal gyrus anteriorly) with simultaneous low voltage electropositive discharges at position 11 (right posterior frontal).

Trauma as an etiology of focal or secondarily generalized epilepsy may have one or more of several mechanisms. Extra-cerebral factors include: fat embolism from long bone fracture producing multifocal cortical lesions; chest injury producing an hypoxic encephalopathy; and neck injury with a carotid dissection giving an ipsilateral stroke with an unaffected contralateral hemisphere. Of these, only the latter etiology would evoke an epilepsy that may benefit from resective surgery.

Direct cranial trauma with depressed skull fracture will create a potentially epileptogenic underlying contusion that is commonly hemorrhagic. If seizures resist antiepileptic medication, partial or complete resection of this traumatic lesion may be possible. Encroachment upon cortical areas still performing valuable functions must be avoided. Scar tissue and bone fragments may prevent subdural electrode placement and thus require ECoG to determine the lesional or perilesional area responsible for seizure generation.

Non-penetrating, "blunt" head injuries may produce temporal pole and orbitofrontal contusions. As the semiology of consequent post-traumatic seizures may reflect either temporal or frontal origin, ECoG may be required if subdural recordings are not physically possible (scar tissue impeding insertion) or are inconclusive. That mild fluid percussion in the rat could produce hippocampal dentate hilar cell loss raises the real possibility that this potentially epileptogenic structure could participate in post-traumatic epilepsy without evidence of its involvement in structural damage (Lowenstein *et al.*, 1992). Thus any ECoG should cover the mesial temporal region when trauma has occurred.

The periphery of lesions are unevenly epileptogenic (Pathak & Blume, 1997), a principle particularly evident with brain tumours. Therefore ECoG for tumour related epilepsy should record from as many aspects of the lesion as possible. Our anecdotal experience indicates that tumour epileptogenesis can range from surprisingly straightforward to bewildering complexity.

■ Indication: precise localization

Despite thorough preoperative investigation, ECoG may be required in the following circumstances.

The most common of these would be when invasive (subdural or depth) recording provides only *approximate* regional localization of neocortical epileptogenesis, *i.e.* somewhere between the 7-12 subdural electrodes per line spaced at 10-15 mm intervals. This relates not only to an inevitable limited spatial sampling but also to the variable relationship of electrodes to patient-specific gyral patterns. Although applicable to many areas, this applies principally to Rolandic cortex where inappropriate surgical intrusion of only a few millimeters may significantly disrupt some aspects of sensorimotor function. Thus, in some circumstances, ECoG may help determine which gyri, or portions thereof, are appropriate or not for resection. Ictal or interictal abnormalities may extend to the edges of a subdural grid or to the end of a subdural line; insertion of subdural electrodes may encounter obstruction in certain areas leading to such unsatisfactory placement. In these circumstances ECoG might be needed to comprehensively assess the extent of an epileptogenic area.

Investigation of patients with intractable limbic seizures without a mesial temporal or other lesion considered epileptogenic may require ECoG if subdural recordings fail to disclose a convincing seizure origin. Such origin may be orbito- frontal, posterior temporal-occipital or cingulate.

■ Recording technique

After craniotomy our centre places on the cortex the same type of electrode strips and/or grids used for subdural recordings, thus steel or platinum placed 10-15 mm apart for strips or 10 mm for grids. Alternatively, an electrode holder-wire-electrode assembly is used. The electrodes are made of silver, platinum or stainless steel with a ball-shaped tip for brain contact. Assure that the entire hookup is complete before proceeding; diffuse monorhythmic potentials or electrical silence can represent an incomplete circuit.

Referential recording to a contralateral scalp or distant normal cortex electrode allows identification of complex electrical spike or seizure fields such as those created by dipoles that commonly appear on ECoG (Figure 1). Referential recording also avoids partial or complete "cancellation" of potentials that may occur with bipolar recording when phenomena are widespread. As voltage of ECoG potentials are about 5-6 times greater than those of scalp recordings, sensitivities usually range from 30 to 70 µV/mm.

If epileptiform potentials occur less often than needed for intra-operative decisions, one can ask an awake patient to hyperventilate for three minutes. If anaesthesia is employed, it could be carefully lightened; isoflurane, fentanyl and propofol all tend to lower spike quantity.

Our EEG machine is placed in the operating theatre so that the electroencephalographer can see and modify electrode placement, particularly in relationship to any cortical structural abnormality. Interchange between the EEGer and the surgical team is also facilitated thereby.

■ ECoG interpretation

Non-epileptiform background activity

The presence or absence of normal background activity for the area of the ECoG should be the first aspect assessed. In an awake patient alpha and lambda may appear posteriorly and beta in the Rolandic region. With most anaesthetic agents beta activity initially increases, then a mixture of theta and delta appears diffusely.

The following features characterize focal abnormal background activity: i) attenuation or loss of higher frequency activity (alpha, beta, theta); ii) conversion from normal rhythmic delta, theta or alpha to arrhythmic waves; iii) greater delta than in other regions; iv) regional attenuation of all activity; v) regional burst-suppression. Focal atrophy, a lesion, a postictal state and surgical trauma may all contribute to the presence of these focal features.

The neurosurgeon should be made aware of areas containing normal as well as those with abnormal background activity; it would be quite unusual to resect areas with normal background activity.

Epileptiform activity (spikes, seizures)

Some data suggest that ECoG spikes would reliably localize epileptogenesis: i) continuous epileptiform discharges (CEDs) are highly specific and sensitive indicators of cortical dysplastic lesions – a common cause of intractable focal epilepsy (Dubeau *et al.* 1998) (*Figure 1*); ii) neocortical resective surgery is more effective when both a lesion and bordering tissue with spikes are resected than either alone (Awad *et al.*, 1991); and iii) effectiveness of frontal resection correlates inversely with post-resection spike quantity (Wennberg *et al.*, 1998).

However, the Awad study also concluded that residual ECoG post-resection spikes did not affect the "definition of completeness of focus resection". Importantly, several studies have found the area of ECoG spikes to exceed that of epileptogenesis (Chatrian, 2003). In frontal lobe procedures Rasmussen (1983) found that the ECoG spiking area substantially exceeded the extent of resection necessary for seizure control. Also, among patients with frontal lobe epilepsy, Quesney (1991) found only 15% with unilateral frontal or focal frontal lobe spiking.

The EEGer may be surprised to find multifocality of ECoG spikes in a patient whose scalp EEGs *apparently* disclosed only unifocal ones. In some instances, further scrutiny of such scalp recordings may reveal slight but distinct variations in spike fields of a single lobe representing the multifocality on ECoG. As a focal epileptic seizure may transiently augment spike incidence, a preoperative attack, precipitated by anxiety and low antiepileptic serum levels, may increase spike quantity and foci. Sustained ECoG spike multifocality may also represent evident or occult dual pathology.

Large spike fields may result from propagation of interictal discharges and from multifocal discharges. Therefore, the EEGer must distinguish between initiating and propagated spikes; two clues can help: i) background activity is more abnormal at the initiating site than the propagated one (Jasper, 1954); and ii) examined closely, initiating spikes often contain one more phase than propagated ones. Note that propagated spikes, issuing from normal or more normal cortex, may have higher voltage than those from areas with abnormal background activity and these latter are more likely the initiators.

Jasper also noted increased abundance of spikes at the periphery of an epileptogenic lesion after removal of a principal spike focus. If the epileptogenic lesion extends to this area or its background activity has been clearly abnormal, further removal should be considered if this area is not a neurologically functional one. However, such peripheral spike activation may be transient, reflecting mild resection trauma or loss of the "surround inhibition" that was generated by the principal epileptogenic area (Li, 1959; Prince & Wilder, 1967).

The EEG technologist and EEGer must be aware of seizures during the procedure for epilepsy localization and immediate patient care purposes. ECoG seizure morphology – with its morphological and frequency evolutions – differs little from scalp seizures except for better display of high-frequency potentials at seizure onset.

■ Electrical stimulation of the cortex

Mapping areas of various cortical functions can be the only purpose of electrical stimulation of the cortex during ECoG; site of after-discharge (AD) generation correlates inadequately with that of spontaneous seizure origin (Jasper, 1954; Blume *et al.*, 2004). The normally varying AD thresholds among cortical areas may require adjustment of stimulus parameters. Appropriate stimulus parameters may range as follows: diphasic pulse duration 0.3-2.0 msec; 50-60 Hz; 1.5-18 mA, beginning at the lowest current. This current is applied between 2 electrodes from a surgeon-held probe for 1-5 seconds (Holmes & Chatrian, 2007). Our 2004 study in patients with epilepsy disclosed that 8% of stimuli elicited ADs that involved more than one electrode position. Therefore, without ECoG monitoring, the occurrence of ADs could mislocalise cortical function.

Acknowlegements

We thank Dr. David Steven who performed the partial right inferior frontal lobectomy and Dr. Richard McLachlan who interpreted the electrocorticogram.

References

- Awad IA, Rosenfeld J, Ahl J, Hahn JF, Luders H. Intractable epilepsy and structural lesions of the brain: mapping, resection strategies, and seizure outcome. *Epilepsia* 1991; 32: 179-86.
- Blume WT, Holloway GM, Wiebe S. Temporal epileptogenesis: localizing value of scalp and subdural interictal and ictal data. *Epilepsia* 2001; 42: 508-14.
- Blume WT, Jones DC, Pathak P. Properties of after-discharges from cortical electrical stimulation in focal epilepsies. *Clin Neurophysiol* 2004; 115 (4): 982-9.
- Blume WT, Wiebe S, Tapsell LM. Occipital lobe epilepsy: lateral *versus* medial. *Brain* 2005; 128: 1209-25.
- Chatrian G-E. Intraoperative electrocorticography. In: Ebersole JS, Pedley TA. *Current Practice of Clinical Electrocorticography*, 3rd ed. Philadelphia: Lippincott Williams & Wilkins, 2003, pp. 681-712.
- Crino P. The pathophysiology of tuberous sclerosis complex. *Epilepsia* 2010; 51 (Suppl 1): 27-9.
- Dubeau F, Palmini A, Fish D, Avoli M, Gambardella A, Spreafico R, Andermann F. The significance of electrocorticographic findings in focal cortical dysplasia: a review of their clinical, electrophysiological and neurochemical characteristics. *Electroencephalogr Clin Neurophysiol Suppl* 1998; 48: 77-96.
- Gambardella A, Palmini A, Andermann F, Dubeau F, DaCosta JC, Quesney LF, et al. Usefulness of focal rhythmic discharges on scalp EEG of patients with focal cortical dysplasia and intractable epilepsy. *Electroencephalogr Clin Neurophysiol* 1996; 98: 243-9.
- Holmes MD, Chatrian G-E. Intraoperative electrocorticography. In: Engel JJr, Pedley TA (eds.). *Epilepsy A Comprehensive Textbook*, 2nd edition. Philadelphia: Lippincott Williams & Wilkins, 2007, pp. 1817-1831.
- Jasper HH. Electrocorticography. In: Penfield W, Jasper H. *Epilepsy and the Functional Anatomy of the Human Brain*. Boston: Little Brown, 1954, pp. 692-736.
- Jiang J, Ang LC, Blume WT. Extent of EEG epileptiform pattern distribution in "focal" cortical dysplasia. *J. Clin Neurophysiol* 2010; 27 (5): 309-11.
- Li C-L. Cortical intracellular potentials and their responses to strychnine. *J Neurophysiol* 1959; 22: 436.
- Lowenstein DH, Thomas MJ, Smith DH, McIntosh TK. Selective vulnerability of dentate hilar neurons following traumatic brain injury: a potential mechanistic link between head trauma and disorders of the hippocampus. *J Neurosci* 1992; 12 (12): 4846-53.
- Palmini A. Electrophysiology of focal cortical dysplasia. *Epilepsia* 2010; 51 (Suppl 1): 23-6.

- Paterson JH, McKissock W. A clinical survey of intracranial angiomas with special reference to their progress and surgical treatment: a report of 110 patients. *Brain* 1956; 79: 233-66.
- Pathale P, Blume WT. Asymmetrical epileptogenicity of brain lesions. *Epilepsia* 1997; 38 (Suppl 8): 64.
- Prince DA, Wilder BJ. Control mechanisms in cortical epileptogenic foci: "Surround inhibition" *Arch Neurol* 1967; 16: 194.
- Quesney LF. Preoperative electroencephalographic investigation in frontal lobe epilepsy: electroencephalographic and electrocorticographic recordings. *Can J Neurol Sci* 1991; 18 (Suppl 4): 559-63.
- Rasmussen T. Characteristics of a pure culture of frontal lobe epilepsy. *Epilepsia* 1983; 24: 482-93.
- So NK. Depth electrode studies in mesial temporal epilepsy. In: Luders HO (ed.). *Epilepsy Surgery.* New York: Raven Press, 1991, pp.371-384.
- Wennberg R, Quesney LF, Olivier A, Rasmussen T. Post-excision residual spiking after frontal lobe removal: outcome. *Electroencephalogr Clin Neurophysiol Suppl* 1998; 48: 97-104.

Event-related ECoG spectra and functional mapping in extratemporal brain regions

Mackenzie C. Cervenka, Nathan E. Crone

Department of Neurology, The Johns Hopkins University School of Medicine, Baltimore, USA

■ Introduction

Electrocorticographic (ECoG) spectral analysis is an emerging technique for mapping cortical function prior to epilepsy surgery that uses task-related fluctuations in EEG power spectra to identify functional activation of cortical areas sampled by intracranial EEG electrodes. ECoG spectral mapping was originally developed as an alternative to electrocortical stimulation mapping (ESM) for identifying "eloquent" cortex in patients undergoing surgical planning for intractable epilepsy. The term "eloquent" is used to describe any cortical region that is essential for linguistic, motor, or sensory function that if resected, will likely result in a deficit. While ESM involves direct stimulation of the cortex to produce a temporary functional deficit, ECoG spectral mapping involves passively recording and analyzing electrographic changes that occur over the surface of the brain. ECoG spectral mapping has been used to study cortical regions involved in sensorimotor functions, special sensory functions (visual and auditory), attention, memory, and language, and recently to control brain-computer and brain-machine interfaces.

The principles of ECoG spectral analysis can be traced back to early studies of scalp electroencephalography (EEG) when neuroscientists first recognized and described event-related changes in background EEG rhythms within discrete frequency ranges, at discrete times, and spatial distributions over the cortex (Adrian, 1934; Chatrian, 1959; Gastaut, 1952; Jasper, 1938). Examples include the posterior dominant rhythm or alpha rhythm seen over the occipital lobes in a resting patient with eye closure, and the mu rhythm seen over the sensorimotor cortex immediately before initiation of a contralateral movement that resolves with movement onset. The physiologic frequency ranges in which event-related changes have been commonly investigated with non-invasive scalp EEG include the theta (4-7 Hz), alpha (8-13 Hz), and beta (13-25 Hz) frequencies. Scalp EEG has also been used to study event-related changes in higher frequencies collectively referred to as gamma (> 30 Hz) frequencies. However, the signal-to-noise ratio of scalp EEG at these higher frequencies is suboptimal because of the small amplitude of this activity in relation to scalp myogenic artifacts. ECoG recordings from the cortical surface provide an opportunity to study event-related changes in high frequencies, as well as in lower, traditional frequency bands, and to use different markers of cortical activation for functional mapping.

Detection of EEG or ECoG spectral changes indexing functional brain activation usually requires signal decomposition into time – and frequency – dependent estimates of signal energy or power. The signal power in a given frequency band is typically averaged over multiple trials of a given task or event. In order to statistically evaluate event-related changes in signal power or energy, signals averaged in the frequency domain are compared to signals obtained during a "baseline" interval where the brain is assumed to be in a "resting", "default", or relatively inactive state (Pfurtscheller, 1999). Results yield an increase or decrease in spectral power within discrete frequency bands, which can then be temporally and spatially correlated to task-related cortical activation or inhibition.

Because EEG signals represent the summed membrane potentials of a large population of neurons and their amplitudes are sensitive to the synchronization of these potentials, fluctuations in the power of these signals have most often been conceptualized in relation to changes in the synchronization of neuronal population activity. This is particularly justifiable when there is a well defined peak in the EEG power spectrum. Gert Pfurtscheller (1977) first used the term event-related desynchronization (ERD) to describe event-related power suppression in frequency bands where well defined EEG rhythms were observed during resting states (a.k.a. "resting rhythms"). These have included the posterior basic rhythm over visual cortex (Adrian, 1934), the central mu rhythm over motor cortex described previously (Chatrian, 1959), and the tau rhythm over auditory cortex (Lehtela, 1997). In these cases, power suppression was interpreted as a loss of synchronization, *i.e.* a desynchronization, within the neuronal generators of resting rhythms during cortical activation. Conversely, band-specific power augmentation has been described as event-related synchronization (ERS). Event-related synchronization (ERS) has been identified, for example, within the beta band over motor cortex immediately following movement onset (Neuper, 1996; Stancak, 1995).

Event-related changes in EEG/ECoG signal power can be interpreted as markers of functional brain activation. For example, power suppression, or ERD, in alpha and beta bands has been demonstrated to reflect functional cortical activation while ERS in these frequency ranges has correlated with cortical inhibition (Pfurtscheller, 1989). However, in higher frequencies (gamma, > 30 Hz) the reverse has been demonstrated. Power augmentation in gamma frequencies typically reflects cortical activation (Crone, 2006), while gamma power suppression may reflect cortical inhibition (Lachaux, 2008).

Power augmentation in higher frequency bands within the gamma range (> 30 Hz) has been observed during functional activation in a variety of functional-anatomic domains. In some cases, the observed power augmentation has been found in well-defined gamma bands, justifying the term ERS (Pfurtscheller, 1994). However, the most consistent power augmentation during cortical activation has been observed in a broad range of gamma frequencies that are usually higher than the gamma frequencies where band-limited gamma augmentation, *i.e.* ERS, has been found most often. Although broadband gamma augmentation has for convenience been commonly referred to as "high-gamma", its frequency range (typically 60-200 Hz) can overlap the frequencies at which band-limited gamma responses are most commonly observed (40-80 Hz).

Electrocortical stimulation mapping (ESM) is currently the "gold standard" for mapping eloquent cortex in preparation for surgery. However, this technique has important limitations. For example, it can provoke pain and seizure discharges and at times it can produce equivocal results. The procedure is time-consuming and labor intensive for medical staff and often all electrodes are not evaluated as a result. In addition, patients occasionally demonstrate postoperative deficits (especially in language function) despite adherence to boundaries designated as regions of eloquent cortex based on ESM findings (Hamberger, 2005; Sinai, 2005). ECoG spectral mapping is a less invasive alternative to ESM. All implanted electrodes can be assessed simultaneously to provide measures of cortical activation, and the passive recording of electrocerebral activity does not require cortical stimulation, eliminating the possibility of provoking pain or seizure discharges. The clinical utility of this technique continues to be evaluated by comparing the results to ESM and to other brain mapping techniques as well as to postoperative outcomes following surgery (Brunner, 2009; Miller, 2007b; Sinai, 2005; Towle, 2008). Advances in ECoG spectral mapping could eventually improve the accuracy of cortical mapping in preparation for surgical intervention, but for now its clinical utility is probably most appropriate as a complement to ESM.

■ ECoG spectral mapping in extratemporal cortex

Electrocorticographic spectral mapping has been used to map human cortical function with excellent spatial and temporal resolution. Although temporal lobe function has been the focus of many of these studies, a variety of other studies have either focused exclusively on extratemporal cortex (e.g. motor, somatosensory, prefrontal, or visual cortex) or have by necessity included extratemporal cortex because the function studied necessarily involved activation of extratemporal cortex (e.g. language function). Functions that have been investigated using ECoG spectral mapping have included vision (Asano, 2009; Lachaux, 2005; Tallon-Baudry, 2005), hearing (Crone, 2001a; Edwards, 2005; Trautner, 2006), planning and execution of movements (Crone, 1998a; Gonzalez, 2006; Miller, 2007b; Miller, 2009; Ohara, 2000; Rektor, 2006; Szurhaj, 2006), somatosensory function (Ray, 2008), and language perception and production (Brown, 2008; Crone, 2001b; Jung, 2008; Lachaux, 2007; Mainy, 2008; Ray, 2003; Sinai, 2005; Sinai, 2009; Tanji, 2005; Towle, 2008). ECoG spectral analysis has also been used to study cortical mechanisms of attention and memory (Axmacher, 2006; Axmacher, 2008; Brovelli, 2005; Howard, 2003; Jung, 2008; Mormann, 2005; Ray, 2008; Sederberg, 2003; Sederberg, 2007a; Sederberg, 2007b).

Areas involved in visual processing have been identified within occipital cortex and fusiform gyrus (Asano, 2009; Lachaux, 2005; Tallon-Baudry, 2005). Regions involved with auditory perception have been identified over the superior temporal gyrus and will not be discussed further as our focus here is on mapping extratemporal cortex. Regions involved in planning and execution of movements have been identified in premotor and primary motor regions of the frontal lobes, even during single trials (Gonzalez, 2006; Miller, 2007b), and with enough spatial resolution to differentiate movements of individual fingers (Miller, 2009). Language perception and production have been shown to involve not only the dominant perisylvian temporal cortex, but also frontal, parietal, and occipital regions, depending on the language task performed and the language modalities assessed (Crone, 2001b; Jung, 2008; Sinai, 2005). Memory tasks have resulted in activation of expected mesial temporal structures, but also prefrontal areas, perisylvian regions, Broca's area, auditory and prefrontal cortex, postcentral gyrus, and fusiform gyrus (Mainy, 2007; Axmacher, 2008).

■ Mapping visual function

ECoG spectral mapping of visual cortex has been performed using a variety of visual stimuli including pictures of faces, discrimination between shapes, and stroboscopic flash-stimuli (Asano, 2009; Lachaux, 2005; Tallon-Baudry, 2005). Epilepsy patients with implanted posterior depth and subdural grid electrodes were studied. Lachaux *et al.* (2005) studied visual responses using a face detection task in four adult epilepsy patients with implanted depth electrodes sampling the parieto-occipital cortex. They identified broad-band (40-200 Hz) gamma activity over the fusiform gyrus, the lateral occipital gyrus and intra-parietal sulcus (Lachaux, 2005). Using this technique, they were able to identify early temporal-occipital changes, followed by parietal activation. They also identified alpha and gamma suppression that temporally correlated with gamma augmentation. Tallon-Baudry *et al.* (2005) also demonstrated gamma activity within the lateral occipital regions and the fusiform gyrus during a visual stimulus discrimination task. Furthermore, they demonstrated that increased attention resulted in an increase in gamma activity prior to stimulus onset within the lateral occipital region and during stimulus presentation in the fusiform gyrus. The authors concluded that the role of gamma activity differs between posterior cortical regions during visual tasks.

Asano *et al.* (2009) evaluated nine children who received intracranial monitoring with subdural electrodes for seizure localization that included coverage of visual cortex. During stroboscopic flash-stimuli, they found broadband high-gamma augmentation (50-150 Hz) first over anterior-medial occipital cortex, followed by lateral-polar occipital cortex. These studies not only identified cortical regions involved in visual perception but also demonstrated the change in localization of activated cortex over time.

■ Mapping of motor function

Motor mapping is often necessary prior to extratemporal epilepsy surgery near frontal and/or parietal cortex to identify eloquent motor cortex, and to avoid resection that will result in postoperative paresis or paralysis. In some instances, the neurosurgeon can avoid eloquent motor cortex by identifying anatomic landmarks such as the central sulcus and precentral gyrus. However, these landmarks may not always be fully exposed during craniotomy and may not be evident, especially if distorted by adjacent tumor or other focal lesions. In these instances, motor mapping is crucial in the operating room or during extra-operative intracranial monitoring to assure accurate identification of eloquent motor cortex.

Intraoperatively, a strip of electrodes can be placed on the cortical surface over the region suspected to contain the central sulcus. Somatosensory evoked potentials (SEPs) can be recorded from median, ulnar, and tibial nerve stimulation to identify the central sulcus (Baumgartner, 1991a; Baumgartner, 1998; Lueders, 1983), but these results may be subject to interpretation (Allison, 1991). The same procedure can be performed extra-operatively with subdural electrodes (Baumgartner, 1992) and can also be performed non-invasively with magnetoencephalography (MEG) (Baumgartner, 1991b). Electrocortical stimulation mapping of motor function is often performed in addition to or in place of SEPs to further define the boundaries of eloquent motor cortex. ECoG spectral analysis provides a complimentary measure of motor activation that has been used to identify the cortical areas activated during different kinds of movement in different body parts.

Many studies have explored the clinical utility of ECoG spectral mapping of sensorimotor function in extratemporal lobe epilepsy patients undergoing surgery (Aoki, 1999; Brunner, 2009; Crone, 1998a; Crone, 1998b; Leuthardt, 2007; Miller, 2007b; Ohara, 2000; Pfurtscheller, 2003; Szurhaj, 2005). ECoG recordings have identified alpha and beta ERD over sensorimotor cortex during movement tasks (Crone, 1998a; Crone, 1998b; Leuthardt, 2007; Toro, 1994). Crone et al. (1998) demonstrated diffuse alpha ERD during initiation of a muscle contraction as well as more somatotopically localized, though less robust beta ERD (Crone, 1998b). Alpha and beta ERD were seen over both contralateral and ipsilateral sensorimotor cortices during unilateral limb movements with overlapping distributions of ERD for different limbs. During the same limb movements, ECoG gamma power increased over more focal cortical regions and high gamma (75-100 Hz) augmentation was observed with a spatial distribution and temporal profile that was even more specific.

Many researchers have studied gamma augmentation as a marker for sensorimotor function through a variety of movement tasks and methods of data analysis while assessing patients with intracranial grid electrodes over motor and premotor cortex (Aoki, 1999; Brovelli, 2005; Leuthardt, 2007; Ohara, 2000; Reddy, 2009; Szurhaj, 2005). Ohara et al. (2000) analyzed gamma activity during self-paced finger and wrist movements and found an increase in gamma power over motor cortex during contralateral movements, and a high temporal correlation to movement onset within a high gamma frequency band (60-90 Hz). Pfurtscheller et al. (2003) demonstrated high gamma (60-90 Hz) ERS over somatotopically-specific regions of the sensorimotor cortex during self-paced tongue and finger movements, with more widespread alpha and beta ERD. Reddy et al. (2009) recently used detection of high gamma augmentation (50-160 Hz) to accurately differentiate hand movements of a joystick in 4 cardinal directions (up, down, left or right) in six patients. Broadband high gamma augmentation (60-200 Hz) has also been demonstrated during motor planning tasks over premotor cortex (Brovelli, 2005). Despite differing techniques and movement tasks used, these studies all revealed gamma and high gamma augmentation that spatially and temporally correlated with movement onset. Furthermore, they suggest that ECoG spectral mapping is a reliable technique for motor mapping prior to cortical resection.

Studies have compared ECoG spectral mapping results to electrocortical stimulation mapping (EMS) of motor activity in order to assess the relative accuracy of ECoG spectral mapping compared to other functional mapping techniques. In a large series of 22 patients, Miller et al. (2007b) compared low (8-32 Hz) and high frequency (76-100 Hz) power changes during a variety of motor tasks with different body parts and demonstrated high gamma power augmentation over a more discrete spatial distribution than low frequency ERD. They then compared the ECoG spectral mapping results to the results of electrocortical stimulation mapping in a subset of these patients and demonstrated a significant increase in high gamma activity in 17 of 20 electrode pairs that inhibited motor activity during ESM. Recently, Brunner et al. (2009) produced a functional cortical map of hand and tongue movements using ECoG spectral analysis in only a few minutes with a low false positive rate of 0.46% for hand movements and 1.10% for tongue movements compared to ESM, and no false negatives. This finding suggests that ECoG functional mapping might be used for real-time mapping of motor cortex with improving accuracy compared to ESM.

ECoG spectral mapping is also being investigated as a tool in the control of brain-computer interfaces (BCI) and brain-machine interfaces to operate prosthetic devices through detection and interpretation of ECoG signal changes. This would allow patients with progressive neuromuscular diseases or other conditions causing paralysis but sparing cortical function to improve mobility and performance of independent activities of daily living (Tai, 2008). ECoG signal changes must be detected rapidly and with excellent spatial accuracy in order to ultimately be translated into the precise movement of a prosthetic device.

Leuthardt et al. (2004) first demonstrated the use of ECoG signals to control vertical computer cursor movements in a single patient. This was performed following a 3-24 minute training period by using imagination of motor and speech actions, through a closed-loop paradigm. Leuthardt et al. (2006) then used this paradigm to study one-dimensional cursor control in four epilepsy patients with electrodes implanted over motor cortex, and demonstrated accuracies between 73-100%. Ramsey et al. (2006) observed gamma augmentation in the dorsolateral prefrontal cortex during mental calculation and proposed that this could be used as input into a BCI application. Miller et al. (Miller, 2007a) showed that high gamma power augmentation could be detected during single trials of a motor task. Miller et al. (2009) then demonstrated the spatial accuracy of ECoG spectral mapping by identifying broadband ECoG changes that differentiated finger tapping movements of individual fingers in ten epilepsy patients. Kubanek et al. (2009) used ECoG changes to decode flexion of individual fingers in four epilepsy patients. Acharya et al. (2010) used low-pass filtered ECoG signals from perirolandic electrodes to decode slow finger and hand movements during a grasping exercise. All of these studies indicate that fine hand and finger movements can be accurately decoded using changes in ECoG spectra. In addition, feasibility studies of long-term implantation of intracranial electrodes in the treatment of pain have demonstrated the potential safety of this procedure (Osenbach, 2006; Rasche, 2006). Experiments are ongoing to use real-time ECoG spectral analysis to assist in controlling prosthetic devices.

■ Mapping of somatosensory function and attention

ECoG spectral mapping has also been used to assess cortical activation of somatosensory cortex, again with a focus on detection of high gamma augmentation. Ray et al. (2008) compared conditions where patients were asked to attend to or ignore a vibrotactile stimulus and found an increase in high gamma activity over somatosensory cortex when subjects were attending to the stimulus, rather than ignoring it. Several studies have been performed using magnetoencephalography (MEG) in healthy subjects to assess high gamma activation during somatosensory tasks (Bauer, 2006; Gross, 2007; Hauck, 2007; Ihara, 2003). Bauer et al. (2006) demonstrated enhanced 60-95 Hz MEG responses in the contralateral primary somatosensory cortex in response to direct attention to tactile stimulation. Gross et al. (2007) also showed an increase in 60-95 Hz oscillatory activity in primary somatosensory cortex during perceived compared to unperceived noxious stimuli of equal intensity using MEG. MEG has been used to assess lower frequency gamma activity but is less sensitive than ECoG in evaluating more broadband gamma responses.

■ Mapping of memory

Although preservation of memory function is of greatest concern when planning epilepsy surgery involving resection of mesial temporal structures (Busch, 2008; Glikmann-Johnston, 2008; Guerreiro, 1999), many extratemporal regions also play a critical role in memory formation (Mainy, 2007; Axmacher, 2008). Studies have investigated the "phonological loop" involved with working memory, including regions within the frontal lobe (prefrontal cortex, precentral gyrus, and Broca's area), and within the parietal lobe (postcentral gyrus), as well as portions of the temporal lobe (Mainy, 2007; Axmacher, 2008). Mainy *et al.* (2007) mapped encoding in working memory in nine epilepsy patients with implanted electrodes and identified an increase in broadband high gamma (50-150 Hz) activity within the phonological loop. Axmacher *et al.* (2008) combined ECoG spectral mapping of gamma activity (51-75 Hz) and fMRI to study visual working memory and demonstrated the role of prefrontal cortex using both measures.

Several studies have also demonstrated ECoG spectral changes during a variety of other memory tasks within extratemporal regions (Axmacher, 2008; Howard, 2003; Mainy, 2007; Mormann, 2005; Sederberg, 2003; Sederberg, 2007a; Sederberg, 2007b). Sederberg *et al.* (2003) asked ten epilepsy patients with implanted subdural grid electrodes to memorize a list of common nouns and found an increase in theta power over discrete regions involving not only the right temporal but also the right frontal cortex and more widespread gamma increases (28-64 Hz) during successful noun encoding compared to unsuccessful encoding. In a subsequent study, Sederberg *et al.* (2007a) examined 39 patients with a total of 2349 surgically implanted electrodes and demonstrated an increase in gamma power within a narrow frequency range of 44-64 Hz over the left frontal cortex as well as the left temporal and mesial temporal structures. In a larger study of 52 epilepsy patients with implanted electrodes, Sederberg *et al.* (2007b) identified greater increases in broadband activity (28-100 Hz) over prefrontal cortex and temporal structures during true than during false memories. Howard *et al.* (2003) also demonstrated a linear correlation between an increase in gamma activity (30-60 Hz) and memory load over a broad cortical distribution. These findings suggest that extratemporal regions play an important role in memory formation and that ECoG spectral mapping is a useful tool in demonstrating the spatial distribution of memory function in epilepsy patients with implanted electrodes.

■ Mapping of extratemporal language function

ECoG spectral mapping has been used extensively to measure cortical activation during a variety of expressive and receptive language tasks including auditory question presentation with responses, visual object naming, reading, signing, lexical decision tasks, word recognition and word repetition (Brown, 2008; Crone, 2001b; Jung, 2008; Mainy, 2008; Ray, 2003; Sinai, 2005; Tanji, 2005; Towle, 2008). High gamma augmentation (> 60 Hz) has been found to be a reliable marker for activation of language cortex. Regions of cortical activation ultimately depend on the types of stimuli presented such as auditory versus visual and whether or not verbal responses were elicited. Only those studies that included activation of extratemporal cortical regions will be reviewed here.

In an early study of cortical activation using ECoG spectral analysis of 80-100 Hz gamma activity, Crone *et al.* (2001b) demonstrated differences in the spatial organization of language cortex recruited for spoken versus signed language. They studied responses to visual object naming, word reading, and word repetition tasks in an epilepsy patient fluent in

English and in American Sign Language. Naming and reading in English produced activation over basal temporo-occipital cortex, spoken responses activated tongue regions within the primary motor cortex, and signed responses produced activation in the hand regions.

Studies have also directly compared ECoG language mapping to language mapping with electrocortical stimulation (Crone, 2001b; Sinai, 2005; Sinai, 2009; Towle, 2008). In their study of cortical activation during English versus American Sign Language, Crone et al. (2001b) reported a correlation between ECoG spectral mapping results and ESM findings in both language modalities and during word reading, auditory word repetition, and object naming tasks. Sinai et al. (2005) compared visual object naming maps using ESM and ECoG spectral mapping of high gamma augmentation (80-100 Hz). They found a specificity of 78% and a sensitivity of 38% for naming with ECoG spectral mapping compared to ESM. In addition, they determined that the specificity for mouth-related motor function was 81% with a sensitivity of 46% for ECoG spectral mapping relative to ESM. Combining naming and mouth-related motor function mapping, the specificities and sensitivities increased to 84% and 43%, respectively. The authors concluded that ECoG language mapping could be used to produce a preliminary map of cortical activation during naming that could help guide ESM, but that the sensitivity of ECoG high gamma was not sufficient to replace ESM.

Towle et al. (2008) used an auditory word repetition task to demonstrate high gamma (70-100 Hz) augmentation within several cortical regions during stimulus presentation and during verbal responses in 12 pediatric and adult epilepsy patients. During stimulus presentation, activation occurred not only in the primary auditory cortex within the temporal lobe, but also in regions within the parietal cortex. Increased high gamma augmentation occurred over lateral frontal and anterior parietal cortex during verbal responses. They also compared ECoG spectral mapping results to ESM and reported a specificity of 57% with a sensitivity of 63%. In a more recent study, Sinai et al. (2009) examined speech comprehension and tone detection in six epilepsy patients with left lateral subdural electrode coverage and evaluated broadband high gamma power changes (60-250 Hz), then compared these results to ESM findings. They demonstrated a high spatial concordance between ESM and broadband high gamma augmentation, with a specificity of 98%, a sensitivity of 67% and a positive predictive value of 67%. These findings suggested that mapping of broadband high gamma activity was more accurate for auditory perceptual function, for which the functional anatomy is likely more densely organized than that of visual object naming.

One potential role for ECoG spectral mapping of language is for use in pediatric patients undergoing epilepsy surgery. ESM and Wada testing are less reliable in pediatric patients than in the adult epilepsy population (Hamberger, 2007; Schevon, 2007). In some pediatric populations, patients are unable to reliably follow instructions in order to obtain interpretable and reproducible results during ESM and Wada testing. Of the 12 patients studied by Towle (2008), 6 were under the age of 18, and ECoG spectral mapping of word repetition produced accurate results in these patients. In addition, Brown (2008) studied three children with intractable seizures and intracranial electrodes implanted over the left hemisphere during a question and answer task. They demonstrated increases in gamma (50-150 Hz) power over auditory cortex during question presentation, over the posterior frontal region between questions and answers, and over the pre- and post- central gyrus immediately preceding and during the delivery of answers. These findings suggest that ECoG spectral mapping is a safe and reliable alternative to ESM for mapping language in children.

■ Conclusions

Epilepsy patients with extratemporal seizure foci may require intracranial monitoring for seizure localization and for accurately mapping functionally important cortical regions prior to resective surgery. Electrocorticographic spectral mapping is an evolving technique that may provide a safer and more efficient means of mapping functional cortex in these patients compared to electrocortical stimulation mapping. Functions that have been mapped in extratemporal regions have included vision, motoric responses, somatosensory responses, attention, memory, and language processing. ECoG spectral mapping has been used to investigate the fine spatial and temporal dynamics of cortical activation associated with these functions. In addition, real-time mapping using ECoG spectral changes is leading to rapid advances in the development of brain-computer and brain-machine interfaces.

References

- Acharya S, Fifer MS, Benz HL, Crone NE, Thakor NV. Electrocorticographic amplitude predicts finger positions during slow grasping motions of the hand. *J Neural Eng* 2010; 7: 046002.
- Adrian ED, Matthews BHC. The Berger rhythm: potential changes from the occipital lobes in man. *Brain* 1934; 57: 355-85.
- Allison T, McCarthy G, Wood CC, Jones SJ. Potentials evoked in human and monkey cerebral cortex by stimulation of the median nerve. A review of scalp and intracranial recordings. *Brain* 1991; 114 (Pt 6): 2465-503.
- Aoki F, Fetz EE, Shupe L, Lettich E, Ojemann GA. Increased gamma-range activity in human sensorimotor cortex during performance of visuomotor tasks. *Clin Neurophysiol* 1999; 110: 524-37.
- Asano E, Nishida M, Fukuda M, Rothermel R, Juhasz C, Sood S. Differential visually-induced gamma-oscillations in human cerebral cortex. *Neuroimage* 2009; 45: 477-89.
- Axmacher N, Mormann F, Fernandez G, Elger CE, Fella J. Memory formation by neuronal synchronization. *Brain Research Reviews* 2006; 52: 170-82.
- Axmacher N, Schmitz DP, Wagner T, Elger CE, Fell J. Interactions between medial temporal lobe, prefrontal cortex, and inferior temporal regions during visual working memory: a combined intracranial EEG and functional magnetic resonance imaging study. *J Neurosci* 2008; 28: 7304-12.
- Bauer M, Oostenveld R, Peeters M, Fries P. Tactile spatial attention enhances gamma-band activity in somatosensory cortex and reduces low-frequency activity in parieto-occipital areas. *J Neurosci* 2006; 26: 490-501.
- Baumgartner C, Barth DS, Levesque MF, Sutherling WW. Functional anatomy of human hand sensorimotor cortex from spatiotemporal analysis of electrocorticography. *Electroencephalogr Clin Neurophysiol* 1991a; 78: 56-65.
- Baumgartner C, Barth DS, Levesque MF, Sutherling WW. Human hand and lip sensorimotor cortex as studied on electrocorticography. *Electroencephalogr Clin Neurophysiol* 1992; 84: 115-26.
- Baumgartner C, Doppelbauer A, Deecke L, Barth D, Zeitlhofer J, Lindinger G, *et al.* Neuromagnetic investigation of somatotopy of human hand somatosensory cortex. *Experimental Brain Research* 1991b; 8: 641-8.

- Baumgartner U, Vogel H, Ellrich J, Gawehn J, Stoeter P, Treede RD. Brain electrical source analysis of primary cortical components of the tibial nerve somatosensory evoked potential using regional sources. *Electroencephalogr Clin Neurophysiol* 1998; 108: 588-99.

- Brovelli A, Lachaux JP, Kahane P, Boussaoud D. High gamma frequency oscillatory activity dissociates attention from intention in the human premotor cortex. *Neuroimage* 2005; 28: 154-64.

- Brown EC, Rothermel R, Nishida M, Juhasz C, Muzik O, Hoechstetter K, *et al*. In vivo animation of auditory-language-induced gamma-oscillations in children with intractable focal epilepsy. *Neuroimage* 2008; 41: 1120-31.

- Brunner P, Ritaccio AL, Lynch TM, Emrich JF, Wilson JA, Williams JC, *et al*. A practical procedure for real-time functional mapping of eloquent cortex using electrocorticographic signals in humans. *Epilepsy Behav* 2009;15: 278-86.

- Busch RM, Chapin JS, Umashankar G, Diehl B, Harvey D, Naugle RI, *et al*. Poor presurgical performance on both verbal and visual memory measures is associated with low risk for memory decline following left temporal lobectomy for intractable epilepsy. *Epileptic Disord* 2008; 10: 199-205.

- Chatrian GE, Petersen MC, Lazarte JA. The blocking of the rolandic wicket rhythm and some central changes related to movement. *Electroencephalography and clinical Neurophysiology* 1959; 11: 497-510.

- Crone NE, Boatman D, Gordon B, Hao L. Induced electrocorticographic gamma activity during auditory perception. *Clin Neurophysiol* 2001a; 112: 565-82.

- Crone NE, Hao L, Hart J, Jr., Boatman D, Lesser RP, Irizarry R, *et al*. Electrocorticographic gamma activity during word production in spoken and sign language. *Neurology* 2001b; 57: 2045-53.

- Crone NE, Miglioretti DL, Gordon B, Lesser RP. Functional mapping of human sensorimotor cortex with electrocorticographic spectral analysis. II. Event-related synchronization in the gamma band. *Brain* 1998a; 121: 2301-15.

- Crone NE, Miglioretti DL, Gordon B, Sieracki JM, Wilson MT, Uematsu S, *et al*. Functional mapping of human sensorimotor cortex with electrocorticographic spectral analysis. I. Alpha and beta event-related desynchronization. *Brain* 1998b; 121: 2271-99.

- Crone NE, Sinai AS, Korzeniewska A. High-frequency gamma oscillations and human brain mapping with electrocorticography. *Prog Brain Res* 2006; 159: 279-302.

- Edwards E, Soltani M, Deouell LY, Berger MS, Knight RT. High gamma activity in response to deviant auditory stimuli recorded directly from human cortex. *J Neurophysiol* 2005; 94: 4269-80.

- Gastaut H. Etude electrocorticographique de la reactivite des rythmes rolandiques. *Rev.Neurol.(Paris)* 1952; 87: 176-82.

- Glikmann-Johnston Y, Saling MM, Chen J, Cooper KA, Beare RJ, Reutens DC. Structural and functional correlates of unilateral mesial temporal lobe spatial memory impairment. *Brain* 2008; 131: 3006-18.

- Gonzalez SL, de Peralta RG, Thut G, Millan JD, Morier P, Landis T. Very high frequency oscillations (VHFO) as a predictor of movement intentions. *Neuroimage* 2006; 32: 170-9.

- Gross J, Schnitzler A, Timmermann L, Ploner M. Gamma oscillations in human primary somatosensory cortex reflect pain perception. *PLoS Biology* 2007; 5: 1168-73.

- Guerreiro C, Cendes F, Li LM, Jones-Gotman M, Andermann F, Dubeau F, *et al*. Clinical patterns of patients with temporal lobe epilepsy and pure amygdalar atrophy. *Epilepsia* 1999; 40: 453-61.

- Hamberger MJ. Cortical language mapping in epilepsy: a critical review. *Neuropsychol Rev* 2007; 17: 477-89.

- Hamberger MJ, Seidel WT, McKhann GM, 2nd, Perrine K, Goodman RR. Brain stimulation reveals critical auditory naming cortex. *Brain* 2005; 128: 2742-9.

- Hauck M, Lorenz J, Engel AK. Attention to painful stimulation enhances gamma-band activity and synchronization in human sensorimotor cortex. *J Neurosci* 2007; 27: 9270-7.
- Howard MW, Rizzuto DS, Caplan JB, Madsen JR, Lisman J, Aschenbrenner-Scheibe R, *et al.* Gamma oscillations correlate with working memory load in humans. *Cereb Cortex* 2003; 13: 1369-74.
- Ihara A, Hirata M, Yanagihara K, Ninomiya H, Imai K, Ishii R, *et al.* Neuromagnetic gamma-band activity in the primary and secondary somatosensory areas. *Neuroreport* 2003; 14: 273-7.
- Jasper HH, Andrews HL. Electro-encephalography. III. Normal differentiation of occipital and precentral regions in man. *Archives of Neurology and Psychiatry* 1938; 39: 96-115.
- Jung J, Mainy N, Kahane P, Minotti L, Hoffmann D, Bertrand O, *et al.* The neural bases of attentive reading. *Hum Brain Mapp* 2008; 29: 1193-206.
- Kubanek J, Miller KJ, Ojemann JG, Wolpaw JR, Schalk G. Decoding flexion of individual fingers using electrocorticographic signals in humans. *J Neural Eng* 2009; 6: 066001.
- Lachaux JP, Fonlupt P, Kahane P, Minotti L, Hoffmann D, Bertrand O, *et al.* Relationship between task-related gamma oscillations and BOLD signal: New insights from combined fMRI and intracranial EEG. *Hum Brain Mapp* 2007 ; 28: 1368-75.
- Lachaux JP, George N, Tallon-Baudry C, Martinerie J, Hugueville L, Minotti L, *et al.* The many faces of the gamma band response to complex visual stimuli. *Neuroimage* 2005; 25: 491-501.
- Lachaux JP, Jung J, Mainy N, Dreher JC, Bertrand O, Baciu M, *et al.* Silence is golden: transient neural deactivation in the prefrontal cortex during attentive reading. *Cereb Cortex* 2008; 18: 443-50.
- Lehtela L, Salmelin R, Hari R. Evidence for reactive magnetic 10-Hz rhythm in the human auditory cortex. *Neurosci Lett* 1997; 222: 111-4.
- Leuthardt EC, Miller K, Anderson NR, Schalk G, Dowling J, Miller J, *et al.* Electrocorticographic frequency alteration mapping: a clinical technique for mapping the motor cortex. *Neurosurgery* 2007; 60: 260-70; discussion 270-1.
- Leuthardt EC, Miller KJ, Schalk G, Rao RP, Ojemann JG. Electrocorticography-based brain computer interface--the Seattle experience. *IEEE Trans Neural Syst Rehabil Eng* 2006; 14: 194-8.
- Leuthardt EC, Schalk G, Wolpaw JR, Ojemann JG, Moran DW. A brain-computer interface using electrocorticographic signals in humans. *J Neural Eng* 2004; 1: 63-71.
- Lueders H, Lesser RP, Hahn J, Dinner DS, Klem G. Cortical somatosensory evoked potentials in response to hand stimulation. *Journal of Neurosurgery* 1983; 58: 885-894.
- Mainy N, Jung J, Baciu M, Kahane P, Schoendorff B, Minotti L, *et al.* Cortical dynamics of word recognition. *Hum Brain Mapp* 2008; 29: 1215-30.
- Mainy N, Kahane P, Minotti L, Hoffmann D, Bertrand O, Lachaux JP. Neural correlates of consolidation in working memory. *Hum Brain Mapp* 2007; 28: 183-93.
- Miller KJ, denNijs M, Shenoy P, Miller JW, Rao RP, Ojemann JG. Real-time functional brain mapping using electrocorticography. *Neuroimage* 2007a; 37: 504-7.
- Miller KJ, Leuthardt EC, Schalk G, Rao RP, Anderson NR, Moran DW, *et al.* Spectral changes in cortical surface potentials during motor movement. *J Neurosci* 2007b; 27: 2424-32.
- Miller KJ, Zanos S, Fetz EE, den Nijs M, Ojemann JG. Decoupling the cortical power spectrum reveals real-time representation of individual finger movements in humans. *J Neurosci* 2009; 29: 3132-7.
- Mormann F, Fell J, Axmacher N, Weber B, Lehnertz K, Elger CE, *et al.* Phase/amplitude reset and theta-gamma interaction in the human medial temporal lobe during a continuous word recognition memory task. *Hippocampus* 2005; 15: 890-900.
- Neuper C, Pfurtscheller G. Post-movement synchronization of beta rhythms in the EEG over the cortical foot area in man. *Neuroscience Letters* 1996; 216: 17-20.

- Ohara S, Ikeda A, Kunieda T, Yazawa S, Baba K, Nagamine T, *et al*. Movement-related change of electrocorticographic activity in human supplementary motor area proper. *Brain* 2000; 123: 1203-15.
- Osenbach RK. Motor cortex stimulation for intractable pain. *Neurosurg Focus* 2006; 21: E7.
- Pfurtscheller G. Graphical display and statistical evaluation of event-related desynchronization (ERD). *Electroencephalography and clinical Neurophysiology* 1977; 43: 757-60.
- Pfurtscheller G. Functional topography during sensorimotor activation studied with event-related desynchronization mapping. *J.Clin.Neurophysiol.* 1989; 6: 75-84.
- Pfurtscheller G, Flotzinger D, Neuper C. Differentiation between finger, toe and tongue movement in man based on 40 Hz EEG. *Electroencephalography and Clinical Neurophysiology* 1994; 90: 456-60.
- Pfurtscheller G, Graimann B, Huggins JE, Levine SP, Schuh LA. Spatiotemporal patterns of beta desynchronization and gamma synchronization in corticographic data during self-paced movement. *Clin Neurophysiol* 2003; 114: 1226-36.
- Pfurtscheller G, Lopes da Silva FH. Event-related EEG/MEG synchronization and desynchronization: basic principles. *Clin Neurophysiol* 1999; 110: 1842-57.
- Ramsey NF, van de Heuvel MP, Kho KH, Leijten FS. Towards human BCI applications based on cognitive brain systems: an investigation of neural signals recorded from the dorsolateral prefrontal cortex. *IEEE Trans Neural Syst Rehabil Eng* 2006; 14: 214-7.
- Rasche D, Ruppolt M, Stippich C, Unterberg A, Tronnier VM. Motor cortex stimulation for long-term relief of chronic neuropathic pain: a 10 year experience. *Pain* 2006; 121: 43-52.
- Ray S, Jouny CC, Crone NE, Boatman D, Thakor NV, Franaszczuk PJ. Human ECoG analysis during speech perception using matching pursuit: a comparison between stochastic and dyadic dictionaries. *IEEE Trans Biomed Eng* 2003; 50: 1371-3.
- Ray S, Niebur E, Hsiao SS, Sinai A, Crone NE. High-frequency gamma activity (80-150 Hz) is increased in human cortex during selective attention. *Clin Neurophysiol* 2008; 119: 116-33.
- Reddy CG, Reddy GG, Kawasaki H, Oya H, Miller LE, Howard MA, 3rd. Decoding movement-related cortical potentials from electrocorticography. *Neurosurg Focus* 2009; 27: E11.
- Rektor I, Sochurkova D, Bockova M. Intracerebral ERD/ERS in voluntary movement and in cognitive visuomotor task. *Event-Related Dynamics of Brain Oscillations* 2006; 159: 311-30.
- Schevon CA, Carlson C, Zaroff CM, Weiner HJ, Doyle WK, Miles D, *et al*. Pediatric language mapping: sensitivity of neurostimulation and Wada testing in epilepsy surgery. *Epilepsia* 2007; 48: 539-45.
- Sederberg PB, Kahana MJ, Howard MW, Donner EJ, Madsen JR. Theta and gamma oscillations during encoding predict subsequent recall. *J Neurosci* 2003; 23: 10809-14.
- Sederberg PB, Schulze-Bonhage A, Madsen JR, Bromfield EB, McCarthy DC, Brandt A, *et al*. Hippocampal and neocortical gamma oscillations predict memory formation in humans. *Cereb Cortex* 2007a; 17: 1190-6.
- Sederberg PB, Schulze-Bonhage A, Madsen JR, Bromfield EB, Litt B, Brandt A, *et al*. Gamma oscillations distinguish true from false memories. *Psychol Sci* 2007b; 18: 927-32
- Sinai A, Bowers CW, Crainiceanu CM, Boatman D, Gordon B, Lesser RP, *et al*. Electrocorticographic high gamma activity versus electrical cortical stimulation mapping of naming. *Brain* 2005; 128: 1556-70.
- Sinai A, Crone NE, Wied HM, Franaszczuk PJ, Miglioretti D, Boatman-Reich D. Intracranial mapping of auditory perception: event-related responses and electrocortical stimulation. *Clin Neurophysiol* 2009; 120: 140-9.
- Stancak A, Jr., Pfurtscheller G. Desynchronization and recovery of beta rhythms during brisk and slow self-paced finger movements in man. *Neuroscience Letters* 1995; 196: 21-4.
- Szurhaj W, Bourriez JL, Kahane P, Chauvel P, Mauguiere F, Derambure P. Intracerebral study of gamma rhythm reactivity in the sensorimotor cortex. *Eur J Neurosci* 2005; 21: 1223-35.

- Szurhaj W, Derambure P. Intracerebral study of gamma oscillations in the human sensorimotor cortex. *Event-Related Dynamics of Brain Oscillations*. Vol 159, 2006: 297-310.
- Tai K, Blain S, Chau T. A review of emerging access technologies for individuals with severe motor impairments. *Assist Technol* 2008; 20: 204-19; quiz 220-1.
- Tallon-Baudry C, Bertrand O, Henaff MA, Isnard J, Fischer C. Attention modulates gamma-band oscillations differently in the human lateral occipital cortex and fusiform gyrus. *Cereb Cortex* 2005; 15: 654-62.
- Tanji K, Suzuki K, Delorme A, Shamoto H, Nakasato N. High-frequency gamma-band activity in the basal temporal cortex during picture-naming and lexical-decision tasks. *J Neurosci* 2005; 25: 3287-93.
- Toro C, Deuschl G, Thatcher R, Sato S, Kufta C, Hallett M. Event-related desynchronization and movement-related cortical potentials on the ECoG and EEG. *Electroencephalography & Clinical Neurophysiology* 1994; 93: 380-9.
- Towle VL, Yoon HA, Castelle M, Edgar JC, Biassou NM, Frim DM, *et al*. ECoG gamma activity during a language task: differentiating expressive and receptive speech areas. *Brain* 2008; 131: 2013-27.
- Trautner P, Rosburg T, Dietl T, Fell J, Korzyukov OA, Kurthen M, *et al*. Sensory gating of auditory evoked and induced gamma band activity in intracranial recordings. *Neuroimage* 2006; 32: 790-8.

Insular and peri-rolandic epilepsy surgery: techniques

Werner Surbeck[1], Alain Bouthillier[1], Dang Khoa Nguyen[2]

[1] *Neurosurgery Service, Notre-Dame Hospital, University of Montreal, Quebec, Canada*

[2] *Neurology Service, Notre-Dame Hospital, University of Montreal, Quebec, Canada*

■ Insular epilepsy surgery

Based on the first reported intracerebral recordings of insular seizures and additional findings from insular cortical stimulation, the Lyon epilepsy group (Isnard *et al.*, 2004) concluded that insular seizures were typically associated with a sensation of laryngeal constriction and paresthesias with or without dysarthria, auditory hallucinations, or motor signs. Further observations of insular seizures documented by our group and others with intracerebral recordings indicate that the clinical spectrum of insular seizures is wider. Seizures originating from the insula may also present as hyper-motor symptoms resembling frontal lobe (FL) seizures (Ryvlin *et al.*, 2006; Afif *et al.*, 2008; Dobesberger *et al.*, 2008; Nguyen *et al.*, 2009), early visceral symptoms or dysphasia suggesting temporal lobe (TL) seizures (Nguyen *et al.*, 2009), and early somatosensory symptoms in the absence of laryngeal constriction mimicking parietal lobe (PL) seizures (Nguyen *et al.*, 2009). Apart from mimicking TL, PL and FL seizures, insular seizures may also co-exist with them (Nguyen *et al.*, 2009). It is possible that some epilepsy surgery failures result from a lack of recognition of insular seizures.

Anatomy of the insula

The Island of Reil – considered the fifth lobe of the brain – is a triangular area enclosed in the depth of the Sylvian fissure (*Figure 1*). Its tip, the apex, is located in its antero-inferior portion and represents the most superficial part of the insula. The insular cortex becomes visible by retraction of the frontal, parietal and temporal opercula which accommodate essential language areas in the dominant hemisphere. The circumference of the insula is outlined by the circular sulcus that can be divided into anterior, superior and inferior components. The oblique central insular sulcus that separates the insular cortex into anterior and posterior portions may lead, in some cases, directly into the rolandic sulcus. The 3 anteriorly-placed short gyri and the 2 posteriorly-placed long gyri form a fan-like pattern. They converge anteriorly and inferiorly towards the vascular entrance of this region, the limen insulae, which contains the uncinate fasciculus in its underlying white matter. Up to 2 short transverse gyri are located at the orbito-frontal junction (Türe et al., 1999). Directly underlying the insular cortex are the extreme capsule and the claustrum. The external capsule (harbouring the arcuate fasciculus), lenticular nucleus and internal capsule follow.

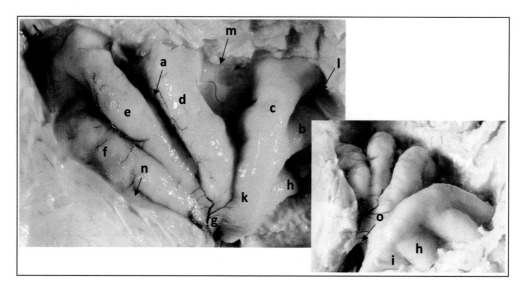

Figure 1. Lateral view of the right insular cortex. The oblique central insular sulcus **a** separates the insular cortex into anterior and posterior portions. The 3 anteriorly-placed short gyri (anterior **b**, middle **c** and posterior **d** short gyri) and the 2 posteriorly-placed long gyri (anterior **e** and posterior **f** long gyri) form a fan-like pattern, converging anteriorly and inferiorly against the limen insulae **g**. Two short transverse gyri are located at the orbito-frontal junction (accessory **h** and transverse gyri **i**). The insular apex **k** represents the most superficial part of this area. The circumference of the insula is outlined by the circular sulcus that can be divided into anterior **l**, superior **m**, and inferior **n** components. The lateral limit of the anterior perforated substance as entry point of the most lateral lenticulostriate arteries is separated from the limen insulae by the limen recess **o**, an area devoid of perforating arteries.

The insular cortex is supplied by perforating arteries arising from the superior, inferior, or middle trunks of the M2 segment, branches of the distal M1 segment originating proximal to the bi- or trifurcation of the middle cerebral artery (MCA), and recurring branches of the opercular M3 segments (Tanriover et al., 2004). Approximately 85% of the tiny insular perforating arteries supply the insular cortex as well as the extreme capsule and the claustrum. Another 10% of these perforators supply the external capsule. Larger-caliber, perforating arteries, which account for approximately 5% of perforator arteries, may reach as far as the corona radiata. The latter are commonly found in the postero-superior portion of the insula. The external capsule and claustrum are considered as the margins of territories supplied by the lateral lenticulostriate arteries (LSA) and the insular arteries. Disagreement exists about the exact limit between the 2 vascular territories (Donzelli et al., 1998). The putamen and internal capsule are vascularised by the LSA and the anterior choroidal artery. Although the most lateral LSA frequently originate from the pre-bifurcation M1 segment, a post-bifurcation origin may sometimes be seen. The lateral limit of the anterior perforated substance, as the entry point of the most lateral LSA, is separated from the limen insulae by the limen recess, an area devoid of perforating arteries (Tanriover et al., 2004). The M2 branch lying within the central sulcus gives rise to the central or anterior parietal artery with approximately equal frequency.

Function of the insula

The cytoarchitecture of the insula is arranged in a centrifugal manner, with the least differentiation rostrally, at the limen insulae (agranular allocortex), and the greatest differentiation caudally (granular isocortex). Between the 2 regions lies a dysgranular transitional zone (Mesulam & Mufson, 1985). Projections to and from the insula link allocortical paralimbic regions and granular isocortical areas as well as the amygdala, thalamus, basal ganglia, and brainstem. These extensive interconnections explain the known or suspected involvement of the insular cortex in the processing of all 5 senses as well as their autonomic, vestibular, motor, language and complex behavioural implications (Flynn et al., 1999; Shelley & Trimble, 2007).

Investigation of suspected insular epilepsy

Considering that insular cortex epilepsy has many faces, increased awareness is necessary to identify patients with insular seizures. In the absence of a clearly-delimited insular epileptogenic lesion, intra-cerebral recordings are usually required to confirm insular seizures when clinical presentation or functional investigations identify the insula as one of the potential areas of epileptogenicity. Insular sampling can be achieved by different implantation methods. The most widely-employed has been frame-based trans-opercular depth electrode implantation via the orthogonal approach described by Talairach and Bancaud (1973). This approach is associated with a relatively low complication rate (Guenot et al., 2001). A drawback of classical perpendicular implantation is the necessity of crossing the frontal, parietal or temporal operculum (which accommodates essential functional areas, particularly in the dominant hemisphere). Other limitations include restricted sampling of superficial peri-Sylvian (frontal, parietal, temporal) neocortices, lower spatial coverage for seizure detection and mapping, and an inadequate number of contacts per trans-opercular electrode actually sampling the insula (2 contacts/electrode). The latter can be enhanced via a sagittal approach, described by the Grenoble Group (Afif et al., 2008), which targets an anterior (trans-frontal) and/or a posterior (trans-parietal) trajectory to guide depth electrodes stereotactically into the insula. To improve the coverage of peri-Sylvian neocortices, our group prefers a combination of depth and subdural (grid/ strip) electrodes to capitalize on the singular advantages of each electrode type (Surbeck et al., 2011). When a unilateral insular epileptic focus is suspected and high-density sampling of the peri-Sylvian areas and/or cortical stimulation are required, a first combined method (Type I) is adopted (Figure 2).

Unilateral fronto-temporo-parietal craniotomy is performed to expose the Sylvian fissure, which is identified by anatomical landmarks and neuronavigation. The Sylvian fissure is then dissected by microsurgical techniques. Care is taken to spare as much of the Sylvian venous structures as possible, especially when the superficial Sylvian system is dominant (Sindou & Auque, 2000). Insular cortical areas of interest (anterior and/or posterior) are exposed, depending on the findings of non-invasive pre-operative investigation. One to 3 electrodes is (or are) placed under direct vision between the M2 branches after a small

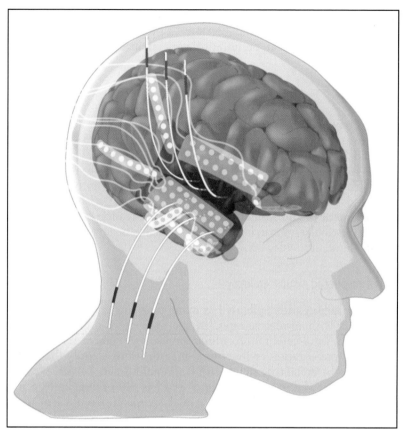

Figure 2. Type I implantation. Accomplishment of a unilateral fronto-temporo-parietal craniotomy. Implantation of 3 insular electrodes under direct vision after micro-dissection of the Sylvian fissure (blue-marked depth electrodes). Orthogonal implantation of 3 additional depth electrodes into mesial temporal structures under frameless stereotaxy (violet-marked depth electrodes) and coverage of the 3 adjacent lobes with subdural strip and grid electrodes.

incision of the pia matter with a microblade. The insular depth electrodes used (Spencer depth electrodes®; Ad-Tech Medical Instrument Corporation, Racine, WI, USA) have a diameter of 1.1 mm and carry 4 contacts along their length, each 2.3 mm in length and spaced 5 mm apart center to center. Two contacts per electrode are entered into the insular cortex. If mesio-temporal sampling is necessary, frameless stereotaxy is undertaken to implant 3 depth electrodes perpendicularly through the middle temporal gyrus (4-contact Spencer depth electrodes®, 1.1 mm diameter, 2.3 mm length, 10 mm spacing), one directed into the amygdala, one into the anterior hippocampus and the last into the posterior hippocampus. In the final stage, subdural strip and/or grid electrodes are placed on the surface of the 3 remaining peri-Sylvian lobes, the inferior surfaces of the FL and TL as well as over inter-hemispheric areas, depending on pre-operative investigation and the need for extra-operative functional mapping *(Figure 3)*. The depth electrodes are attached to the subdural electrodes by sutures to prevent later displacement. All electrode leads are tunnelled through the dura and skin, and purse-string sutures are placed around their exit site on the skin to minimize cerebrospinal fluid (CSF) leakage. Duroplasty may be necessary for adequate closure of the dural opening. The bone flap is not replaced until electrode removal and – if the epileptogenic zone is identified – the resective procedure.

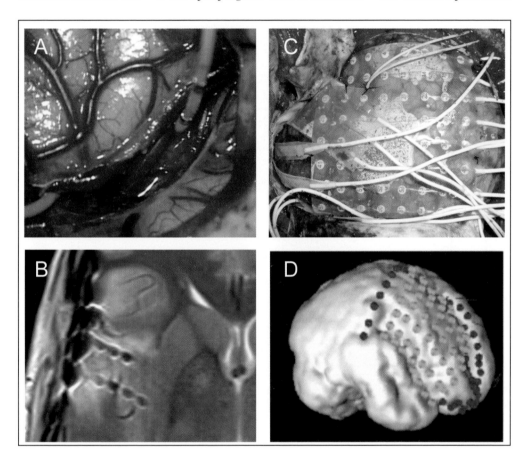

Figure 3. Type I implantation in a patient with FL-like epilepsy. **A.** Insertion of depth electrodes in the insular cortex under direct vision after microdissection of the Sylvian fissure. **B.** Axial MRI view of the insular electrodes. **C-D.** Intra-operative view and 3-dimensional visualization of intra-cranial electrode arrangement.

When bilateral implantation of temporo-mesial and insular structures is necessary, a second combined method (Type II) is undertaken *(Figure 4)*. After induction of general anaesthesia and fixation of the Cosman-Roberts-Wells stereotactic frame (Integra Radionics, Burlington, MA, USA), a CT scan is obtained. Image fusion is achieved with high-resolution magnetic resonance imaging (MRI) and Treon navigation software (Medtronic, Minneapolis, MN, USA). Intra-insular electrodes (10-contact Spencer depth electrodes®; 1.1 mm diameter, 2.3 mm length, 10 mm spacing) are implanted via an anterior (trans-frontal) approach and a posterior (trans-parietal) trajectory, as described by Afif *et al.* (2008).

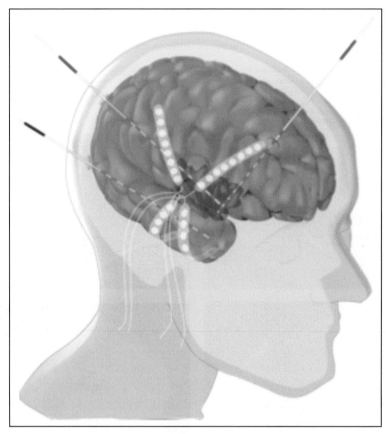

Figure 4. Type II implantation. Depth electrode implanted sagittally into the insula, with an anterior trans-frontal and a posterior trans-parietal trajectory (blue-marked depth electrodes), and the hippocampus with an occipito-temporal trajectory parallel to the hippocampal long axis (violet-marked depth electrode). Subsequent subdural strip electrode insertion through a parietal burr hole.

Taking into account the pyramidal shape of the insula, the trans-frontal and trans-parietal trajectories are not strictly "sagittal" but rather oblique, running medio-laterally and targeting the apex insulae. By doing so, it is possible to place all insular contacts close to the insular surface without passing through the Sylvian fissure. The hippocampus and amygdala are sampled by parieto-occipitally-introduced electrodes with a trajectory following the hippocampal long axis, as described by Spencer (1987). Because they sometimes penetrate the ventricular system, and thereby potentially distort brain anatomy, hippocampal electrodes are implanted after the insular ones. After tunneling, purse-string sutures are placed around the exit site of the electrodes on the skin. Coverage of the remaining peri-Sylvian lobes is achieved by subdural strip electrodes inserted through extended burr holes (*Figure 5*). As with any intra-cranial electrode procedure, great care should be taken to minimize the potential for CSF leakage and associated infections upon closure in both described techniques. Prophylactic antibiotics during long-term intra-cranial electroencephalography (EEG) recordings are not administered routinely in our institution as they do not clearly reduce the rate of infections (Wyler *et al.*, 1991). Steroids are habitually utilized to reduce post-operative discomfort and withdrawn after 3 to 4 days (Sahjpaul *et al.*, 2003). Post-implantation, high-resolution MRI is performed to determine the exact position of the electrodes.

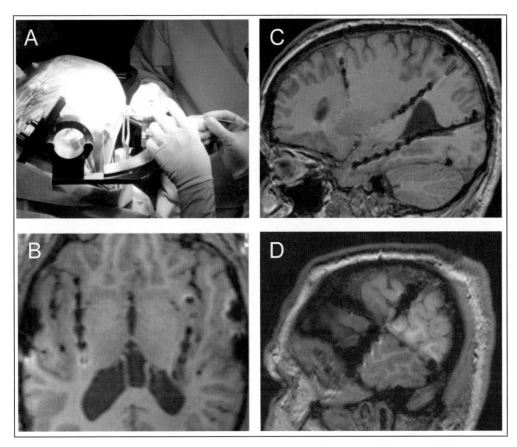

Figure 5. Type II implantation in a patient with early somatosensory ictal symptoms, left temporal lobe seizures on scalp EEG and right hippocampal atrophy. **A.** Frame-guided insertion of depth electrodes in a sagittal plane. **B.** Axial MRI view of posterior insular electrodes. **C.** Sagittal MRI view of the anterior and posterior insular electrodes as well as of the amygdalo-hippocampal electrode. **D.** Sagittal MRI view of subdural electrodes inserted through a burr hole.

Type I implantation provides less insular, but better peri-sylvian coverage than the Type II procedure. In 16 patients implanted by the former method at our institution, microdissection of the sylvian fissure and implantation of the insular electrodes resulted in 2 reversible complications (contralateral foot drop due to the migration of an insular depth electrode into the internal capsule and dysphasia from temporal opercular retraction). Three other complications in this group were attributed to a grid electrode (transient dysphasia from oedema in 2 patients and asymptomatic venous haemorrhage). With Type II implantation (4 patients), no complications occurred.

Surgery

The techniques and outcome of insular surgery for tumours and vascular malformations have been repeatedly published since the introduction of microsurgical techniques. The surgical strategy in epilepsy surgery differs in that the target consists of superficial epileptogenic gray matter. Deep-seated structures are rarely involved in resective procedures. Only a few reports of insular surgery for chronic intractable epilepsy exist in the literature. In the early 1950s, Penfield suggested that seizures originating in the insular cortex were able to mimic TL seizures to such a degree that confusion between the 2 types of seizures might explain some temporal lobectomy failures (Penfield & Faulk, 1955). Consequently, insular resection was added to temporal lobectomy when residual epileptiform activity in the insula was noted after removal of the TL. These first attempts of insular ablation were abandoned after Silfvenius et al. (1964) showed that additional resection of the insula significantly increased surgical morbidity without providing further benefit over seizure control. Almost half a century later, the first series of insulectomies performed predominantly for refractory epilepsy since Penfield, was reported by our group (Malak et al., 2009).

Operative technique

Insulectomy is either performed as an isolated operation or as part of more extensive cortical resection when the epileptogenic zone includes, but is not limited to, the insular cortex. Craniotomy extension should be adapted to the intended area of resection. For isolated insulectomy, we execute a fronto-temporal craniotomy to expose the sylvian fissure. The fissure should be widely dissected by microsurgical techniques to evade brain injury due to opercular retraction. The identification of sylvian vascularisation is crucial to avoid harmful vascular injury. The exposed insular cortex is inspected for macroscopic abnormalities. Anatomical landmarks are flagged by direct vision and neuronavigation. The abnormal insular cortex is removed by resecting tissue between the sylvian M2 branches (see video 1). Larger-caliber perforating arteries, which are mainly located in the posterior half of the insula, may reach as far as the corona radiata and should therefore be identified and preserved (Tanriover et al., 2004). Resection is limited to the cortex to avoid injuries to the LSA with resulting infarction of the putamen and internal capsule. Overall extension of insular resection should be based on all available data (Figure 6). The supplementary use of intra-operative electrocorticography (ECoG) is controversial. Interictal spikes may be modified by anaesthesia, rare, absent, widespread and multifocal. Furthermore, they may consist of propagated spikes, injury spikes' due to surgical manipulation, or post-excisional activation spikes (Chatrian & Quesney, 1997). We, therefore, rarely employ it in insular epilepsy surgery but rather rely on non-invasive pre-operative workup and extra-operative ictal depth electrode recordings. When the opercular cortex is part of the epileptogenic focus, dissection of the sylvian fissure can be avoided: the opercular and consecutively insular cortex can be removed in a subpial fashion (Figure 7). Operculo-insulectomy in the dominant hemisphere should only be performed when language areas are clearly identified by pre-operative stimulation mapping and can be spared during the procedure. In patients undergoing insulectomy in addition to adjacent lobectomy, the already-exposed insula can by subtracted by subpial resection post-lobectomy.

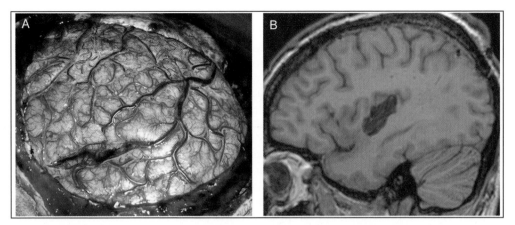

Figure 6. Isolated insulectomy in a patient with seizures caused by cortical dysplasia of the right insula. **A.** Intra-operative view after partial insulectomy. **B.** Sagittal MRI view of the removed insular cortex.

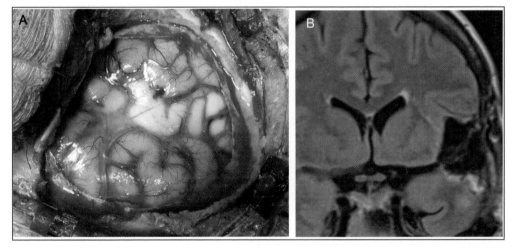

Figure 7. Operculo-insulectomy in a patient suffering from seizures deriving from insular and temporo-opercular dysplasia. **A.** Intra-operative view after delimitation of the temporo-opercular cortex to be removed. **B.** Coronal MRI view after subpial operculo-insular resection.

Risks and complications

The risks and complications of insular surgery have been reported almost exclusively in the context of oncologically-motivated surgery. Epilepsy surgery of the insular region may be slightly less dangerous as only the cortex need be removed, sparing deep-seated structures.

1. Risks to *motor function* arise from vascular injury to the lateral LSA and the larger-caliber perforating arteries with consecutive vascular insult of the internal capsule or the corona radiata. Vascular insult of the primary motor cortex may result from injury to the central artery which often runs within the central insular sulcus. The risk of direct injury to the internal capsule in epilepsy surgery is negligible in contrast to the above-mentioned tumour surgery. Silfvenius *et al.* (1964) initially reported that additional resection of the insula significantly increased surgical morbidity from 3% to 21% (mainly hemiparesis) without

providing further benefit over seizure control. However, most patients recovered in the early post-operative phase, and only 7% of those in the insulectomy group had motor deficits at discharge. Unfortunately, longer follow-up data are unavailable to determine if further recovery ensued. Analyzing data from the 11 largest series of insular surgeries (mainly for tumour resection) between 1988 and 2007, we found that hemiparesis occurred in 17% but was permanent in only 3% (Malak et al., 2009). Our group recently reported our experience with 7 insular surgeries undertaken for non-tumoural refractory epilepsy (Malak et al., 2009). Since then, 3 additional cases have been operated. Aetiologies included cortical dysplasia (3 patients), Rasmussen's encephalitis (1 patient), gliosis (2 patients), and tuber (1 patient). Three cases had no MRI-identifiable lesion. Three procedures were conducted on the dominant side and 7 on the non-dominant side. Cortectomy restricted to the insular lobe was performed in 1 case. In all others, parts of the FL (6), TL (4) or PL (2), including the opercular cortex, were resected in addition to the insula. Insulectomy was complete in 4 patients and partial in 6 (Figures 6 and 7). Post-operatively, 5 of 10 patients suffered from minor hemiparesis of variable duration (days to weeks). There was no permanent new weakness.

2. Risk to *language function* in the dominant hemisphere could arise from injury to the opercular cortex, the arcuate fasciculus running within the external capsule and the putamen. Resection, extensive retraction and vascular deprivation of eloquent opercular areas must be avoided. Delimitation of opercular speech function by cortical stimulation mapping helps in achieving this goal. Lesion of the arcuate fasciculus can generate conduction aphasia (Tanabe et al., 1987), while left putaminal damage may induce non-fluent dysphasia by disturbing voluntary control of the laryngeal muscles (D'Esposito & Alexander, 1995; Lee et al., 1996). Due to the more superficial nature of epilepsy surgery, the risk for these complications is low. Since electrical stimulation of the left insula before or during epilepsy surgery was reported to induce language disturbances (Ojemann & Whitaker, 1978; Ostrowsky et al., 2000), surgical removal of the dominant insular cortex was not recommended by these authors, as it was judged to be essential for speech. Speech disturbance by electrical stimulation of the non-dominant side has also been observed (Afif et al., 2010). We noted speech arrest during left-side insular cortical stimulation in a patient with refractory non-lesional insular cortex epilepsy. The patient subsequently underwent isolated resection of the posterior left insula with complete recovery from the slight post-operative dysphasia within 1 week. Because of seizure persistence, the remaining insular cortex was ablated by gamma knife surgery with subsequent seizure freedom and no phasic problems. This suggests that insulectomy can be compensated by peri-insular language areas. The contralateral hemisphere may also be implicated in language compensation (Vikingstad et al., 2000). We feel that insulectomy is safe, if structural and functional imaging of the opercular cortices harbouring the peri-insular language network is normal. No speech deficit occurred in relation to insular resective procedures in the 3 patients of our series operated on the dominant side. In the above-mentioned review of the literature on insular surgery (Malak et al., 2009), transient dysphasia was reported in 16% of patients who underwent surgery in the dominant hemisphere, but persisted in only 1.4%.

3. Risk to *higher cognitive functions* ascribed to pure insular cortical resection is unknown. Manes et al. (1999), who examined the neuropsychiatric impact of isolated insular strokes, discerned that patients with right insular lesions had a greater frequency of subjective anergia, under-activity, and tiredness compared to patients with non-insular or left insular lesions. These findings were attributed to a disconnection between the insula and the

frontal lobe or the anterior cingulate cortex, structures that have been associated with willed action and motor behaviour (Agustine, 1996). We did not observe any loss of cognitive function in our patients, but more detailed neuropsychological re-examination of our series is in progress.

Outcome

In our series, an Engel I outcome was reached in 9 out of 10 patients (Engel *et al.*, 1993). Successful epilepsy surgery (Engel I outcome) with insular cortex resection was also reported by Isnard *et al.* (2004) and Kaido *et al.* (2006) for 2 patients each and by Dobesberger *et al.* (2008) in 1 patient. For patients with tumoural insular epilepsy, lesionectomy also appears to be very efficient in controlling seizures (Malak *et al.* (2009): on average, 87% of patients who presented with epilepsy had an Engel Class I or II outcome at follow-up.

Conclusion

With the identification of an increasing number of cases, the many faces of insular cortex epilepsy are being slowly characterized. There is now evidence that some surgical candidates with drug-resistant epilepsy have an epileptogenic zone that involves the insula, and failure to recognize it may be responsible for unsuccessful epilepsy surgery. As resection of insular seizure foci is possible with acceptable risks, increased awareness and further understanding of this seizure entity may hopefully lead to improved epilepsy surgery outcomes.

■ Peri-rolandic epilepsy surgery

Peri-rolandic epilepsy surgery consists of surgical removal or transection of epileptogenic foci involving the pre-central and/or post-central gyrus with or without the adjacent cortex. It is generally associated with a high risk of persistent neurological deficit and an unfavourable rate of seizure control due to the high eloquence of this primary somatosensorimotor area (Pilcher *et al.*, 1947; Pondal-Sardo *et al.*, 2006). Incomplete removal of epileptogenic tissue results in epilepsy surgery failure, whereas extensive resection may cause harmful neurological deficits through injury of functional cortical or sub-cortical structures. The impact on patients' lives by functional damage of the region is far-reaching, as stated by Penfield and Rasmussen: "Viewed through the eyes of his patient, the worst sin the neurosurgeon can commit is to produce aphasia or paralysis of leg or arm. After that come the more dispensable functions of vision in one half-field and sensory discrimination in the hand" (Penfield & Rasmussen, 1957). Recent advances of structural and functional imaging techniques have improved the detection and delineation of epileptogenic tissue and clearer discrimination from the neighbouring functional cortex. Their use during neuronavigation, combined with the results of pre- and/or intra-operative electrophysiological data, has generated promising reports in the recent literature (Lehmann *et al.*, 1994; Cohen-Gadol *et al.*, 2003; Marnet *et al.*, 2008).

Anatomy of the rolandic region

The French scientist Francois Leuret gave credit to Luigi Rolando, for observing the central sulcus (CS) in the early 19th century (Rolando, 1829), by naming the anatomical landmark after him: "Between these two convolutions (pre-central and post-central gyri) exists a furrow that separates them...; it is as constant as the sylvian fissure. I have called this furrow the fissure of Rolando, because it was this anatomist who first described it in man..." (Leuret, 1839). The sinusoid-shaped CS or rolandic sulcus extends downward and slightly forward on the lateral surface of the hemispheres toward the sylvian fissure from which it is usually (in 81-95% of hemispheres) separated by the sub-central gyrus, a small gyral bridge connecting the lower ends of the pre-central and post-central gyri (Cunningham, 1892; Cushing, 1908). In nearly 90% of cases, the CS extends onto the medial surface of the hemisphere, intersecting the upper hemispheric border 2 cm posterior to the midpoint between the nasion and the inion (Wilkins, 1996; Rhoton, 2002). The adjacent pre- and post-central gyri compose the central or rolandic region. Irregular limbs of the pre- and post-central sulci may open into the CS, in which case the pre- and post-central gyri are divided into upper and lower or multiple segments (Rhoton, 2002). The supplementary motor area is a limited part of the mesial portion of the superior frontal gyrus located anteriorly to the pre-central gyrus and above the cingulate gyrus, whereas the pre-motor area occupies the posterior parts of the superior, middle and inferior frontal gyri over the cerebral convexity. Both areas are not part of the rolandic cortex. The central region on the lateral surface of the brain is supplied by cortical branches of the MCA. While the pre-central gyrus is mostly supplied by the central artery, the post-central gyrus is supplied by both the central and post-central arteries. The medial part of the central area is mainly supplied by the calloso-marginal artery and, in a minority of cases, by the peri-callosal artery, both of which are branches of the anterior cerebral artery (Foix & Levy, 1927; Ugur et al., 2005). Whether single or double, the central artery(s) course(s) over the sub-central gyrus (if present) before entering the CS. The artery(arteries) then run(s) upward in the depths of the CS before coming to the surface. When single, the central artery almost always bifurcates and, thus, there are a minimum of 2 terminal branches of this vessel (Salamon et al. 1975). No CS artery was found in 16% of specimen by Marrone and Lopes (1993). The lateral surface of the central region is drained by the pre-central, central and post-central veins into the superior sagittal sinus, and by the fronto-sylvian and parieto-sylvian veins into the superficial sylvian vein. The large anastomotic vein of Trolard crosses the cortical surface of the FL and/or PL between the superior sagittal sinus and the sylvian fissure. In 75% of hemispheres, this vein is located over the pre-central, central, or post-central sulcus, most often at the level of the post-central sulcus (Rhoton, 2002). The vein of Trolard is larger in the non-dominant hemisphere (DiChiro, 1962; Auque & Civit, 1996).

Function of the rolandic region

The central region represents the neocortical, primary somatomotor and somatosensory cortex, respectively. While the pre-central gyrus receives most of its afferent information from the basal ganglia and the cerebellum via the ventral lateral nucleus of the thalamus, the post-central gyrus receives sensory information from the body, head and face via the ventral posterior nucleus of the thalamus. The main efferent output of the rolandic region is the corticospinal tract. Intra-operative electrical stimulation under local anaesthesia to map sensorimotor areas has been performed since the pioneering era of epilepsy surgery (Cushing, 1909; Horsley, 1909; Krause, 1912; Foerster, 1934). Synthesis of stimulation results from the Montreal Neurological Institute gave birth to the somatotopic "homunculus," which cartoons the relative size and order of the cortical sensorimotor representation (Penfield & Boldrey, 1937). They also noted an overlap in function of the pre-central "motor" and post-central "sensory" gyri so that 80% of the total motor response were obtained from pre-central stimulation and 20% from post-central stimulation

(Penfield & Jasper, 1954). Based on these observations and experimental work, it has been estimated that ~30% of the corticospinal tract is composed of axons deriving from neurons whose cell bodies lie within the PL, including the post-central gyrus (Lassek, 1954). Conversely, the pre-central cortex harbours not only motor but also a significant amount of sensory function (Penfield & Jasper, 1954). The homunculus has to be understood as a simplified teaching tool that does not represent complete reality. In fact, since the original data presented by Penfield and Boldrey (1937), neurophysiological studies on monkeys and functional imaging in humans show a large overlap of cortical zones related to movement and sensation of different body parts. These observations support the hypothesis of functional mosaicism of sensorimotor cortical regions (Schieber & Hibbard 1993; Farrell et al., 2007). Furthermore, Duffau et al. (2001) noted that multiple cortical representations for hand and forearm movements exist in the primary motor cortex. From a practical point of view, the pre-central gyrus can be divided into 3 regions: the lateral third represents the face area, the middle third represents the hand and upper extremity areas, and the medial third represents the trunk and the hip (Haines, 2008).

Investigation of suspected peri-rolandic epilepsy

As with any epileptic condition, the primary form of treatment is long-term anticonvulsant drug therapy. If peri-rolandic seizures are suspected and drug therapy fails, cortical ictal recordings and detailed mapping of the sensorimotor cortex are frequently necessary, especially in the absence of a congruent and clearly-delimited epileptogenic lesion on brain imaging. Cortical structures to be explored by subdural electrodes are chosen based on the pre-surgical workup, including a detailed questionnaire and physical examination, a neuropsychological evaluation, high-resolution cerebral MRI, video EEG recording of seizures, ictal single-photon emission computed tomography, 18F fluorodeoxyglucose positron emission tomography, and functional MRI (Figure 8). The CS can be identified on MRI according to well-known anatomical guidelines: 1. It can be distinguished on the axial plane as the sulcus running parallel and immediately posterior to the pre-CS. The latter is identified by its characteristic "T" intersection with the superior frontal sulcus. 2. The CS can be identified in the mid-sagittal plane as the sulcus immediately anterior to termination of the marginal ramus of the cingulate sulcus. 3. A characteristic omega-shaped "knob" can be seen over the somatosensory hand region of the post-central gyrus, bordering the CS (Yousry et al., 1997).

A generous craniotomy is performed for subdural electrode placement, and the rolandic fissure is identified by anatomical landmarks and neuronavigation. The pre-central gyrus can be confirmed by direct cortical stimulation in non-curarised patients. Cold Ringer's lactate should always be available to stop stimulation-induced seizures (Sartorius & Berger, 1998). Detailed intra-operative mapping of the rolandic cortex is not necessary, as patients will be evaluated by extra-operative cortical stimulation. Somatosensory evoked potential recording from median nerve electrical stimulation can identify the CS indirectly by determining inversion polarity (phase reversals) (Benfila et al., 2009). The lateral central cortex is usually covered by a 8 × 8 subdural grid electrode. Inter-hemispheric and adjacent cortical regions are covered by subdural strip and/or grid electrodes, depending on pre-operative investigation. The subdural electrodes are attached to the borders of the dura to avoid later displacement. Supplemental depth electrodes can also be positioned under frameless stereotaxy. An image of the final operative field with electrode placement is captured by digital camera (Figure 9). All electrode leads are tunnelled through the skin,

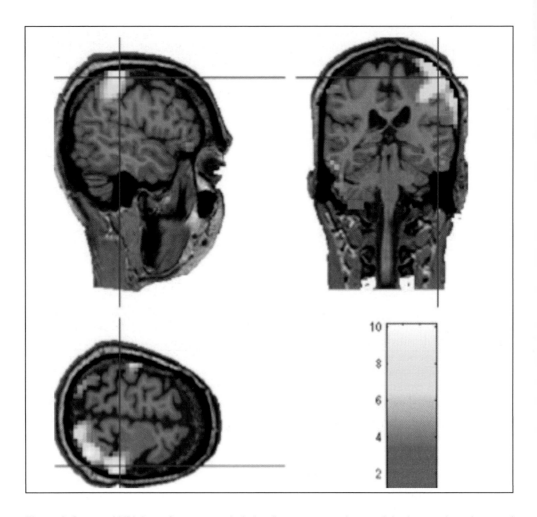

Figure 8. Functional MRI during finger tapping (right hand) in a patient with cortical dysplasia involving the central region. Activation partly overlying the posterior portion of dysplasia is shown with no clear evidence of functional reorganization.

and purse-string sutures are tied around their exit site to further minimize the potential for CSF leakage. Duroplasty is often necessary for adequate closure of dural opening. The bone flap is not replaced until electrode removal and the resective procedure. Post-operative sub-galeal drains are always placed and a head dressing is applied. Steroid administration to reduce procedure discomfort is stopped after 3 to 4 days (Sahjpaul *et al.*, 2003). Post-implantation MRI is performed to determine the exact position of the electrodes (*Figure 10*). Once sufficient data on the functional cortex and the region of epileptogenicity have been obtained, surgical strategy is discussed and the patient is returned to the operating room for subdural electrode removal and therapeutic procedures.

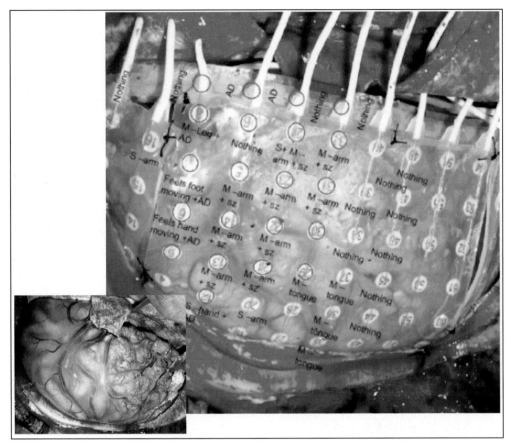

Figure 9. Functional cortical mapping. Operative field with subdural electrodes covering the fronto-parietal convexity in a patient with cortical dysplasia involving the right central region (see *Figure 1*). Sensorimotor responses during extra-operative mapping are marked. The dysplasic cortex harbours important sensorimotor function of the hand, arm and leg regions with no evidence of major functional reorganization.

Surgery

Because patients usually undergo detailed extra-operative mapping of the central region, awake craniotomy is unnecessary in the great majority of cases. The first step after re-opening of the craniectomy is re-identification of the CS and pre- and post-central gyri with additional information obtained from extra-operative mapping. Furthermore, the epileptogenic lesion is delimited by macroscopic features, texture and the results of non-invasive and invasive workup. There is ongoing controversy regarding the value of ECoG in guiding the operative procedure (Chatrian & Quesney, 1997), as discussed previously. Subpial resection of the epileptogenic cortex is undertaken to preserve the draining veins and arteries of the surrounding essential cortex. The hand and leg representation areas are generally considered as "untouchable", whereas resections of the cortex representing the face can be performed without long-lasting sequela. Identification of the central artery is crucial in avoiding unintentional damage to this vessel. Obliteration of the bridging veins to the superior sagittal sinus in the central region is risky, although frequently-caused contralateral hemiparesis is often transient (Sindou & Auque, 2000). Recovery of the

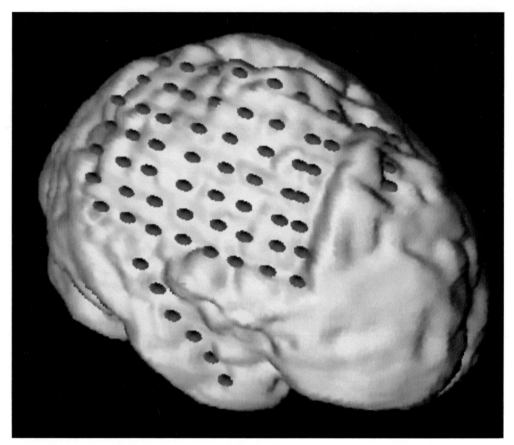

Figure 10. Three-dimensional representation of the exact position of electrodes with respect to the patient's brain by post-operative MRI with Gridview software (Stellate Systems Inc., Montreal, Quebec, Canada).

deficit is attributed to diffuse anastomoses between the cortical veins (Rhoton, 2002). In patients without previous intra-cranial study, mapping of neurological function at risk can be achieved by intra-operative cortical stimulation. Electromyography (EMG) during intra-operative monitoring has been adopted by some centers as EMG responses are evoked at smaller currents than observed movements (Yingling *et al.*, 1999). With this method, it is also easier to detect the effect of face area stimulation.

Multiple subpial transections (MST) to eliminate horizontal cortical seizure-propagating pathways while preserving vertical functional pathways can be performed in isolation or in addition to the resective procedure. MST are indicated when important functional responses are obtained within the epileptogenic cortex, and the risk to neurological function is judged too high to allow cortical resection (*e.g.* resection in the primary motor or sensory hand cortex while functional re-organization is not proven; see *Figure 11*). After closure of the dural opening, the bone flap is replaced and the wound is closed. Sub-galeal drains are used, and a head dressing is applied. MRI is undertaken after surgery to determine the extent of resection.

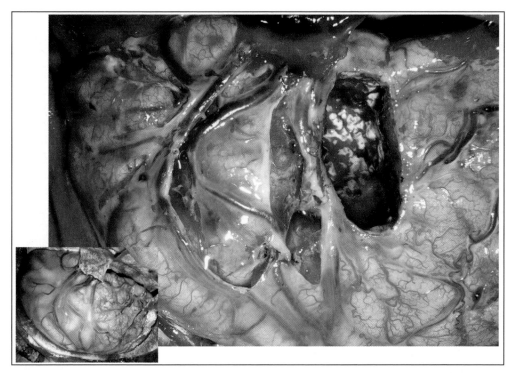

Figure 11. Post-operative image after surgery for right frontal cortical dysplasia involving the central region (see *Figures 7 and 8*). As the dysplasic cortex harboured important sensorimotor function of the hand, arm and leg regions and functional reorganization could not be proven either by functional imaging or extra-operative cortical stimulation, the risk to neurological function was judged too high to allow cortical resection in the central region. Therefore, multiple subpial transections were performed in addition to pre-central resection.

Risks and complications

1. Risk to *motor function* arises from resection or vascular deprivation of the eloquent motor cortex. Total removal of pre-central representation of the extremities results in complete paralysis, subsequent spasticity, and occasionally partial recovery of gross movements over time. Furthermore, a slight decrease in 2-point discrimination can be observed. Partial removal of the pre-central arm area produces diffuse weakness of the whole extremity rather than restricted paralysis but leaves only mild weakness over time (Penfield & Rasmussen, 1957). Removal of the pre-central gyrus below hand representation produces minor paresis of the lower portion of the face, interfering transiently with mastication, pharyngeal movement, and word articulation. Most often, there are no long-lasting post-operative deficits in this region, even in the dominant side for language (Penfield & Rasmussen, 1957; Lehman *et al.*, 1994; Cukiert *et al.*, 2001). High rates of post-surgical, permanent motor deficits (30-63%) are reported in larger, unselected series of peri-rolandic epilepsy surgery, including lesions in the middle and medial third of the pre-central gyrus (Pilcher *et al.*, 1947; Lehman *et al.*, 1994; Pondal-Sardo *et al.*, 2006; Benfila *et al.*, 2009). Marnet *et al.* (2004) described a series of 17 patients operated on for intractable epilepsy caused by Taylor-type focal cortical dysplasias (TTFCD) in the central region. They noted permanent motor deficits in only 23% of patients, a fact that may be explained by the absence of motor responses to cortical stimulation within the dysplasic cortex. Similar

observation of an absent functional cortex within TTFCD was made by others (Marusic *et al.*, 2002). Transient motor deficits can be found in almost all patients operated on in the central region or in its immediate vicinity (Cukiert *et al.*, 2001; Cohen-Gadol *et al.*, 2003; Marnet *et al.*, 2008). Post-operative functional recovery after resection of epileptogenic foci within the central region may be explained by activation of latent alternative representations, as suggested by Duffau (2001), cerebral plasticity, including abnormal functional organization in patients harbouring long-standing epileptogenic lesions (Burneo *et al.* 2004), and growth or displacement of the primary sensorimotor area (Bittar *et al.*, 2000). Weakness in the contralateral extremity, after resection of the post-central gyrus with the possibility of full recovery (Benfila *et al.*, 2009), is due to the above-mentioned contribution of this gyrus to the corticospinal tract (Lassek, 1954).

2. Risk to *sensory function* arises from resection or vascular deprivation of the eloquent sensory cortex. Removal of the post-central gyrus culminates in astereognosis in the opposite extremities with its maximum in the distal parts of the limbs. The loss of sense of movement and position in space is due to the loss of muscle-tendon sensory input and 2-point discrimination. Removal of the post-central gyrus below the hand representation produces a non-disabling, partial discriminatory sensory defect in the contralateral side of the face and tongue. Although attenuation of sensory discrimination in the hand has an important impact on patients' lives, it is judged to be less handicapping than weakness (Penfield & Rasmussen, 1957).

Outcome

The reported good outcome (Engel I and II) after peri-rolandic epilepsy surgery ranges from 43% to 94% with a tendency for better results in studies reporting cortical resection without MST, those with surgeries involving mostly the face area, and in the presence of TTFCD (Pilcher *et al.*, 1947; Cukiert *et al.*, 2001; Otsubo *et al.*, 2001; Cohen-Gadol *et al.*, 2003; Devinsky *et al.*, 2003; Pondal-Sordo *et al.*, 2006; Marnet *et al.*, 2008; Behdad *et al.*, 2009; Benfila *et al.*, 2009; DuanYu *et al.*, 2010). As the functional risks with surgery below hand representation are low, more aggressive resections can be performed, leading to better seizure outcome. Favourable seizure outcome has been repeatedly reported for TTFCD, especially in extratemporal areas (Urbach *et al.*, 2002; Siegel *et al.*, 2006; Marnet *et al.*, 2008). MST, developed as a palliative surgical procedure for focal seizures arising in the eloquent cortex, is less effective than resective techniques for seizure control. Several groups have observed unfavourable outcomes in patients undergoing MST exclusively, with > 95% seizure reduction ranging from 0 to 10% (Schramm *et al.*, 2002; Pondal-Sordo *et al.*, 2006). A meta-analysis of 211 patients undergoing MST at 6 centers revealed, however, that as much as two-thirds of patients had > 95% seizure reduction with only MST (Spencer *et al.*, 2002). The results were better when MST was added to cortical resections (68-87% with > 95% seizure reduction).

Conclusion

Peri-rolandic epilepsy surgery may be performed with acceptable risks for the benefit of seizure control. The high eloquence of this primary somatosensorimotor cortical area necessitates careful workup, including functional stimulation mapping. While extensive resection may cause harmful neurological deficits, incomplete removal of the epileptogenic zone will lead to persisting seizures. MST should be considered when the risk to neurological function is judged too high to allow cortical resection. High seizure frequency and progressive cognitive decline as well as long-standing pre-operative motor or sensory deficit may raise the acceptance of potential post-operative deficits.

References

- Afif A, Chabardes S, Minotti L, Kahane P, Hoffmann D. Safety and usefulness of insular depth electrodes implanted via an oblique approach in patients with epilepsy. *Neurosurgery* 2008; 62: 471-9.

- Afif A, Minotti L, Kahane P, Hoffmann D. Middle short gyrus of the insula implicated in speech production: intracerebral electric stimulation of patients with epilepsy. *Epilepsia* 2010; 51: 201-13.

- Agustine JR. Circuitry and functional aspects of the insular lobe in primates including humans. *Brain Res Rev* 1996; 22: 229-44.

- Auque J, Civit Th. Les veines superficielles. *Neurochirurgie* 1996; 42 (Suppl 1): 88-108.

- Behdad A, Limbrick DD, Jr., Bertrand ME, Smyth MD. Epilepsy surgery in children with seizures arising from the rolandic cortex. *Epilepsia* 2009; 50: 1450-61.

- Benfila M, Sala F, Jane J, Otsubo H, Ochi A, Drake J, *et al*. Neurosurgical management of intractable rolandic epilepsy in children: role of resection in eloquent cortex. *J Neurosurg Pediatrics* 2009; 4: 199-216.

- Bittar RG, Olivier A, Sadikot AF, Andermann F, Reutens DC. Cortical motor and somatosensory representation: effect of cerebral lesions. *J Neurosurg* 2000; 92: 242-8.

- Burneo JG, Kuzniecky RI, Bebin M, Knowlton RC. Cortical reorganization in malformations of cortical development: a magnetoencephalographic study. *Neurology* 2004; 63: 1818-24.

- Chatrian GE, Quesney LF. Intraoperative electrocorticography. In: Engel J, Jr., Pedley TA, eds. *Epilepsy: a Comprehensive Textbook*. Philadelphia: Lippincott-Raven Publishers, 1997, 1749-65.

- Cohen-Gadol AA, Britton JW, Collignon FP, Bates LM, Cascino GD, Meyer FB. Nonlesional central lobule seizures: use of awake cortical mapping and subdural grid monitoring for resection of seizure focus. *J Neurosurg* 2003; 98: 1255-62.

- Cukiert A, Buratini JA, Machado E, Sousa A, Vieira J, Forster C, *et al*. Seizure's outcome after cortical resections including the face and tongue rolandic areas in patients with refractory epilepsy and normal MRI submitted to subdural grids' implantation. *Arq Neuropsiquiatr* 2001; 59: 717-21.

- Cunningham DJ. *Contribution to the Surface Anatomy of the Cerebral Hemisphere*. Dublin: Royal Irish Academy, 1892, 306-55.

- Cushing H. Surgery of the head. In: Keen WW, ed. *Surgery – its Principles and Practice*. Philadelphia: W.B. Saunders Co., 1908, 17-248.

- Cushing H. A note upon the faradic stimulation of the postcentral gyrus in conscious patients. *Brain* 1909; 32: 44-53.

- D'Esposito M, Alexander MP. Distinct profiles following left putaminal hemorrhage. *Neurology* 1995; 45: 38-41.

- Devinsky O, Romanelli P, Orbach D, Pacia S, Doyle W. Surgical treatment of multifocal epilepsy involving eloquent cortex. *Epilepsia* 2003; 44: 718-23.

- DiChiro G. Angiographic patterns of cerebral convexity veins and superficial dural sinuses. *AJR Am J Roentgenol* 1962; 87: 308-21.

- Dobesberger J, Ortler M, Unterberger I, Walser G, Falkenstetter T, Bodner T, *et al*. Successful surgical treatment of insular epilepsy with nocturnal hypermotor seizures. *Epilepsia* 2008; 49 (1): 159-62.

- Donzelli R, Marinkovic S, Brigante L, de Divitiis O, Nikodijevic I, Schonauer C, et al. Territories of the perforating (lenticulostriate) branches of the middle cerebral artery. Surg Radiol Anat 1998; 20: 393-8.

- DuanYu N, GuoJun Z, Liang Q, LiXin C, Tao Y, YongJie L. Surgery for perirolandic epilepsy: epileptogenic cortex resection guided by chronic intracranial electroencephalography and electric cortical stimulation mapping. Clin Neurol Neurosurg 2010; 112 (2): 110-7.

- Duffau H. Acute functional reorganisation of the human motor cortex during resection of central lesions: a study using intraoperative brain mapping. J Neurol Neurosurg Psychiatry 2001; 70: 506-13.

- Duffau H, Bauchet L, Lehéricy S, Capelle L. Functional compensation of the left dominant insula for language. Neuroreport 2001; 12: 2159-63.

- Engel J, Jr., Van Ness PC, Rasmussen TB, Ojemann LM. Outcome with respect to epileptic seizures. In: Engel J, Jr., ed. Surgical Treatment of Epilepsies. New York: Raven Press, 1993, 609-21.

- Farrell DF, Burbank N, Lettich E, Ojemann GA. Individual variation in human motor-sensory (rolandic) cortex. J Clin Neurophysiol 2007; 24 (3): 286-93.

- Flynn FG, Benson DF, Ardila A. Anatomy of the insula: functional and clinical correlates. Aphasiology 1999; 13: 55-78.

- Foix CH, Levy M. Les ramollissement sylviens, syndromes et de lésions en foyer du territoire de l'artère sylvienne et de ses branches. Rev Neurol 1927; 48: 1-51.

- Foerster O. Über die Bedeutung und Reichweite des Lokalisationsprinzips im Nervensystem. Verh Dtsch Ges Inn Med 1934; 46: 117-211.

- Guenot M, Isnard J, Ryvlin P, Fischer C, Ostrowsky K, Mauguiere F, et al. Neurophysiological monitoring for epilepsy surgery: The Talairach SEEG method. stereoelectroencephalography. Indications, results, complications and therapeutic applications in a series of 100 consecutive cases. Stereotact Funct Neurosurg 2001; 77: 29-32.

- Haines DH. Neuroanatomy: An Atlas of Structures, Sections, and Systems, 7th ed. Baltimore: Lippincott Williams & Wilkins, 2008.

- Horsley V. The function of the so-called motor area of the brain (Linacre Lecture). BMJ 1909; 11: 125-32.

- Isnard J, Guenot M, Sindou M, Mauguière F. Clinical manifestations of insular lobe seizures: a stereo-electroencephalographic study. Epilepsia 2004; 45 (9): 1079-90.

- Kaido T, Otsuki T, Nakama H, Kaneko Y, Kubota Y. Complex behavioral automatism arising from insular cortex. Epilepsy & Behav 2006; 8: 315-9.

- Krause F. Surgery of the Brain and Spinal Cord Based on Personal Experience. New York: Rebman, 1912.

- Lassek AM. The Pyramidal Tract: its Status in Medicine. Springfield: Charles C. Thomas, 1954.

- Lee MS, Lee SB, Kim WC. Spasmodic dysphonia associated with a left ventrolateral putaminal lesion. Neurology 1996; 47: 827-8.

- Lehman R, Andermann F, Olivier A, Tandon PN, Quesney LF, Rasmussen TB. Seizures with onset in the sensorimotor face area: clinical patterns and results of surgical treatment in 20 patients. Epilepsia 1994; 35: 1117-24.

- Leuret F. Anatomie comparée du système nerveux. Paris: Baillière 1839; 1: 397-8.

- Malak R, Bouthillier A, Carmant L, Cossette P, Giard N, Saint-Hilaire J-M, et al. Microsurgery of epileptic foci in the insular region. J Neurosurg 2009; 110 (6): 1153-63.

- Manes F, Paradiso S, Robinson RG. Neuropsychiatric effects of insular stroke. J Nerv Ment Dis 1999; 187: 707-12.

- Marnet D, Devaux B, Chassoux F, Landré E, Mann M, Turak B, et al. Surgical resection of focal cortical dysplasias in the central region. Neurochirurgie 2008; 54: 399-408.

- Marrone AHC, Lopes DK. Microsurgical study of the pre-central, central and post-central arteries of the human brain cortex. *Funct Dev Morphol* 1993; 3: 185-8.
- Marusic P, Najm IM, Ying Z, Prayson R, Rona S, Nair D, *et al*. Focal cortical dysplasias in eloquent cortex: functional characteristics and correlation with MRI and histopathologic changes. *Epilepsia* 2002; 43: 27-32.
- Mesulam MM, Mufson E. The insula of Reil in man and monkey. Architectonics, connectivity and function. In: Peters A, Jones EG, eds. *Cerebral Cortex*, volume 4. New York: Plenum Press, 1985, 179-226.
- Nguyen DK, Nguyen DB, Malak R, Leroux JM, Carmant L, Saint-Hilaire JM, *et al*. Revisiting the role of the insula in refractory partial epilepsy. *Epilepsia* 2009; 50: 510-20.
- Ojemann GA, Whitaker HA. Language localization and variability. *Brain Lang* 1978; 6: 239-60.
- Ostrowsky K, Isnard J, Ryvlin P, Guénot M, Fischer C, Mauguière F. Functional mapping of the insular cortex: clinical implication in temporal lobe epilepsy. *Epilepsia* 2000; 41: 681-6.
- Otsubo H, Chitoku S, Ochi A, Jay V, Rutka JT, Smith ML, *et al*. Malignant rolandic-sylvian epilepsy in children: diagnosis, treatment, and outcomes. *Neurology* 2001; 57: 590-6.
- Penfield W, Boldrey E. Somatic motor and sensory representation in the cerebral cortex of man as studied by electrical stimulation. *Brain* 1937; 60: 389-443.
- Penfield W, Faulk ME. The insula: further observations on its function. *Brain* 1955; 78: 445-70.
- Penfield W, Jasper H. *Epilepsy and the Functional Anatomy of the Human Brain*. Boston: Little, Brown & Co., 1954.
- Penfield W, Rasmussen T. *The Cerebral Cortex of Mman: Excision of Cortical Regions*. New York: MacMillan, 1957, 183-201.
- Pilcher C, Meacham WR, Holbrook TJ. Partial excision of the motor cortex in treatment of Jacksonian convulsions. Results of forty-one cases. *Arch Surg* 1947; 54: 633-43.
- Pondal-Sordo M, Diosy D, Tellez-Zenteno JF, Girvin JP, Wiebe S. Epilepsy surgery involving the sensory-motor cortex. *Brain* 2006; 129: 3307-14.
- Rhoton AL. The cerebral veins. *Neurosurgery* 2002; 51[Suppl 1]: 159-205.
- Rolando L. Della strutura degli Emisferi Cerebrali. *Memorie della Regia Accademia delle Scienze di Torino* 1829; 35: 103-45.
- Ryvlin P, Minotti L, Demarquay G, Hirsch E, Arzimanoglou A, Hoffman D, *et al*. Nocturnal hypermotor seizures, suggesting frontal lobe epilepsy, can originate in the insula. *Epilepsia* 2006; 47: 755-65.
- Sahjpaul RL, Mahon J, Wiebe S. Dexamethasone for morbidity after subdural electrode insertion – a randomized controlled trial. *Can J Neurol Sci* 2003; 30: 340-8.
- Salamon G, Raybaud C, Michotey P, Grisoli F, Farnarier P. Angiographic study of cerebral convolutions and their area of vascularization. *Rev Neurol* 1975; 131: 259-84.
- Sartorius CJ, Berger MS. Rapid termination of intraoperative stimulation-evoked seizures with application of cold Ringer's lactate to the cortex. Technical note. *J Neurosurg* 1998; 88: 349-51.
- Schieber MH, Hibbard LS. How somatotopic is the motor cortex hand area? *Science* 1993; 261: 489-93.
- Schramm J, Aliashkevich AF, Grunwald T. Multiple subpial transections: outcome and complications in 20 patients who did not undergo resection. *J Neurosurg* 2002; 97: 39-47.
- Shelley BP, Trimble MR. The insular lobe of Reil – its anatomico-functional behavioural and neuropsychiatric attributes in humans: a review. *World J Biol Psychiatry* 2007; 5 (4): 176-200.
- Siegel AM, Cascino GD, Meyer FB, Marsh WR, Scheithauer BW, Sharbrough FW. Surgical outcome and predictive factors in adult patients with intractable epilepsy and focal cortial dysplasia. *Acta Neurol Scand* 2006; 113: 65-71.
- Silfvenius H, Gloor P, Rasmussen T. Evaluation of insular ablation in surgical treatment of temporal lobe epilepsy. *Epilepsia* 1964; 5: 307-20.

- Sindou M, Auque J. The intracranial venous system as a neurosurgeon's perspective. In: Cohadon F, ed. *Advances and Technical Standards in Neurosurgery*, vol 26. Vienna: Springer-Verlag, 2000, 131-216.
- Spencer DD. Depth electrode implantation at Yale University. In: Engel J, Jr., ed. *Surgical Treatment of Epilepsies*. New York: Raven, 1987; 603-8.
- Spencer SS, Schramm J, Wyler A, O'Connor M, Orbach D, Krauss G, et al. Multiple subpial transection for intractable partial epilepsy: an international meta-analysis. *Epilepsia* 2002; 43: 141-5.
- Surbeck W, Bouthillier A, Weil AG, Crevier L, Carmant L, Lortie A, et al. The combination of subdural and depth electrodes for intracranial EEG investigation of suspected insular (perisylvian) epilepsy. *Epilepsia* 2011; 52: 458-66.
- Talairach J, Bancaud J. Stereotaxic approach to epilepsy. Methodology of anatomo-functional stereotaxic investigations. *Progr Neurol Surg* 1973; 5: 297-354.
- Tanabe H, Sawada T, Inoue N, Ogawa M, Kuriyama Y, Shiraishi J. Conduction aphasia and arcuate fasciculus. *Acta Neurol Scand* 1987; 76: 422-7.
- Tanriover N, Rhoton AL, Jr., Kawashima M, Ulm AJ, Yasuda A. Microsurgical anatomy of the insula and the sylvian fissure. *J Neurosurg* 2004; 100: 891-922.
- Türe U, Yasargil DC, Al-Mefty O, Yasargil MG. Topographic anatomy of the insular region. *J Neurosurg* 1999; 90: 720-33.
- Ugur HC, Kahilogullari G, Coscarella E, Unlu A, Tekdemir I, Morcos JJ, et al. Arterial vascularization of primary motor cortex (precentral gyrus). *Surg Neurol* 2005; 64: 48-52.
- Urbach H, Scheffler B, Heinrichsmeier T, von Oertzen J, Kral T, Wellmer J, et al. Focal cortical dysplasia of Taylor's balloon cell type: a clinicopathological entity with characteristic neuroimaging and histopathological features, and favorable postsurgical outcome. *Epilepsia* 2002; 43: 33-40.
- Vikingstad EM, Cao Y, Thomas AJ, Johnson AF, Malik GM, Welch KMA. Language hemispheric dominance in patients with congenital lesions of eloquent brain. *Neurosurgery* 2000; 47: 562-70.
- Wilkins RH. Principles of neurosurgical operative technique. In: Wilkins RH, Rengachary SS, eds. *Neurosurgery*, volume 1, 2nd edition. New York: McGraw-Hill, 1996, 517-29.
- Wyler AR, Walker G, Somes G. The morbidity of long-term seizure monitoring using subdural strip electrodes. *J Neurosurg* 1991; 74: 734-7.
- Yingling CD, Ojemann S, Dodson B, Harrington MJ, Berger MS. Identification of motor pathways during tumor surgery facilitated by multichannel electromyographic recording. *J Neurosurg* 1999; 91: 922-7.
- Yousry TA, Schmid UD, Alkadhi H, Schmidt D, Peraud A, Buettner A. Localization of the motor hand area to a knob on the precentral gyrus: a new landmark. *Brain* 1997; 120: 141-57.

Video 1. Partial posterior insulectomy.
Videos of this chapter available at: www.etle.surgery.jle.com

Surgical treatment
of hypothalamic hamartomas

Ramez Malak, Elisabeth M.S. Sherman, Walter J. Hader

*Calgary Epilepsy Programme, Department of Clinical Neurosciences,
University of Calgary, Alberta, Canada*

■ Introduction

Gelastic epilepsy associated with hypothalamic hamartomas (HH) is now a well characterized clinical syndrome consisting of gelastic seizures starting in infancy which become
refractory to medications and may progress to include the development of multiple seizures
types in association with evidence of severe behavioural and developmental decline (Berkovic, 2003; Brandberg, 2004). The hypothalamic hamartoma-gelastic epilepsy syndrome
was initially felt to be the result of a progressive epileptic encephalopathy (Berkovic, 1988;
2003) or more recently due to secondary epileptogenesis (Kerrigan, 2005). Subsequent
confirmation of the intrinsic epileptogenesis of hypothalamic hamartomas (Kahane, 2003;
Kuzniecky, 1997; Munari, 1995) and its association with gelastic seizures has led to the
belief that not only the seizures themselves but the accompanying encephalopathy may be
potentially reversible with surgical treatment of the HH. Treatment of hypothalamic hamartomas by a variety of surgical approaches (Arita, 1998; Parrent, 1999; Fohlen, 2003; Harvey,
2003; Régis, 2006; Homma, 2007; Mathieu, 2006; Ng, 2006; 2008; Schulze-Bonhage, 2008)
has demonstrated that cessation of the seizures can occur and improvement in behaviour
and cognitive dysfunction is possible, supporting the concept that hypothalamic hamartomas
may be associated with an element of reversible encephalopathy.

■ Hypothalamic hamartomas

Hypothalamic hamartomas are rare non-neoplastic developmental lesions of the inferior
hypothalamus, which are composed of cytologically normal neurons abnormally distributed
within the hypothalamus (Coons, 2007). Hamartomas are found in the hypothalamus
attached to the tuber cinereum or more commonly to one or both mamillary bodies.
Grossly, they are light brown, avascular lesions with granular texture and firm consistency.
Microscopically, the abnormally distributed but cytologically normal neurons and glia
predominate in a nodular pattern comprised of hundreds of small to intermediate size
neurons. The neuronal size suggests that they may be interneurons which may contribute

to the basic intrinsic epileptogenicity of HH (Coons, 2007). The majority of cases are sporadic, but about 5% of cases may be associated with Pallister-Hall syndrome, which is an autosomal dominant disorder associated with a frameshift mutation in the GLI3 gene (Boudreau, 2005). Patients with Pallister-Hall present with panhypopituitarism and multiple dysmorphic features, including postradial polydactyly, bifid epiglottis and imperforate anus. The hamartomas in Pallister-Hall patients are histologically indistinct from sporadic cases and although gelastic seizures may occur, the course is generally more benign than that seen in sporadic cases of gelastic epilepsy with hypothalamic hamartoma (Boudreau, 2005).

■ Anatomy of the third ventricle and hypothalamus

The third ventricle is located in the center of the head, below the corpus callosum and the body of the lateral ventricle, above the sella turcica, pituitary gland, optic chiasm, and midbrain, and between the cerebral hemispheres, the two halves of the thalamus, and the two halves of the hypothalamus (Figure 1). It is intimately related to the circle of Willis and its branches and the great vein of Galen and its tributaries (Rhoton, 2002). The third ventricle communicates at its anterosuperior margin with each lateral ventricle through the foramen of Monro and posteriorly with the fourth ventricle through the aqueduct of Sylvius. The roof of the third ventricle extends from the foramen of Monro to the suprapineal recess and is formed by four layers: the fornix, the vascular layer containing the internal cerebral veins and choroidal arteries coursing in the velum interpositum between the two membranes of the tela choroidea., and finally the choroid plexus of the third ventricle which forms the deepest layer of the roof.

The floor of the third ventricle is formed anteriorly by the optic chiasm and the hypothalamus (the infundibulum, tuber cinereum and mamillary bodies) and posteriorly by the mesencephalon. The anterior margin of the third ventricle is formed, by the columns of the fornix, foramina of Monro, anterior commissure, lamina terminalis, optic recess, and by the optic chiasm. The posterior wall consists of the suprapineal recess, the habenular

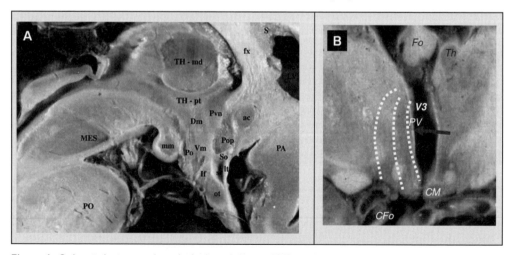

Figure 1. Cadaveric brain cuts through the hypothalamus. **A)** Sagittal paramedian cut showing the cranio-caudal disposition of the hypothalamic nuclei. **B)** Coronal cut showing the mesio-lateral disposition of the hypothalamic nuclei.

commissure, the pineal body and its recess, the posterior commissure, and the aqueduct of sylvius. The lateral walls are formed by the hypothalamus inferiorly and the thalamus superiorly, separated by the hypothalamic sulcus. The foramen of Monro is bounded anteriorly by the junction of the body and the columns of the fornix and posteriorly by the anterior pole of the thalamus. Lateral to the foramen on each side are the genu of the internal capsule. The structures that pass through the foramen are the choroid plexus, the distal branches of the medial posterior choroidal arteries, and the thalamostriate, superior choroidal, and septal veins (Rhoton, 2002).

■ Hypothalamus

The hypothalamus is situated in the anteroinferior portion of third ventricle. It is the center for integrating emotional and visceral information by controlling both endocrine and autonomic functions, in addition to receiving information from the limbic system. Hypothalamic nuclei can be grouped in a medial to lateral and in an anterior to posterior fashion. There are three medio-lateral zones: the periventricular zone, the medial zone and the lateral zone. The periventricular zone contains the nuclei that interact with the pituitary gland such as the arcuate nucleus that control the release of hormones from the adenohypophysis, and the paraventricular nucleus that produces oxytocin and the antidiuritic hormone (ADH). The medial zone contains autonomic centers, and the lateral zone is a limbic integration centers. There are also three zones from anterior to posterior (anterior, middle and posterior) *(Figure 2)*.

■ Clinical presentation

Hypothalamic hamartomas may be identified incidentally, in association with precocious puberty alone or with a syndrome of intractable gelastic epilepsy, and in some cases severe behavioural and intellectual impairment. Gelastic seizures, the initial manifestation of the hypothalamic hamartomas, often date back to the first years of life (Choi, 2004; Feiz-Erfan, 2005) although they may not be seen until late childhood or even adulthood (Mullatti, 2003; Striano, 2005). Seizures typically are characterized by brief episodes of inappropriate

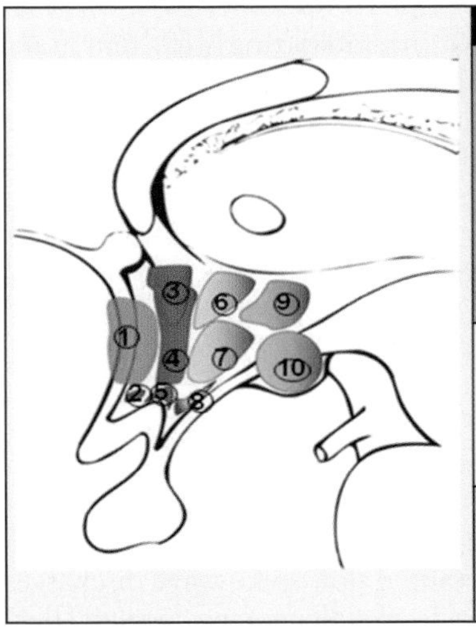

Groupe	Nucleus	Function
Anterior	1) Preoptic N	Autonomic: HR and BP, thermoregulation
	2) Suprachiasmatic N	Circadian rythms
	3) Paraventricular N	ADH, ocytocin
	4) Anterior N	Thermoregulation
	5) Supraoptic N	ADH, ocytocin
Middle	6) Dorsomedial N	Behavioral and hunger
	7) Ventromedial N	Behavioral and hunger
	8) Arcuat N (infundibular, tuberal)	Adnohypophysis inhibitory and release factors
Posterior	9) Posterior N	Autonomic: HR and BP, thermoregulation
	10) Mamillary body	Limbic system

Figure 2. Hypothalamic nuclei.

laughter after which facial contractions in the form of a smile or grimace may be seen; in the latter case, they have been referred to as dacrystic seizures (*i.e.*, crying seizures). Autonomic features such as flushing, tachycardia and changes in respiration may occur with the seizure (Harvey, 2007). The gelastic seizures may subside completely over time or persist in adulthood in a more benign form as simply a "pressure to laugh", becoming difficult to diagnose as a seizure at all (Mullatti, 2003; Sturm, 2000; Striano, 2005). Invariably, the seizures evolve and the typical gelastic seizure may be associated with loss of contact and focal motor phenomenon suggestive of frontal or temporal epilepsy foci (Berkovic, 2003; Sartori, 1999). Gelastic seizures have been reported, although rarely, in patients with temporal and frontal lobe epilepsy (Boudreau, 2005; Sturm, 2000), but HH remains the chief and most common cause. Evolution of the gelastic epilepsy to include multiple seizure types including generalized tonic clonic, tonic and atonic seizures as part of a generalized encephalopathy with diffuse EEG changes, intellectual deterioration and behavioural impairment may occur (Berkovic, 2003). Behavioural impairment, often characterized by difficulty controlling anger outbursts or "rage attacks" accompanied by disinhibition or difficulties with conduct and/or aggression are common; many pediatric patients meet criteria for oppositional defiant disorder or attention deficit hyperactivity disorder (Weissenberger, 2001). The severity of the seizure disorder, contrary to previous notions, does not appear to have an obvious correlation with the behavioural traits observed (Valdueza, 1994).

Neuropsychological manifestations

Cognitive dysfunction associated with hypothalamic hamartoma is considered a hallmark of the intractable gelastic epilepsy syndrome. Cognitive problems may be progressive in nature and deterioration may parallel the development of clinical and electroencephalographic features of secondary generalized epilepsy (Berkovic, 1988). Cognitive deterioraton may be a direct effect of the seizures on the developing nervous system and signal the development of an acquired epileptic encephalopathy (Berkovic, 1988; Berkovic, 2003). While severe cognitive impairments are often present in patients with multiple seizure types and evidence of secondary epileptogenesis (Prigatano, 2007; Quiske, 2006; 2007) global cognitive impairments have been demonstrated prior to the onset of epilepsy in some patients suggesting that the hamartoma itself may be interfering with important integrative functions essential for learning (Prigatano, 2007). In addition, it has become clear that a spectrum of neuropsychological impairments exists (Prigatano, 2007). For instance, normal cognitive function may be seen in patients with milder forms of gelastic epilepsy (Mullatti, 2003; Striano, 2005). Prigitano *et al.* (2007) in an assessment of 58 patients with hypothalamic hamartomas and gelastic epilepsy, determined that larger hamartomas and the presence of early onset of seizures were important predictors of cognitive dysfunction.

EEG

Interictal EEG recordings in infants with gelastic seizures and hypothalamic hamartomas may be normal and often ictal recordings of the brief infantile seizures may not be associated with any EEG change (Berkovic, 2003; Harvey, 2007). Later in childhood, as seizures evolve into multiple types, a background of generalized slow spike-wave discharges without focal abnormalities suggestive of secondary generalized epilepsy may develop (Berkovic, 1988; 2003). Independent epileptiform discharges may be seen and even focal ictal cortical abnormalities have been identified on intracranial EEG (Kahane, 2003). Early focal surgical resections aimed at these cortical abnormalities suggesting seizure origin in temporal or frontal structures led to disappointing results (Berkovic, 2003; Palmini, 2002; Cascino, 1993). Converging lines of evidence has since demonstrated that it is the intrinsic epileptogenicity of HH that is the origin of gelastic seizure. These include: 1) recordings of the implanted depth electrode into the hamartoma during the gelastic seizures (Kahane, 2003; Kuzniecky, 1997; Munari, 1995); 2) the reproduction of laughter and gelastic seizures following stimulation of the HH (Kahane, 2003; Kuzniecky, 1997); 3) the observation of ictal hyperperfusion and hypermetabolism of the hamartoma with SPECT (Kuzniecky, 1997) and PET imaging; and ultimately by 4) the resolution or the improvement of seizures following resection, ablation or radiation treatment of HH (Rosenfeld, 2001; Ng, 2006; 2008). Lastly, pacemaker-like activity may be found within clusters of cells in resected hamartomas, supporting the notion that epileptic properties are indeed intrinsic to the hamartomas themselves (Wu, 2005).

MR imaging

High resolution MR imaging remains the procedure of choice for identification of hypothalamic hamartomas which may be as little as a few millimeters to few centimeters in size. Identification of a HH on MR imaging in the context of a patient with the hallmarks of the gelastic epilepsy syndrome is sufficient neuroimaging for consideration of surgical management of the hamartoma. Hamartomas are usually isointense to gray matter on T1 and hyperintense or isointense on T2 weighted imaging and do not enhance after gadolinium administration. The anatomic relationship with the hypothalamus, like its clinical manifestations is variable. The hamartomas may be "pedunculated" or "parahypothalamic" (Arita, 1998), in which the hamartoma is attached to the floor by a narrow or wide peduncle in the absence of distortion of the overlying hypothalamus. This location is most common in association with a clinical presentation of precocious puberty (Arita, 1998), which after surgical removal has proved curative in small case series (Luo, 2002; Northfield, 1967). Conversely, hamartomas which predominate in patients with gelastic epilepsy directly involve and distort the hypothalamus (Arita, 1998; Freeman, 2003) and have been described as being "sessile" or "intrahypothalamic". The sessile's HH association with gelastic epilepsy maybe due the juxtaposition to the hypothalamus proper and central connections (Rosenfeld, 2001). Several classifications for HH have been proposed based on the pre operative MRI scan, in an effort to select the most appropriate surgical approach and to predict surgical outcome (Arita, 1999; Fohlen, 2003; Palmini, 2002; Régis, 2007; Valdueza, 1994,). Criteria common to the various schemes include: sessile vs pedunculated, degree of protrusion, orientation of protrusion towards the third ventricle vs the interpeduncular fossa, unilateral vs. bilateral location and the size of the hamartoma. Classification into four types that has been proposed by Delalande and Fohlen (2003) (Figure 3) separates lesions into types most likely to take into consideration the surgical approach amenable for resection while understanding that a continuum of lesions likely exist (Kerrigan 2005).

Type I	Horizontal implantation plane and may be lateralized on one side	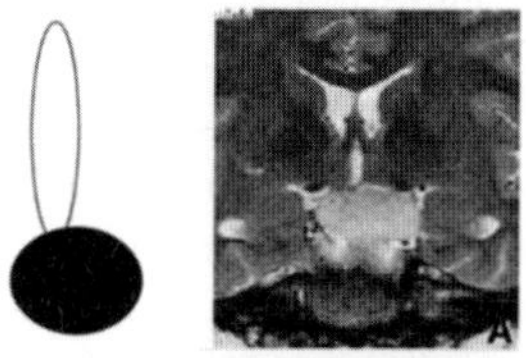
Type II	Vertical insertion plane and intraventricular location	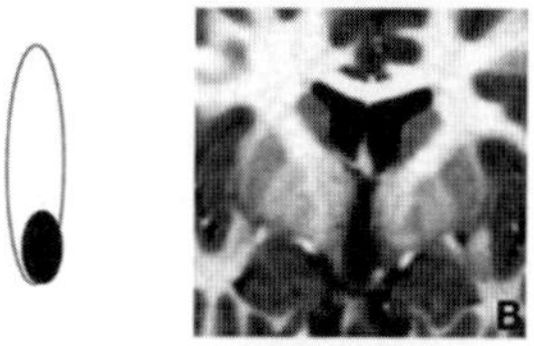
Type III	Combination of Types I and II	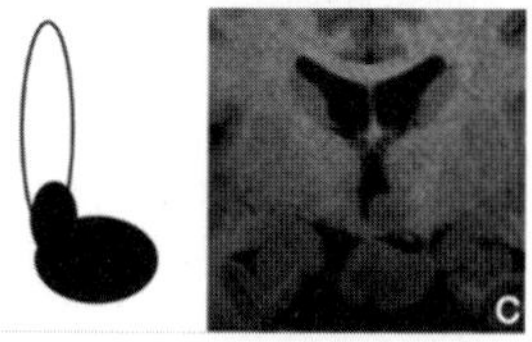
Type IV	Giant hamartomas	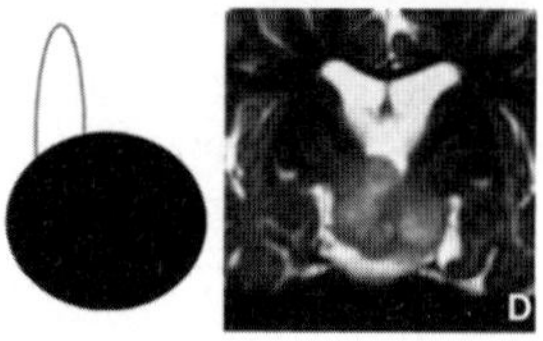

Figure 3. Delalande and Fohlen's Topographic classification of hypothalamic hamartomas. (From Delalande & Fohlen. *Neurol Med Chir* 2003; 43: 61-68).

■ Surgical management of hypothalamic hamartomas

The first case of surgically treated HH was reported by Northfield and Russell (Northfield, 1967, cited in Machado 1991). Although they did not recognize the gelastic seizures, they described one patient as having signs of mental retardation and precocious puberty and "frequently laughed and giggled". Surgical removal of HH for the treatment of precocious puberty was demonstrated in several additional case series subsequent to the original description (Alvarez-Garijo, 1983; Takeuchi, 1979; Kammer, 1980; Luo, 2002). In some patients who had associated gelastic seizures, surgery improved or cured the epilepsy and even led to improvement of cognitive functions (Takeuchi, 1979; Sato, 1985; Nishio, 1989). Based on those observations, successful direct surgical resection of a HH specifically for the treatment of gelastic seizures, was completed in a child in 1991 by Hoffman at the Hospital for Sick Children (Machado, 1991).

■ Surgical approach

A variety of surgical approaches have now been described for the management of gelastic epilepsy associated with HH. They can be divided broadly into four categories: basal, transcallosal interforniceal, endoscopic, and stereotactic approaches. The goal of surgery by any modality ideally would be complete safe removal or treatment with cessation of seizures originating from the hamartoma and improvement of secondary encephalopathic features. It is not clear, however, if complete or subtotal treatment of HH is needed to achieve seizure freedom as reports have suggested that seizure freedom can be achieved with both strategies (Freeman, 2003; Ng, 2006). The chance of complete removal, however, appears dependant on the size and the location of the HH: the larger the lesion the less likely the chance of complete resection, and the closer the attachment to the mamillary bodies the harder and the riskier the complete resection will be (Rosenfeld, 2007). As a result, surgical disconnection has been proposed as an alternative to removal by Fohlen (2003) in cases where the tumor is large, and complete and safe resection is not possible. This is believed by some to be the optimal surgical strategy required to achieve a good seizure outcome with minimal risk (Fohlen, 2003; Procaccini, 2006; Rosenfeld, 2007). Disconnection with or without resection from the mamillary bodies and the hypothalamus, however, may be as technically challenging as removal since the plane for such a disconnection may not be well-defined.

■ Basal

Various standard basal neurosurgical approaches for removal of hypothalamic hamartomas have been reported including subfrontal, subtemporal, pterional, fronto-temporal as well as orbito-zygomatic (Fohlen, 2003; Palmini, 2002; Valdueza, 1994). Results of surgical interventions for hypothalamic hamartomas from two larger series, in which either the pterional or fronto-temporal approach was used, confirmed that improvement in the gelastic epilepsy, and associated cognitive or behavioural manifestations was possible with direct treatment of hypothalamic hamartomas (Palmini, 2002; Fohlen, 2003). In those series, two out of 13 (Palmini, 2002) and three out of 14 patients (Fohlen, 2003) were rendered completely seizure free while the remainder achieved either a significant or complete reduction of drop attacks and generalized tonic-clonic seizures. The major disadvantage of those basal approaches where the lesion is reached "from below" is that the boundary between normal hypothalamic tissue and hamartoma tissue is not readily visible especially during the resection of sessile hamartomas; therefore, complete resection is often impossible (Feiz-Erfan, 2005). In addition, 7 patients in one of the series experienced serious complications (Palmini, 2002) including cranial nerve paresis, strokes and even death. As a result of the modest seizure freedom achieved with basal surgical approaches, alternative approaches have been developed in order to obtain a greater degree of hamartoma resection or treatment while limiting complications.

■ Transcallosal interforniceal

The transcallosal interforniceal approach was first reported by Rosenfeld in 2001 as an alternative to traditional basal approaches for the surgical removal of hypothalamic hamartomas associated with gelastic epilepsy. Initial results were promising with seizure freedom reported in three of five patients (Rosenfeld, 2001). Advantages of the transcallosal approach over basal approaches to the third ventricle include limited brain retraction and manipulation of major vessels and cranial nerve responsible for most of the complications in the basal approaches (Fohlen, 2003; Palmini, 2002; Rosenfeld, 2004). In addition the approach offered a better view of the HH in the third ventricle allowing more complete microsurgical resection from within the lesion (Harvey, 2003) with the possibility of following the HH into the interpeduncular fossa and prepontine cistern, if necessary. A third advantage is the ability to debulk and/or disconnect the HH and spare the mamillary bodies if they can be identified, as well as preservation of the pituitary stalk and the optic chiasm. Further experience led to modifications of the original approach to the anterior transcallosal transseptal interforniceal approach in order to minimize forniceal retraction and reduce the risk of memory disturbances (Rosenfeld, 2004). Compared to the classic interforniceal approach (Apuzzo, 1998), the entry to the third ventricle is between the two columns of the fornix between the foramen of Monro and the anterior commissure; so there is no need to divide the body of the fornix *(Figure 4)*. Additionally, avoidance of injury to more posteriorly placed vascular structures including the tela choroidea, choroid plexus and internal cerebral veins and their tributaries, is possible. The disadvantage is that the most anterior and posterior margins of the floor of the third ventricle are difficult to visualize (Rosenfeld, 2004).

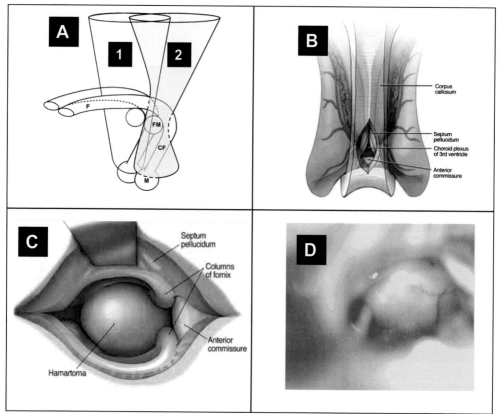

Figure 4. The anterior transcallosal transseptal interforniceal approach. **A)** Trajectory for (1) standard transcallosal interforniceal (2) and the anterior transseptal interforniceal approach. **B)** The corpus callosum is divided and leaves of the septum pellucidum are separated. **C)** The HH is evident and the fornices are retracted laterally. **D)** intraoperative view of hamartoma.
(From: Feiz-Erfan et al., J Neurosurg 2005; 103 (4 Suppl): 325-32; and Rosenfeld et al., J Clin Neuroscience 2004; 11 (7): 738-44).

Technique

The patient is placed in a supine position with the head slightly elevated and flexed. Alternatively the patient the patient can be placed in the lateral decubitus position with the non dominant side down, so that gravity alone retracts the hemisphere away from the falx and the third ventricle can be entered in a transverse plane (Rosenfeld, 2004). Either a U-shaped or a bicoronal incision behind the hairline is performed. A moderate sized (4-5 cm) precoronal parasagittal craniotomy is made just adjacent to the midline. Careful examination of the preoperative magnetic resonance images can help in assessing the best location for the craniotomy to avoid bridging veins draining into the superior sagittal sinus. On very rare occasions, the craniotomy is done on the dominant side because of particular parasagittal venous anatomy.

After the dural opening, the interhemispheric fissure is dissected and the two hemispheres are separated using soft cotton balls and/or self-retaining retractors. Image guidance helps direct the approach through to the anterior corpus callosum. At the bottom of the falx cerebri, the two cingulate gyri are often adherent and it is important to stay in the interpial midline plane during the dissection. The corpus callosum is finally identified by its white glistening color and by the presence of the pericallosal arteries. A longitudinal 10 to 15 mm midline incision into the corpus callosum is made using a sharp dissector, coagulation and aspiration, or the ultrasonic aspirator. After the initial exposure and limited anterior callosotomy, dissection of the leaves of the septum pellucidum is performed between the mesial surface of the frontal horns of the lateral ventricles (*Figure 4*). The third ventricle is entered between the forniceal columns at the anterior border of the foramen of Munro. Upon entering the anterior end of the roof of the third ventricle, the HH is removed using the microtip and the ultrasonic aspirator at a low setting; surgery may then proceed beyond the floor of the third ventricle into the interpeduncular cistern if necessary. When the tumor is large with significant inferior projections into the basal cisterns, combined or staged transcallosal approach with an additional basal transsylvian approach may be utilized. The detailed clinical and operative anatomy of the anterior transcallosal transseptal interforniceal approach can be reviewed in detail (Rosenfeld, 2004; Siwanuwatn, 2005).

Seizure outcome

Results from the two largest series to date have reported seizure freedom in 14 (54%) of 26 patients (Ng, 2006) in one series and 15 (52%) of 29 patients (Harvey, 2003) in the second series of patients with a mean follow-up of 20 and 30 months, respectively. An additional 35% and 24% of patients had greater than 90% reduction in their seizures, respectively. The likelihood of seizure freedom was associated with younger age, shorter duration of epilepsy, smaller HH volume and complete HH resection. Presence or absence of developmental delay and seizure type (gelastic only *versus* multiple seizure types) did not appear to correlate with seizure freedom. In addition to reduction in seizure frequency after resection, significant improvements in behavior, reduced aggression, increased concentration and improved mood have been reported. Ng and associates (Ng, 2006) reported subjective improvement in behavior in 88% of patients and in cognition in 58% of patients as reported by parents as early as the first few weeks following surgery. This improvement has been attributed to the decreased frequency of interictal spike-wave activity and may relate to the reversal of the epileptic encephalopathy observed in some of these patients (Freeman, 2003; Harvey, 2007).

Complications

Injuries to the hypothalamus with attempted complete removal of hamartomas comprise the most common complications reported with the transcallosal interforniceal and anterior transcallosal transseptal interforniceal approches. Asymptomatic hypernatraemia without polyuria was the most common endocrine complication observed in up to 55% of patients in one series (Freeman, 2003a). More overt diabetes insipidus may develop and has been reported in up to 15% of patients, but it is usually transient with no need for long-term antidiuretic hormone therapy. The most common reported complaint after resection was difficulty with short term memory which was seen in almost half of patients (Harvey, 2003) and noted to be persistent at 3 months in almost one third of patients. Weight gain or hypothalamic obesity, a known complication of operations on the hypothalamus including tumor resections and endoscopic third ventriculostomy for hydrocephalus, (Hader, 2008) was seen in the early postoperative period in 45% of patients treated by the transcallosal approach. Additionally, partial or complete panhypopituitarism has been described with low thyroxine and growth hormone levels in which replacement therapy may be required. Excessive sleepiness and hyperthermia are may also observed in the early postoperative period. Injury to structures beneath the hypothalamus with transcallosal resection of large lesions or in combination with basal approaches may result in cranial nerve paresis (Ng, 2006; Rosenfeld, 2007) and hemiparesis (Ng, 2006; Andrew, 2008) secondary to thalamic infarcts, although the frequency appears less than previously seen with basal approaches (Palmini, 2002).

■ Endoscopic

Transventricular endoscopic resection has been demonstrated to be a good treatment option for small intrahypothalamic HH (less than 10 mm) that are ideally attached to only one wall of the third ventricle and exhibit definite intraventricular extension (Freeman, 2004; Hader, 2008; Ng, 2005; Ng, 2008; Procaccini, 2006) (Figure 5). Use of the endoscopic approach may be preferred over the transcallosal approach in adults where the septum pellucidum leaves are hard to separate which increase the potential risk to lose the midline orientation and cause injury to the columns of the fornix. The primary challenge with the endoscopic approach remains that in most patients with HH the lateral and third ventricles are of normal size. Rigid fixation of the endoscope with the ability for micromanipulation is essential in order to safely access the ventricular system and remove the hamartoma. A distance of at least 6 mm from the lesion to the foramen of Monro is needed to allow safe manipulation of the endoscopic instruments within the third ventricle during removal.

Technique

Removal of the hamartoma is best achieved through the foramen of Monro which is contralateral to the hypothalamic attachment. The operation is done under general anesthesia with the patient in a supine position and head slightly flexed. A 3 cm parasagittal incision is placed immediately anterior to the coronal suture and 2 cm off midline. Frameless stereotactic neuronavigation is utilized to accurately approach the foramen of Monro for entry into the third ventricle, particularly when ventricular size is normal. Rigid fixation of the endoscope is essential with a pneumatic arm with capabilities for micromanipulation of the scope to prevent trauma to the fornix and choroid plexus. The

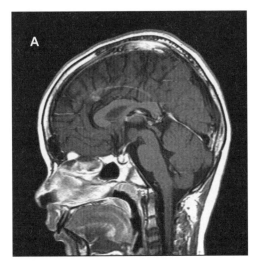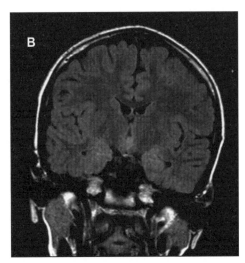

Figure 5. Intraventricular hypothalamic hamartoma. **A)** Sagittal T1MRI shows intraventricular HH. **B)** Coronal Flair MRI shows HH attached to mamillary body.

trajectory can be changed by releasing the rigid fixation of the endoscope without disconnecting the endoscope-scope holder unit *(Figure 6)*. Alternatively, a robotic arm can be used for trajectory planning, positioning of the endoscope and holding the endoscope steady at the target (Procaccini, 2006). After entering the lateral ventricle, the endoscope is moved anterior to the choroid plexus, which is retracted posteriorly to allow entry to the third ventricle. The HH is usually easily identified from the surrounding hypothalamus

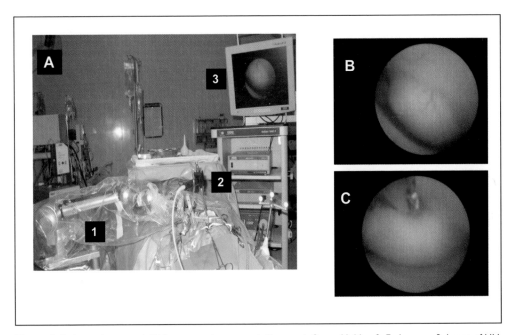

Figure 6. Endoscopic removal. **A)** Intraoperative set up; 1. Pneumatic Scope Holder; 2. Endoscope; 3. Image of HH. **B)** Endoscopic view of HH. **C)** Plane of dissection along ventricular wall.

as a mass projecting into the third ventricle and displaying a light brown color and relatively avascular surface. An endoscopic micropituitary rongeur or cupped biopsy forcep is introduced through a working channel, and the interface between the hamartoma and surrounding normal brain is dissected circumferentially in a piecemeal fashion, followed by debulking of the center of the hamartoma until the pial surface or the ependymal surface of the floor of the third ventricle is identified. Ringer's lactate solution at body temperature is used to irrigate the ventricle during resection. Great care should be taken to preserve the pial surface of the interpeduncular cistern to avoid disruption of posterior cerebral perforating arteries and subsequent thalamic infarcts (Ng, 2008). Minimal bleeding usually responds to gentle irrigation or pressure with the endoscope, and coagulation should be avoided as much as possible especially close to the pial surface. Intraoperative interdissection MR imaging has proven to be a useful adjunct for resection of hamartomas particularly when the boundary between the hamartoma and normal hypothalamus are indistinct. A ventriculostomy can be placed in the lateral ventricle at the end of the intervention.

Seizure outcome

Seizure freedom was attained in 18 (49%) of 37 patients with minimum one-year follow-up from the largest series of patients who underwent endoscopic resection of their hamartomas from the Barrow Institute. This outcome was similar to that seen with an open transcallosal approach at the same center in which 54% of patients were seizure free (Ng, 2006). Significant improvement in behavioural and cognitive disturbances after endoscopic resection was also noted. Compared with an open transcallosal approach patients who had an endoscopic resection experienced a clinically and statistically shorter hospital stay (Ng, 2007). Assessment of outcome as measured by quality of life has been rated as very good not only in patients seizure free after surgery but in patients with an incomplete response to endoscopic surgical removal (Hader, 2008) who demonstrated significant improvements in behaviour and cognition.

Complications

Although considered as a minimally invasive procedure, transient serious complications have been reported in up to 25% of patients who undergo endoscopic resections; these are permanent in 7% of patients (Ng, 2008). As with surgical removal via a transcallosal approach, the most common complication after endoscopic removal was difficulty with short-term memory, occurring in 6 patients (14%) and persisting three months after surgery in 3 patients (8%). (Ng, 2008) Details of the underlying factors causing memory disturbance were not provided. However, injury to the fornix upon entry into the third ventricle after endoscopic removal in addition to resection of the hamartoma from the mamillary bodies have been implicated as playing a role in memory problems after endoscopic removal (Hader, 2008). While the approach through the contralateral ventricle is ideal for the resection of the hamartoma, a greater risk of significant memory disturbance may exist with injury to the fornix in the language-dominant hemisphere (Hader, 2008). In the largest series (Ng, 2008), hemiparesis presumably due to thalamic perforator injury occurred in 3 patients and was felt to be related to penetration of the interpeduncular cistern at the time of the procedure. Transient weight gain greater than 10% of body weight was also identified in up to 10% of patients (Ng, 2008).

■ Stereotactic approaches

Radiosurgery

The safety and efficacy of radiosurgical treatment for patients with intractable epilepsy has previously been demonstrated in a European multicenter trial of patients with mesial temporal lobe epilepsy (Régis, 2004). Long-term follow-up suggests that the success of radiosurgery for intractable mesial temporal lobe epilepsy may be similar to that with standard microsurgical resection (Bartolomei, 2008). Successful radiosurgical lesioning of hypothalamic hamartomas by gamma knife radiosurgery for the treatment of intractable gelastic epilepsy was first described in 1998 by Arita and associates (Arita, 1998) and has subsequently been reported in several small case series both with Gamma Knife (Mathieu, 2006; Unger, 2000) and LINAC radiosurgical technology (Selch, 2005). In the largest series (Régis, 2006) with 27 patients and a minimum of 3 years follow up, seizure freedom was achieved in 10 patients (37%) and a significant improvement in seizure frequency in another 6 (22%). Less frequent preoperative gelastic seizures and the ability to deliver optimal doses to lesion margins, particularly for small intrahypothalamic or intraventricular lesion were good predictors of therapeutic response. Improvements in seizures appear to follow a temporal sequence with an early initial response to treatment followed by transient worsening and then resultant reduction and remission of seizures (Régis, 2006). Similar to open surgical procedures, patients who experienced good seizure outcome also showed behavioral and cognitive improvement. Repeat radiosurgery was possible in patients not responding to initial therapy and an improved response can be seen. In addition, surgical resection is possible after radiosurgery and has been utilized with larger lesions. Unarguably the major advantage of radiosurgery in the treatment of HH is its safety. Compared with other treatment options vascular and neurological complications including cognitive complications have not been reported with radiosurgical treatment of HH.

Interstitial brachytherapy

Interstitial radiosurgery, formally called brachytherapy, involves the temporary direct or stereotactic placement of single or multiple radioactive sources into the target volume. Energy delivery is carried out using ^{125}I, by which a high energy (up to 200 Gy isodose) is delivered to the target with a steep fall off to the periphery, leading to central necrosis, and injury to the surrounding tissue layer subsequently resulting in a programmed cell death (*Figure 7*). In spite of the high energy delivered, there is minimal radiation injury

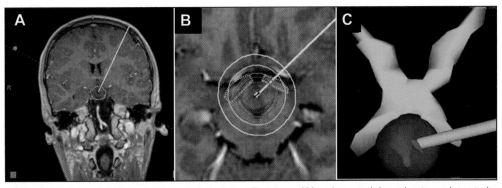

Figure 7. Brachytherapy. Stereotactic seed implantation: Trajectory **(A)** and marginal dose planning with particular regard to the close proximity of the optic tracts **(B)**. 3D reconstruction of HH and optic pathways **(C)**. (From Schulze-Bonhage, *Neurology* 2008; 71: 277-82).

outside the target. The treatment is delivered over a period of 3 weeks, with a low-dose rate (1-15 cGy/h). Such a small dose allows the surrounding structures to recover from the radiation exposure, and therefore minimizing the risk to surrounding vital structures including optic nerves and tracts, mamillary bodies and brainstem. In the single large series to date of 24 patients with HH and intractable epilepsy, Engel Class I or II outcome was achieved in 37% and 17% of patients respectively, with a mean follow-up of 24 months (Schulze-Bonhage, 2008). Reimplantation of seeds was repeated in 13 patients, and was generally offered at 1 year if seizure control was insufficient. No immediate perioperative morbidity was seen. Five patients (21%) developed headaches and lethargy and were noted to have developed perilesional edema on follow up MRI at 3 months. Symptoms were treated with oral corticosteroids and subsequent imaging demonstrated resolution of the edema. Weight gain from 5 to 24 kg was seen in 4 patients (17%), in all whom diet failed to reverse the post treatment increases. Neuropsychological assessment was available in most patients. Subjective improvement in attention and ability to concentrate was reported however 5 patients (21%) showed a significant decrease in verbal memory (more than 1 SD change) and 6 patients (25%) had a significant decrease in visual memory. When compared to radiosurgical procedures, interstitial radiosurgery has the advantage of a short time to produce therapeutic effect ranging between 2 and 8 weeks, compared to LINAC or gamma knife surgery which in the short term seizures may worsen seizures and where a minimum of two years are required to observe sustained reductions in seizure frequency (Régis, 2006).

Radiofrequency thermocoagulation

Several reports with small numbers of patients have demonstrated the safety and efficacy of stereotactic radiofrequency thermocoagulation (SRT) for HH (Homma, 2007; Kuzniecky, 1997; Parrent, 1999). Homma and associates (Homma, 2007) reported on 5 patients with HH who underwent a stereotactic radiofrequency thermocoagulation for the treatment of intractable epilepsy. In all cases the hamartoma was intraventricular and less than 15 mm in diameter. In 3 patients, a depth electrode was placed in the lesion using a leksell stereotactic system® (ELEKTA, Sweden) and recording from the hamartoma confirmed the ictal onset. Following the recording the depth electrode was replaced using the lesion electrode. Up to 74° C for 60 seconds were used as tolerated by the patients. Following a mean follow up period of 50.6 months, three patients were seizure free and the remaining 2 patients have more than 90% improvement in seizure frequency. Transient low grade fever developed in 3 patients and no patient was reported to have a permanent complication related to the procedure.

In a recent Japanese series of 25 patients with gelastic epilepsy and HH, thirty-one SRT procedures were performed, requiring an average of 4 tracks (1 to 8) and 7 lesions (1 to 18) per procedure (*Figure 8*) (Kameyama, 2009) Complete seizure freedom was achieved in 19 patients (76.0%), however, follow up was short with only a minimum follow up of 6 months. In addition there was an improvement in behavioral problems and IQ results post SRT. Detailed results of memory performance were not reported but 2 patients (8%) were noted to have transient short-term memory disturbances postoperation. Other post operative complications included hyperthermia (16%), hyperphagia (8%), hyponatremia (16%), Horner's syndrome (12%), and transient personality change (8%). In addition there was one case of asymptomatic chronic subdural hematoma, and another asymptomatic

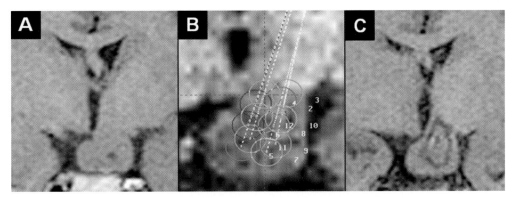

Figure 8. Stereotactic radiofrequency thermocoagulation. A, T1-weighted MRI scan showing a large HH. B, target localization (12 lesions) via 4 tracks C, MRI 3 months after SRT. (From Kameyama *et al.*, *Neurosurgery* 2009; 65: 438-49).

subacute epidural hematoma (Kameyama, 2009). The results while promising were too soon after treatment to be conclusive for the long term effectiveness of a multi-lesion strategy.

Deep brain stimulation

Electrical stimulation of the anterior nucleus of the thalamus has recently been confirmed in a multicenter double-blind randomized trial to reduce seizures in patients with medically refractory epilepsy (Fisher, 2010). A single case report has demonstrated the utility of high frequency deep brain stimulation of the mammillothalamic tract in two pediatric patients with intractable epilepsy and HH. One patient followed for 23 months post op, was seizure free for the last 10 months, and the second had a significant reduction in seizure frequency (Khan, 2009). No complications resulted and improvement in mood and quality of life was reported by caregivers in both instances.

■ Conclusions

Surgical management of hypothalamic hamartomas associated with gelastic epilepsy, has been demonstrated to improve seizures, behaviour and quality of life through a variety of approaches in the majority of patients. Partial treatment of the lesion as demonstrated by subtotal resection or treatments with less invasive stereotactic methods that are not intended to completely obliterate the lesion may be similarly effective to direct surgical approaches with a more favourable side effect profile (*Table I*). The optimum timing of surgery for gelastic epilepsy remains unclear, however, early intervention prior to the onset of secondary epilepsy may result in better seizure outcome and prevention of behavioural and cognitive decline related to the progressive epileptic encephalopathy that may be seen in some patients. Demonstration of the normalization of severe cognitive impairments after resection of hypothalamic hamartoma supports the notion that a reversible component of cognitive dysfunction may exist in some patients with gelastic epilepsy.

Table I. Outcome following surgical treatment of hypothalamic hamartoma

Approach	Series	N	Engel I	Memory deficit [a]		Endocrine deficit	Hyperphagia	Infarct [b]	Hemiparesis	
				trans	perm				trans	perm
Basal	Palmini, 2002	13	15%	NR	NR	8%	8%	30%	23%	8%
	Fohlen, 2003	14	21%	NR	NR	35%	7%	14%	7%	7%
Transcallosal	Rosenfeld, 2004	45	52%	36%	13%	20%	34%	7%	7%	0%
	Ng, 2006	26	54%	58%	8%	15%	19%	4%	4%	0%
Endoscopic	Procaccini, 2006	26	42%	NR	NR	12%	12%	0%	0%	0%
	Ng, 2008	37	49%	14%	8%	0%	14%	30%	11%	0%
Radiosurgery	Regis, 2006	27	37%	NR	NR	0%	0%	0%	0%	0%
Brachytherapy	Schulze, 2008	24	38%	21%	8%	0%	17%	0%	0%	0%
SRT	Kameyama, 2009	25	76%	8%	NR	0%	8%	0%	0%	0%

SRT: Stereotactic radiofrequency thermocoagulation; trans: transient; perm: permanent; NR: Not reported; [a] Memory deficit: Subjective short term; [b] Infarct: radiological (CT, or MRI).

References

- Alvarez-Garijo JA, Albiach VJ, Vila MM, Mulas R, Esquembre V. Precocious puberty and hypothalamic hamartoma with total recovery after surgical treatment. Case report. *J Neurosurg* 1983; 58: 583-5.

- Andrew M, Parr JR, Stacey R, Rosenfeld JV, Hart Y, Pretorius P, *et al.* Transcallosal resection of hypothalamic hamartoma for gelastic epilepsy. *Childs Nerv Syst* 2008; 24: 275-9.

- Apuzzo M, Amar A. Transcallosal interforniceal approach. In: Apuzzo M. (ed.) *Surgery of the Third Ventricle*, 2nd ed. Baltimore: Williams and Wilkins, 1998, pp. 421-452.

- Arita K, Kurisu K, Iida K, Hanaya R, Akimitsu T. Hibino S, *et al.* Subsidence of seizure induced by stereotactic radiation in a patient with hypothalamic hamartoma. Case report. *J Neurosurg* 1998; 89: 645-8.

- Arita K, Ikawa F, Kurisu K, Sumida M, Harada K, Uozumi T, *et al.* The relationship between magnetic resonance imaging findings and clinical manifestations of hypothalamic hamartoma. *J Neurosurg* 1999; 91: 212-20.

- Bartolomei F, Hayashi M, Tamura M, Rey M, Fischer C, Chauvel P, Régis J. Long-term efficacy of gamma knife radiosurgery in mesial temporal lobe epilepsy. *Neurology* 2008; 70: 1658-63.

- Berkovic SF, Andermann F, Melanson D, Ethier RE, Feindl W, Gloor P. Hypothalamic hamartomas and ictal laughter: evolution of a characteristic epileptic syndrome and diagnostic value of magnetic resonance imaging. *Ann Neurol* 1988; 23: 429-39.

- Berkovic SF, Arzimanoglou A, Kuzniecky R, Harvey AS, Palmini A, Andermann F. Hypothalamic hamartoma and seizures: a treatable epileptic encephalopathy. *Epilepsia* 2003; 44: 969-73.

- Boudreau EA, Liow K, Frattali CM, Wiggs E, Turner JT, Feuillan P, *et al.* Hypothalamic hamartomas and seizures: distinct natural history of isolated and Pallister-Hall syndrome cases. *Epilepsia* 2005; 46: 42-7.

- Brandberg G, Raininko R, Eeg-Olofsson O. Hypothalamic hamartoma with gelastic seizures in Swedish children and adolescents. *Eur J Pediatr Neurol* 2004; 8: 35-44.

- Cascino GD, Andermann F, Berkovic SF, *et al.* Gelastic seizures and hypothalamic hamartomas: evaluation of patients undergoing chronic intracranial EEG monitoring and outcome of surgical treatment. *Neurology* 1993;43: 747-50.

- Choi JU, Yang KH, Kim TG, Chang JH, Chang JW, Lee BI, Kim DS. Endoscopic disconnection for hypothalamic hamartoma with intractable seizure. Report of four cases. *J Neurosurg* 2004; 100 (5 Suppl): 506-11.

- Coons SW, Rekate HL, Prenger EC, Wang N, Drees C, Ng YT, *et al.* The histopathology of hypothalamic hamartomas: study of 57 cases. *J Neuropathol Exp Neurol* 2007; 66: 131-41.

- Delalande O, Fohlen M. Disconnecting surgical treatment of hypothalamic hamartoma in children and adults with refractory epilepsy and proposal of a new classification. *Neurol Med Chir* 2003; 43: 61-8.

- Feiz-Erfan I, Horn EM, Rekate HL, Spetzler RF, Ng YT, Rosenfeld JV, Kerrigan JF. Surgical strategies for approaching hypothalamic hamartomas causing gelastic seizures in the pediatric population: transventricular compared with skull base approaches. *J Neurosurg* 2005; 103 (4 Suppl): 325-32.

- Fisher R, Salanova V, Witt T, Worth R, Henry T, Gross R, *et al.* and the SANTE Study Group. Electrical stimulation of the anterior nucleus of thalamus for treatment of refractory epilepsy. *Epilepsia* 2010; 51: 899-908.

- Fohlen M, Lellouch A, Delalande O. Hypothalamic hamartoma with refractory epilepsy: surgical procedures and results in 18 patients. *Epileptic Disord* 2003; 5: 267-73.

- Freeman JL, Harvey AS, Rosenfeld JV, Wrennall JA, Bailey CA, Berkovic SF. Generalized epilepsy in hypothalamic hamartoma: evolution and postoperative resolution. *Neurology* 2003; 60: 762-7.

- Freeman JL, Zacharin M, Rosenfeld JV, Harvey AS. The endocrinology of hypothalamic hamartoma surgery for intractable epilepsy. *Epileptic Disord* 2003a; 5: 239-47.

- Freeman JL, Coleman LT, Welland RM, Kean MJ, Rosenfeld JV, Jackson GD, *et al.* MR imaging and spectroscopic study of epileptogenic hypothalamic hamartomas: analysis of 72 cases. *Am J Neuroradiol* 2004; 25: 450-62.

- Hader WJ, Ozen L, Hamiwka L, Sherman E. Neuropsychological and quality of life outcome after endoscopic resection of hypothalamic hamartomas. *Can J Neurol Sci* 2008; 35: S73 (Abstract).

- Hader WJ, Walker RL, Myles ST, Hamilton M. Complications of endoscopic third ventriculostomy in previously shunted patients. *Neurosurgery* 2008; 63 (Suppl 1): 168-74.

- Harvey AS, Freeman JL, Berkovic SF, Rosenfeld JV. Transcallosal resection of hypothalamic hamartomas in patients with intractable epilepsy. *Epileptic Disord* 2003; 5: 257-65.

- Harvey AS, Freeman JL. Epilepsy in hypothalamic hamartoma: clinical and EEG features. *Semin Pediatr Neurol* 2007; 14: 60-4.

- Homma J, Kameyama S, Masuda H, Ueno T, Fujimoto A, Oishi M, Fukuda M. Stereotactic radiofrequency thermocoagulation for hypothalamic hamartoma with intractable gelastic seizures. *Epilepsy Res* 2007; 76: 15-21.

- Kahane P, Ryvlin P, Hoffman D, Minotti L, Benabid AL. From hypothalamic hamartoma to cortex: what can be learnt from depth recordings and stimulation? *Epileptic Disord* 2003; 5: 205-17.

- Kameyama S, Murakami H, Masuda H, Sugiyama I. Minimally invasive magnetic resonance imaging-guided stereotactic radiofrequency thermocoagulation for epileptogenic hypothalamic hamartomas. *Neurosurgery* 2009; 65 (3): 438-49.

- Kammer KS, Perlman K, Humphreys RP, Howard NJ. Clinical and surgical aspects of hypothalamic hamartoma associated with precocious puberty in a 15-month-old boy. *Child's Brain* 1980; 7: 150-7.

- Kerrigan JF, Ng YT, Chung S, Rekate HL. The hypothalamic hamartoma: a model of subcortical epileptogenesis and encephalopathy. *Semin Pediatr Neurol* 2005; 12: 119-31.

- Khan S, Wright I, Javed S, Jardine P, Carter M, Gill SS. High frequency stimulation of the mamillothalamic tract for the treatment of resistant seizures associated with hypothalamic hamartoma. *Epilepsia* 2009; 50 (6): 1608-11.

- Kuzniecky R, Guthrie B, Mountz J, Bebin M, Faught E, Gilliam F, Liu HG. Intrinsic epileptogenesis of hypothalamic hamartomas in gelastic epilepsy. *Ann Neurol* 1997; 42: 60-7.

- Luo S, Li C, Ma Z, Zhang Y, Jia G, Cheng Y. Microsurgical treatment for hypothalamic hamartoma in children with precocious puberty. *Surg Neurol* 2002; 57: 356-62.

- Machado HR, Hoffman HJ, Hwang PA. Gelastic seizures treated by resection of a hypothalamic hamartoma. *Childs Nev Syst* 1991; 7: 462-5.

- Mathieu D, Kondziolka D, Niranjan A, Flickinger J, Lunsford LD. Gamma knife radiosurgery for refractory epilepsy caused by hypothalamic hamartomas. *Stereotact Funct Neurosurg* 2006; 84: 82-7.

- Mullatti N, Selway R, Nashef L, Elwes R, Honavar M, Chandler C, *et al.* The clinical spectrum of epilepsy in children and adults with hypothalamic hamartoma. *Epilepsia* 2003; 44: 1310-9.

- Munari C, Kahane P, Francione S, Hoffmann D, Tassi L, Cusmai R, *et al.* Role of the hypothalamic hamartoma in the genesis of gelastic fits (a video-stereo-EEG study). *Electroencephalogr Clin Neurophysiol* 1995; 95: 154-60.

- Ng YT, Rekate HL, Prenger EC, Chung SS, Feiz-Erfan I, Wang NC, *et al.* Transcallosal resection of hypothalamic hamartoma for intractable epilepsy. *Epilepsia* 2006; 47: 1192-202.

- Ng YT, Rekate HL, Prenger EC, Wang NC, Chung SS, Feiz-Erfan I, *et al.* Endoscopic resection of hypothalamic hamartomas for refractory symptomatic epilepsy. *Neurology* 2008; 70 (17): 1543-8.

- Nishio S, Fujiwara S, Aiko Y, Takeshita I, Fukui M. Hypothalamic hamartoma. Report of two cases. *J Neurosurg* 1989; 70: 640-5.

- Northfield DW, Russell DS. Pubertas praecox due to hypothalamic hamartoma: report of two cases surviving surgical removal of the tumor. *J Neurol Neurosurg Psychiatry* 1967; 30: 166-73.

- Palmini A, Chandler C, Andermann F, Costa Da Costa J, Paglioli-Neto E, Polkey C, *et al.* Resection of the lesion in patients with hypothalamic hamartoma and catastrophic epilepsy. *Neurology* 2002; 58: 1338-47.

- Parrent AG. Stereotactic radiofrequency ablation for the treatment of gelastic seizures associated with hypothalamic hamartoma. Case report. *J Neurosurg* 1999; 91: 881-4.

- Prigatano GP. Cognitive and behavioral dysfunction in children with hypothalamic hamartoma and epilepsy. *Semin Pediatr Neurol* 2007; 14: 65-72.

- Procaccini E, Dorfmuller G, Fohlen M, Bulteau C, Delalande O. Surgical management of hypothalamic hamartomas with epilepsy: the stereoendoscopic approach. *Operative Neurosurg* 2006; 59: 336-44.

- Quiske A, Frings L, Wagner K, Unterrainer J, Schulze-Bonhage A. Cognitive functions in juvenile and adult patients with gelastic epilepsy due to hypothalamic hamartoma. *Epilepsia* 2006; 47: 153-8.

- Quiske A, Unterrainer J, Wagner K, Frings L, Breyer T, Halsband U, *et al.* Assessment of cognitive functions before and after stereotactic interstitial radiosurgery of hypothalamic hamartomas in patients with gelastic seizures. *Epilepsy Behav* 2007; 10: 328-32.

- Régis J, Rey M, Bartolomei F, Vladyka V, Liscak R, Schröttner O, Pendl G. Gamma knife surgery in mesial temporal lobe epilepsy: a prospective multicenter study. *Epilepsia* 2004; 45: 504-15.

- Régis J, Scavarda D, Tamura M, Nagayi M, Villeneuve N, Bartolomei F, *et al.* Epilepsy related to hypothalamic hamartomas: surgical management with special reference to gamma knife surgery. *Childs Nerv Syst* 2006; 22: 881-95.

- Rhoton AL. The lateral and third ventricles. *Neurosurgery* 2002; 51 (Suppl 1): 207-71.

- Rosenfeld JV, Harvey AS, Wrennall J, Zacharin M, Berkovic SF. Transcallosal resection of hypothalamic hamartomas, with control of seizures, in children with gelastic epilepsy. *Neurosurgery* 2001; 48: 108-18.

- Rosenfeld JV, Freeman JL, Harvey AS. Operative technique: the anterior transcallosal transseptal interforniceal approach to the third ventricle and resection of hypothalamic hamartomas. *J Clin Neurosci* 2004; 11: 738-44.

- Rosenfeld JV, Feiz-Erfan I. Hypothalamic hamartoma treatment: surgical resection with the transcallosal approach. *Semin Pediatr Neurol* 2007; 14: 88-98.

- Sartori E, Biraben A, Taussig D, Bernard AM, Scarabin JM. Gelastic seizures: video-EEG and scintigraphic analysis of a case with frontal focus; review of the literature and pathophysiological hypotheses. *Epileptic Disord* 1999; 1: 221-8.

- Sato M, Ushio Y, Arita N, Mogami H. Hypothalamic hamartoma: report of two cases. *Neurosurgery* 1985; 16: 198-206.

- Schulze-Bonhage A, Trippel M, Wagner K, Bast T, Deimling FV, Ebner A, *et al.* Outcome and predictors of interstitial radiosurgery in the treatment of gelastic epilepsy. *Neurology* 2008; 71: 277-82.

- Selch MT, Gorgulho A, Mattozo C, Solberg TD, Cabatan-Awang C, DeSalles AA. Linear accelerator stereotactic radiosurgery for the treatment of gelastic seizures due to hypothalamic hamartoma. *Minim Invasive Neurosurg* 2005; 48: 310-4.

- Siwanuwatn R, Deshmukh P, Feiz-Erfan I, Rekate HL, Zabramski JM, Spetzler RF, Rosenfeld JV. Microsurgical anatomy of the transcallosal anterior interforniceal approach to the third ventricle. *Neurosurgery* 2005; 56 (2 Suppl): 390-6.

- Striano S, Striano P, Sarappa C, Boccella P. The clinical spectrum and natural history of gelastic epilepsy-hypothalamic hamartoma syndrome. *Seizure* 2005; 14: 232-9.

- Sturm JW, Andermann F, Berkovic SF. "Pressure to laugh": an unusual epileptic symptom associated with small hypothalamic hamartomas. *Neurology* 2000; 54: 971-3.
- Takeuchi J, Handa H, Miki Y, Munemitsu H, Aso T. Precocious puberty due to a hypothalamic hamartoma. *Surg Neurol* 1979; 11: 456-60.
- Unger F, Schröttner O, Haselsberger K, Körner E, Ploier R, Pendi G. Gamma knife radiousurgery for hypothalamic hamartomas in patients with medically intractable epilepsy and precocious puberty. *J Neurosurg* 2000; 92: 726-31.
- Valdueza JM, Cristante L, Dammann O, Bentele K, Vortmeyer A, Saeger W, *et al*. Hypothalamic hamartomas: with special reference to gelastic epilepsy and surgery. *Neurosurgery* 1994; 34: 949-58.
- Weissenberger AA, Dell ML, Liow K, Theodore W, Frattali CM, Hernandez D, Zametkin AJ. Aggression and psychiatric comorbidity in children with hypothalamic hamartomas and their unaffected siblings. *J Am Acad Child Adolesc Psychiatry* 2001; 40: 696-703.
- Wu J, Xu L, Kim DY, Rho JM, St John PA, Lue LF, Coons S, *et al*. Electrophysiological properties of human hypothalamic hamartomas. *Ann Neurol* 2005; 58: 371-82.

Hemispherectomy in the treatment of intractable epilepsy

Violette Renard Recinos, Pablo F. Recinos, George I. Jallo

Division of Pediatric Neurosurgery, Johns Hopkins University School of Medicine, Baltimore, Maryland, USA

■ Introduction

Hemispherectomy for the treatment of intractable, unilateral hemispheric seizures is a well described, effective surgical intervention that has the potential to significantly improve the quality of life for patients suffering from this disorder. Since it was first performed by Dandy in 1928 (Dandy, 1928), the procedure has evolved from anatomical hemispherectomy, whereby the entire abnormal hemisphere is removed, to variations including functional hemispherectomy and hemispherotomy, where the goal is to disconnect the damaged hemisphere by performing a partial anatomical resection while preserving many brain structures. In this chapter, we will discuss the history of the evolution of hemispherectomy surgery, review the common epilepsy syndromes associated with hemispheric seizures, discuss the indications for the procedure, and explore in detail the variations and modifications of the hemispherectomy and hemispherotomy techniques.

■ History

In 1928, Walter Dandy performed the first resection of an entire hemisphere in the treatment of a patient with a hemispheric glioma (Dandy, 1928). The patient had survived the operation and was in good clinical condition until eventually succumbing to his disease. That same year, Lhermitte published a report on the physiological features associated with the surgery (Lhermitte, 1928). Five years later, Garner published the first modification of the procedure, in which he spared the basal ganglia by preserving the lenticulostriate branches and the artery of Hubner (Gardner, 1933). In 1938, McKenzie successfully treated a child with infantile hemiplegia and intractable epilepsy with anatomical hemispherectomy (McKenzie, 1938). This procedure, which was initially seen as a treatment for hemispheric gliomas, was gaining popularity as a treatment for drug-resistant hemispheric epilepsy. In 1950, Krynauw became the first to publish his results on a series of 12 children who underwent the procedure for intractable seizures with good outcomes. He demonstrated that not only did the surgery result in complete or nearly complete seizure control, it also showed a significant motor and cognitive improvement post-operatively. Because of these encouraging results, anatomical hemispherectomy became a more widely considered treatment option for hemispheric epilepsy.

In the 1960s, however, as with many new techniques that initially gain popularity quickly, reports of late complications caused a rapid decline in interest of the anatomical hemispherectomy. In 1966, Oppenheimer and Griffith reported on chronic intracranial hemorrhages, thought secondary to vascular tearing by dislocation of the residual brain tissue (Oppenheimer & Griffith, 1966). This was believed to result in cerebral hemosiderosis, which potentially caused late neurological deterioration. Other reports commented on obstructive hydrocephalus and chronic subdural fluid collections, also thought secondary to the chronic intracranial hemorrhages with a mortality rate as high as 25% of cases (Oppenheimer & Griffith, 1966; Falconer & Wilson, 1969). This prompted neurosurgeons to almost completely abandon the anatomical hemispherectomy procedure and examine other variants of the technique which would allow for excision of the epileptogenic areas in the hemisphere while reducing the volume of the resection cavity.

Several new variants of the hemispherectomy were described including modified anatomical hemispherectomy, functional hemispherectomy, hemidecortication and hemispherotomy. In 1973, Rasmussen described a functional hemispherectomy procedure where he excised portions of the temporales and centrales regions and disconnected the remaining cerebral cortex, which was left behind (Rasmussen, 1973). This and other techniques garnered early acceptance as an alternative to the traditional anatomical hemispherectomy.

Support of the anatomical hemispherectomy was revived in the 1980s with the advent of advanced neuroimaging with computed tomography (CT) and magnetic resonance imaging (MRI). Using CT and MRI, surgeons were able to identify the occurrence of progressive hydrocephalus as the main cause of the neurological deterioration described in the earlier anatomical hemispherectomy surgeries. Although hydrocephalus was suspected earlier by clinical presentation prior to the availability of cerebral imaging, with the advent of CT and MRI it was now more readily apparent and recognized early, allowing for prompt intervention and minimizing complications. In recent decades, reports of cerebral hemosiderosis disappeared in the scientific literature although it continues to be quoted as one of the factors to support functional hemispherectomy *versus* anatomical hemispherectomy (Davies *et al.*, 1993; Fountas *et al.*, 2006; Kossoff *et al.*, 2002a; Peacock *et al.*, 1996). However it should be noted that there have been reports of long term follow-up of anatomical hemispherectomy that attribute the delayed complications to post-operative hydrocephalus rather than cerebral hemosiderosis.

Variants of the techniques continued to be introduced, all with the goal of minimizing the resection cavity and the occurrence of postoperative hydrocephalus. Hemidecortication and hemicortisectomy were introduced and added to the growing surgical options available to neurosurgeons in controlling hemispheric epilepsy (Ignelzi & Bucy, 1968). Overall, advances in neuroimaging as well as consideration of the various pros and cons of each variant of hemispheric resection have allowed the neurosurgeon to tailor his or her surgery to the specific needs of each patient.

■ Epilepsy syndromes associated with hemispheric lesions

Hemispherectomy and its variants are now commonly accepted surgical procedures for the treatment of hemispheric epilepsy. The general criteria for considering a patient for hemispheric epilepsy surgery includes the presence of symptomatic, drug-resistant seizures in a patient with hemiplegia secondary to the unilaterally damaged hemisphere. These hemispheric lesions are often the result of a congenital or acquired lesion. Here we will review the most common disorders.

The most common congenital syndromes include infantile spasms, hemiconvulsion-hemiplegia epilepsy syndrome (HHE), Sturge-Weber Syndrome, hemimegalencephaly and other nonhypertrophic migrational disorders, and cortical dysplasia.

Infantile spasms, also known as West syndrome, are most commonly seen in the first year of life and are associated with a typical electroencephalographic (EEG) pattern of hypsarrhythmia. Clinically, they are associated with developmental delay, regression and medically refractory seizures. The seizures are often clusters of spasms resembling a flexion and extension pattern whereby the child's body bends forward while the arms and legs are extended. These clusters often occur upon awakening or after feeding, and they can occur several times a day with up hundreds of spasms associated with each cluster. These seizures generally resolve by age 5 but may be replaced with other seizure disorders. Many conditions can cause infantile spasm including birth injury, congenital brain malformations, metabolic and degenerative diseases, and hypoxic brain insults (Çataltepe, 2010).

HHE syndrome is an uncommon sequela of prolonged, hemiconvulsive seizures in infancy and early childhood. It is most frequently seen within the first two years of life, and is characterized by three phases. The initial phase is a unilateral, prolonged hemiconvulsive seizure that occurs without antecedent, that involves the face, arm and leg. The second phase is a resulting hemiplegia. The third phase that ensues is partial epileptic seizures, which eventually progresses to chronic epilepsy within several years. The cause of HHE syndrome is still poorly understood, but may be the result of cerebral atrophy from persistent hemiconvulsive seizures and hemiplegia (Çataltepe, 2010).

Sturge-Weber syndrome, also called encephalotrigeminal angiomatosis, is a rare congenital disorder associated with pial angiomatosis usually involving a unilateral hemisphere, facial angiomas (port-wine stains), developmental delay and various ophthalmologic problems. The complex leptomeningeal angiomas result in abnormal hemodynamic vasculature that induces hypoxia in the surrounding brain tissue, eventually causing damage to the brain parenchyma and secondary seizures. Seizures, in fact are usually the earliest symptom which may occur as early as the newborn period. They are usually refractory to medications and patients may develop hemiplegia or hemianopsia after a prolonged period of seizure activity. Hemispherectomy is the main treatment modality, with many advocating early intervention (usually within the first one to two years of life) to prevent refractory seizures, developmental delay and persistent hemiplegia (Çataltepe, 2010; Graveline et al., 1999; Kossoff et al., 2002b).

Hemimegalencephaly is a rare congenital disorder caused by abnormal neuronal migration, resulting in a unilaterally enlarged hemisphere that is characterized by wide, thickened and flattened cortex and shallow gyri. Many patients develop medically intractable seizures in infancy, which, if not well controlled, may result in hemiparesis, hemianopsia, and mental retardation. These patients also may experience high mortality rates in the first months of life due to continuous seizures. Hemispherectomy is the most effective treatment to control seizures, and may contribute to improved psychomotor development when performed early (Çataltepe, 2010).

Cortical dysplasia is the most common underlying pathology in children undergoing surgical resection for refractory epilepsy *(Figure 1)*. Like hemimegalencephaly, it is a congenital disorder caused by abnormal neuronal migration, which results in disruption of the normal lamination of the cortex and can vary in severity. When anticonvulsants fail to control seizure activity, hemispherectomy or multilobar resections are frequently the best treatment options for these patients (Hamiwa, 2010).

The most common acquired lesions include Rasmussen Syndrome, porencephalic cysts, and other sequelae of vascular insults, traumatic injury, or meningoencephalitis. Rasmussen Syndrome was first described by Theodore Rasmussen in 1958 (Rasmussen, 1958). Although the etiology is unknown, it is thought to be an inflammatory encephalitis, likely autoimmune in nature which may be triggered by a viral infection. It is characterized by slowly progressive neurological dysfunction and seizures in children. The seizures first start with a generalized tonic-clonic seizure, but they usually continue as simple partial motor seizures. Progressive hemiparesis and mental retardation are common and thus hemispherectomy is advocated early to help stop the seizures and prevent developmental delay (Kossoff et al., 2002a; Bien et al., 2005; Pardo et al., 2004; Vining, 2006).

Vascular insults or traumatic injury can cause large hemispheric porencephalic cysts characterized by a unilaterally enlarged ventricle and severe brain atrophy. When associated with medically refractory seizures and hemiplegia, they are optimally treated with a hemispherectomy-like procedure with good outcomes.

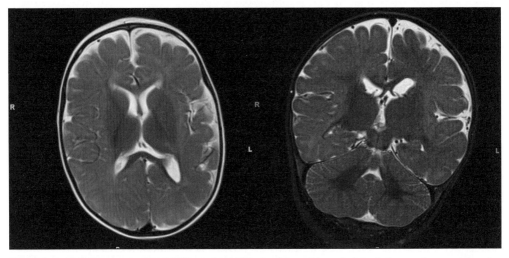

Figure 1. Axial (left) and coronal (right) T2-weighted MRI of a patient with cortical dysplasia secondary to a migration defect. It is notable that the left hemisphere has less volume globally as well as decreased definition of the syri and grey-white matter junction.

■ Indications and preoperative assessment

As in all cases of epilepsy surgery, careful consideration of the indications for the procedure, as well a thorough assessment of the risks and benefits is of utmost importance in selecting the ideal candidates. While hemispherectomy surgery can have a profoundly positive impact on the quality of life for many patients, it is associated with significant risks which need to be justified by the patient's clinical status.

Using various assessment tools, imaging and techniques, the epilepsy surgery team needs to evaluate several pre-operative criteria in order to deem a patient an acceptable surgical candidate. The first question to be answered is "Are the seizures medically intractable?" This first step requires a detailed epileptic history detailing the onset of seizure activity, the frequency and quality of the seizures, the types of medications used and the development of drug resistance. Often in the case of hemispheric seizures, by virtue of their particular lesion or disorder, children rarely need exhaustive medical trials to prove that their seizures are intractable. Specifically in cases of Rasmussen syndrome, Sturge-Weber Syndrome and cortical dysplasia, the natural history of the disease often is enough to warrant earlier surgical intervention after a failed trial of medical management.

Another important criteria in the hemispherectomy decision making process is the presence of contralateral hemiplegia. Usually, secondary to the unilateral hemispheric damage, these patients experience some degree of hemiparesis or hemiplegia, with at least partial hemianopsia as well. On physical examination, the hemiparesis is often in distal extremity strength, while proximal function is somewhat preserved. This is because of the functional neuroanatomy involved, where fine finger movements and repeated alternating movements are a cortical function, while gross motor movements such as joint positioning occur on a subcortical matter and have ipsilateral input as well (De Ribaupierre & Delalande, 2008; Villemure & Daniel, 2006). It is important to note that the criteria for hemiparesis is not absolute; in progressive syndromes such as Rasmussen where there is a known natural history that will eventually result in cognitive and motor function, early intervention may still be warranted. Even though these patients may not yet be experiencing weakness, early surgery may prevent the developmental, cognitive and psychomotor decline (Graveline et al., 1999; Peacock, 1995).

In addition to the history and physical, when the epilepsy patient arrives at the clinic office for pre-operative evaluation of candidacy for hemispherectomy the patient will likely be scheduled for a number of other diagnostic tests and evaluations. As mentioned earlier, these patients often have some degree of hemianopsia. This requires a thorough ophthalmological examination to document baseline status as well as assist in preoperative counseling and postoperative follow-up.

The patient should also be scheduled for preoperative electroencephalographic (EEG) assessment to document if the abnormality is indeed widespread and involving the whole hemisphere, or if the epileptogenic focus is limited to a particular area where a smaller cortical resection may be sufficient to accomplish seizure control. Several EEG characteristics are associated with good outcomes for hemispheric resection; the presence of multifocal epileptogenic abnormalities limited to the damaged hemisphere with ipsilateral suppression of electrical activity, bilateral synchronous discharges spreading from the affected hemisphere without contralateral slowing, and the absence of abnormal signals from the unaffected hemisphere such as independent interictal sharp wave spiking, generalized discharges and abnormal background activity. Although some abnormal activity in the "normal" hemisphere is not an absolute contraindication, it may be a prognostic indicator for potentially unfavorable outcome (Peacock et al., 1996; Çataltepe, 2010; Peacock, 1995; Gonzalez-Martinez et al., 2005).

Detailed neuroimaging, both anatomical and functional with MRI, positron emission tomography (PET), angiography and single photoemission computed tomography (SPECT) scans are critical in understanding the anatomy, diagnosing particular syndromes, assessing contralateral hemisphere, and overall surgical planning. A thorough understanding of the anatomical details including ventricular size, thickness of the corpus callosum, presence of abnormalities in the arterial or venous structures, the characteristics of the sylvian fissure and distortion of anatomical landmarks is of paramount importance to the neurosurgeon.

Confirming functional and anatomical integrity of the contralateral hemisphere is another important criterion needed when considering a patient for hemispherectomy surgery. Review of the anatomy can be accomplished with the imaging mentioned above. Wada testing, when possible, is an important tool in verifying that the "good" hemisphere will be sufficient to sustain the necessary language and memory functions after the procedure. This is accomplished by performing the Wada test on the damaged hemisphere only in order to avoid any risk of ischemic injury to the normal side.

Neuropsychological evaluation is also a routine part of the preoperative assessment as it helps to determine the patient's baseline function, and evaluate the functionality of the normal hemisphere. The goal of the evaluation is to assess the developmental level in infants or children and test cognitive and behavioral skills in the older children. Among the skills tested is language function. Language is localized to one hemisphere by 5 years of age and complete shift in laterality of language is very difficult after this time. Thus, age of onset of hemispheric insult is important to ascertain because it will help to counsel parents regarding postoperative expectations.

In summary, in an ideal situation, the anatomical and functional studies should demonstrate that the remaining hemisphere is structurally normal, free from seizures, and fully capable of accommodating new function. As this unfortunately is not always the case, it is up to the epilepsy team to carefully assess each patient and evaluate the risks and benefits to make the most appropriate recommendations.

■ Surgical planning

Once the preoperative assessment is complete and the patiente determined a good candidate for hemispherectomy, the epilepsy team, the patient and the family need to be prepared for the upcoming procedure. The goals and timing of surgery need to be addressed, as well as the expected seizure outcome and neurological status. Families need also be prepared as to what the risks are and have reasonable expectations postoperatively. The goal of the surgery is usually not only seizure control, but also prophylactic prevention of further neurological deterioration from multiple seizures and side effects from anti-epileptic medications. There has been increasing evidence to suggest that early surgical intervention in patients with catastrophic epilepsy is preferred as one considers the burden of epilepsy on the immature brain and the plasticity of the young developing brain. The young brain has been shown to have the best opportunity for functional recovery from insults (Çataltepe, 2010; Graveline et al., 1999; Peacock, 19995).

Even if operating on a young child, the concern always arises as to whether or not there will be new neurological deficit from the surgery, and if so, if this will be transient or long-term. Generally, if the child is less than 3 years of age, no new permanent deficit is expected but this may vary on a case by case basis. Families need to be prepared for the risks of post operative deficits including complete hemiplegia of the contralateral extremities and visual field loss. Finally, once surgical intervention is decided upon, the next step is determining the surgical technique. As previously described, the procedure has been modified through the years and there are various techniques to accomplish the stated goals. These will be described in detail below.

■ Surgical technique

Anesthesia and perioperative monitoring

Regardless of technique used, hemispheric surgery requires an anesthesia team well versed in pediatric neuroanesthesiology. Often, they will use opioids along with low-dose isoflurane or sevoflurane as their anesthetic protocol. The opiods allow for sedation and analgesia, while also reducing the oxygen cerebral metabolic rate and intracranial pressure without significantly changing the cerebral perfusion pressure. After the patient undergoes induction and is endotracheally intubated, the anesthesia team then will likely insert a central venous catheter along with peripheral intravenous catheters, and an arterial line. A transurethral catheter is also inserted to help monitor urine output and volume status. Throughout the surgery, monitoring includes pulse oximetry, end-tidal CO_2, blood pressure, central venous pressure, and core body temperature. Lab values are sent at regular intervals throughout the case, including hematocrit, blood chemistry, acid-base status, coagulation and fibrinogen levels. As there may be significant blood loss, especially in the younger children, cross-matched blood should be available in the room prior to skin incision. Antibiotics, steroids and mannitol should be administered pre-incision.

Anatomical hemispherectomy

The term anatomical hemispherectomy is the surgical procedure involving the removal of an entire cerebral hemisphere, with or without sparing of the basal ganglia, in either en bloc resection or piece meal fashion. As previously discussed, anatomical hemispherectomy has enjoyed a revival of interest in the last decade as recent series with long-term follow-up has shown a much smaller complication rate than previously described. The best candidates are those patients who suffer from intractable, catastrophic epilepsy caused by a diffuse lesion of one cerebral hemisphere (Di Rocco et al., 2010; 2000).

After the patient is properly anesthetized and prepped with the appropriate lines, the patient is positioned on the operating table in the supine position with a roll under the ipsilateral shoulder and head turn 90 degrees with the affected hemisphere up. The head is secured with Mayfield pins or in a padded horseshoe secured with adhesive tape. The incision is planned to maximize exposure to the entire hemisphere. The most common incisions are either a large question-mark fashion or a T-shaped incision. The question mark incision starts just above the zygomatic arch up to the level of the pinna, extends posteriorly to the occipital protuberance and then curves anteriorly up to midline where it terminates frontally, just behind the hairline. The T-shaped incision involves a midline saggital incision that extends from just behind the hairline anteriorly to the occipital protuberance posteriorly. Another transverse incision is made from the midline incision, approximately 2 cm behind the coronal suture, to the zygomatic arch. To reduce bleeding, the skin in first infiltrated with a mixture of lidocaine or bupivacaine with epinephrine. Upon incision, careful cauterization and Raney clips may prove crucial to obtaining the hemostasis necessary when operating on infants and young children. As the skin flap is elevated, the temporalis muscle may be incised along with the skin in a myocutaneous flap to prevent damage to the frontalis branch of facial nerve.

Once the skin flap is elevated and the cranium exposed, burr holes are placed for the craniotomy. Using an air driven skull perforator, midline burr holes are placed either on or slightly contralateral to the saggital sinus. Additional burr holes are placed frontally, usually at the most anterior extent of the exposure and another in the frontal keyhole. Others may be placed above the root of the zygoma, in the temporal squama laterally and the lambdoid suture posteriorly. The dura is carefully dissected away from the bone with a #3 Penfield dissector and a craniotome with footplate is used to complete the craniotomy by connecting the burr holes. Hemostatic agents such as gelfoam, surgical, floseal and surgical clips should be readily available in the event of bleeding from the sagittal sinus or large draining veins. The bone flap should be elevated with a periosteal elevator under direct visualization to minimize underlying dural injury. Once the dura is exposed, a temporal craniectomy can be performed to maximize exposure to the temporal lobe. Dural tack-up stitches are then placed using 4-0 Nurolon suture. The dura is opened in either a starlike fashion or curved fashion and reflected with the base toward the midline.

The hemispherectomy begins with the anterior vascular deafferentation of the hemisphere. Under microscopic guidance, the sylvian fissure is dissected with microsissors, arachnoid knife and Rhoton dissectors. The frontal and temporal lobes are gently retracted to help expose the internal carotid artery and its distal branches. The middle cerebral artery is identified and it is sectioned just proximal to its bifurcation, thus sparing the perforating branched to the basal ganglia. The anterior cerebral arteries (ACA) on both sides and the anterior communicating artery are then identified to avoid inadvertent clipping of the contralateral ACA. Once identified, the ipsilateral ACA is divided proximal to the origin of the callosomarginal artery. Next the arachnoid is divided along the basal surface of the frontal lobe up to the level of the olfactory tract and along the temporal lobe up to visualize the tentorial notch. If the Sylvian fissure is fused or if the anatomy is distorted, a standard temporal or frontal lobectomy may be performed in order to access the deep vessels.

Once these vessels have been ligated allowing for anterior and mesial devascularization of the hemisphere, attention is turned to the medial surface of the hemisphere, toward the falx, where the bridging cortical veins are dissected, coagulated and divided to reach the corpus callosum. The ipsilateral pericallosal artery is identified and sectioned. Sometimes, the contralateral pericallosal artery may be difficult to identify, therefore it is important to proceed with caution when performing the corpus callosotomy. In order to avoid damage to the contralateral vessel, the corpus callosotomy is accomplished mainly by suctioning and limited bipolar cautery until the contralateral pericallosal artery is properly identified and protected. The corpus callosotomy is extended from the genu to the splenium. Once the lateral ventricle is entered, a cottonoid or large cotton ball is placed in the foramen of Monroe to prevent blood from entering the contralateral ventricle. The frontobasal white matter is divided through an intraventricular ependymal incision lateral and anterior to the basal ganglia. The frontal lobe disconnection can then be completed by extending the ependymal incision up to the sylvian fissure and performing a cortisectomy on the cortical surface from the sylvian fissure to midline.

The posterior cerebral artery (PCA) is then identified. It is divided at the level of the P3 segment, devascularizing the temporo-occipital basal areas. The disconnection of the temporal lobe can then be completed by extending the intraventricular ependymal incision posteriorly up to the trigonal area and temporal horn. The parieto-occipital lobe can be removed by dissecting the bridging veins medially and laterally, and dissecting the posterobasal white matter inferiorly. The amygdalohippocampectomy can be completed after the temporal horn is entered, or it can be subpially dissected with suctioning after the temporal lobe is removed. The disconnected hemisphere can be removed en bloc or it can be removed piece meal throughout the disconnection procedure if necessary.

If structures in the basal ganglia are believed to be diseased and contributing to seizure etiology, the basal nuclei and thalamus may be excised. Otherwise, these nuclei are usually spared as they may support post-operative motor activity.

Once the hemispherectomy is completed, meticulous hemostasis must be obtained. Additionally, cauterization of the choroid plexus is recommended as it may help prevent postoperative hydrocephalus. The foramen of Monroe is plugged with gelfoam or a small piece of muscle and fibrin glue. The remnant tissue and dural surfaces can be covered with Surgicel for further hemostasis. Dural closure is obtained by reapproximating the dural leafs and running or interrupted 4-0 Nurolon suture in a watertight fashion. Several dural tack up sutures should be applied to hold the dura up against the craniotomy to prevent an epidural collection. The bone flap is secured with sutures, resorbable plates or a titanium plating system. The temporalis muscle and fascial edges are reapproximated with 0 or 3-0 vicryl sutures, followed by galea closure. The skin is sutured with either running 3-0 nylon, staples, or an absorbable running suture such as 4-0 caprosyn. A subgaleal drain may be left in place prior to skin closure, which should be monitored closely for postoperative CSF accumulation (Di Rocco et al., 2010).

Hemidecortication

Hemidecortication, also known as hemicortectomy, describes a variant of the anatomical hemispherectomy where the cortical gray matter and hippocampus are removed, but the white matter over the anterior horn and body of the lateral ventricle, and nearly all subcortical gray structures are left intact (Carson et al., 1996; Hartmann et al., 2010). This technique was first described by Ignelzi and Bucy in 1968, and several modifications to the techniques have followed (Kossoff et al., 2002a; Ignelzi & Bucy, 1698; Carson et al., 1996). In 1992, Winston et al. described a technique that they referred to as a "de-gloving" of the entire cerebral cortex, and in 1996 Carson et al. published their series on this technique (Carson et al., 1996; Winston et al., 1992). This maneuver reduces the size of the hemispherectomy cavity, minimizing the mixing of bloody material and debris from the surgery with the ventricular CSF, thereby reducing the risk of postoperative hydrocephalus.

As hemidecortication is a variant to the anatomical hemispherectomy, much of the preoperative planning, anesthesia, positioning, craniotomy and dural opening are the same. After the hemisphere is exposed as described above in the anatomical hemispherectomy section, a devascularization is performed in a similar manner. The sylvian fissure is dissected and the MCA is ligated proximal to its bifurcation, sparing the lenticulostriate branches as in the anatomical procedure. Next, the bridging veins are dissected and divided. Decortication then performed using suction and bipolar coagulation to remove the gray matter in a piecemeal fashion while leaving a mantle of white matter over the ependymal surface. Usually, the temporal lobe is decorticated first, followed by the frontal, parietal, and occipital lobes. Branches of the ACA and PCA are clipped and divided as they are encountered during the decortication procedure. Some surgeons have undermined and removed large slabs of cortex, rather than proceeding piecemeal with suction or ultrasonic aspirator, while others have attempted to reduce the volume of the hemispherectomy cavity further by plicating the dura.

By preserving the white matter over the ependymal surface, the ventricular system remains mostly intact with the exception of the ventricular surface in the trigonal region which is violated secondary to the temporal lobectomy *(Figure 2)*. This area is reconstructed with Gelfoam and Surgicel to prevent cerebral spinal fluid eggression. The insular cortex is resected last because of reports that in young children, manipulation of this area appears to be associated with cardiovascular instability (Carson *et al.*, 1996). Meticulous hemostasis is obtained and closure is performed in a similar fashion to the anatomical hemispherectomy.

Functional hemispherectomy

As anatomical hemispherectomy fell out of favor in the late 1960s, functional hemispherectomy became popularized as it was associated with a smaller resection cavity and fewer delayed complications. Since its first description by Rasmussen in 1973 (Rasmussen, 1973), it has become the most commonly performed hemispherectomy technique. It is best defined as a subtotal anatomical resection with a full disconnection of the damaged hemisphere producing a physiologically complete hemispherectomy. The originally described method required the excision of portions of the central and temporal regions including resection of the amygdala and hippocampus, and disconnection of the residual frontal and parieto-occipital lobes medially, corpus callosotomy and an insulectomy. Modifications of this technique reduce the volume of tissue excised in the central region and perform a hemispheric disconnection with minimal resection.

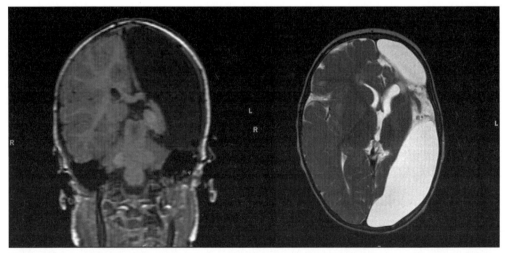

Figure 2. Postoperative axial T2-weighted (left) and coronal T1-weighted (right) MRI of a patient who underwent left hemidecortication. Note that the ventricular system is mostly intact with the exception of the small violation in the trigone region. The preservation of the integrity of the ventricular system may help decrease risk of hydrocephalus development.

There have been several modifications of the functional hemispherectomy techniques which have evolved over time. As for all the hemispherectomy procedures described in this chapter, additional subtle variations may be found in the vast growing literature on the topic. Here we describe the general surgical technique for functional hemispherectomy as performed by several high volume centers (Lam & Mathern, 2010).

The opening is a standard craniotomy as described for the previous hemispherectomy procedures. Some authors prefer an osteoplastic craniotomy where the temporalis muscle is left intact and not dissected off of the bone. After the majority of burr holes are connected with the craniotome, the bone flap is fractured between the frontal and temporal burr holes underlying the preserved temporalis muscle and the flap is subsequently elevated still attached to the temporal muscle and reflected anteriorly. The dura is opened in either a curved fashion with a pedicle in the frontal-temporal area or it is opened in a stellate fashion.

The first resection involves removal of a central opercular block of tissue. The resection begins with a cortical incision perpendicular to the anterior sylvian fissure. The branches of the MCA are identified and ligated as the cerebral cortex is dissected on the frontal and temporal side of the sylvian fissure. The bottom of the sylvian fissure is exposed and the frontal and temporal edges of the circular sulcus of the insula are identified as the anterior border of the central operculum dissection. The cortical incision is extended to follow the middle frontal gyrus around in a c-shape to the middle temporal gyrus. The cortisectomy is deepened along the white matter tracts down to the level of the ependyma. The ventricle is usually opened at the widest spot near the trigone and this opening is extended anteriorly and posteriorly along the lateral and temporal ventricular horn. Once the ventricle is open, the anterior resection margin identified earlier at the circular sulcus of the insula is deepened to the level of the ventricles. Small perforating branches from the ACA are encountered which need to be cauterized and divided. This central operculum block is gently lifted to allow for the disconnection of the base of the block from the lateral ependymal wall of the ventricle. This block of tissue is undercut, staying parallel to the choroid plexus in the frontal and temporal horns, and transects the internal capsule, thalamus, globus pallidus and caudate nucleus. The opercular block can then be removed en bloc, exposing the underlying ventricular system. The amygdala is subpially dissected and suctioned to expose the anterior temporal horn, and most of the medial caudate nucleus is removed to expose the anterior frontal ventricular system. Two additional cortical excisions are made on either side parallel to the proximal sylvian fissure, disconnecting the orbital frontal cortex and the anterior temporal pole to the level of the ventricle.

The next step in the procedure involves the mesial dissections disconnecting the two cerebral hemispheres from each other and the mesial frontal lobe from the thalamus. Using gentle retraction over the roof of the lateral ventricle, the corpus callosum is exposed and resected using suction and bipolar coagulation. As the corpus callosum is resected anteriorly around its genu, the ACA is identified and followed until the floor of the orbital frontal resection is reached. Once the anterior dissection is complete, the corpus callosum dissection is continued posteriorly to the splenium. The hippocampus is then visualized and resected, and the final disconnection involves resection of the white matter and cortex from the posterior hippocampal resection to the splenium.

Meticulous hemostasis is then obtained. Some authors advocate leaving an intraventricular catheter in the resection cavity to clear out post-operative blood. The dura is closed in the usual fashion, and the bone flap replaced as described above.

Hemispherotomy

In the broad terminology of hemispherectomy surgery, hemispherotomy can be viewed as a variation of the functional hemispherectomy. In 1992, Delalande *et al.* introduced the term hemispherotomy to describe the newer surgical techniques to further minimize the amount of brain resected while still disconnecting the entire hemisphere (Delalande *et al.*, 2007). The main differences between the various techniques involve the amount of resected brain, the approach to the lateral ventricle, the hippocampal dissection, the question of resection of the insular cortex, and the level of preservation of the vascular structures in the peri-insular area. The most recently described techniques are grouped into either vertical or lateral approaches.

The technique described by Delalande *et al.*, the transventricular vertical hemispherotomy is the most commonly used vertical approach technique (Delalande *et al.*, 2007). In this approach, a paramedian, linear incision is made parallel to the sagittal suture, and a small 3 × 5 cm craniotomy is made one to two centimeters lateral to the midline with one-third anterior to the coronal suture and two-thirds behind it. The hemispherotomy involves a corpus callosotomy performed by first entering the lateral ventricle through a paramedian cortisectomy. The body and splenium of the corpus callosum is transected followed by a cut in the posterior column of the fornix at the level of the trigone. Further divisions are made by intraventricular disconnections lateral to the thalamus. The callosotomy is completed by dividing the genu and the rostrum of the corpus callosum until just above the anterior commissure. The gyrus rectus is also subpially dissected down to the level of the ACA and optic nerve. Following the ACA, the final step is a disconnection through the caudate nucleus from the rectus gyrus to the anterior temporal horn.

Lateral hemispherotomy approaches include the perisylvian transcortical transventricular hemispherical deafferentation described by Schramm *et al.* in 1995 (Schramm *et al.*, 1995). In this approach, the goal is the deafferentation of all the cortical structures from its connection to the basal ganglia and the contralateral hemisphere. In 2001, Schramm *et al.* described a modification to this technique called the transylvian keyhole functional hemispherectomy where he replaced the anteromesial temporal lobectomy with a selective amygdalohippocampectomy (Schramm *et al.*, 2001). Another lateral approach is the peri-insular hemispherotomy, first described by Villemure and Mascott in 1995 (Villemure & Mascott, 1995). This technique, as along with the various modifications maintain the fundamental concept of isolation of the cerebral hemisphere by disconnection of the medial temporal structures, internal capsule, corpus callosum, and horizontal frontal fibers.

■ Complications

Regardless of the preferred surgical technique, hemispherectomy surgery is a complicated procedure associated with substantial risks and potential complications. There are special considerations regarding each of the surgical approaches, which may make them more or less favorable to individual epilepsy teams.

The anatomical hemispherectomy, while regaining popularity in recent years due to decreased complication rates, is still associated with substantial risk when compared to other techniques. It is associated with higher blood loss, longer hospital stays, higher rate of hydrocephalus and increased risk of sagittal sinus thrombosis secondary to extensive midline exposure (Davies *et al.*, 1993; Cook *et al.*, 2004; Devlin *et al.*, 2003). However, of all the approaches, anatomical hemispherectomy has had the lowest reoperation rate for persistent seizures in some series (Carreno *et al.*, 2001). It also may be the procedure of choice in certain patients with multilobar cortical dysplasia, hemimegalencephaly and Rasmussen's patients secondary to their distorted anatomy, making it more difficult to perform a disconnection procedure. Hemidecortication, compared with anatomical hemispherectomy has also been associated with complications including a higher blood loss, higher infection rates, and higher risk of incomplete disconnection (Kossoff *et al.*, 2002a; Carson *et al.*, 1996; Schramm *et al.*, 1995). However, the preservation of the integrity of the ipsilateral ventricular system may help decrease the risk of hydrocephalus (Carson *et al.*, 1996).

Functional hemispherectomy techniques are advantageous in that while they limit cortical resection, they still provide for a considerable brain resection volume, allowing more space to avoid complications from postoperative edema. The various hemispherotomy techniques also have several benefits including smaller incision and craniotomy, decreased risk of infection, and lower hydrocephalus rates (Delalande *et al.*, 2007; Schramm *et al.*, 2001; Villemure *et al.*, 2000). However these techniques are associated with smaller exposure, difficult anatomical orientation in some cases of cortical dysplasia and hemimegalencephaly, worse risk of postoperative brain swelling, and higher reoperation rate (Çataltepe, 2010). Thus, hemispherotomy procedures are more favorable in patients with atrophic hemispheres and enlarged ventricles, but can still be performed safely in all hemispheric epilepsy patients by experienced surgeons.

All cases of hemispherectomy procedures have the potential for intraoperative complications involving fluid and electrolyte imbalances and bleeding. Aggressive fluid, electrolyte, and hemostatic management is absolutely necessary during these procedures, including blood and clotting factor transfusions to treat associated coagulopathies. A frequent postoperative complication following hemispherectomies is aseptic meningitis, which is likely secondary to the blood products entering the CSF. Leaving a ventricular catheter for several days to drain the blood products out of the ventricular system may help counteract this phenomenon.

Although many patients present preoperatively with hemiparesis, the patients may have worsening motor function following the surgery. While most patients participate in aggressive physical therapy and recover at least some degree of motor function, distal extremity weakness may persist. Additionally, a complete hemianopsia is expected following the procedure which is unlikely to improve.

Delayed hydrocephalus, not related to superficial cerebral hemosiderosis has been reported in up to 30% of patients following an anatomic hemispherectomy and up to 18% in the patients following functional hemispherectomy (De Ribaupierre & Delalande, 2008; Delalande *et al.*, 2007). The need for shunting has varied in different series (Carson *et al.*, 1996; Hartman *et al.*, 2010). These patients require close follow up with high suspicion for hydrocephalus should their clinical picture so suggest. Persistent high intracranial pressures are indicative of inadequate absorption of the CSF and advocates for prompt shunting to avoid long-term sequelae.

Mortality rates have been reported between 0 and 6% secondary to early postoperative brain shift, brainstem lesions, hemodynamic instability, brain swelling and infection as the main causes of death (Davies *et al.*, 1993; Çataltepe, 2010; Villemure & Daniel, 2006; Peacock, 1995; Delalande *et al.*, 2007). These complications occur at a much lower rate as a result of the advances in anesthesia and surgical techniques.

■ Outcomes

All of the hemispherectomy techniques are associated with good seizure control rates and favorable outcomes. A review of outcome results at major epilepsy centers have shown that the most common factor affecting outcome is the etiology of the hemispheric lesion with best outcomes seen in patients with Sturge-Weber syndrome and Rasmussen syndrome. Patients with the lowest seizure-free outcome are seen in the cortical dysplasia group (Çataltepe, 2010; Holthausen et al., 1997).

It has been difficult to compare outcomes between the various surgical techniques secondary to differences in experience level of the surgeons and the varying pathologies. The largest review of the outcomes is a combined patient pool from multiple centers which reviewed 333 hemispherectomy cases. In this particular review, the highest seizure-free outcome was 85.7% in the hemispherotomy group, followed by the modified anatomical hemispherectomy technique as described by Adams (78.3%), the functional hemispherectomy group (66.1%), the anatomical hemispherectomy group (64.3%) and the hemidecortication group (60.7%) (Holthausen et al., 1997).

■ Conclusions

Hemispherectomy surgery and its variations in surgical techniques throughout the years have proven to be a highly effective treatment option for intractable hemispheric epilepsy. All techniques have been reported to provide good seizure control with a relatively low complication rate. The choice of which hemispheric procedure to perform is largely dependent upon the surgeon's training and experience in a particular technique. Evaluating outcomes based on technique is difficult secondary to variability in patient pathology and surgeon experience. The most common reason for surgical failure is incomplete disconnection, but the most significant factor in surgical outcome appears to be pathology. With proper preoperative screening and patient selection, hemispherectomy surgery can be a rewarding procedure associated with dramatic improvement in the quality of life of patients suffering from hemispheric epilepsy.

References

• Bien CG, Granata T, Antozzi C, et al. Pathogenesis, diagnosis and treatment of Rasmussen encephalitis: a European consensus statement. Brain 2005; 128: 454-71.

• Carreno M, Wyllie E, Bingaman W, Kotagal P, Comair Y, Ruggieri P. Seizure outcome after functional hemispherectomy for malformations of cortical development. Neurology 2001; 57: 331-3.

• Carson BS, Javedan SP, Freeman JM, et al. Hemispherectomy: a hemidecortication approach and review of 52 cases. J Neurosurg 1996; 84: 903-11.

• Çataltepe O. Hemispherectomy and hemispherotomy techniques in pediatric epilepsy surgery: an overview. In: Çataltepe O, Jallo G, eds. Pediatric Epilepsy Surgery: Preoperative Assessment and Surgical Treatment. New York: Thieme, 2010: 205-14.

• Cook SW, Nguyen ST, Hu B, et al. Cerebral hemispherectomy in pediatric patients with epilepsy: comparison of three techniques by pathological substrate in 115 patients. J Neurosurg 2004; 100: 125-41.

- Dandy W. Removal of right cerebral hemisphere for certain tumors with hemiplegia. JAMA 1928; 90: 823-5.
- Davies KG, Maxwell RE, French LA. Hemispherectomy for intractable seizures: long-term results in 17 patients followed for up to 38 years. J Neurosurg 1993; 78: 733-40.
- De Ribaupierre S, Delalande O. Hemispherotomy and other disconnective techniques. Neurosurg Focus 2008; 25: E14.
- Delalande O, Bulteau C, Dellatolas G, et al. Vertical parasagittal hemispherotomy: surgical procedures and clinical long-term outcomes in a population of 83 children. Neurosurgery 2007; 60: ONS19-32; discussion ONS.
- Devlin AM, Cross JH, Harkness W, et al. Clinical outcomes of hemispherectomy for epilepsy in childhood and adolescence. Brain 2003; 126: 556-66.
- Di Rocco C, Fountas K, Massimi L. Anatomical hemispherectomy. In: Çataltepe O, Jallo G, eds. Pediatric Epilepsy Surgery: Preoperative Assessment and Surgical Treatment. New York: Thieme, 2010: 215-24.
- Di Rocco C, Iannelli A. Hemimegalencephaly and intractable epilepsy: complications of hemispherectomy and their correlations with the surgical technique. A report on 15 cases. Pediatr Neurosurg 2000; 33: 198-207.
- Falconer MA, Wilson PJ. Complications related to delayed hemorrhage after hemispherectomy. J Neurosurg 1969; 30: 413-26.
- Fountas KN, Smith JR, Robinson JS, Tamburrini G, Pietrini D, Di Rocco C. Anatomical hemispherectomy. Childs Nerv Syst 2006; 22: 982-91.
- Gardner W. Removal of the right cerebral hemisphere for infiltrating glioma. JAMA 1933; 12: 154-64.
- Gonzalez-Martinez JA, Gupta A, Kotagal P, et al. Hemispherectomy for catastrophic epilepsy in infants. Epilepsia 2005; 46: 1518-25.
- Graveline C, Hwang P, Fitzpatrick T, Jay V, Hoffman H. Sturge-Weber syndrome: implications of functional studies on neural plasticity, brain maturation, and timing of surgical treatment. In: Kotagal P, Luders H, eds. The Epilepsies: Etiologies and Prevention. San Diego: Academic Press, 1999: 61-70.
- Hamiwka L, Grondin R, Madsen J. Surgical approaches in cortical dysplasia. In: Çataltepe O, Jallo G, eds. Pediatric Epilepsy Surgery: Preoperative Assessment and Surgical Treatment. New York: Thieme, 2010: 185-95.
- Hartman A, Frazier J, Jallo G. Hemidecortication and intractable epilepsy. In: Çataltepe O, Jallo G, eds. Pediatric Epilepsy Surgery: Preoperative Assessment and Surgical Treatment. New York: Thieme, 2010: 225-9.
- Holthausen H, May T, Adams T, Andermann F, Villemure J, Wyllie E. Seizures post hemispherectomy. In: Tuxhorn I, Holthausen H, Boenigk H, eds. Pediatric Epilepsy Syndromes and Their Surgical Treatments. London: John Libbey, 1997: 749-73.
- Ignelzi RJ, Bucy PC. Cerebral hemidecortication in the treatment of infantile cerebral hemiatrophy. J Nerv Ment Dis 1968; 147: 14-30.
- Kossoff EH, Buck C, Freeman JM. Outcomes of 32 hemispherectomies for Sturge-Weber syndrome worldwide. Neurology 2002b; 59: 1735-8.
- Kossoff EH, Vining EP, Pyzik PL, et al. The postoperative course and management of 106 hemidecortications. Pediatr Neurosurg 2002a; 37: 298-303.
- Lam S, Mathern G. Functional hemispherectomy at UCLA. In: Çataltepe O, Jallo G, eds. Pediatric Epilepsy Surgery: Preoperative Assessment and Surgical Treatment. New York: Thieme, 2010: 230-40.
- Lhermitte J. L'abaltion complète de l'hémisphère droit dans les cas de tumeur cérébrale localisée conpliquée d'hémiplégie. La décérébration supra-thalamique unilatérale chez l'homme. Encéphale 1928; 23: 314-23.

- McKenzie K. The present status of a patient who had the right cerebral hemisphere removed. *JAMA* 1938; 111: 168-83.
- Oppenheimer DR, Griffith HB. Persistent intracranial bleeding as a complication of hemispherectomy. *J Neurol Neurosurg Psychiatry* 1966; 29: 229-40.
- Pardo CA, Vining EP, Guo L, Skolasky RL, Carson BS, Freeman JM. The pathology of Rasmussen syndrome: stages of cortical involvement and neuropathological studies in 45 hemispherectomies. *Epilepsia* 2004; 45: 516-26.
- Peacock WJ, Wehby-Grant MC, Shields WD, *et al.* Hemispherectomy for intractable seizures in children: a report of 58 cases. *Childs Nerv Syst* 1996; 12: 376-84.
- Peacock WJ. Hemispherectomy for the treatment of intractable seizures in childhood. *Neurosurg Clin N Am* 1995; 6: 549-63.
- Rasmussen T, Olszewski J, Lloydsmith D. Focal seizures due to chronic localized encephalitis. *Neurology* 1958; 8: 435-45.
- Rasmussen T. Postoperative superficial hemosiderosis of the brain, its diagnosis, treatment and prevention. *Trans Am Neurol Assoc* 1973; 98: 133-7.
- Schramm J, Behrens E, Entzian W. Hemispherical deafferentation: an alternative to functional hemispherectomy. *Neurosurgery* 1995; 36: 509-15; discussion 15-6.
- Schramm J, Kral T, Clusmann H. Transsylvian keyhole functional hemispherectomy. *Neurosurgery* 2001; 49: 891-900; discussion -1.
- Villemure JG, Daniel RT. Peri-insular hemispherotomy in paediatric epilepsy. *Childs Nerv Syst* 2006; 22: 967-81.
- Villemure JG, Mascott CR. Peri-insular hemispherotomy: surgical principles and anatomy. *Neurosurgery* 1995; 37: 975-81.
- Villemure JG, Vernet O, Delalande O. Hemispheric disconnection: callosotomy and hemispherotomy. *Adv Tech Stand Neurosurg* 2000; 26: 25-78.
- Vining EP. Struggling with Rasmussen's Syndrome. *Epilepsy Curr* 2006; 6: 20-1.
- Winston KR, Welch K, Adler JR, Erba G. Cerebral hemicorticectomy for epilepsy. *J Neurosurg* 1992; 77: 889-95.

Multiple subpial transections

Marcin Zarowski[1], Mohamad Z. Koubeissi[2], Joseph Madsen[3], Tobias Loddenkemper[4]

[1] *Division of Epilepsy and Clinical Neurophysiology,
Department of Neurology, Harvard Medical School, Children's Hospital
Boston, USA & Polysomnography and Sleep Research Unit,
Department of Developmental Neurology,
Poznan University of Medical Sciences, Poznan, Poland*
[2] *Department of Neurology, University Hospitals Case Medical Center,
Case Western Reserve University, Cleveland, USA*
[3] *Department of Pediatric Neurosurgery, Harvard Medical School,
Children's Hospital Boston, USA*
[4] *Division of Epilepsy and Clinical Neurophysiology, Department
of Neurology, Harvard Medical School, Children's Hospital Boston, USA*

■ Introduction

Overlap between epileptogenic and functional areas of speech, movement, primary sensation, or memory limits the extent and effectiveness of resective surgical treatment. In such cases, resection of the epileptogenic zone may leave the patient with permanent, unacceptable sensorimotor, language or other cognitive deficits. Morrell *et al.* devised a new surgical approach for patients with overlap between eloquent areas and the epileptogenic zone and termed this technique multiple subpial transections (MST) (Morrell *et al.*, 1989).

■ Background

MST is based on the observation that the bulk of the functionally important connections of a cortical territory were arranged in vertical columns (Asanuma, 1975; Morrell *et al.*, 1989; Sperry *et al.*, 1955) but horizontal fibers are necessary to generate epileptic activity (Morrell *et al.*, 1989). If the columnar cortical organization is preserved, the horizontal fibers may be sectioned without functional loss. The slow propagation of epileptic activity is dependent on the horizontal fiber system (Morrell, 1961; Morrell, 1969). A larger continuous cortical segment is more likely to support epileptiform activity. The "Critical Mass" of cerebral cortex to sustain synchronous spiking has been determined to be 12.5 mm^2 (Lüders *et al.*, 1981; Tharp, 1971). Cortical islands greater than 5 mm in width, or horizontal connections of greater than 5 mm, can support epileptic spikes (Dichter & Spencer,

1969b; Lüders *et al.*, 1981; Tharp, 1971). Observations from several laboratories show that independent epileptic regions can become synchronous when they are placed 4 mm apart from each other. Conversely, if the two foci are 6.7 mm apart, spike activity remains independent (Dichter & Spencer, 1969a; Dichter & Spencer, 1969b; Lüders *et al.*, 1981; Tharp, 1971). These anatomic and functional considerations and physiological observations in animal models provoked the initial attempt to transect the cortex in 5 mm intervals perpendicular to the longitudinal axis of the gyrus. Prior to performing the procedure on the human brain, Morrell and colleagues tested this technique in a monkey model. These animal experiments did not cause any neurological deficits and demonstrated improvement of seizures (Morrell *et al.*, 1989).

■ Surgical technique

The MST technique utilizes a series of shallow cuts limited to the grey matter. The procedure is designed to sever horizontally coursing intracortical transverse fibers longer than 5 mm while preserving vertically directed incoming and outgoing neural elements subserving the integrity of the functional columns (Morrell *et al.*, 1989).

Bipolar electrocauterizaton is used to disconnect small pial points spaced approximately 5 mm apart along the epileptogenic focus either at the location of the gyrus or at the crest (Wyler, 2000). Subsequently the pia mater is sharply penetrated at this site. A right angle blunt dissector is introduced through the incised pial hole and it is subpially directed towards the margin of the sulcus, making a cut to a depth of 5 to 7 mm in an axis perpendicular to the gyrus (Morrell *et al.*, 1989; Morrell *et al.*, 1995; Tovar-Spinoza & Rutka, 2010). The blade of the MST knife is maintained in a strictly vertical orientation to avoid undercutting the cortex (Tovar-Spinoza & Rutka, 2010). MST parallel cuts are then made from this cut until the entire proposed epileptogenic zone has been transected (spaced 5 mm apart). Special care needs to be taken to avoid disrupting the pia matter or injuring sulcal vessels during this transection procedure (Benifla *et al.*, 2006).

The efficacy of the procedure is evaluated intraoperatively by electrocorticography before and after MSTs to evaluate interictal activity (Benifla *et al.*, 2006; Tovar-Spinoza & Rutka, 2010). The MST surgical technique is not standardized, and may or may not include resection of adjacent cortex. Surgeons perform MSTs with some variations and this may also explain some variation in results (Tovar-Spinoza & Rutka, 2010).

■ Indications

The main indication for MSTs is an epileptogenic zone located in eloquent cortex (Tovar-Spinoza & Rutka, 2010). Eloquent cortex encompasses regions of cortex that are responsible for language, motor, sensory, memory, and other higher functions. MST provides an opportunity to abolish or reduce seizures without causing a functional deficit (Devinsky *et al.*, 1994) and may be performed in combination with cortical resection or as a standalone procedure (Tovar-Spinoza & Rutka, 2010).

Morrell *et al.* published his experience on the first 32 patients in 1989 (Morrell *et al.*, 1989). In this series he distinguished four groups based on the cerebral location: i) precentral gyrus (16 cases); ii) postcentral gyrus (6 cases); iii) Broca's area (5 cases); and iv) the posterior temporo-parietal area including Wernicke's area, the angular gyrus, and the supramarginal gyrus (5 cases). None of these 32 patients suffered a clinically significant neurological deficit.

Wyler et al. reported 6 patients with complex partial seizures arising from the primary sensorimotor cortex undergoing MSTs (Wyler et al., 1995). This series included four patients with non-lesional MRIs. All patients had seizure onset zones within the central sulcus as determined by subdural ictal onset recordings.

MST can be performed in combination with cortical resection (Tovar-Spinoza & Rutka, 2010). Shimizu and Maehara presented a series of 31 patients, and MST was combined with lobectomy in 11, cortical excision in 5, lesionectomy in 5, and other resections in 4 cases (Shimizu & Maehara, 2000). MST was applied when the epileptic focus was located in eloquent cortex such as language or motor areas.

MSTs have also been successfully used in epilepsia partialis continua due to *Rasmussen encephitis* (Sawhney et al., 1995). Sawhney et al. reported six patients with Rasmussen syndrome who had been subjected to MST (Sawhney et al., 1995). Three patients showed improvement (recovery of speech or seizure reduction grades I or II, or seizure reduction grade III with decreased severity). One of these patients relapsed briefly with increased seizures after 18 months, but then experienced lasting remission. Seizure frequency remained unchanged in two patients with Rasmussen syndrome and increased in another. Two subsequently underwent hemispherectomy and became seizure free. Molyneux et al. first reported a patient who underwent MST for intractable epilepsia partialis continua due to cortical dysplasia (Molyneux et al., 1998). The seizure control was good and the patient was spared the hemiparesis that would have resulted from resection of the motor cortex.

Landau-Kleffner syndrome (LKS) has been considered as one of the main indications for MSTs in children (Morrell et al., 1995). The surgical treatment of LKS was first discussed by Morrell in 1995 (Morrell et al., 1995).

Landau-Kleffner syndrome is characterized by acquired aphasia and behavioral changes. These changes may be related to underlying regional epileptic activity and seizures that regress over time (Landau & Kleffner, 1957). In some patients Landau-Kleffner syndrome may be associated with electrical status epilepticus in slow wave sleep (ESES) (Cross and Neville, 2009). Outcome of language and behavior following pharmacological treatment is variable and difficult to predict (Grote et al., 1999). The etiology, prognosis and optimal treatment are unknown. Previous treatment interventions utilized anticonvulsants or steroids.

MST has been used in 19 cases of Landau-Kleffner syndrome associated with ESES (Cross and Neville, 2009; Irwin et al., 2001; Morrell et al., 1995; Vendrame & Loddenkemper, 2010). The results of 14 children with aphasia, seizures and a severely abnormal EEG in whom MST was applied were published by Morrell et al in 1995 (Morrell et al., 1995). Seven of the 14 patients (50%) have recovered age-appropriate speech. Four of the 14 (29%) have shown marked improvement. Eleven patients (79%) became seizures free after a follow up period of 13 to 78 months.

Irvin et al. reported 5 children with Landau-Kleffner syndrome (Irwin et al., 2001). All five had ESES before surgery and this pattern resolved after the procedure. Seizure frequency and behavior improved dramatically after MST in all children.

Table I. Multiple subpial transections (MST) for the treatment of medically uncontrolled epilepsy

Reference	N	Age (y)	MSTs only	MSTs with resection	Follow-up	Outcome: seizure freedom	Neurologic deficits
Blount et al., 2004	30	11.7 ± 4.4	4	26	> 30 mo	12/30 seizure free	No permanent motor deficit
Chuang et al., 2006	2	2-3	2	–	1-6 no	2/2 significant seizure reduction	No permanent motor deficit
Devinsky et al., 1994	3	28-47	–	3	9-12 mo	2/3 seizure free 1/3 > 70% seizure reduction	2/1 mild speech deficits
Devinsky et al., 2003	13	0.5-40	–	13	42-98 mo	4/13 seizure free 6/13 > 50% seizure reduction	9/13 no neurological deficit
D'Giano et al., 2001	1	6	1	–	12 mo	1/1 seizure free	Stable cognition
Grote et al., 1999	14	5.2-13.1	14	–	6-79 mo	No data	
Hufnagel et al., 1997	22	7-45	6	16	No data	4/6 > 50% seizure reduction (MSTs only) 9/16 seizure free (MSTs with resection)	5/22 subtle neurological deficits
Irwin et al., 2001	5	7.5-16	5	–	30 mo	4/5 seizure free	Stable cognition; Improved behavior
Lui et al., 1995	50		32		6-40 mo	32/50 seizure free 13/50 > 50% seizure reduction	No functional deficits
Molyneaux et al., 1998	1	19	1	–	9 mo	1/1 seizure free	No neurological deficit
Morrell et al., 1989	20	No data	20	–	60-264 mo	11/20 seizure free	No significant neurological deficit
Morrell et al., 1995	14	5-13	14	–	78 mo	11/14 seizure free	11/14 improved speech
Mulligan et al., 2001	12	No data	5	7	6-36 mo	5/12 > 75% reduction in seizure frequency	1/12 persistent neurologic deficit

Orbach et al., 2001	54	No data	3	51	28-89 mo	26/54 Engel class I or II	No data
Sawhney et al., 1995	21	6-47	9	12	10-60 mo	11/21 worthwhile decrease in seizure frequency	1/21 chronic neurological deficits
Shimizu et al., 2000	31	No data	6	25	>12 mo	10/31 Engel class I or II	No mortality or morbidity was encountered
Smith, 1998	100	No data	32	68	No data	59/100 seizure free 14/100; 90% seizure reduction	7/100 persistent neurologic deficit
Wyler et al., 1995	6	12-40	6	-	18-22 mo	5/6 > 70% seizure reduction	6/6 mild deficits
Yandet et al., 2007	12	No data	-	12	3-36 no	8/12 Engel class I or II	No permanent complication
Zhao et al., 2003	200	2.5-55	80	120	12-96 mo	100/200 seizure free 32/200 > 75% seizure reduction	No functional deficits

Y: years; mo: months

Nass et al. report seven patients with autism or autistic epileptiform regression who responded in varying MSTs after failed medical management (Nass et al., 1999). In all seven patients, seizure control or EEG improved after MST. All of these seven children demonstrated at least modest improvement. Improvements in receptive language were greater than in expressive language function. Social and overall behavior improved to a moderate degree, although improvements were not always sustained.

Grote et al. reported speech and language outcome of 14 children who underwent MST for treatment of Landau-Kleffner syndrome (Grote et al., 1999). Eleven out of 14 children demonstrated significant improvement on measures of receptive or expressive vocabulary after surgery.

This data suggests that MST surgery may provide substantial and long-lasting improvements in language functioning in selected children with Landau-Kleffner syndrome (Grote et al., 1999). However, some results indicate that a secondary epileptic focus can be organized in the contralateral hemisphere or subcortical structures even if focal epileptic activity was inhibited after MST (Hashizume & Tanaka, 1998).

■ Presurgical evaluation

MST is reserved for patients with severe intractable epilepsy and confirmed localization of the epileptogenic zone in eloquent cortex. The technique usually serves as a complementary procedure to cortical resection or lesionectomy. Therefore the presurgical assessment of patients is similar to other epilepsy surgery candidates (Benifla *et al.*, 2006). A multicenter survey from 20 centers from Europe, Australia and the United States (Harvey *et al.*, 2008) reported using scalp EEG, video EEG, and MRI during the presurgical evaluation at all centers. Additionally, 17 used 2-[18F]fluoro-2-deoxyglucose positron emission tomography (FDG-PET), 16 used ictal single-photon emission computerized tomography (SPECT), 14 used fMRI (usually for language localization), 7 used magnetoencephalography and magnetic source imaging (MEG/MSI), and 10 performed intracarotid amobarbital procedures (IAP; Wada tests). Only three centers used all presurgical tests (ictal-SPECT, FDG-PET, fMRI, MEG, and IAP). In US centers more patients had ictal-SPECT, FDG-PET, and IAP studies and fewer patients had exclusively scalp EEG studies prior to surgery. Invasive video-EEG monitoring with subdural grid electrodes (SDG) also plays an important role in defining the epileptogenic zone during the presurgical evaluation. Subdural grids are individually placed for each patient based on data collected from the seizure semiology, interictal and ictal scalp EEG during the noninvasive part of the presurgical evaluation (Benifla *et al.*, 2006). In MST patients, intraoperative ECoG usually complements the workup to provide information on cortical spike frequency prior to and after the procedure.

■ Outcome after MST

In Morrell's original series follow up information was available in 20 patients. These patients were evaluated with respect to seizure control including a follow-up period of 5 years or more (5 to 22 years). Complete control of seizures was achieved in 11 (55%) patients. In 18 of the 20 cases, MST resulted in immediate cessation of electrical abnormality in the transected zone. Nine patients (45%) developed recurrent seizures and all of these patients were found to have an underlying progressive etiology five patients had Rasmussen encephalitis, three had tumors, and one had subacute sclerosing panencephalitis (Morrell *et al.*, 1989).

Only one (16.7%) of six patients in Wyler's series did not benefit from MSTs without additional resection. Except for one instance of transient hand paresis, there was no subjective or objective deterioration of function after MST (Wyler *et al.*, 1995). Rougier *et al.* reported 7 cases of MST without associated cortical resection (Rougier *et al.*, 1996). The follow-up period ranged from 1 to 4 years. Five (71.4%) patients had a decrease in seizure frequency. Two patients experienced a temporary sensory-motor deficit and recovered completely within one month after MST.

The use of MST without resection has also been described by Schramm *et al.* In this series 20 consecutive patients with drug-resistant focal epilepsy were treated with MST without cortical resection (Schramm *et al.*, 2002). This series included 13 non-lesional cases based on MRI. Outcome after 49.3 ± 18.3 months was Engel Class I in 10%, Engel class II in 5% and Engel Class III in 30%. Outcome was found to be better in patients with non-lesional MRI, and worse in patients with large MST areas. There were no permanent neurological deficits but there were seven patients with transient deficits.

Devinsky *et al.* presented three patients with medically refractory partial epilepsy (Devinsky *et al.*, 1994). Two patients had anterior temporal lobectomy (ATL) and MSTs in the posterior language cortex. One patient had MSTs only over the fronto-parietal convexity, including frontal and parietal language areas. All three patients were mapped with extra-operative stimulation using subdural grids. Both patients with ATL and MST in the posterior language cortex remained seizure-free after 1 year. Both had postoperative language dysfunction and this improved significantly within 9 months after surgery. Of 25 MST cases presented by Shimizu and Maehara, surgical outcomes after > 1 year follow-up showed Engel Class I or II in 10 cases, Class III in 12, and Class IV in 3. No mortality or morbidity was encountered during surgery or postoperatively (Shimizu & Maehara, 2000).

In 2002 Spencer et al. published a meta-analysis to elucidate the indications and outcome of MSTs (Spencer et al., 2002). Two hundred eleven patients were included. Fifty-three patients underwent MST without resection. For the patients who underwent MST without resection, the rate of excellent outcome (> 95% reduction in seizure frequency) was 71% for generalized, 62% for complex partial, and 63% for simple partial seizures. In patients with MST plus resection, excellent outcome was obtained in 87% of patients for generalized seizures, 68% for complex partial seizures, and 68% for simple partial seizures. Overall, new neurologic deficits were found in 47 patients, and this was comparable in patients with MST plus resection (23%) or pure MST (19%). This data suggest that MST can be considered as a feasible and effective treatment approach in patients with uncontrolled seizures arising from functionally important cortical areas (Spencer et al., 2002).

Orbach et al. analyzed the long-term outcome after MST in 54 patients after a mean of 56 months (range 28-89) (Orbach et al., 2001a; Orbach et al., 2001b). Three patients had MSTs only and 51 patients with lesions partially localized in eloquent and non-eloquent cortex had both resections and MST. Twenty seven (50%) of 54 patients became entirely seizure free. Forty-three (79.6%) of the 54 had a consistent reduction in seizure frequency. However, ten (18.5%) patients experienced an increase in seizure frequency several years (between 2 and 5 years) after showing initial postoperative improvement.

■ Limitations

Many clinical cases series demonstrated that MSTs improve seizure control with minimal or no neurological impairment (Devinsky et al., 1994; Morrell et al., 1989; Morrell et al., 1995; Orbach et al., 2001a; Rougier et al., 1996; Schramm et al., 2002; Wyler et al., 1995). There is no consensus on the benefit of MST. The most common two indications for MST are overlap between epileptogenic zone and eloquent areas and pharmacologically intractable seizures in patients with LKS. However, patient selection may in part explain variable outcomes (Tovar-Spinoza & Rutka, 2010). Another reason for variable results may include lack of a standardized surgical technique. Efficacy for seizure control and neurologic outcome has been difficult to evaluate because MST is frequently combined with resection.

■ Outlook

Current data suggest that MST is likely more effective when combined with cortical resection compared with its application as a stand-alone procedure. Prospective studies are needed to assess the full potential of MST as stand-alone therapy although these studies may be difficult to conduct due to difficulties with identification of ideal controls. MSTs may have limited indications in patients where the epileptogenic zone overlaps with eloquent cortex.

References

- Asanuma H. Recent developments in the study of the columnar arrangement of neurons within the motor cortex. *Physiol Rev* 1975; 55: 143-56.
- Benifla M, Otsubo H, Ochi A, Snead OC, 3rd, Rutka JT. Multiple subpial transections in pediatric epilepsy: indications and outcomes. *Childs Nerv Syst* 2006; 22: 992-8.
- Cross JH, Neville BG. The surgical treatment of Landau-Kleffner syndrome. *Epilepsia* 2009; 50 (Suppl 7): 63-7.
- Devinsky O, Perrine K, Vazquez B, Luciano DJ, Dogali M. Multiple subpial transections in the language cortex. *Brain* 1994; 117 (Pt 2): 255-65.
- Dichter M, Spencer WA. Penicillin-induced interictal discharges from the cat hippocampus. I. Characteristics and topographical features. *J Neurophysiol* 1969a; 32: 649-62.
- Dichter M, Spencer WA. Penicillin-induced interictal discharges from the cat hippocampus. II. Mechanisms underlying origin and restriction. *J Neurophysiol* 1969b; 32: 663-87.
- Grote CL, Van Slyke P, Hoeppner JA. Language outcome following multiple subpial transection for Landau-Kleffner syndrome. *Brain* 1999; 122 (Pt 3): 561-6.
- Harvey AS, Cross JH, Shinnar S, Mathern BW. Defining the spectrum of international practice in pediatric epilepsy surgery patients. *Epilepsia* 2008; 49: 146-55.
- Hashizume K, Tanaka T. Multiple subpial transection in kainic acid-induced focal cortical seizure. *Epilepsy Res* 1998; 32: 389-99.
- Irwin K, Birch V, Lees J, Polkey C, Alarcon G, Binnie C, et al. Multiple subpial transection in Landau-Kleffner syndrome. *Dev Med Child Neurol* 2001; 43: 248-52.
- Landau WM, Kleffner FR. Syndrome of acquired aphasia with convulsive disorder in children. *Neurology* 1957; 7: 523-30.
- Lüders HO, Bustamante LA, Zablow L, Goldensohn ES. The independence of closely spaced discrete experimental spike foci. *Neurology* 1981; 31: 846-51.
- Molyneux PD, Barker RA, Thom M, van Paesschen W, Harkness WF, Duncan JS. Successful treatment of intractable epilepsia partialis continua with multiple subpial transections. *J Neurol Neurosurg Psychiatry* 1998; 65: 137-8.
- Morrell F. Microelectrode studies in chronic epileptic foci. *Epilepsia* 1961; 2: 81-8.
- Morrell F. Cellular pathophysiology of focal epilepsy. *Epilepsia* 1969; 10: 495-505.
- Morrell F, Whisler WW, Bleck TP. Multiple subpial transection: a new approach to the surgical treatment of focal epilepsy. *J Neurosurg* 1989; 70: 231-9.
- Morrell F, Whisler WW, Smith MC, Hoeppner TJ, de Toledo-Morrell L, Pierre-Louis SJ, et al. Landau-Kleffner syndrome. Treatment with subpial intracortical transection. *Brain* 1995; 118 (Pt 6): 1529-46.
- Nass R, Gross A, Wisoff J, Devinsky O. Outcome of multiple subpial transections for autistic epileptiform regression. *Pediatr Neurol* 1999; 21: 464-70.
- Orbach D, Romanelli P, Devinsky O, Doyle W. Late seizure recurrence after multiple subpial transections. *Epilepsia* 2001a; 42: 1316-9.
- Orbach D, Romanelli P, Devinsky O, Doyle W. Late seizure recurrence after multiple subpial transections. *Epilepsia* 2001b ; 42: 1130-3.
- Rougier A, Sundstrom L, Claverie B, Saint-Hilaire JM, Labrecque R, Lurton D, Bouvier G. Multiple subpial transection: report of 7 cases. *Epilepsy Res* 1996; 24: 57-63.
- Sawhney IM, Robertson IJ, Polkey CE, Binnie CD, Elwes RD. Multiple subpial transection: a review of 21 cases. *J Neurol Neurosurg Psychiatry* 1995; 58: 344-9.
- Schramm J, Aliashkevich AF, Grunwald T. Multiple subpial transections: outcome and complications in 20 patients who did not undergo resection. *J Neurosurg* 2002; 97: 39-47.

- Shimizu H, Maehara T. Neuronal disconnection for the surgical treatment of pediatric epilepsy. *Epilepsia* 2000; 41 (Suppl 9): 28-30.
- Spencer SS, Schramm J, Wyler A, O'Connor M, Orbach D, Krauss G, *et al.* Multiple subpial transection for intractable partial epilepsy: an international meta-analysis. *Epilepsia* 2002; 43: 141-5.
- Sperry RW, Miner N, Myers RE. Visual pattern perception following sub-pial slicing and tantalum wire implantations in the visual cortex. *J Comp Physiol Psychol* 1955; 48: 50-8.
- Tharp BR. The penicillin focus: a study of field characteristics using cross-correlation analysis. *Electroencephalogr Clin Neurophysiol* 1971; 31: 45-55.
- Tovar-Spinoza Z, Rutka JT. Multiple Subpial Transections in children with refractory epilepsy. In : Cataltep O, Jallo G, eds. *Pediatric Epilepsy Surgery. Preoperative Assessment and Surgical Treatment.* New York Stuttgart: Thieme, 2010, 268-73.
- Vendrame M, Loddenkemper T. Surgical treatment of refractory status epilepticus in children: candidate selection and outcome. *Semin Pediatr Neurol* 2010; 17: 182-9.
- Wyler AR. Multiple subpial transections in neocortical epilepsy: Part II. *Adv Neurol* 2000; 84: 635-42.
- Wyler AR, Wilkus RJ, Rostad SW, Vossler DG. Multiple subpial transections for partial seizures in sensorimotor cortex. *Neurosurgery* 1995; 37: 1122-7; discussion 1127-8.

Vagus nerve stimulation: techniques and outcome

James W. Wheless

Le Bonheur Comprehensive Epilepsy Program, Le Bonheur Children's Hospital and The University of Tennessee Health Science Center, Memphis, USA

Although the use of neurostimulation therapies for the treatment of refractory epilepsy is growing at a remarkable pace, vagus nerve stimulation therapy (VNS therapy') is currently the only Food and Drug Administration (FDA)-approved neurostimulation therapy for this life-long and life-limiting disorder. VNS therapy first received CE Mark approval in 1994 for the adjunctive treatment of seizures in patients whose epilepsy is dominated by partial seizures with or without secondary generalization or generalized seizures that are refractory to antiepileptic drugs (AEDs). In the United States, VNS therapy was approved in 1997 for use by the FDA as an adjunctive treatment to reduce the frequency of seizures in adults and adolescents aged 12 years and over with partial onset seizures that are refractory to AEDs. To date, VNS therapy is approved for distribution in more than 70 countries, with more than 60,000 patients treated with VNS therapy worldwide.

■ Evolving treatment approaches

Despite the fact that more than 12 new AEDs have been approved globally over the past two decades, no noticeable decrease has been seen in the number of patients with refractory epilepsy. Therefore, the treatment approach for epilepsy in this subset of patients is evolving as evidenced by the publication of the International League Against Epilepsy (ILAE) consensus statement outlining the definition of drug-resistant epilepsy (Kwan *et al.*, 2010). The ILAE defines difficult-to-treat epilepsy as the failure of adequate trials of two tolerated and appropriately chosen and used AED schedules (whether as monotherapies or in combination) to achieve sustained seizure freedom. A suggested epilepsy treatment sequence is shown in *Figure 1*. Making a clear distinction between newly diagnosed epilepsy and refractory epilepsy is critical to improving patient care by ensuring that patients receive optimal and timely care as well as to facilitating clinical research for this difficult-to-treat population. The risk of delaying more effective treatment options is a growing concern. Non-pharmacological treatment options like vagus nerve stimulation (VNS) therapy are a unique complement to standard AED therapy and have distinct advantages over drug therapy *(Figure 2)*. VNS therapy also had been shown to be of benefit among patients with failed epilepsy surgery without exacerbating the burdens of AED polytherapy (Amar *et al.*, 2004; Vale *et al.*, 2011).

■ Mechanism of action

Neurostimulation therapy for epilepsy is not a new idea. Clinical research linking the cessation of seizures with the application of peripheral stimulation to specific areas of the body or with electrical stimulation to specific nerves or internal structures of the brain dates back centuries (Vonck *et al.*, 2001; Ben-Menachem, 2002a). The effect of VNS on central nervous system (CNS) activity was documented in the 1880s with early attempts linking electrical vagal nerve and cervical sympathetic stimulation and carotid artery compression to the treatment of seizures (Lanska, 2002). Although the precise mechanism of action (MOA) of VNS therapy is not completely understood, numerous studies have been completed to create a better understanding of the anti-seizure affects of VNS.

The basic hypothesis on the MOA is based on the knowledge that VNS aims at inducing action potentials within the different types of fibers that constitute the vagus nerve at the cervical level (Vonck, 2008a) The vagus nerve is a mixed cranial nerve that has an extensive distribution of projections throughout the body and within the brain including the locus coeruleus, the nucleus of solitary tract (NTS), the thalamus, and limbic structures. Composed of both afferent and efferent fibers, it is the afferent fibers, which make up approximately 80% of the vagus nerve, that make the vagus nerve such a successful

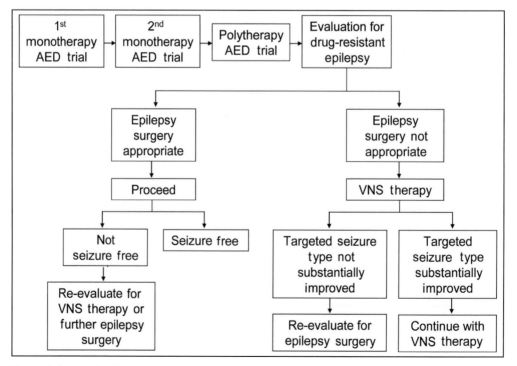

Figure 1. Suggested epilepsy treatment sequence.

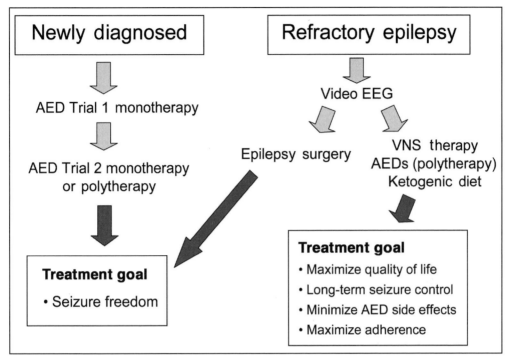

Figure 2. Identifying refractory epilepsy earlier in the treatment process allows for timely consideration of other treatment options, which can have broader lifestyle implications.

pathway to the brain for neuromodulation treatments. The afferent fibers of the vagus nerve project from the viscera to the nucleus tractus solitarius (NTS), which in turn has widespread projections to higher centers in the brain and the brainstem (Vonck et al., 2001; Ben-Menachem et al., 2002a) These diffuse pathways allow VNS to influence higher brain structures, including the amygdala and thalamus, which are important areas for epileptogenesis. Based on in vivo cortical recordings, it has been proposed that slow hyperpolarization may be one of the mechanisms underlying the seizure-reducing effect of VNS by means of reducing the excitability of neurons involved in seizure propagation (De Herdt et al., 2010).

A 27-patient SPECT study conducted to correlate changes in regional cerebral blood flow (rCBF) with long-term clinical efficacy after initial stimulation and after chronic treatment showed that, during the acute stimulation period, the left thalamus exhibited decreased rCBF (Vonck et al., 2008b). These findings may reflect a lowered state of activity in certain cortical areas preventing the propagation of epileptic activity. This study also suggested that acute limbic hyper-perfusion and chronic thalamic hypo-perfusion correlate with positive clinical efficacy. These findings are consistent with the theory that VNS interferes with the epileptic network.

Another area under investigation in understanding the MOA of VNS surrounds the identification of the potential involvement of specific neurotransmitters (Vonck et al., 2008a). The intracranial effect of VNS may be based on local or regional GABA increases or glutamate and aspartate decreases or may involve other neurotransmitters that have been shown in the past to have a seizure threshold regulating role such as serotonine and norepinephrine. A SPECT study in humans before and after 1 year of VNS showed a normalization of GABA(A) receptor density in the individuals with a clear therapeutic response to VNS (Marrosu *et al.*, 2003). An increased norepinepherine concentration after VNS also has been measured in the hippocampus and the amygdale (Vonck *et al.*, 2008a, Roosevelt *et al.*, 2006; Hassert *et al.*, 2004; Borovikova *et al.*, 2000).

By producing long-term changes in cerebral blood flow and influencing neurotransmission in the brain, VNS may indeed establish a true and long-term antiepileptic effect rather than only desynchronizing abnormal synchronous epileptic activity (Vonck *et al.*, 2003). However, clear predictive outcome factors and patient selection criteria for VNS, as with most epilepsy treatments, remain elusive.

■ The VNS therapy system

Components

The VNS therapy System (Cyberonics, Inc; Houston, Texas) is composed of the implantable components, which include a programmable pulse generator and a bipolar lead that transmits the stimulation currents from the generator to the vagus nerve, and non-implantable components. The non-implantable components include a programming wand and handheld computer with software for adjusting the level and frequency of the delivered stimulation, a tunneling tool, and hand-held magnets that can both stop and start stimulation. Over time, the implanted components evolved from a generator with a dual-pin lead (the Model 100 and 101), to a single-pin design lead and thinner and more lightweight generators (the Model 102 and 103). Although the dual-pin lead is no longer distributed, the dual pin version (Model 300) is still present in some previously implanted patients. As a result, the newer generators are also available with dual-pin headers (the Model 102R and 104) to accommodate end-of-service re-implants. The newest generations of leads, which have replaced the Model 300 worldwide and the 302 in the US, are known as the Perennia leads (PerenniaDURA [Model 303] and PerenniaFLEX [304]). All VNS therapy leads are available in two sizes (2.0 mm and 3.0 mm) to account for different sizes of vagus nerves.

These design changes to the generators (shown in *Figure 3*) and the lead simplify implantation of the device as well as provide an improved cosmetic appearance and increased comfort to the patient, particularly in the pediatric population, as well as more durability.

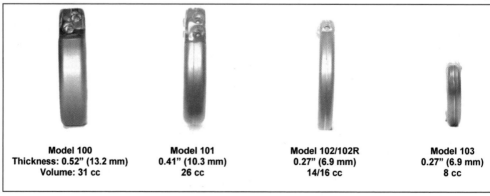

Model 100	Model 101	Model 102/102R	Model 103
Thickness: 0.52" (13.2 mm)	0.41" (10.3 mm)	0.27" (6.9 mm)	0.27" (6.9 mm)
Volume: 31 cc	26 cc	14/16 cc	8 cc

Figure 3. The VNS therapy generators have evolved into models that are thinner, lighter, and have less volume, making them easier to implant.

Surgical procedure

Implantation of the device is typically done as an outpatient or observation procedure, which is about 1 hour and is performed under general, local, or regional anesthesia (Amar et al., 1998). The implantation procedure uses a similar surgical approach to carotid endarterectomy. Typically, two incisions are made, one in the left neck area to attach the lead to the vagus nerve and one in the upper left chest area for the placement of the generator. However, an alternative surgical technique using a single cervical incision and sub-pectoral placement of the generator also has been used successfully, particularly for children who have a reduced muscular mass (Zamponi et al., 2002; Rychlicki et al., 2006a). For electrode placement, a transverse incision is recommended to "hide" the scar in neck (Figure 4). The lead is placed around the left vagus nerve, which has less cardiac innervation than the right vagus nerve (Figures 5-7). Excessive handling of the nerve should be avoided to prevent injury and preserve branches off the vagus as well as to prevent the nerve from drying out.

The generator is generally placed in a subcutaneous pocket in the subclavicular or anterior axillary region of the chest (Figure 8). Alternatively, an intrascupular placement of the generator can be used, particularly with patients with developmental disabilities, in an effort to reduce the risk of wound tampering. The tunneling tool is used to pass the electrode from the nerve to the generator pocket (Figure 9), and the pin attached to the electrode is then attached to the generator (Figure 10). Typically, the lead is tunneled subcutaneously from the neck incision to the pocket incision before placement of the electrodes around the nerve and tethering of the strain relief. However, particularly when implanting a PerenniaDURA Model 303 lead which is less flexible than the other lead Models, tunneling after electrode placement may be desirable to minimize manipulation

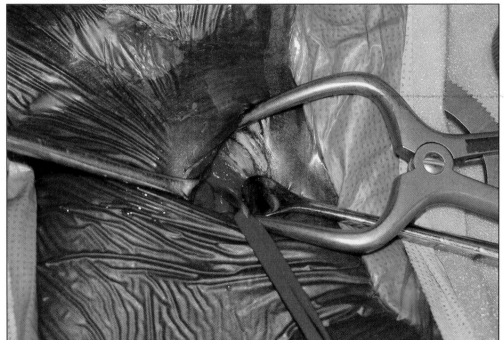

Figure 4. Neck incision with the vagus nerve isolated.

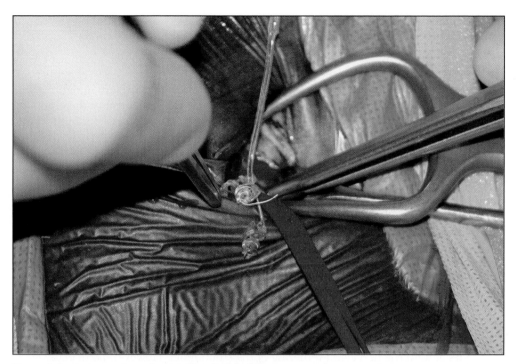

Figure 5. Lead wire starting to be placed on the left vagus nerve.

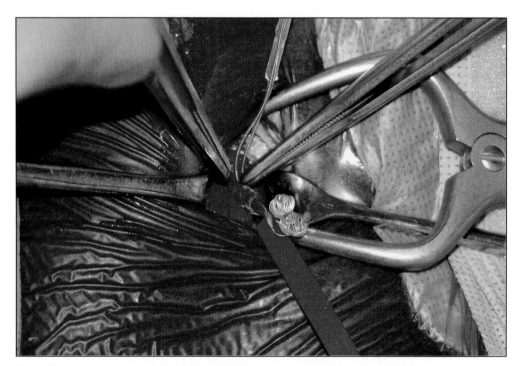

Figure 6. Lead wire electrode on the left vagus nerve.

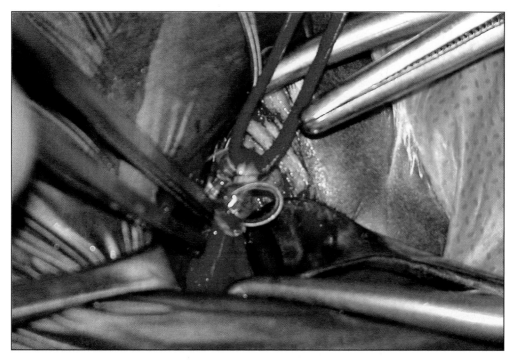

Figure 7. Lead wire, both electrodes on vagus nerve, and anchor tether.

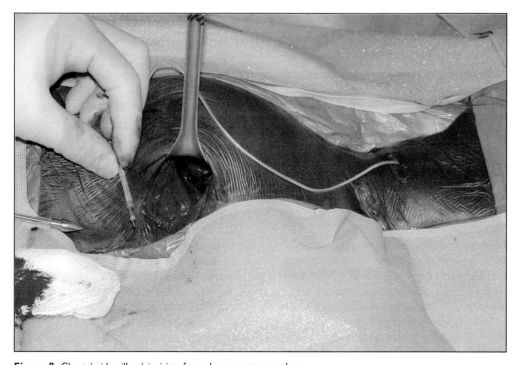

Figure 8. Chest (mid-axillary) incision for pulse generator pocket.

of the nerve. Care should be taken to ensure that an adequate strain relief bend (at least 3 cm) and loop are created before tethering the lead in place *(Figures 11-12)*. Tie downs should be secured to nearby fascia rather than muscle.

Neck and chest incisions after subcutaneous closure are shown in *Figures 13 and 14*. Before conclusion of the surgery, intraoperative testing is performed using the hand held computer and dosing wand to ensure system integrity *(Figure 15)*. A neck incision after final closure with Durabond is shown in *Figure 16*.

Implantation of the VNS device is typically performed as a day surgery. Patients experiencing any unusual discomfort or adverse effects during the intraoperative test of the device may be kept in the hospital for overnight observation. Surgical complications with VNS are rare (Cohen-Gadol *et al.*, 2003). Studies show that the most frequently reported surgical complications are infection, which is estimated to occur in up to 3% of cases, temporary vocal cord paralysis, and hoarseness (Ben-Menachem *et al.*, 2002a). Generally, infections at the implant site can be treated with antibiotics, but explantation of the device has been necessary in approximately 1% of the cases (Ben-Menachem *et al.*, 2002a). Initiating antibiotics before the implant surgery and using them during the recovery period also helps to reduce the rate of infections following surgery (Rychlicki *et al.*, 2006a). In rare cases, other adverse events resulting from the surgical procedure include nerve damage and intraoperative instances of bradycardia or asystole during the lead test (Cohen-Gadol *et al.*, 2003). Early temporary left vocal cord paralysis has occurred in less than 1% of cases both as a result of manipulating the vagus nerve during surgery and of the stimulation (Rychlicki *et al.*, 2006a; Cohen-Gadol *et al.*, 2003).

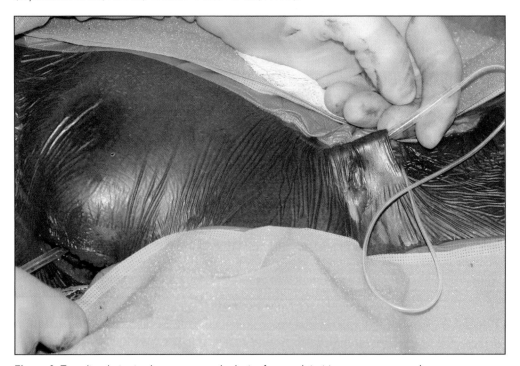

Figure 9. Tunneling device in place to connect lead wire from neck incision to generator pocket.

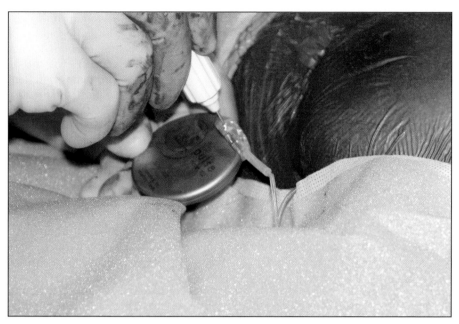

Figure 10. VNS therapy Generator (Model 102) being attached to lead wire.

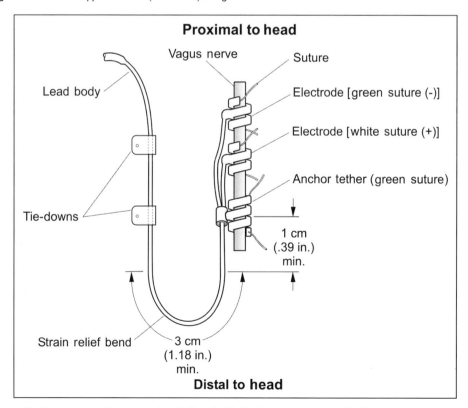

Figure 11. Placement of adequate strain relief bend with tie downs to tether the lead in place.

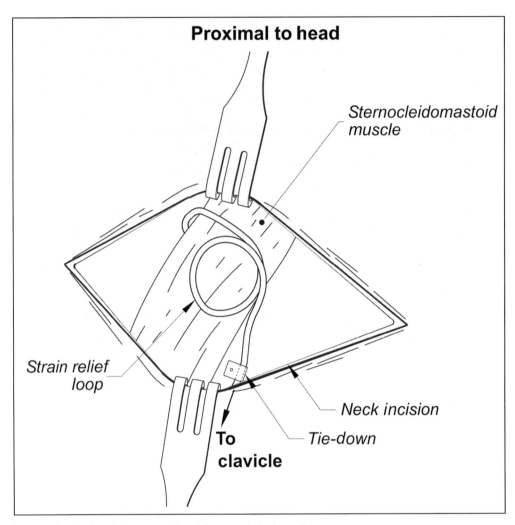

Figure 12. Creation of adequate strain relief loop with tie down placement.

A correct technical procedure, which requires a thorough knowledge of vagus nerve anatomy, will minimize the side effects associated with VNS therapy (Rychlicki *et al.*, 2006a).
When necessary, either owing to lack of efficacy or device malfunction, both the generator
and the lead, including the spiral electrodes around the vagus nerve, can be safely removed
even after a prolonged period of implantation among both children and adults (Rychlicki
et al., 2006a). If removal of the entire system is not possible owing to fibrotic encapsula-
tion, no more than 4 cm of the lead wire should be left remaining.

Dosing

As with dose adjustments for AED therapy, the goal of adjusting the dose of VNS therapy
is to maximize the therapeutic effect while minimizing side effects. VNS therapy is dosed
by adjusting any of five stimulation parameters within a pre-established range of settings,
shown in *Table I*, to achieve an optimal response for each patient (Tecoma & Iragui,

2006). Each parameter controls the total "dose" of stimulation each patient receives by varying the dose amount (stimulation strength [mA]), the dosing frequency (stimulation on/off time [seconds/minutes]), and the side effect burden (stimulation pulse width [μsec] and frequency [Hz]). While there is a broad array of options to adjust when dosing VNS therapy, investigations have been done to better understand how to most effectively dose VNS therapy based on the anatomy and neurophysiology of the vagus nerve.

Table I. Dosing VNS therapy is achieved by adjusting any of five different parameter settings to optimize outcomes for each patient

Parameters	Range	Typical	Suggested
Output current	0-3.5 mA	1.25 mA	> 1.50 mA
Signal frequency	1-30 Hz	30 Hz	20 Hz
Pulse width	130-1,000 μsec	500 μsec	250 μsec
On time	7-60 sec	30 sec	7 (14) sec
Off time	0.2-180 min	5 min	0.3 (0.5) min
Magnet Settings			
Output current	0-3.5 mA	1.5 mA	>1.75 mA
Pulse width	130-1,000μsec	500 μsec	250 μsec
On time	7-60 sec	60 sec	14 sec

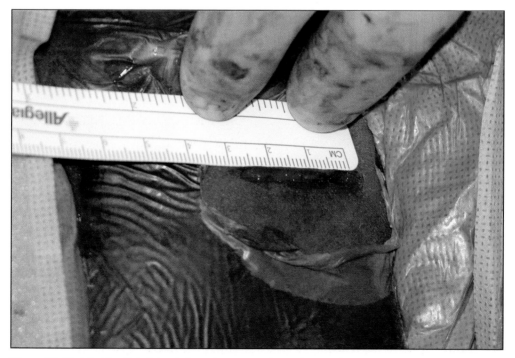

Figure 13. Neck incision (1 inch long) after subcutaneous closure in operating room.

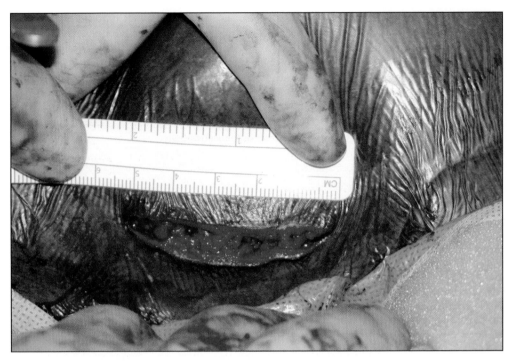

Figure 14. Chest (mid-axillary) incision after subcutaneous closure (5 cm long).

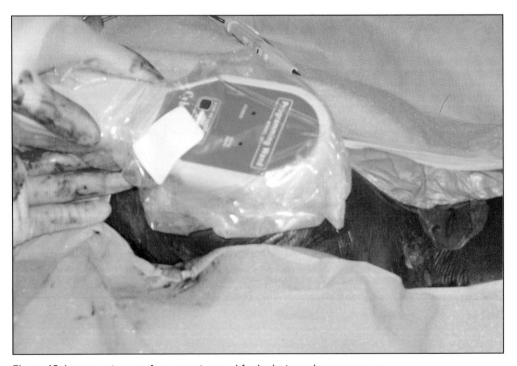

Figure 15. Intraoperative use of programming wand for lead wire and generator test.

The vagus nerve consists of 80% C-fibers that are non-myelinated and 20% A- and B-fibers that are myelinated. C-fiber activation is not believed to be involved in the efficacy of VNS (Krahl et al., 2001). A fundamental concept of neurostimulation is the need to deliver a sufficient stimulus to a nerve to cause depolarization and thus create an action potential. As input stimulus is increased, more fibers are recruited; however, there is a point of diminishing returns where a greater amount of stimulus does not yield greater fiber recruitment and excitation. Armed with the knowledge that a certain level of stimulus is needed to deliver effective therapy and that the output current and pulse width, combined, determine the strength of the stimulus, a physician can begin to efficiently optimally dose a patient. Attaining full activation of the vagus nerve requires selecting the right combination of VNS therapy parameter settings.

The dosing frequency is described using the term duty cycle. The term standard cycling refers to parameter settings in which the on time is 21 or 30 seconds, and the off time is 3 or 5 minutes. Rapid cycling denotes settings with an on time of less than 30 seconds and off times of less than 1 minute. Rapid cycling parameters that use shorter on and off times are used for some patients, but rapid cycling settings will decrease battery life and therefore should be used only when standard parameter settings are not effective.

The device manufacturer (Cyberonics, Inc; Houston, Texas) recommends waiting 2 weeks after implantation before turning the device on to allow for surgical recovery. However, stimulation has been initiated successfully in the operating room at low (e.g., 0.25 mA) settings at many centres (Labiner & Ahern, 2007). Stimulation settings are then adjusted over the following weeks until a therapeutic setting that is comfortable to the patient is reached (Figure 17). Optimum therapeutic settings vary by patient and, therefore, stimulation parameters must be adjusted on a patient-by-patient basis to achieve maximum therapeutic effectiveness for each individual (Labiner & Ahern, 2007). Studies of device parameters among children indicate that children may require higher stimulus currents or longer pulse widths than adults to achieve a therapeutic effect owing to higher stimulation thresholds and lower conduction velocity (Tecoma & Iragui, 2006).

For patients who receive a reimplant for battery replacement at end of service, stimulus parameters should be started back at a lower level than what they were receiving preoperatively because patients cannot always tolerate the same level of stimulation they were receiving before reimplant (Tatum et al., 2004; Vonck et al., 2005). Reports also indicate that some patients may not experience the same level of seizure control after an end-of-service reimplant, particularly if the patients go for an extended period of time (e.g., several months) without stimulation (Tatum et al., 2004; Vonck et al., 2005). To ensure continuity in treatment response, many physicians advocate battery replacement before end of service occurs. Clinical signs indicating the need for battery replacement include an increase in seizure frequency or intensity, the occurrence of irregular stimulation, and the loss of other benefits of VNS such as a return of depressive symptoms (Tecoma & Iragui, 2006).

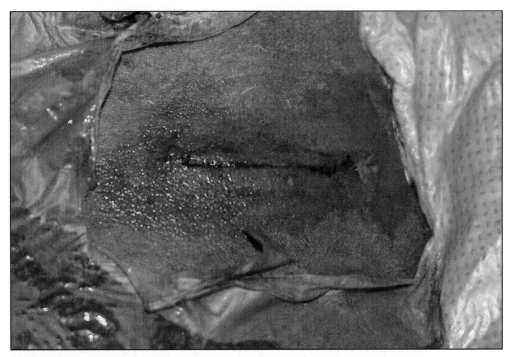

Figure 16. Neck incision after final closure with Durabond®.

■ Safety

With more than 60,000 patients implanted with VNS therapy worldwide, the safety and tolerability of VNS therapy in epilepsy is well documented. The side effects associated with VNS therapy typically occur only during stimulation, decrease over time, can often be addressed by changes in the stimulation parameter settings, and rarely result in discontinuation of treatment. The most common side effects among the clinical study patients include voice alteration/hoarseness (19.3%), cough (5.9%), and shortness of breath (3.2%) (Morris 3rd & Mueller, 1999; Ben-Menachem, 2001). No changes were seen in autonomic function and VNS therapy has not been associated with disease-specific treatment-emergent serious adverse events (Morris 3rd & Mueller, 1999; Ben-Menachem, 2001). Moreover, no teratogenic effects have been reported with VNS therapy and reports of to-term pregnancies are available in the literature (Ben-Menachem, 2001; Danielsson & Lister, 2009; Husain et al., 2005). VNS therapy is not associated with excess mortality. A reduction in sudden unexplained death in epilepsy (SUDEP) has been reported after long-term (2 years) use of VNS therapy (Cohen-Gadol et al., 2003). Additionally, rates of SUDEP for VNS therapy patients have been shown to be less than half the rates in the comparable non-VNS epilepsy patient population (4.1 vs. 9.3 per 1,000 patient years) (Annegers et al., 2000). Data also show that all-cause mortality rates for VNS therapy patients with epilepsy are less than half the rates in the comparable non-VNS epilepsy patient population (6.8 vs. 14-19 per 1,000 patient years) (Sperling et al., 1999; Ryvlin & Kahane, 2003).

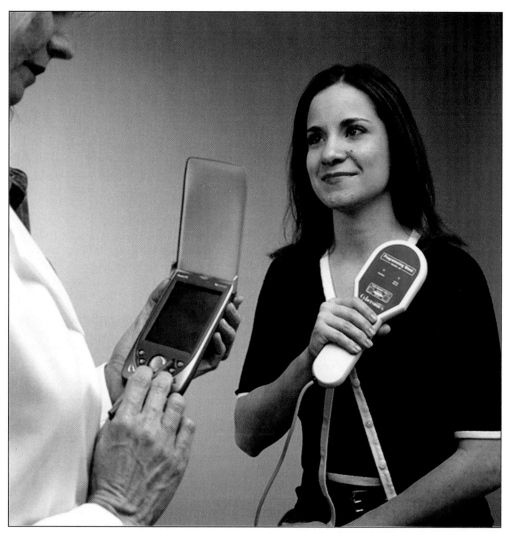

Figure 17. A patient receiving VNS is having the stimulus settings adjusted by the physician during a follow-up office visit.

Patients who have undergone a bilateral or left cervical vagotomy are not candidates for VNS therapy. Also, patients with a history of cardiac dysfunction should be evaluated by a cardiologist before initiating VNS therapy. Care also should be used when treating patients with a history of apnea or swallowing difficulties as there have been rare reports of an increase in apnea and aspiration among children when the device is on (Ben-Menachem, 2001). Diathermy, which is contraindicated for patients receiving VNS therapy, and full-body magnetic resonance imaging (MRI) scans could cause the implanted components of the VNS therapy system to heat to unsafe levels, which could result in either temporary or permanent tissue or nerve damage. A 1.5 Tesla (T) brain MRI of patients who have a VNS therapy system implanted is recognized as a safe procedure when a transmit/receive (T/R) head coil is used. For MRIs, the generator output current should be set to 0 mA and the device tested and reprogrammed to the original settings after the scan. In Europe, testing with 3.0 T MRI machines has been approved by the regulatory authorities; however, it has not been approved yet in the US. A recent study showed that safe clinical MRI head scanning of patients with VNS therapy was possible on a GE Signa Excite 3T MRI system using one specific T/R head coil under highly controlled conditions in 17 patients (Gorny et al., 2010). Diagnostic ultrasounds are not contraindicated for VNS patients.

■ Effectiveness

Five clinical studies, including two randomized, controlled, double-blind, pivotal studies, were performed to evaluate the safety and effectiveness of VNS therapy among patients partial or generalized seizures that were not well controlled by AED therapy (Morris et al., 1999; Labar et al., 1999; The Vagus Nerve Stimulation Study Group, 1995; Ramsay et al., 1994; Handforth et al., 1998; Uthman et al., 1990; George et al., 1994; Ben-Menachem et al., 1994). The two controlled pivotal studies (EO3 and EO5) showed statistically significant mean reductions in seizure frequency between patients receiving high stimulation (active treatment group) and low stimulation (control group) (The Vagus Nerve Stimulation Study Group, 1995; Handforth et al., 1998). These findings were seen independent of AEDs and no factors were identified that predicated response.

Long-term follow-up of these patients showed that response to VNS therapy improves over time and is sustained long-term (Morris 3rd & Mueller, 1999), a finding that has been confirmed in numerous other outcome studies (De Herdt et al., 2007; Elliott et al., 2011a; Elliott et al., 2011b; Vonck et al., 1999; Vonck et al., 2004; Uthman et al., 2004; Labar, 2004; Bialer et al., 2006). In addition to the increase in seizure frequency reductions over time, these studies show a decrease in side effects as well as high continuation and reimplant rates for VNS therapy (Ben-Menachem, 2002a). These clinical study findings indicate that VNS therapy is well tolerated and is not associated with a tolerance to effect over time (Bialer et al., 2006). The high durability of response seen with VNS therapy despite the refractory nature of the disorder among this patient population makes VNS therapy a valuable non-pharmacological treatment option to enhance AED therapy regimens.

Studies show that VNS therapy is well tolerated among patients of various ages and with different seizure types and syndromes (Tecoma & Iragui, 2006; Ben-Menachem et al., 1999). Studies among patients with idiopathic and symptomatic generalized epilepsy showed similar or greater rates of seizure frequency reduction than studies among patients with partial seizures (Tecoma & Iragui, 2006; Benbadis et al., 2004; Holmes et al., 2004; Labar et al., 1998). LGS has shown predominantly effective results, particularly for tonic seizures and atypical absences, and noted improvements in quality of life, particularly in alertness (Tecoma & Iragui, 2006; Frost et al., 2001; Karceski, 2001; Aldenkamp et al., 2001; Majoie et al., 2001). Similar findings also have been reported among patients over the age of 50 as well as among patients with developmental disabilities (Tecoma & Iragui, 2006; LaRoche & Helmers, 2003; Gallo, 2006; Sirven et al., 2000).

Studies among children and adolescents show equal if not superior results with VNS therapy compared with adult study outcomes (Rychlicki et al., 2006a; Tecoma & Iragui, 2006; Alexopoulos et al., 2006; Rychlicki et al., 2006b). As in adult studies, clinical response progressively improves over time, and, of particular interest in this age group, patients tend to function at a higher level and show considerable quality-of-life and neuropschological performance improvements (Rychlicki *et al.*, 2006b). Two recent studies showed that VNS was more effective among patients implanted when they were less than 12 years of age (Alexopoulos *et al.*, 2006; Rychlicki *et al.*, 2006b). *Table II* shows outcome data from various studies published since VNS therapy approval.

Table II. Vagus nerve stimulation therapy: real world results

Reference	Study type	Study population	Follow-up	Seizure frequency reduction	Overall responder rate
Elliott, *et al.* 2011	Retrospective	N = 436 Mean age: 29 yrs	Mean: 5 yrs	56%	64%
Shahwan, *et al.* 2009	Retrospective	N = 26 Median age: 11.8 yrs	Median: 3 yrs		54%
Rossignol, *et al.* 2009	Retrospective	N = 28 Age range: 3.5-21 yrs	24 mos	53%	68%
Kostov, *et al.* 2009	Retrospective	N = 30 with LGS Median: 13 yrs	Median: 52 mos	61%	67%
De Herdt, *et al.* 2007	Retrospective	N = 138 Mean age: 32 yrs	Mean: 44 mos	51%	59%
You, *et al.* 2007	Retrospective	N = 28 Mean age: 9.3 yrs	Mean: 31.4 mos		54%
Alexopoulos, *et al.* 2006	Retrospective	N = 46 Median age: 12.1 yrs	Median: 2 yrs	83%	59%
Rychlicki, *et al.* 2006	Prospective	N = 34 (N = 29 at 12 mos) Mean age: 11.5 yrs	Mean: 30.8 yrs (Outcomes shown for 12 mos)	49%	55%
Huf, *et al.* 2005	Prospective	N = 40 Mean age: 36.6 yrs	2 yrs	26%	28%
Labar 2004	Retrospective	N = 269 Mean age: 32 yrs	12 mos	58%	57%
Vonck, *et al.* 2004	Prospective	N = 118 Mean age: 32 yrs	Mean: 33 mos		51%
Park 2003	Retrospective	N = 59 Mean age: 12.4 yrs	12 mos	55%	58%
Frost, *et al.* 2001	Retrospective	N = 50 (N = 24 at 6 mos) Median age: 13 yrs	6 mos	58%	58%

Helmers, et al. 2001	Retrospective	N = 125 (N = 56 at 6 mos) Median age: 12 yrs	6 mos	51%	57%
Patwardhan, et al. 2000	Retrospective	N = 38 Median: 8 yrs	Median: 12 mos	66%	68%
Sirven 2000	Retrospective/ Prospective	N = 45 (N = 31 at 1 year) Age range: 50->70 yrs	12 mos		67%
Labar, et al. 1999	Prospective	N = 25 Median: 18 yrs	3 mos	46%	
Morris, et al. 1999	Prospective	N = 440 (5 clinical studies) Mean age: 30.8 yrs	36 mos	44%	43%

■ Cost effectiveness

The annual costs of diagnosing and treating patients with epilepsy are high and vary markedly among patients with various levels of severity of the disorder. Griffiths et al. (1999) showed that average annual cost of care for third-party payers was almost twice as much among patients receiving more than three AEDs versus only one AED. This difference in treatment cost was observed for all services combined as well as for each specific type of service, and was not solely attributable to the increase in medication costs. These findings are similar to those reported in other epilepsy cost studies. Nonadherence to AEDs, which is highly prevalent in the epilepsy population, also diminishes treatment effectiveness and further increases mortality as well as significantly increases healthcare utilization (Faught et al., 2009; 2008) In contrast to these studies, however, substantial savings in healthcare utilization and costs have been shown over time with VNS therapy.

The most recent healthcare utilization study to include VNS therapy, published by Bernstein et al. (2006) retrospectively analyzed the utilization of medical services and direct and indirect costs by 138 patients with VNS therapy in Kaiser Permanente, a large staff-model health maintenance organization. The average quarterly rates for 1 year before and 4 years after initiation of VNS were compared. This study showed significant decreases in outpatient visits, emergency department visits, hospital length of stay, and number of hospital admissions through 4 years of VNS therapy. Cost studies from Europe, the United Kingdom, and Canada all have shown similar results, including significant reductions in annual epilepsy-related direct medical costs among patients receiving VNS therapy compared with patients receiving standard (non-surgical) treatments (Boon et al., 2002; Ben-Menachem et al., 2002b) These savings in treatment costs, when amortized over the life of the device, can equal or exceed the initial costs of VNS therapy (e.g., the purchase price of the device and cost of implant surgery) (Ben-Menachem et al., 2002b).

■ Conclusions

In the treatment of refractory epilepsy, consideration of non-pharmacological treatment options earlier in the treatment process can have broader lifestyle implications for patients. VNS therapy is the only neurostimulation treatment currently FDA approved for the treatment of refractory epilepsy. Although VNS therapy is not a first-line treatment option, it should be considered as an adjunctive treatment option after two AEDs fail to control seizures, are not tolerated, and when epilepsy surgery is not an option. VNS therapy has been shown to have distinct advantages over polytherapy, including localized rather than systemic effects, no pharmacological side effects or drug-drug interactions, a reduction in lifetime treatment costs, no adherence issues, and oftentimes perceived improvements in overall quality of life. Studies and observational reports show that VNS is well tolerated, effective in a variety of seizure types and syndromes over the long-term. The safety and effectiveness of VNS therapy for the treatment of refractory epilepsy along with these benefits are changing the way physicians treat refractory epilepsy.

References

- Aldenkamp AP, Van de Veerdonk SH, Majoie HJ, *et al.* Effects of 6 months of treatment with vagus nerve stimulation on behavior in children with Lennox-Gastaut syndrome in an open clinical and nonrandomized study. *Epilepsy Behav* 2001; 2: 343-50.

- Alexopoulos AV, Kotagal P, Loddenkemper T, *et al.* Long-term results with vagus nerve stimulation in children with pharmacoresistant epilepsy. *Seizure* 2006; 15: 491-503.

- Amar AP, Apuzzo ML, Liu CY. Vagus nerve stimulation therapy after failed cranial surgery for intractable epilepsy: results from the vagus nerve stimulation therapy patient outcome registry. *Neurosurgery* 2004; 55: 1086-93.

- Amar AP, Heck CN, Levy ML, *et al.* An institutional experience with cervical vagus nerve trunk stimulation for medically refractory epilepsy: rationale, technique, and outcome. *Neurosurgery* 1998; 43: 1265-76; discussion 1276-80.

- Annegers JF, Coan SP, Hauser WA, Leestma J. Epilepsy, vagal nerve stimulation by the NCP system, all-cause mortality, and sudden, unexpected, unexplained death. *Epilepsia* 2000; 41: 549-53.

- Benbadis SR, O'Neill E, Tatum WO, Heriaud L. Outcome of prolonged video-EEG monitoring at a typical referral epilepsy center. *Epilepsia* 2004; 45: 1150-3.

- Ben-Menachem E, Hellstrom K, Verstappen D. Analysis of direct hospital costs before and 18 months after treatment with vagus nerve stimulation therapy in 43 patients. *Neurology* 2002a; 59 (6 Suppl 4): S44-S47.

- Ben-Menachem E, Hellstrom K, Waldton C, Augustinsson LE. Evaluation of refractory epilepsy treated with vagus nerve stimulation for up to 5 years. *Neurology* 1999; 52: 1265-7.

- Ben-Menachem E, Manon-Espaillat R, Ristanovic R, *et al.* Vagus nerve stimulation for treatment of partial seizures: 1. A controlled study of effect on seizures. First International Vagus Nerve Stimulation Study Group. *Epilepsia* 1994; 35: 616-26.

- Ben-Menachem E. Vagus nerve stimulation, side effects, and long-term safety. *J Clin Neurophysiol* 2001; 18: 415-8.

- Ben-Menachem E. Vagus-nerve stimulation for the treatment of epilepsy. *Lancet Neurology* 2002b; 1: 477-82.

- Bialer M, Johannessen SI, Kupferberg HJ, *et al.* Progress report on new antiepileptic drugs: A summary of the Eigth Eilat Conference (EILAT VIII). *Epilepsy Res* 2007; 73: 1-52.

- Boon P, D'Have M, Van Walleghem P, et al. Direct medical costs of refractory epilepsy incurred by three different treatment modalities: a prospective assessment. Epilepsia 2002; 43: 96-102.
- Borovikova LV, Ivanova S, Zhang M, et al. Vagus nerve stimulation attenuates the systemic inflammatory response to endotoxin. Nature 2000; 405: 458-62.
- Cohen-Gadol AA, Britton JW, Wetjen NM, et al. Neurostimulation therapy for epilepsy: current modalities and future directions. Mayo Clin Proc 2003; 78: 238-48.
- Danielsson I, Lister L. A pilot study of the teratogenicity of vagus nerve stimulation in a rabbit model. Brain Stimul 2009; 2: 41-9.
- De Herdt V, Boon P, Ceulemans B, et al. Vagus nerve stimulation for refractory epilepsy: a Belgian multicenter study. Eur J Paediatr Neurol 2007; 11: 261-9.
- De Herdt V, De Waele J, Raedt R, et al. Modulation of seizure threshold by vagus nerve stimulation in an animal model for motor seizures. Acta Neurol Scand 2010; 121: 271-6.
- Elliott RE, Morsi A, Kalhorn SP, et al. Vagus nerve stimulation in 436 consecutive patients with treatment-resistant epilepsy: long-term outcomes and predictors of response. Epilepsy Behav 2011; 20: 57-63.
- Elliott RE, Morsi A, Tanweer O, et al. Efficacy of vagus nerve stimulation over time: Review of 65 consecutive patients with treatment-resistant epilepsy treated with VNS > 10 years. Epilepsy Behav 2011; 20: 478-83.
- Faught E, Duh MS, Weiner JR, et al. Nonadherence to antiepileptic drugs and increased mortality: findings from the RANSOM Study. Neurology 2008; 71: 1572-8.
- Faught RE, Weiner JR, Guerin A, et al. Impact of nonadherence to antiepileptic drugs on health care utilization and costs: findings from the RANSOM study. Epilepsia 2009; 50: 501-9.
- Frost M, Gates J, Helmers SL, et al. Vagus nerve stimulation in children with refractory seizures associated with Lennox-Gastaut syndrome. Epilepsia 2001; 42: 1148-52.
- Gallo BV. Epilepsy, surgery, and the elderly. Epilepsy Res 2006; 68 (Suppl 1): 83-6.
- George R, Salinsky M, Kuzniecky R, et al. Vagus nerve stimulation for treatment of partial seizures: 3. Long-term follow-up on first 67 patients exiting a controlled study. First International Vagus Nerve Stimulation Study Group. Epilepsia 1994; 35: 637-43.
- Gilliam FG, Barry JJ, Hermann BP, et al. Rapid detection of major depression in epilepsy: a multicentre study. Lancet Neurol 2006; 5: 399-405.
- Gorny KR, Bernstein MA, Watson RE Jr. 3 Tesla MRI of patients with a vagus nerve stimulator: initial experience using a T/R head coil under controlled conditions. J Magn Reson Imaging 2010; 31: 475-81.
- Griffiths RI, Schrammel PN, Morris GL, et al. Payer costs of patients diagnosed with epilepsy. Epilepsia 1999; 40: 351-8.
- Handforth A, DeGiorgio CM, Schachter SC, et al. Vagus nerve stimulation therapy for partial-onset seizures: a randomized active-control trial. Neurology 1998; 51: 48-55.
- Hassert DL, Miyashita T, Williams CL. The effects of peripheral vagal nerve stimulation at a memory-modulating intensity on norepinephrine output in the basolateral amygdala. Behav Neurosci 2004; 118: 79-88.
- Helmers SL, Wheless JW, Frost M, et al. Vagus nerve stimulation therapy in pediatric patients with refractory epilepsy: retrospective study. J Child Neurol 2001; 16: 843-8.
- Holmes MD, Silbergeld DL, Drouhard D, et al. Effect of vagus nerve stimulation on adults with pharmacoresistant generalized epilepsy syndromes. Seizure 2004; 13: 340-5.
- Huf RL, Mamelak A, Kneedy-Cayem K. Vagus nerve stimulation therapy: 2-year prospective open-label study of 40 subjects with refractory epilepsy and low IQ who are living in long-term care facilities. Epilepsy Behav 2005; 6: 417-23.
- Husain MM, Stegman D, Trevino K. Pregnancy and delivery while receiving vagus nerve stimulation for the treatment of major depression: a case report. Ann Gen Psychiatry 2005; 4: 16.

• Karceski S. Vagus nerve stimulation and Lennox-Gastaut syndrome: a review of the literature and data from the VNS patient registry. *CNS Spectr* 2001; 6: 766-70.

• Kostov K, Kostov H, Tauboll E. Long-term vagus nerve stimulation in the treatment of Lennox-Gastaut syndrome. *Epilepsy Behav* 2009; 16: 321-4.

• Krahl SE, Senanayake SS, Handforth A. Destruction of peripheral C-fibers does not alter subsequent vagus nerve stimulation-induced seizure suppression in rats. *Epilepsia* 2001; 42: 586-9.

• Kwan P, Arzimanoglou A, Berg AT, *et al*. Definition of drug-resistant epilepsy: consensus proposal by the ad hoc Task Force of the ILAE Commission on Therapeutic Strategies. *Epilepsia* 2010; 51: 1069-77.

• Labar D, Murphy J, Tecoma E. Vagus nerve stimulation for medication-resistant generalized epilepsy. E04 VNS Study Group. *Neurology* 1999; 52: 1510-2.

• Labar D, Nikolov B, Tarver B, Fraser R. Vagus nerve stimulation for symptomatic generalized epilepsy: a pilot study. *Epilepsia* 1998; 39: 201-5.

• Labar D. Vagus nerve stimulation for 1 year in 269 patients on unchanged antiepileptic drugs. *Seizure* 2004; 13: 392-8.

• Labiner DM, Ahern GL. Vagus nerve stimulation therapy in depression and epilepsy: therapeutic parameter settings. *Acta Neurol Scand* 2007; 115: 23-33.

• Lanska DJ. J.L. Corning and vagal nerve stimulation for seizures in the 1880s. *Neurology* 2002; 58: 452-9.

• LaRoche SM, Helmers SL. Epilepsy in the elderly. *Neurologist* 2003; 9: 241-9.

• Majoie HJ, Berfelo MW, Aldenkamp AP, *et al*. Vagus nerve stimulation in children with therapy-resistant epilepsy diagnosed as Lennox-Gastaut syndrome: clinical results, neuropsychological effects, and cost-effectiveness. *J Clin Neurophysiol* 2001; 18: 419-28.

• Marrosu F, Serra A, Maleci A, *et al*. Correlation between GABA(A) receptor density and vagus nerve stimulation in individuals with drug-resistant partial epilepsy. *Epilepsy Res* 2003; 55: 59-70.

• Morris GL 3rd, Mueller WM. Long-term treatment with vagus nerve stimulation in patients with refractory epilepsy. The Vagus Nerve Stimulation Study Group E01-E05. *Neurology* 1999; 53: 1731-5.

• Park YD. The effects of vagus nerve stimulation therapy on patients with intractable seizures and either Landau-Kleffner syndrome or autism. *Epilepsy Behav* 2003; 4: 286-290.

• Patwardhan RV, Stong B, Bebin EM, *et al*. Efficacy of vagal nerve stimulation in children with medically refractory epilepsy. *Neurosurgery* 2000; 47: 1353-7; discussion 1357-8.

• Ramsay RE, Uthman BM, Augustinsson LE, *et al*. Vagus nerve stimulation for treatment of partial seizures: 2. Safety, side effects, and tolerability. First International Vagus Nerve Stimulation Study Group. *Epilepsia* 1994; 35: 627-36.

• Roosevelt RW, Smith DC, Clough RW, *et al*. Increased extracellular concentrations of norepinephrine in cortex and hippocampus following vagus nerve stimulation in the rat. *Brain Res* 2006; 1119: 124-32.

• Rossignol E, Lortie A, Thomas T, *et al*. Vagus nerve stimulation in pediatric epileptic syndromes. *Seizure* 2009; 18: 34-7.

• Rychlicki F, Zamponi N, Cesaroni E, *et al*. Complications of vagal nerve stimulation for epilepsy in children. *Neurosurg Rev* 2006a; 29: 103-7.

• Rychlicki F, Zamponi N, Trignani R, *et al*. Vagus nerve stimulation: clinical experience in drug-resistant pediatric epileptic patients. *Seizure* 200b; 15: 483-90.

• Ryvlin P, Kahane P. Does epilepsy surgery lower the mortality of drug-resistant epilepsy? *Epilepsy Res* 2003; 56: 105-20.

• Shahwan A, Bailey C, Maxiner W, Harvey AS. Vagus nerve stimulation for refractory epilepsy in children: More to VNS than seizure frequency reduction. *Epilepsia* 2009; 50: 1220-8.

- Sirven JI, Sperling M, Naritoku D, *et al*. Vagus nerve stimulation therapy for epilepsy in older adults. *Neurology* 2000; 54: 1179-82.
- Sperling MR, Feldman H, Kinman J, *et al*. Seizure control and mortality in epilepsy. *Ann Neurol* 1999; 46: 45-50.
- Tatum WO 4th, Ferreira JA, Benbadis SR, *et al*. Vagus nerve stimulation for pharmacoresistant epilepsy: clinical symptoms with end of service. *Epilepsy Behav* 2004; 5: 128-32.
- Tecoma ES, Iragui VJ. Vagus nerve stimulation use and effect in epilepsy: what have we learned? *Epilepsy Behav* 2006; 8: 127-36.
- The Vagus Nerve Stimulation Study Group. A randomized controlled trial of chronic vagus nerve stimulation for treatment of medically intractable seizures. *Neurology* 1995; 45: 224-30.
- Uthman BM, Reichl AM, Dean JC, *et al*. Effectiveness of vagus nerve stimulation in epilepsy patients: a 12-year observation. *Neurology* 2004; 63: 1124-6.
- Uthman BM, Wilder BJ, Hammond EJ, Reid SA. Efficacy and safety of vagus nerve stimulation in patients with complex partial seizures. *Epilepsia* 1990; 31 (Suppl 2): S44-S50.
- Vale FL, Ahmadian A, Youssef ASTWOBSR. Long-term outcome of vagus nerve stimulation therapy after failed epilepsy surgery. *Seizure* 2011; 20: 244-8.
- Vonck K, Boon P, D'Have M, *et al*. Long-term results of vagus nerve stimulation in refractory epilepsy. *Seizure* 1999; 8: 328-34.
- Vonck K, Boon P, Goossens L, *et al*. Neurostimulation for refractory epilepsy. *Acta Neurol Belg* 2003; 103: 213-7.
- Vonck K, De Herdt V, Boon P. Vagal nerve stimulation - a 15-year survey of an established treatment modality in epilepsy surgery. In: Pickard JD, ed. *Advances and Technical Standards in Neurosurgery*. Wien: Springer-Verlag, 2008a.
- Vonck K, De Herdt V, Bosman T, *et al*. Thalamic and limbic involvement in the mechanism of action of vagus nerve stimulation, a SPECT study. *Seizure* 2008b; 17: 699-706.
- Vonck K, Dedeurwaerdere S, Groote LD, *et al*. Generator replacement in epilepsy patients treated with vagus nerve stimulation. *Seizure* 2005; 14: 89-99.
- Vonck K, Thadani V, Gilbert K, *et al*. Vagus nerve stimulation for refractory epilepsy: a transatlantic experience. *J Clin Neurophysiol* 2004; 21: 283-9.
- Vonck K, Van Laere K, Dedeurwaerdere S, *et al*. The mechanism of action of vagus nerve stimulation for refractory epilepsy: the current status. *J Clin Neurophysiol* 2001; 18: 394-401.
- Wheless JW. Neurostimulation therapy for epilepsy. In: Wheless JW, Willmore LJ, Brumback RA, eds. *Advanced Therapy in Epilepsy*. Hamilton: BC Decker, 2009: 393-401.
- You SJ, Kang HC, Kim HD, *et al*. Vagus nerve stimulation in intractable childhood epilepsy: a Korean multicenter experience. *J Korean Med Sci* 2007; 22: 442-5.
- Zamponi N, Rychlicki F, Cardinali C, *et al*. Intermittent vagal nerve stimulation in paediatric patients: 1-year follow-up. *Childs Nerv Syst* 2002; 18: 61-6.

Deep brain stimulation in extratemporal epilepsy

Vicenta Salanova[1], Robert Worth[2], Thomas Witt[2], Dragos Sabau[1]

[1] *Departments of Neurology, Comprehensive Epilepsy Program, University Hospital, Indianapolis, USA*

[2] *Department of Neurosurgery, Comprehensive Epilepsy Program, University Hospital, Indianapolis, USA*

■ Introduction

Epilepsy affects 3 million people in The United States and 60 million world-wide and at least one-third of these patients are refractory to medical treatment (Engel Jr, 1996). Many of these patients benefit from resective epilepsy surgery, however, a large number of patients are not surgical candidates. Furthermore, some patients with extratemporal epilepsy are unable to have resective surgery, or do not have a favorable surgical outcome due to large epileptogenic areas, adjacent to eloquent cortex (Salanova, 1992; 1993; 1994; 1995).

The vagal nerve stimulation (VNS) is an option for some of these patients; the VNS was approved for the treatment of patients with refractory partial epilepsy who are not candidates for surgical resection. In clinical trials, 30% to 40% of patients with medically refractory partial epilepsy had a reduction in seizures of at least 50% (VNS study group, 1995).

Over the last several decades several targets have been used in an attempt to suppress seizures with high frequency electrical stimulation, including the cerebellum, the caudate nucleus, and the centromedian nuclei of the thalamus. (Fisher, 1998).

More recent studies have concentrated on the role of high frequency electrical stimulation of the subthalamic nucleus (STN), and anterior thalamic nucleus (ATN) in the treatment of refractory epilepsy (Chabardes, 2002; Fisher, 2010). The reason for this being that there is anatomic and physiologic evidence supporting the role of the thalamus in epilepsy. The thalamus has general effects on cortical excitability mediated by diffusely projecting nonspecific thalamic nuclei such as the anterior and intralaminar nuclei. The anterior nucleus of the thalamus projects largely to the cingulate gyrus, and via the cingulate gyrus, to limbic structures and wide regions of neocortex (Fisher, 1998).

Experimental studies have shown that high frequency stimulation of the subthalamic nucleus (STN), suppress seizures in animal models of epilepsy (Usui, 2005).

Mirski et al. (1997), reported that high- frequency stimulation (50-100 Hz) of the anterior nucleus (AN) of the thalamus increased the seizure threshold in rats with pentylenetetrazol-induced seizures. They also demonstrated the anticonvulsant effect of anterior thalamic high- frequency stimulation in the rat and found that low- frequency stimulation (8 Hz) was pro-convulsant. They postulated that the disruption of corticothalamic transmission with AN stimulation would prevent normal recruitment and synchronization into a generalized seizure.

Human studies also support the role of the thalamus in epilepsy. Henry (2002) reported changes in the thalamus using positron emission tomography (PET) scanning in patients with refractory epilepsy and showed that seizures improved most in patients who had bilateral thalamic activation induced by VNS in long-term PET studies. He stated that these results supported earlier evidence from acute VNS- activation PET studies that altered thalamic processing contributes to anti-seizure effects of VNS.

■ Deep brain stimulation in epilepsy

Recently several epilepsy centers have reported pilot studies of patients with refractory partial epilepsy treated with DBS. Hodaie et al. (2002) reported five patients with medically refractory epilepsy who had stereotactic placement of bilateral deep brain stimulation (DBS) electrodes in the AN of the thalamus, and were treated with intermittent high frequency stimulation. Bipolar stimulation was initiated by using 100 Hz, 90-microseconds pulse width, cycling 1 minute on with 5 minutes off, alternating left and right. Voltage was increased by 1 V/min to a maximum of 10 V. The authors stated that "these initial parameters were chosen based on the available experimental evidence, indicating high frequency (100 Hz) stimulation to be the most important parameter". Electroencephalography (EEG) recording through the thalamic electrodes showed interictal spikes in all patients and ictal electrographic changes shortly after seizure onsets. They reported a mean reduction in seizure frequency of 54%.

They also reported that the benefits did not differ between stimulation-on and stimulation-off periods. Patients had a decrease in seizure frequency immediately after implantation of the DBS electrodes, although stimulation did not start until four weeks after implantation. Hodaie (2002) postulated that "there may be and initial lesioning or so called microthalamotomy effect, similar to that seen with DBS implantation in other thalamic nuclei".

Andrade et al. (2006) reported on the long- erm follow-up (2 to 7 years) of these five patients plus one new patient receiving AN stimulation and two patients who had centro-median thalamic stimulation. Five patients with AN implantation had greater than 50% seizure reduction. They reported that "activation of the pulse generators and the multiple subsequent changes made to stimulation parameters or contacts stimulated over the subsequent months and years could not be linked to any further benefit in seizure control".

Kerrigan et al. (2004), reported an open-label pilot study of intermittent electrical stimulation of the AN of the thalamus in five patients with intractable partial epilepsy; four of these patients also had secondarily generalized seizures. The stimulation parameters were

100 cycles per second, pulse width of 90 microseconds, and voltages ranging between 1 and 10 V. Four of the five patients showed significant improvement in the severity of the seizures and the frequency of the secondarily generalized seizures. The authors noted that "in four patients in whom ANT stimulation was stopped, an immediate increase in seizure frequency and intensity occurred. These patients improved when the stimulation was resumed. These observations tend to argue that intermittent electrical stimulation of ANT is the active factor in achieving the therapeutic effect rather than a lesion effect within the ANT caused by physical placement of the electrode".

■ The SANTE trial

Fisher (2010) reported the results of a multicenter, double-blind, randomized trial of bilateral Stimulation of the anterior nuclei of the thalamus for treatment of localization-related epilepsy (the SANTE trial). Patients were 18-65 years old, with partial seizures including secondarily generalized seizures, at least 6 per month. Patients had failed at least three antiepileptic drugs (AEDs), prior to base line, and were taken 1-4 AEDs at the time of the study. Patients with an IQ less than 70, and inability to take neuropsychological tests were excluded from the study. Those patients who had a vagal nerve stimulation (VNS) had the VNS removed at the time of the DBS implantation. DBS were implanted in AN bilaterally using a stereotactic technique. Lead positions were verified postoperatively with MRI.

Fisher (2010) stated that "the selection of the anterior nuclei (AN) was based on several factors, which include the initial positive results in the studies of Cooper et al. (1980); three open-label pilot trials before, and subsequently, three after the randomized study, which showed approximately 50% seizure reduction. Stimulation of AN, which projects both to superior frontal and temporal lobe structures commonly involved in seizures, produces EEG changes (Kerrigan et al., 2004) and inhibits chemically-induced seizures in laboratory models (Mirski et al., 1997)."

One hundred and ten patients were randomized. The baseline monthly seizure frequency was 19.5. Half of the patients received stimulation and half no stimulation during a three-month blinded phase; then all received stimulation. The authors reported a greater reduction for the stimulated group compared to the control group, "unadjusted median declines at the end of the blinded phase were 14.5% in the control and 40% in the stimulated group" (Fisher, 2010). Furthermore, complex partial and, the most severe, usually secondarily generalized, were significantly reduced by stimulation. There was continuous improvement, by two years there was a 56% median reduction in seizure frequency, and 14 patients were seizure-free for at least 6 months. This is significant since the patients in the study had very severe epilepsy; 44.5% had been previously treated with the VNS and 24.5% had previous resective epilepsy surgery.

There were no symptomatic or clinically significant hemorrhages, but 5 hemorrhages (4.5%) were detected incidentally by neuroimaging. They reported two patients with acute, transient stimulation associated seizures. They also reported that "cognition and mood showed no group differences, but participants in the stimulated group were more likely to report depression or memory problems as adverse events" (Fisher, 2010). Patients with prior implantation of a VNS or with prior resective epilepsy surgery showed improvements comparable to those without these prior therapies.

On the SANTE trial patients with temporal lobe epilepsy had greater benefit of stimulation during the blinded phase, compared to those patients with seizures from other lobes or seizures multifocal in origin. As discussed by Fisher (2010), "benefit to those with temporal seizure foci may reflect participation of mesial temporal lobe along with the anterior nuclei of thalamus in the limbic Circuit of Papez" (Papez, 1937).

The authors concluded that "this study demonstrated a beneficial and sustained effect on seizure frequency of bilateral anterior nucleus deep brain stimulation", they also stated that "our results do not definitively rule out a contribution from a micro-lesion effect. However, the micro-lesion hypothesis cannot account for the improvement in the stimulated group versus the control group during the blinded phase, nor can a micro-lesion effect account for the progressive reduction in seizure frequency over time that we observed during long term follow-up. The control group improved after month 4 with initiation of stimulation, suggesting an effect of stimulation independent of the earlier implantation surgery" (Fisher, 2010).

The mechanism of thalamic DBS stimulation and the best parameters during electrical stimulation in patients with epilepsy are unknown. Zumsteg et al. (2006) investigated the effects of high-frequency anterior thalamic DBS stimulation in a patient with intractable epilepsy undergoing presurgical evaluation with depth electrodes in both temporal lobes and reported that "the hippocampal inhibition was clearly related to the voltage (> 7) and frequency (> 70 Hz) of the thalamic stimulus and occurred with a delay of approximately 60 seconds after stimulus onset". The authors stated that "our findings that inhibition of ipsilateral hippocampal structures was positively related to the voltage (increasing inhibition with increasing voltage) and frequency (reaching a plateau of about 70 Hz) of the AN are in accordance with the results from previous investigations in movement disorders)". They further stated that "their findings were in keeping with the assumption that the effects of DBS are a stimulation induced modulation of pathologic network activity, and that the DBS of AN might override the activity within a pathologic thalamo-cortical or corticocortical network in patients with epilepsy, thus resulting in a inhibition of distant cortical or limbic structures".

■ Cortical stimulation in epilepsy

Animal data and preliminary reports of patients with refractory partial epilepsy have demonstrated reduction in seizure frequency following cortical stimulation. Velasco (2001) reported that subacute hippocampal stimulation (SAHCS) blocks intractable temporal lobe epileptogenesis with no additional damage to the stimulated hippocampal tissue. SAHCS was applied to 10 patients with nonlesional temporal lobe epilepsy and unilateral focus, before an anterior temporal lobectomy (Velasco, 2000). They reported that "the most evident and fastest antiepileptic response was found in 5 patients in whom stimulation contacts were located at either the anterior pes-hippocampus near the amygdaloid nucleus or at the anterior parahippocampal gyrus near the entorhinal cortex". They also reported that "chronic hippocampal stimulation persistently blocked temporal lobe epileptogenesis in one patient under open protocol during 24 months with no apparent additional alterations in recent memory" (Velasco, 2000).

Tellez-Zenteno et al. (2006) reported four patients with refractory mesial temporal lobe epilepsy (MTLE), who underwent implantation of a chronic stimulating depth electrode along the axis of the left hippocampus. They found that hippocampal stimulation produced a median reduction in seizures of 15% and that all but one patient's seizures improved; however, the results did not reach significance.

Vonck (2002) evaluated long-term amygdalo-hippocampal stimulation in three patients with complex partial seizures and reported that "after a mean follow-up of 5 months all patients had a greater than 50% reduction in seizure frequency, none of the patients reported adverse effects".

■ The Neuro-Pace, RNS trial for epilepsy

Martha Morrell (2009) and the RNS System Pivotal Investigators reported the results of a multicenter double blinded randomized controlled pivotal investigation of the RNS System for treatment of intractable partial epilepsy in adults at the American Epilepsy Society meeting in Boston in December 2009. The RNS System is a cranially implanted responsive neurostimulator being evaluated as an adjunctive therapy for adults with intractable partial onset epilepsy. Patients were 18 to 70 years of age, had an average of 3 disabling partial seizures a month, had failed 2 or more antiepileptic medications and had seizure foci localized to one or two regions. Patients had very severe epilepsy; 34% had been previously treated with a VNS, and 33% with epilepsy surgery; 16% had been treated with both VNS and surgery, and 60% of patients had prior intracranial monitoring for localization of the epileptic focus.

The RNS System is designed to continuously monitor brain activity and, after identifying a patient's unique "signature" indicating that a seizure is starting, deliver brief and mild electrical stimulations to suppress the seizure, and to limit spread. The pivotal trial included 191 patients with medically refractory partial onset epilepsy enrolled at 31 epilepsy programs in the USA.

The blinded evaluation period of the trial began eight weeks after the RNS was implanted and lasted an additional 12 weeks. Half the patients were randomly assigned to have responsive stimulation activated and half had responsive stimulation remain inactive. Five months after the RNS System was implanted, which is when the double- blinded portion of the trial was completed; stimulation was activated for all the patients in the trial.

The trial demonstrated a statistically significant reduction in seizure frequency in the treatment group (responsive stimulation active) as compared to the sham stimulation group (responsive stimulation inactive). In the open label period of the trial, 47% of patients experienced a 50% or greater reduction in their seizure frequency based on their most recent 12 weeks of data, as compared to their baseline. The results indicated that the device became even more effective over time.

■ Conclusions

Animal and human studies demonstrate that high frequency DBS and cortical electrical stimulation may reduce the frequency of seizures. Fisher (2010) reported the results of the multicenter, double-blind, randomized trial of bilateral stimulation of the anterior nuclei of the thalamus for treatment o f refractory epilepsy, and found that "complex partial seizures and most severe seizures were significantly reduced by stimulation". The benefit was sustained, by two years, there was a 56% median percent reduction in seizure frequency; 54% of patients had a seizure reduction of at least 50%, and 14 patients were seizure-free for at least 6 months. The patients in the trial had very severe epilepsy, as 24.5% of patients had previous epilepsy surgery and 44.5% had a VNS implant, and as stated by Fisher, 2010 "improvements were seen in some participants previously not helped by multiple AEDs, VNS, or epilepsy surgery".

Martha Morell (2009) presented the results of a multicenter double blinded randomized controlled pivotal investigation of the RNS System neurostimulator at the American Epilepsy Society and reported that the trial demonstrated a statistically significant reduction in seizure frequency in the treatment group. The patients on the trial also had very severe epilepsy; 34% had been previously treated with a VNS and 33% with epilepsy surgery; 16% had been treated with both VNS and surgery, and 60% of patients had prior intracranial monitoring for localization of the epileptic focus.

The results of these trials are very significant, for they may lead to important new treatment modalities for patients who do not qualify for resective surgery (more than one epileptogenic area, epileptogenic areas adjacent to eloquent cortex, patients at risk of verbal memory deficits following temporal lobectomies) and for patients who have had epilepsy resective surgery but who continue to have seizures.

Acknowledgment and disclosures

Dr Salanova is currently involved in both the SANTE and Neuro-Pace trials and is the principal investigator for the Indiana University site. Dr Worth and Dr Witt are the neurosurgeons currently involved in both trials, and are co-investigators for the Indiana University site. Dr Sabau is a sub-investigator.

References

- Andrade DM, Zumsteg D, Hamani C, Hodai M, Sarkissian S, Lozano MD, et al. Long term follow- up of patients with thalamic deep brain stimulation for epilepsy. Neurology 2006; 66: 1571-3.

- Chabardes S, Kahane P, Minotti L, Koudsie A, Hirsch E, Benabid AL. Deep brain stimulation in epilepsy with particular reference to the subthalamic nucleus. Epileptic. Disord 2002; 4 (Suppl): S83-S93.

- Cooper IS, Upton AR, Amin I. Reversibility of chronic neurologic deficits. Some effects of electrical stimulation of the thalamus and internal capsule in man. Appl Neurophysiol 43: 244-58.

- Engel JR. Surgery for seizures. N Engl J Med 1996, 334: 647-52.

- Fisher RS, Mirski M, Krauss GL: Brain stimulation. In: Engel JR, Pedley TA, eds. Epilepsy. A Comprehensive Textbook, vol 2. New York: Lippincott Raven, 1998: 1867-75.

- Fisher R, Salanova V, Witt T, Worth R, Henry T, Gross R, et al. Electrical stimulation of the anterior nucleus of thalamus for treatment of refractory epilepsy. Epilepsia 2010; 51: 899-908.

- Henry TR. Therapeutic mechanisms of vagus nerve stimulation. Neurology 2002; 59 (Suppl 4): S3-S14.

- Hodai M, Wennberg RA, Dostrovsky JO, Lozano AM. Chronic anterior thalamic stimulation for intractable epilepsy. Epilepsia 2002, 43: 603-8.

- Kerrigan JF, Litt B, Fisher RS, Cranstoun S, French JA, Blum DE, et al. Electrical stimulation of the anterior nucleus of the thalamus for the treatment of intractable epilepsy. Epilepsia 2004, 45: 346-54.
- Mirski MA, Rossell LA, Terry JB, Fisher RS. Anticonvulsant effect of anterior thalamic high frequency electrical stimulation in the rat. Epilepsy Res 1997; 28: 89-100.
- Morrell M and the RNS System Pivotal Investigators. Results of a multicenter double blinded randomized controlled pivotal investigation of the RNS system for treatment of intractable partial epilepsy in adults. Presented at the American Epilepsy Society (AES) Epilepsia 2009, Abstract 1.102.
- Papez J. A proposed mechanism of emotion. Arch Neurol Psychiatry 1937; 38: 725-43.
- Salanova V, Andermann F, Olivier A, Rasmussen T and Quesney LF. Occipital lobe epilepsy: electroclinical manifestations, electrocorticography, cortical stimulation and outcome in 42 patients treated between 1930 and 1991. Brain 1992; 115: 1655-80.
- Salanova V, Morris H, Van Ness PC, Luders H, Dinner D. Wyllie E. Comparison of scalp electroencephalogram with subdural electrocorticogram recordings and functional mapping in frontal lobe epilepsy. Arch. Neurol 1993; 50: 294-9.
- Salanova V, Quesney LF, Rasmussen T, Andermann F, Olivier A. Reevaluation of surgical failures and the role of reoperation in 39 patients with frontal lobe epilepsy. Epilepsia 1994; 35 (1): 70-80.
- Salanova V, Andermann F, Rasmussen T, Olivier A, Quesney LF. Parietal lobe epilepsy. Clinical manifestations and outcome in 82 patients treated surgically between 1929 and 1988. Brain 1995; 118: 607-27.
- The vagus nerve stimulation study group: A randomized controlled trial of chronic vagus nerve stimulation for treatment of medically intractable seizures. Neurology 1995; 45: 224-30.
- Tellez-Zenteno JF, McLachlan RS, Parrent A, Kubu CS, Wiebe S. Hippocampal electrical stimulation in mesial temporal lobe epilepsy. Neurology 2006; 66: 1490-4
- Usui N, Maesawa S, Kajita Y, Endo O, Takebayashi S, Yoshida J. Suppression of secondary generalization of limbic seizures by stimulation of subthalamic nucleus in rats. J Neurosurg 2005; 102: 1122-9.
- Velasco F, Velasco M, Velasco L. Subacute electrical stimulation of the hippocampus blocks intractable temporal lobe seizures and paroxysmal EEG activities. Epilepsia 2000; 41: 158-69.
- Velasco M, Velasco F, Velasco AL. Centromedian-Thalamic and hippocampal electrical stimulation for the control of intractable epileptic seizures. J Clin Neurophysiol 2001; 18: 495-513.
- Vonck K, Boon P, Achten E. Long term amygdale-hippocampa l stimulation for refractory temporal lobe epilepsy. Ann Neurol 2002; 52: 556-65.
- Zumsteg D, Lozano AM, Wennberg RA. Mesial temporal inhibition in a patient with deep brain stimulation of the anterior thalamus for epilepsy. Epilepsia 2006; 47: 1958-62.

SEEG-guided RF-thermocoagulation of extratemporal epileptic foci: a therapeutic alternative for drug-resistant inoperable partial epilepsies

Marc Guénot[1, 3, 4, 5], **Jean Isnard**[2, 3, 4, 5], **Hélène Catenoix**[2, 3, 4, 5], **François Mauguière**[2, 3, 4, 5], **Marc Sindou**[1, 3, 4]

[1] *Dept of Functional Neurosurgery, Pierre-Wertheimer Hospital, Hospices Civils de Lyon, Bron, France*
[2] *Dept of Functional Neurology and Epileptology, Pierre-Wertheimer Hospital, Hospices Civils de Lyon, Bron, France*
[3] *University of Lyon, Lyon, France*
[4] *Institut Fédératif des Neurosciences de Lyon, Lyon, France*
[5] *Inserm, U879, Bron, France*

■ Introduction

Performing stereotactic lesions of the brain in order to relieve, or even cure, epilepsy is not a new idea. Prior literature comprises numerous reports of acute stereotactic ablation for epilepsy. Most reports focus on amygdalotomies or amygdalohippocampotomies (Anderson, 1970; Balasubramanian, 1976; Binnie, 1994; Blume, 1997; Bohbot, 1998; Bouvier, 1980; Exley, 1967; Flanigin,1976; Heimburger, 1966; 1978; Hood, 1983; Marossero, 1980; Mempel, 1980; Nadvornik, 1975; Narabayashi, 1980; Parrent, 1999; Schwab, 1965; Schumann, 1987; Small, 1977; Vaernet, 1972), some focus on various extra-limbic targets (Bouchard, 1976; Ciganek, 1976; Crow, 1972; Hullay, 1976; Nadvornik, 1974; Ojeman, 1975; Patil, 1995a, b; Schaltenbrand, 1966), and others deal with stereotactic ablation of epileptogenic lesions, especially hamartomas of the hypothalamus (Parrent, 1999).

Between 1965 and 1987, 21 studies were conducted to assess the efficiency of stereotactic lesioning of various cerebral targets for the control of intractable seizures. These studies included 5 to 107 patients, of whom 15 patients underwent stereotactic lesioning of the amygdalo-hippocampal structures solely. The rate of improvement, in terms of seizure frequency, was reported to vary from 50 to 85%. However, many of these studies were initially performed to assess the effect of stereotactic amygdalotomy for the control of unmanageable behavior, and it was secondarily found that some of the patients had a bonus relief from seizures. This explains why, in those early studies, literature pertaining to stereotactic amygdalotomy, hippocampotomy or fornicotomy displays results, which are difficult to interpret given the surgical techniques and outcome assessment used. Presurgical assessment was less rigid, it was rare to be able to verify the site and size of the lesion and follow-up data were poor being short and inacccurate. Finally, the relationship of outcome to the surgery was often indeterminate.

In 1999, Parrent & Blume (Parrent, 1999) carried out a single study to assess the safety and efficacy of stereotactic ablation of the amygdala and hippocampus for the treatment of medial temporal lobe epilepsy. Twenty-two stereotactic amygdalohippocampotomies were performed in 19 patients with unilateral temporal lobe seizures. Two lesion groups were defined. In group I, discrete lesions were made, encompassing the amygdala and anterior hippocampus. In group II, a large number of confluent lesions were made encompassing the amygdala and a larger part of the hippocampus. In five group I patients, one (20%) experienced a favourable seizure outcome. Of 15 group II patients, nine (60%) experienced a favourable seizure outcome, with two seizure free. They conclude that extensive amygdalohippocampal ablation improved seizure outcome compared with more limited ablation, but that these results were not so good as those from temporal lobectomy in a similar patient group.

Two different review articles dealing with stereotactic ablation for refractory epilepsy were then published by Parrent (2000), and by Polkey (2003). Both concluded that these technique, although being well tolerated with fewer adverse effects than observed with conventional surgical procedures, and although current image-guided technology offers the opportunity to revisit some of these techniques, have a definitively less favourable outcome than that of standard surgery (Bien, 2001; Sindou, 2006; Wiebe, 2001).

This might be related with several causes, such as the variability of the reported targets and indications (which often mixed behavioural disorders and epilepsy), or the small size of the lesions. Moreover, despite the recent use of image-guided technology, the risk of intra-cerebral bleeding due to the stereotactic positioning of the lesioning probe is a real risk. Finally, the rather disappointing benefit/risk ratio of previously published stereotactic lesioning for epilepsy does explain that this technique, popular in the1960s and 1970s, has been largely abandoned, and was not widely performed up to now.

Irrespective to this matter of fact, invasive presurgical EEG recordings of seizures may be required in many patients suffering from drug-resistant partial epilepsy to define the optimal cortical resection (Behrens, 1994; Binnie, 1994; Cossu, 2005; Guenot, 2002; Munari, 1994). In many epilepsy surgery centers, as in ours, such invasive explorations are carried out using stereoelectroencephalography (SEEG), according to the method first developed in the 1960s by Talairach and Bancaud (Talairach, 1973). Principles and methodology of SEEG have been reported in detail in previous publications (Cossu, 2005; Guenot, 2002). Briefly, SEEG consists of stereotactic implantation of depth electrodes in the brain, in order to identify the exact location(s) of the epileptogenic area(s), as well as the pathways of discharge propagation. The sites of implantation depend, for each particular patient, upon the outcome of prior non-invasive presurgical investigations. Because MRI is coupled with angiography, each electrode can reach its implantation site without injuring cerebral vessels. Each electrode is made of stainless steel, and has 5 to 18 contacts. The dimensions of each contact are 2 mm in length, and 0.8 mm in diameter. From 5 to 16 electrodes are implanted per patient (mean of 11). On the average, 150 contacts per patient reflect local

EEG activity in the depth of the sulci, as well as the medial aspects of the hemispheres (*Figure 1*). This electrode coverage allows a very accurate three-dimensional exploration of the epileptic network, and in our hands provides a map superior to that given by subdural grid electrodes recordings, particularly, if the epileptogenic area is deeply situated. The electrodes are left in place for up to 21 days, or until sufficient information is obtained on localization of seizure onset and propagation.

Most often, the video-SEEG recording of spontaneous seizures leads to "a tailored resection" of the epileptogenic zone (EZ). Some patients, however, are not eligible for surgery after this invasive procedure because the EZ are multiple and/or located close to or inside highly eloquent cortical areas (primary language, motor or visual zones).

In this context, in addition to passive recording, the use of these SEEG electrodes to generate focal lesions of the epileptogenic zone and of seizures propagation pathways seemed to us worth to be investigated. Such lesions can be produced by thermocoagulation, using a radiofrequency (RF) generator connected to the electrode contacts. This is named SEEG-guided RF-thermocoagulation of the epileptogenic foci.

Based on a personal experience of this method in a 41 patients series, this chapter aims: i) at presenting the feasibility and safety of multiple cortical RF-thermolesions made by means of chronically implanted SEEG electrodes; and ii) at reporting the results obtained in 41 consecutive patients who, among those referred to our department for surgical treatment of drug-resistant partial epilepsy between 2003 and 2007, have accepted this procedure as a first therapeutic step before surgery, or as a palliative treatment when surgery was not possible.

■ Technical data

Advantages of the technique

The advantages of using SEEG electrodes for performing multiple RF-thermolesions are supported by several lines of evidence (Guenot, 2004; 2008):

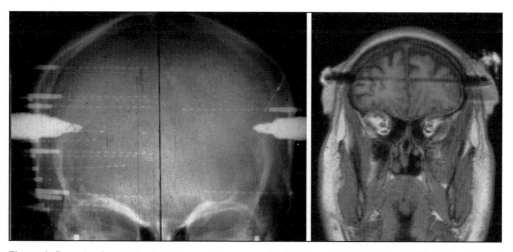

Figure I. Example of a post-implantation control antero-porterior X-ray (left) and MRI scan, T1 weighted, frontal slice (right). The depth electrodes are implanted orthogonally, according to the Talairach's SEEG methodology. 16 depth electrodes are implanted in this particular case, each of them having from 5 to 15 contacts.

1. The high number of implanted electrodes offers the possibility for producing several thermolesions.

2. Confluent lesions can be generated by contiguous placement of multiple thermolesions.

3. The clinical and electrophysiological status of the patient can be monitored in real-time before, during, and after the lesion is performed. Such monitoring allows interruption of the procedure as soon as a sensation of heat is reported. Heat perception can be due to proximity of the lesion site and pericerebral cisternea, and can be a warning against unintentional injury to the optic tract or brainstem.

4. As electrical stimulations are systematically performed during video-SEEG recording sessions, the possible side-effects of a lesion can be anticipated in detail. Consequently, there is no need for supplementary stimulation or a temporary lesion to test for adverse effects during the SEEG-guided-RF-thermolesion procedure.

5. The SEEG-guided-RF-thermolesion procedure does not require anesthesia.

6. Placement of thermolesions does not preclude subsequent conventional surgery in case of failure.

7. The bleeding risk is nil, as the electrodes are already in place, for recording purpose.

8. As revealed by our experience, these lesions are well-tolerated by the patient.

Patient's selection

Obviously, not all the patients who benefited from a SEEG during the same period (n = 132), underwent a SEEG-guided RF thermocoagulation procedure. RF thermocoagulation is only considered as soon as one or more of the implanted electrodes fullfills the following conditions:

1. To be located in the cortex areas showing either a low amplitude fast pattern or spike-wave discharges at the onset of the seizures. Interictal paroxysmal activities were not considered for planning thermo-coagulation sites.

2. All targets are first functionally evaluated using electrical stimulation. Only those showing no clinical response to stimulation are selected for thermo-lesion, including sites located inside or near primary functionnal area.

The SEEG-guided RF thermocoagulation procedure is always performed at the very end of the video-SEEG recording session, which usually lasts between 2 and 3 weeks.

Placement of the lesion (Guenot, 2004)

All SEEG-guided-RF-thermolesion procedures are performed without anesthesia. Lesions are made using a radiofrequency lesion generator system model RFG-5 manufactured by Radionics® (Radionics Medical Products, Inc. 22 Terry Av. Burlington, MA 01803 USA). The SEEG electrodes are manufacured by Dixi® (Dixi Medical, 4, chemin de Palente, BP 889, 25025 Besancon, France). The lesions are produced between two contiguous contacts of the selected electrodes. Temperature can not be monitored *in vivo* at electrode contacts, so the lesions are made using a 50 V, 120 mA current, which was found *in vitro* to increase the local temperature to 78°-82° C within a few seconds, thus producing a lesion around the electrode contact in 10-30 seconds (*Figure 2*). A depth EEG recording is performed during the procedure at the relevant contacts after each coagulation, which shows the absence of focal epileptiform activity at the lesion site after thermolesion. For each patient, several (2 to 31, median: 12 in our experience) bipolar lesions can be performed in one or more anatomical targets. The electrical activity recorded at the contact pairs used for RF thermocoagulation immediately after the procedure shows either a voltage reduction or a frequency slowing consistently associated to a decrease or a disappearance of interictal spikes.

The SEEG electrodes are removed at the end of the SEEG-guided-RF-thermolesion procedure, and the patient is discharged 24 h after its completion.

Postoperative MRI scans, with T1 and T2 sequences in horizontal, frontal and sagittal planes are performed three months after placement of the lesions, in order to assess the anatomical extent of the lesions.

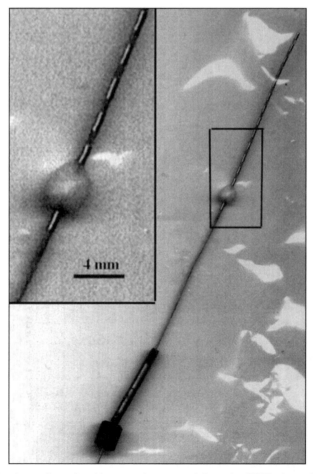

Figure 2. Picture of a chronically implantable stereoelectroencephalography (SEEG) electrode. *In vitro* thermocoagulation in egg white. The coagulated zone, 5 mm in diameter, is visible between the two selected contacts of the electrode.

Our experience (Catenoix 2008, Guenot 2008)

Patients

Forty-one patients (16 female, 25 male; mean age, 28 ± 8.6 years, range: 8 to 46), investigated by SEEG in the department of Functional Neurosurgery of Lyon, France, underwent multiple SEEG-guided RF thermocoagulation between 2003 and 2007.

All patients benefited from presurgical non-invasive investigation, including continuous video-EEG recordings, high resolution magnetic resonance imaging (MRI), [18]fluorodeoxyglucose positron emission tomography (PET) scan and sometimes ictal and interictal single photon emission computerised tomography (SPECT). In all these patients, data obtained from the non-invasive pre-surgical investigations were not sufficiently congruent for localizing reliably the EZ. Intracerebral recording of spontaneous seizures (*i.e.* video-SEEG recording) was thus undertaken before any surgical decision. All electrodes were implanted according to pre-surgical diagnostic necessities, so that the RF thermocoagulation procedure had no incidence on the number of electrodes and did not increase the risk of the stereotactic implantation. All patients were fully informed and gave their consent. They were also informed that, whenever possible, they will be offered conventional EZ surgical resection if they estimated RF thermocoagulation results as insufficient.

Targets, follow-up and results

The data obtained from this unique clinical series may be exposed as follows:

Choice of targets: The choice of targets has been explicated in the previous chapter (patient'selection). It depended upon data from video-SEEG recordings regarding the localization of the epileptogenic focus. All targets were located in the cortex areas showing either a low amplitude fast pattern or spike-wave discharges at the onset of the seizures. Interictal paroxysmal activities were not considered for planning thermo-coagulation sites. Only those showing no clinical response to stimulation were selected for thermo-lesion.

Follow-up: The frequency of seizures and the possible adverse effects of RF thermocoagulation procedure were collected during consultations made at one month, three months, six months, and then once a year after RF thermocoagulation.

The median follow-up after the RF thermocoagulation procedure, until the last consultation or the surgery, was 19 months (mean: 25 ± 21; range: 8 to 72). 21 of the 28 patients who were eligible for surgical resection have been operated a few months (mean: 8.9 ± 5; range: 4 to 28) after the RF thermocoagulation procedure. In the 13 patients who were not eligible for surgery, the mean follow-up duration was 43 months ± 18 (range: 15 to 72) between RF thermocoagulation and the last consultation.

The anatomic localization and extent of the thermo-lesions were assessed in every patient by a brain MRI scan performed 3 months after RF thermocoagulation. MRIs depicted isolated or multiple areas of coagulation necrosis, which were clearly visible along the electrode trajectories. The diameter of lesions ranged from 5-7 mm. The total length of lesioned area, made of confluent discrete lesions along the electrode path, varied according to the number of electrode contacts used for bipolar coagulations (*Figure 3*).

Antiepileptic drugs treatment was left unchanged during the six months following RF thermocoagulation. In some patients, the antiepileptic drug regimen was modified after the first six months of follow-up, but in no patient these changes modified the seizure outcome.

Patients were classified as responders if the decrease in seizures frequency was of 50% or more, and non-responders if not. Groups were compared with the non parametric Mann-Whitney test for continuous data (age, number of RF thermocoagulation, follow-up) because of small sample sizes. For categorical data (etiology, epileptogenic focus and RF thermocoagulation localization), Chi squared or Fisher's exact test was applied. A p-value less than 0.05 was considered as statistically significant.

Results: Regarding the seizure outcome *(Table I)*, the results are as follows:
– 20 patients (48.7%) experienced a seizure frequency decrease of at least 50% that was over 80% in eight of them. One patient was seizure-free after RF thermocoagulation.
– In 21 patients, no significant reduction of the seizure frequency was observed.
– No patient showed any increase of seizure frequency.
– Improvement of the epilepsy was observed at the first evaluation one month after RF thermocoagulation in 32 patients (78%). In 11 of them, this initial clinical benefit disappeared rapidly *i.e.* 3.8 ± 3 months after RF thermocoagulation and in one at 12 months. Beyond this lapse of time, the effect remained stable.

Among the characteristics of the disease (age and sex of the patient, lobar localisation of the EZ) and the characteristics of the thermocoagulations (topography, lateralization, number, morphology of the lesions on MRI) no factor was significantly linked to the outcome. However, the best results were clearly observed in epilepsies symptomatic of a cortical development malformation (CDM), with 67% of responders in this group of 20 patients (p = 0.052).

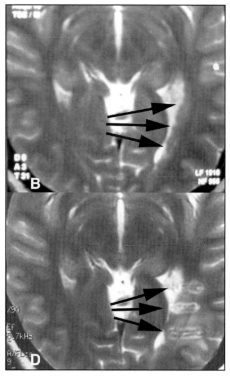

Figure 3. Example of pre- (above) and post- (below) SEEG-guided thermolesions MRI (horizontal slices, T2 sequences). The lesions (arrows, lower picture) were placed in a left periventricular heterotopia (arrows, upper picture).

**Table I. Seizure outcome according to the etiology
of the epilepsy and the localization of the epileptogenic focus**

	Responders (> 50% seizure reduction)	Non-responders (< 50% seizure reduction
Etiologies		
Cortical displasias	12 (1 seizure-free)	7
Heterotopia	3	0
Cryptogenic	4	8
Hippocampal sclerosis	2	4
Post-traumatic	0	1
Localization		
Temporal	12	11
Frontal	3	3
Occipital	3	2
Parietal	1	2
Insula	2	2

In the group of non eligible patients for resective surgery (n = 13), due either to the insular topography of the epileptogenic focus, or to the high probability of a post-surgical visual deficit, or to bilateral epileptic foci, or to an EZ localization inside primary motor zone or language areas, 9 presented with CDM, and 6 of them were responders to SEEG-guided RFTC. One of them was seizure free.

No permanent neurological or cognitive impairment occurred after any of the procedures. Three patients showed transient adverse effects: mouth dysesthesiae during a few days and two months after intra-insular RF thermocoagulation in two patients, motor apraxia in the left hand after RF thermocoagulation within the right supplementary motor area that completely disappeared after six months. In one case, one of the coagulations was interrupted because it produced a slightly painful heat sensation in the ipsilateral side of the head. This sensation disappeared immediately after cessation of the radiofrequency current. In this particular case, the coagulation site was located in the temporo-mesial area, very close to the choroidal fissure.

■ Discussion

Multiple SEEG-guided RF thermocoagulation finally provides a therapeutic capability to a technique (*i.e.* SEEG) previously devoted to a diagnostic purpose only.

As a matter of fact, the use of SEEG electrodes for performing multiple RF-thermolesions appears to provide a unique opportunity to have large access to the epileptogenic network without additional risk from the implantation of lesioning electrodes.

Whenever it is feasible, lobectomy, cortectomy, or hemispherotomy, based on precise localization of the EZ remains the most efficient treatment of partial drug-refractory epilepsies (Clusmann, 2002; Kumlien, 2002; Schramm, 2002). Some palliative procedures, such as multiple subpial trans-sections, callosotomy, or vagus nerve stimulation, can be efficient to decrease, sometimes strongly, seizure frequency. Based on this principle, SEEG-guided RF thermocoagulation is a technique, which aims at causing a partial damage of the EZ, as tailored in each individual patient by the SEEG exploration.

Complications are minor, rare and reversible in all cases. No long-term side effects, particularly on cognitive function, are observed. The fact that RF thermocoagulation is guided by SEEG recordings and carried out only in cortical sites where focal stimulation did not elicit any clinical response probably accounts for the small number, and complete reversibility, of post RF thermocoagulation focal deficits. Thus it is possible to treat targets located very near to cortical areas with high functional value (language or primary visual zone), or poorly accessible to conventional surgical procedure (insular cortex).

The benefit-risk ratio of the SEEG-guided RF thermocoagulation procedure proves particularly favourable for the patients in whom surgery is not feasible or risky. Such was the case for 13 of our 41 patients, of whom seven benefited from RF thermocoagulation with a reduction of 50% or more in seizure frequency in six cases and a complete seizures control in one. In these cases, SEEG-guided RF thermocoagulation proved to be a safe therapeutic option, the results of which compare favourably to those of other palliative therapeutic procedures such as vagus nerve stimulation, multiple subpial transection, callosotomy, or deep intracerebral stimulations (Clusmann, 2002).

Conversely RF thermocoagulation's results in patients eligible for cortectomy proves inferior to those of surgery. Indeed, 21 of our 28 patients went through conventional surgery in a second step, of whom 19 are in Engel's class I and four are awaiting surgery. These results show that the SEEG-guided RF thermocoagulation procedure is not an alternative to resection surgery and incited us to stop proposing RF thermocoagulation to patients eligible to conventional surgery, and especially to patients eligible for temporo-mesial resection, which bears the best surgical prognosis (Sindou, 2006; Wiebe, 2001). This can partially be explained by the relatively small size of the thermocoagulation lesions, as compared to the extent of the epileptogenic area.

The best results of RF thermocoagulation are observed in epilepsies symptomatic of cortical development malformations that are not accessible to surgery. Indeed, a seizure frequency reduction over 50% is noted in 67% of patients suffering from epilepsy symptomatic of dysplasia or heterotopia, of whom one remains seizure free with a follow-up of 40 months. Thus, the favourable outcomes that we observe cannot be explained by a complete lesion of the epileptogenic area, as assumed after surgical cortectomy. SEEG-guided RF-thermocoagulations, when efficient, may instead cause a partial volume reduction of the epileptogenic cortex and disturb its synaptic circuitry and electrophysiological organization, sufficiently to stop, or to reduce, the occurrence of seizures.

■ Conclusion

Despite its limits, the SEEG-guided RF-thermolesion procedure we describe here appears to be feasable, reliable, well-tolerated, and safe. Its risk-benefit ratio remains favorable, so that we advocate it as a first step, even if a standard curative surgery is needed in a second step. Our experience suggests that SEEG-guided RF thermocoagulation should be dedicated to drug-resistant epileptic patients for whom conventional resection surgery is risky or contra-indicated on the basis of invasive pre-surgical evaluation, particularly those suffering from epilepsy symptomatic of cortical development malformation. Knowing the excellent congruence between the completeness of the lesion resection and the favourable evolution of the epileptic disease in cortical development malformations, we now tend, for such patients, to increase the number of electrodes implanted in the lesion itself in order to produce the greatest possible number of thermo-lesions inside the malformation.

References

- Anderson R. Psychological differences after amygdalotomy. *Acta Neurol Scand* 1970; 46 (Suppl 43): 94.
- Balasubramanian V, Kanaka TS. Stereotactic surgery of the limbic system in epilepsy. *Acta Neurochir* 1976; 23: 225-34.
- Behrens E, Zentner J, Van Roost D, Hufnagel A, Elger CE, Schramm J. Subdural and depth electrodes in the presurgical evaluation of epilepsy. *Acta Neurochir* 1994; 128: 84-7.
- Bien CG, Kurthen M, Baron K, Lux S, Helmstaedter C, Schramm J, Elger CE. Long-term seizure outcome and antiepileptic drug treatment in surgically treated temporal lobe epilepsy patients: a controlled study. *Epilepsia* 2001; 42: 1416-21.
- Binnie CD, Elwes RDC, Polkey CE, Volans A. Utility of stereoelectroencephalography in preoperative assessment of temporal lobe epilepsy. *J Neurol Neurosurg Psychiatry* 1994; 57: 58-65.
- Blume WT, Parrent AG, Kaibara M. Stereotactic amygdalohippocampotomy and medial temporal spikes. *Epilepsia* 1997; 38: 930-6.
- Bohbot VD, Allen JJ, Nadel L. Memory deficits characterized by patterns of lesions to the hippocampus and parahippocampal cortex. *Ann NY Acad Sci* 2000; 911: 355-68.
- Bohbot VD, Kalina M, Stepankova K, Spackova N, Petrides M, Nadel L. Spatial memory deficits in patients with lesions to the right hippocampus and to the right parahippocampal cortex. *Neuropsychologia* 1998; 36 (11): 1217-38.
- Bouchard G. Basic targets and the different epilepsies. *Acta Neurochir* 1976; 23: 193-9.
- Bouvier G, Saint-Hilaire JM, Maltais R, Belique R, Desrochers P. Stereotactic lesions in primary epilepsy of the limbic system. *Acta Neurochir* 1980; 30: 151-9.
- Catenoix H, Mauguiere F, Guenot M, Ryvlin P, Bissery Y, Sindou M, Isnard J. SEEG-guided thermocoagulations: a palliative treatment of nonoperable partial epilepsies. *Neurology* 2008; 71 (21): 1719-26.
- Ciganek L, Sramka S, Nadvornik P, Fritz G. Effects of stereotactic operations in the treatment of epilepsies, neurological aspects. *Acta Neurochir* 1976; 23: 201-4.
- Cossu M, Cardinale F, Castana L, Citterio A, Francione S, Tassi L, *et al.* Stereoelectroencephalography in the presurgical evaluation of focal epilepsy: a retrospective analysis of 215 procedures. *Neurosurgery* 2005; 57: 706-18.
- Crow HJ, Cooper R. Stimulation, polarization and coagulation using intracerebral implanted electrodes during the investigation and treatment of psychiatric and other disorders. *Med Prog Technol* 1972; 1 (2): 92-102.
- Clusmann H, Schramm J, Kral T, Hemstaedter C, Ostertun B, Fimner R, Haun D, Elger CE. Prognostic factors and outcome after different types of resection for temporal lobe epilepsy. *J Neurosurg* 2002; 97: 1131-41.
- Exley KA, Parsonage MJ, Wall AL. Electrocoagulation of the amygdalae in an epileptic patient. *Electrencephalogr Clin Neurophysiol* 1967; 43 (Suppl) 31: 172.
- Flanigin HF, Nashold BS. Stereotactic lesions of the amygdala and hippocampus in epilepsy. *Acta Neurochir* 1976; 23: 235-9.
- Guenot M, Isnard J. Multiple SEEG-guided RF-thermocoagulesions of epileptic foci. *Neurochirurgie* 2008; 54 (3): 441-7.
- Guenot M, Isnard J, Ryvlin P, Fischer C, Mauguiere F, SindouM. SEEG-guided RF-thermocoagulation of epileptic foci: feasibility, safety, and preliminary results. *Epilepsia* 2004; 45 (11): 1368-74.
- Guenot M, Isnard J, Ryvlin P, Fischer C, Ostrowsky K, Mauguiere F, Sindou M. Neurophysiological monitoring for epilepsy surgery: the Talairach SEEG method. *Stereotact Funct Neurosurg* 2002; 73: 84-7.

- Heimburger RF,Whitlock CC, Kalsbeck JE. Stereotactic amygdalotomy for epilepsy with agressive behavior. JAMA 1966; 198: 741-5.
- Heimburger RF, Small IF, Milstein V, Moore D. Stereotactic amygdalotomy for convulsive and behavioral disorders. Appl Neurophysiol 1978; 41: 43-51.
- Hood TW, Siegfried J, Wieser HG. The role of stereotactic amygdalotomy in the treatment of temporal lobe epilepsy associated with behavioral disorders. Appl Neurophysiol 1983; 46: 19-25.
- Hullay J, Gombi R, Velok G. Surgical and stereotactic attempts in intractable epilepsy. Acta Med Acad Sci Hung 1976; 33 (2): 119-24.
- Kumlien E, Doss RC, Gates JR. Treatment outcome in patients with mesial temporal sclerosis. Seizure 2002; 11: 413-7.
- Marossero F, Ravagnati L, Sironi VA, Miserocchi G, Franzini A, Entorre G, Cabrini GP. Late results of stereotactic radiofrequency lesions in epilepsy. Acta Neurochir 1980; 30: 145-9.
- Mempel E, Witkiewicz B, Stadnicki R. The effect of medial amygdalotomy and anterior hippocampotomy on behavior and seizures in epileptic patients. Acta Neurochir 1980; 30: 161-7.
- Munari C, Hoffman D, Francione S, Kahane P, Tassi L, Lo Russo G, Benabid AL. Stereoelectroencephalography methodology: advantages and limits. Acta Neurol Scand 1994; (Suppl 152): 56-67.
- Nadvornik P, Sramka M. Anatomical considerations for the stereotaxic longitudinal hippocampectomy. Confin Neurol 1975; 36: 177-81.
- Nadvornik P, Sramka M, Gajdosova D. Critical remarks on the stereotaxic treatment of epilepsy. J Neurosurg Sci 1974; 18: 133-5.
- Narabayashi H. From experiences of medial amygdalotomy on epileptics. Acta Neurochir 1980; 132 (suppl 30): 75-81.
- Ojeman GA, Ward AA. Stereotactic and other procedures for epilepsy. Adv Neurol 1975; 8: 241-63.
- Parrent AG. Stereotactic radiofrequency ablation for the treatment of gelastic seizures associated with hypothalamic hamartoma. Case report. J Neurosurg 1999; 91 (1): 881-4.
- Parrent AG, Blume WT. Stereotactic amygdalohippocampotomy for the treatment of medial temporal lobe epilepsy. Epilepsia 1999; 40 (10): 1408-16.
- Parrent AG, Lozano AM. Stereotactic surgery for temporal lobe epilepsy. Can J Neurol Sci 2000; 27 (1): 79-84.
- Patil AA, Andrews R, Torkelson R. Stereotactic volumetric radiofrequency lesioning of intracranial structures for control of intractable seizures. Stereotact Funct Neurosurg 1995a; 64 (3): 123-33.
- Patil AA, Andrews R, Torkelson R. Minimally invasive surgical approach for intractable seizures. Stereotact Funct Neurosurg 1995b; 65: 86-9.
- Polkey CE. Alternative surgical procedures to help drug-resistant epilepsy, a review. Epileptic Disord 2003; 5: 63-75.
- Schaltenbrand G, Spuler H, Nadjmi M, Hopf HC, Wahren W. The stereotactic treatment of symptomatic epilepsy. Munch Med Wochenschr 1966; 108 (35): 1707-11.
- Schwab RS, Sweet WH, Mark VH, Kjellberg RN, Ervin FR. Treatment of intractable temporal lobe epilepsy by stereotactic amygdala lesions. Trans Am Neurol Assoc 1965; 90: 12-9.
- Schramm J, Kral T, Kurthen M, Blumcke I. Surgery to treat focal frontal lobe epilepsy in adults. Neurosurgery 2002; 51: 644-54.
- Schumann G, Nadvornik P, Schroder T. Results of stereotactic treatment of drug-resistant epilepsy. Psychiatr Neurol Med Psychol 1987; 39: 38-43.
- Sindou M, Guenot M, Isnard J, Ryvlin P, Fischer C, Mauguiere F. Temporo-mesial epilepsy surgery: outcome and complications in 100 consecutive adult patients. Acta Neurochir 2006; 148 (1): 39-45.

- Small IF, Heimburger RF, Small JG, Milstein V, Moore DF. Follow-up of stereotaxic amygdalotomy for seizure and behavior disorders. *Biol Psychiatry* 1977; 12 (3): 401-11.
- Talairach J, Bancaud J. Stereotactic approach to epilepsy. Methodology of anatomo-functional stereotactic investigations. *Prog Neurol Surg* 1973; 5: 297-354.
- Vaernet K. Stereotactic amygdalotomy in temporal lobe epilepsy. *Confin Neurol* 1972; 34: 176-80.
- Wiebe S, Blume WT, Girvin JP, Eliasziw M. A randomized, controlled trial of surgery for temporal lobe epilepsy. *N Eng J Med* 2001; 345: 311-8.

Seizure outcome in extratemporal lobe epilepsies

Américo C. Sakamoto[1], Eliana Garzon[2]

*[1] Department of Neurosciences and Behavioral Sciences, Ribeirão
Preto School of Medicine, University of São Paulo, Brazil; Director,
Epilepsy Surgery Center
University Hospital, Ribeirão Preto School of Medicine, University
of São Paulo, Brazil
[2] Electroencephalography Section, Division of Neurology, University
Hospital, São Paulo School of Medicine, University of São Paulo, Brazil*

▪ Introduction

More than a century ago the so-called modern era of epilepsy surgery was in fact inaugurated by one case of extratemporal surgery performed in England. Despite of this historical landmark epilepsy surgeries since then have been mainly performed in adults with pharmacoresistant temporal lobe epilepsy (TLE). Excepted for the pediatric group extratemporal lobe epilepsy (ETLE) surgeries represent an overwhelming minority of the cases across all centers. In the largest single institution series published so far, encompassing 2,449 resections performed between 1976 and 2006 at the Montreal Neurological Institute, 60.5% of the surgeries were temporal, 16.8% frontal, 3.1% parietal, 1.1% occipital, 3.3% central, and 4.4% multilobar resections (Tanriverdi *et al.*, 2009).

In a large multicenter survey recently performed in France (17 centers) the authors looked at the relationship between age groups and location of the surgeries. When comparing adults and children they reported temporal resections in 72% and 43%, frontal in 12% and 28%, parietal in 2% and 14%, occipital in 2% and 2%, and central in 2% and 11%, respectively (Devaux *et al.*, 2008). Besides being more prevalent, TLE constitutes a more homogeneous group regarding clinical semiology, risk factors, and etiology. Consequently, presurgical evaluation is more straightforward and standardized. In contrast, ETLE is a more heterogeneous group regarding age distribution, clinical semiology, frequency and severity of the seizures, and especially etiological profile, rendering its evaluation much more complex, more tailored to individual cases, and sometimes controversial. Moreover, there is no consensus on how to approach these ETLE patients, in terms of the presurgical evaluation, indications and strategies of invasive procedures, and surgical approaches.

Extratemporal resections for surgical treatment of medically intractable epilepsies, although less frequently performed, are unequivocally effective for the treatment of carefully evaluated and properly selected cases. Overtime epilepsy surgery centers are progressively targeting an increasing number of extratemporal cases, especially in the pediatric population, most likely due to improvements in diagnostic methodologies, especially modern imaging technologies that are now able to detect even very subtle cortical lesions. Between all distinct factors that characterize the extratemporal epilepsies the etiological profile and the localization of the epileptogenic lesions are more relevant for the definition of the diagnostic and surgical strategies, and more determinant for the outcome results. Contrarily to hippocampal sclerosis which is a localized and well-defined lesion, easily detected by MRI, the two most important etiologies of extratemporal epilepsies, namely, cortical dysplasia and gliosis, are poorly defined and imprecisely delimited epileptogenic lesions, frequently distributing over more than one lobe and often overlapping to eloquent cortex. These distinct critical issues affect surgical planning and treatment, and not infrequently prompt the discussion on how far and complete should be the resection, how much deficit is acceptable, cost-benefit considerations of the procedures, etc., and obviously all these aspects affect the post-surgical outcome.

There are many reports in the literature addressing the post-surgical outcome of extratemporal surgeries. However, most of them are cross-sectional studies and frequently involve small number of patients. Larger studies frequently include patients operated on through decades, many of them selected before the advent of modern diagnostic methodologies. In a recently published meta-analysis the authors reported that the post-surgical seizure-free status was observed in 34% of the non-lesional, and 66% of the lesional extratemporal epilepsies. Regarding the age distribution, 46% of the children became seizure-free in the non-lesional, and 73% in the lesional group while in adults 36% in the non-lesional and 72% in the lesional group reached seizure-free status. Overall, the odds of being seizure-free were 2.5 times higher in those who had a lesion on MRI or histopathology (Téllez-Zenteno et al., 2010). In order to analyze the post-surgical seizure outcome in ETLE, in this chapter we will restrict the analysis to the most recent series, comprising large group of patients exclusively investigated according to current diagnostic methodologies, and applying modern statistical models such as multivariate and logistic regression analysis targeting specifically the search for independent predictors of seizure outcome. We prioritized studies focused on pure culture of frontal, parietal and occipital lobe epilepsies, but we also considered reports analyzing together all posterior cortex epilepsies as an individualized group of patients.

■ Frontal lobe epilepsy

Although largely surpassed by temporal lobe resections, frontal lobe epilepsy surgeries are the most frequent type of extratemporal surgeries and consequently, the second most common type of epilepsy surgery. Post-surgical seizure outcome is consensually considered poorer than that observed for temporal lobe surgeries, but the vast majority of previous reports are cross-sectional studies and only included limited number of patients. There are very few series involving large number of patients who were evaluated according to current diagnostic standards and analyzed with utilization of modern statistical methods, including multivariate and logistic regression analysis (see *Table I*).

One of the first studies with significant number of patients evaluated and analyzed according to contemporary approaches was reported by Mosewich et al. (2000). They analyzed 68 patients with FLE operated between 1987 and 1994, and followed-up for 48.7 months (mean). Engel Class I outcome was observed in 58.8% of their patients and only two presurgical variables were predictive of good outcome: absence of history of febrile seizures, and presence of MRI lesion. The only post-surgical variable predictive of outcome was

Table I. Summarized data of most recent and large reports on post-surgical outcome of extratemporal epilepsies

Authors	Lobe	Years	N of patients	Engel Class I	Follow-up	Pre-op predictors	Post-op predictors
Schramm et al., 2002	Frontal lobe epilepsy	1989-1999	68	54%	28.4 months	Not addressed	Not addressed
Jeha et al., 2007	Frontal lobe epilepsy	1995-2003	70	30.1% (5 yrs)	49.2 months	1. MRI negative for MCD 2. Extrafrontal MRI abnormality 3. Generalized/ non-localized ictal EEG	1. Acute PO sz 2. Incomplete resection
Elsharkawy et al., 2008	Frontal lobe epilepsy	1991-2005	97	47.0% (5yrs)	82.8 months	Focal lesion on MRI	Persistence of aura
Trottier et al., 2008	Frontal lobe epilepsy	1990-2005	96	67.3% (5yrs)	66.0 months	Not addressed	Not addressed
Kim et al., 2004	Parietal lobe epilepsy	1994-2001	38	39.5%	50.7 months	No predictor	Not addressed
Binder et al., 2009	Parietal lobe epilepsy	1990-2004	40	57.5%	45.0 months	None	Not addressed
Lee et al., 2005	Occipital lobe epilepsy	1994-2001	26	61.5%	> 24 months	Not addressed	Not addressed
Binder et al., 2008	Occipital lobe epilepsy	1990-2005	29	72.4%	86.1 months	1.Duration of epilepsy (< 20 yrs) 2. Female sex	Not addressed
Dalmagro et al., 2005	Posterior cortex epilepsies	1994-2003	44	65.1%	39.7 months	Duration of epilepsy Normal neurological status	Not addressed
Yu et al., 2009	Posterior cortex epilepsies	2001-2006	43	60.5%	33.6 months	No predictor	Not addressed
Elsharkawy et al., 2009	Posterior cortex epilepsies	1991-2006	80	52.9% (5 yrs)	87.6 months	Absence of GTC seizure	1. Incomplete resection 2. Interictal discharges on post-op EEG
Jehi et al., 2009	Posterior cortex epilepsies	1994-2006	57	65.8% (2-5 years)	39.6 months	1. Etiology other than tumor or dysplasia 2. Lesionectomy only 3. Ipsilateral temporal spiking on scalp EEG	1. Ipsilateral spiking on post-op EEG

seizure control during the first postoperative year, which predicted the long-term outcome. However, multivariate and logistic regression analysis, although planned, was not applied due to the small number of patients with history of febrile seizures.

In another large series also involving 68 adult patients with frontal lobe resections and mean follow-up of 28.4 ± 23.3 months Schramm et al. (2002) reported Engel Class I post-surgical seizure outcome in 54%, Engel Class II in 19%, Engel Class III in 15%, and Engel Class IV in 12% of the patients. In a more recent longitudinal study Jeha et al. (2007) analyzed a group of 70 patients with drug-resistant frontal lobe epilepsy with the specific objectives of defining long-term post-surgical prognostic factors. They reported complete seizure-freedom in 55.7% of the patients at one year follow-up, 45.1% at 3 years follow-up, and 30.1% at 5 years follow-up. Although 80% of seizure recurrences had occurred within the first 6 postoperative months, late recurrences also occurred, and outcome results in general were poorer the longer the follow-up period. They encountered the following independent predictors of seizure recurrences: MRI-negative for malformation of cortical development (risk ratio = 2.2), extrafrontal MRI abnormality (risk ratio = 1.75), generalized/non-localized ictal EEG (risk ratio = 1.83), acute postoperative seizure (risk ratio = 2.17), and incomplete resection (risk ratio = 2.56).

In another recent study involving a larger number of patients Trottier et al. (2008) analyzed the longitudinal outcome in a cohort of 96 patients with frontal lobe epilepsy operated between 1990 and 2005, with follow-up ranging from 2 to 17 years, mean of 5 1/2 years. All patients had MRI and stereoelectroencephalography (SEEG) before surgery. Overall Engel Class I outcome was observed in 71% of the patients, being 80% in cases of lesion-related frontal lobe epilepsies, and 45% in patients with no lesion on imaging or neuropathology of the surgical specimen. Engel Class I outcome was observed in 78.4% of the patients at one year follow-up, 67.3% at five years, and in 57.1% at ten years, thus confirming the occurrence of late relapses negatively impacting the long-term outcome. Dysplastic lesions were observed in 44% (42/96) of the patients, Engel Class I was observed in 86%, Class III in 3% and Class IV in 10% of these patients.

In another large study involving 97 consecutive adult patients with pure frontal lobe epilepsy and addressing surgery outcome and prognostic factors Elsharkawy et al. (2008a) Engel Class I in 54.6% at 6 months post-surgery, 49.5% at 2 years, 47% at 5 years, and 41.9% at 10 years. They observed that patients who remained seizure-free at 2 years had 86% probability of seizure-free at 10 years. On univariate analysis presurgical predictive factors of poor outcome were incomplete resection, use of subdural grids, tonic seizures and unspecific aura, while post-surgical predictors were occurrence of aura and presence of interictal discharges in the postoperative EEG. However, on multivariate and logistic regression analysis only the presence of well-circumscribed focal lesion on preoperative MRI and persistent postoperative aura predicted seizure relapse. In a similar study involving 71 patients Lee et al. (2008) came to different conclusions and observed that the only two predictors of post-surgical outcome were the presence of MRI lesion and the and seizure frequency.

There are scarce data in the literature concerning frontal lobe epilepsy surgery in the pediatric and adolescent population and no report covered large number of patients. Kral et al. (2001) reported a series of 32 children and adolescents operated between 1989 and 2000 and observed that 65.6% became seizure-free after a minimal follow-up of 12 months, outcome similar to adult frontal lobe surgeries.

In summary, post-surgical seizure outcome is poorer in frontal lobe epilepsy surgery, and follows the general trend to further deteriorate overtime. When localized lesions are identified, and their complete resection is feasible, outcome figures are much better and closer to the results observed for temporal lobe surgeries. When compared to older series (Rasmussen 1975, Tailarach *et al.* 1992) results have been progressively improving in the last decades, probably as the result of the advances in imaging and electrophysiological methodologies, especially the development of high resolution MRI scans and utilization of sophisticated invasive EEG techniques. Results are improving even when comparing surgical series of a single center in different times (Elsharkawy *et al.*, 2008b).

■ Parietal lobe epilepsy

Parietal lobe epilepsy (PLE) accounts for only a minority of cases within the extratemporal epilepsies. There are very few surgical series addressing exclusively PLE, in fact only two series were published in the last ten years with number of patients superior to thirty cases (Kim *et al.*, 2004; Binder *et al.*, 2009). A larger series was previously reported but included patients collected over many decades, heterogeneously investigated through use of diagnostic methods and approaches that varied overtime, many of them before the introduction of modern imaging techniques (Salanova *et al.*, 1995).

In a series of 38 surgically treated PLE operated on between 1994 and 2001 Kim *et al.* (2004a) reported Engel Class I in 39.5%, Engel Class II in 13.2%, Engel Class III in 34.2%, and Engel Class IV in 13.2% of their patients. Most of them were invasively evaluated (37/38), and cortical dysplasia was the etiology in the overwhelming majority of the cases (94.3%). Most of their patients (22/38), however, had resection of parts of other lobes in addition to the parietal lobe. The same center published a smaller series of 27 surgical cases and reported that the presence of localized MRI lesions was the only predictor of post-surgical seizure outcome (Kim *et al.*, 2004b).

More recently Binder *et al.* (2009) reported a series of 40 patients with PLE operated on between 1990 and 2004. After a mean follow-up of 45 months post-surgical seizure outcome was classified in Engel Class I in 57.5%, Engel Class II in 10%, Engel Class III in 27.5%, and Engel Class IV in 5% of the patients. The main etiologies were low-grade tumors (16 patients), cortical dysplasias (11 patients), gliotic scars (9 patients), cavernous vascular malformations (2 patients), granulomatous inflammation (1 patient), no histopathological diagnosis (1 patient). In order to search for independent predictors of seizure outcome a backward stepwise logistic regression was performed and demonstrated no predictors (see *Table I*).

■ Occipital lobe epilepsy

Occipital lobe surgeries encompass a small group of epilepsy surgeries. There is no large contemporary series on pure occipital lobe epilepsy (OLE) surgery. The largest one was reported by Salanova *et al.* (1992) involving 42 patients operated on between 1930 and 1991 at the Montreal Neurological Institute, but most patients were operated before modern imaging methodologies became available.

Recently Lee *et al.* (2005) reported on 26 cases of OLE followed-up for at least 24 months. They obtained post-surgical seizure-free status in 61.5% of their patients but did not address the question of the existence of independent predictors of post-surgical seizure outcome.

More recently Binder *et al.* (2008) reported on 52 patients with predominant occipital lobe resections but divided in two groups: pure occipital lobe epilepsies (29 patients, 9.9% of their total extratemporal cases) and extended occipital lobe epilepsies (23 patients). In the pure OLE the main etiologies were gliosis (9 cases, 31%), tumor (8 cases, 27.5%), vascular malformation (7 cases, 24.1%) and dysplasia (5 cases, 17.2%). After a mean follow-up of 86.1 months they observed Engel Class I outcome in 21 patients (72.4%), Engel Class II in 2 patients (6.9%), Engel Class III in 3 patients (10.3%), and Engel Class IV in another 3 patients (10.3%). After logistic regression analysis the only variables that remained as independent predictors of good outcome when comparing favorable (Engel I/II) and unfavorable (Engel III/IV) were early onset of seizures and shorter epilepsy duration, but when comparing seizure-free and not seizure-free groups only shorter epilepsy duration and female sex appeared as independent predictors (see *Table I*).

■ Posterior cortex epilepsies

Due to difficulties in defining precise boundaries for the temporo-parieto-occipital region, and due to the fact that epileptogenic lesions in this area frequently involves more than one lobe, epilepsies affecting these structures are frequently grouped together under the denomination of posterior cortex epilepsies.

In a previous study at our center we specifically target the search for predictors of post-surgical seizure outcome in posterior cortex epilepsies (Dalmagro *et al.*, 2005). Out of 1,537 patients included in our database we selected a group of 81 consecutive cases with posterior cortex epilepsies (PCE) (5.3% of the patients), 44 of them were treated surgically, and 37 only medically. Although this was not a randomized study surgical treatment emerged as highly efficient when compared to pharmacological treatment alone. Somewhat distinct from other series in the literature, gliosis and malformations of cortical development were the main etiologies (34.6% and 33.3%, respectively), while tumor accounted for only 8.6% of the cases. In the surgical group complete seizure control (Engel Class I) was obtained in 65.1% of the patients and the independent predictors of good outcome were shorter duration of epilepsy and absence of neurological abnormalities on clinical examination.

A recent longitudinal study addressing the long-term post-surgical seizure outcome and its predictors has been published (Jehi *et al.*, 2009), involving 57 patients. Resections were performed in the parietal lobe (32 patients, 56.1%), occipital (9 patients, 15.8%), and parietooccipital region (16 patients, 28.1%). The main etiologies were tumor (22 cases, 39%) and malformation of cortical development (19 cases, 34%), and the main surgical approaches were lesionectomies (27 cases, 48%), lobectomies (19 cases, 33%) and multilobar resections (11 cases, 19%). The post-surgical seizure outcome at last follow-up, after mean follow-up of 39.6 months, were 65.8% seizure-free at one year follow-up, 65.8% between 2 and 5 years, and 54.8% beyond 6 years of follow-up. Most recurrences (75%) occurred within the first 6 postoperative months. Independent predictors of seizure outcome on multivariate analysis were etiology other than tumor or dysplasias (risk ratio = 2.29), limiting resection to lesionectomy (risk ratio = 2.06), ipsilateral temporal spiking on pre-op scalp EEG (risk ratio = 2.06), and spiking on postoperative EEG (risk ratio = 2.7).

Approximately at the same time Elsharkawy *et al.* (2009) reported their experience in 80 consecutive adult patients with lesional posterior cortex epilepsies. Engel Class I outcome in their series was 66.3% at 6 months, 52.5% at 2 years, 52.9% at 5 years, and 47.1% at 10 years of post-surgical follow-up. Many variables were predictors of poor outcome in univariate analysis including presence of somatosensory aura, history of generalized tonic-clonic seizure, extraregional spikes, incomplete resection, interictal discharges in the post-op EEGs, incomplete resection and presence of focal cortical dysplasia. Others variables were predictors of good outcome including childhood onset epilepsy, short epilepsy duration, ipsilateral spikes, visual aura, presence of well-circumscribed MRI lesion. However, on multivariate analysis only absence of generalized tonic-clonic seizures was predictor of good outcome, and incomplete resection (post-op MRI) and presence of interictal discharges at 6 months post-op EEG were predictors of poor outcome in the short-term and long-term, respectively.

In another recent study Yu *et al.* (2009) reported post-surgical outcome on 43 patients with posterior cortex epilepsies (11 parietal lobe epilepsies, 13 occipital lobe epilepsies, and 19 parieto-occipital-temporal epilepsies). After a post-op follow-up of 2.8 ± 1.4 years they observed Engel Class I in 60.5%, Engel Class II in 2.3%, Engel Class III in 2.3%, and Engel Class IV in 16.3% of the patients. They found no preoperative predictors of seizure outcome in their sample (see *Table I*).

■ Final remarks

Despite all distinct features involving extratemporal epilepsies that impact presurgical evaluation, surgical strategy and post-surgical seizure outcome, overall results of extratemporal surgeries although poorer than temporal lobe surgeries are still a highly rewarding therapeutic option. Because of the small number of patients operated in most of the epilepsy centers it is difficult to obtain realistic outcome figures and to define independent predictors of seizure outcome. Results are quite variable in the literature, mainly because of selection criteria, variable presurgical strategies regarding utilization of invasive procedures, distinct etiological profile, heterogeneous surgical techniques and variable length of follow-up. Nevertheless, when we restrict the analysis to large and recent series including only patients evaluated through utilization of modern diagnostic methodologies, and properly analyzed from the statistical standpoint (see *Table I*), we can observe that seizure-free status can be obtained in 30.1 to 67.3% of frontal lobe surgeries, in 39.5 to 57.5% of parietal lobe surgeries, in 61.5 to 72.4% of occipital lobe surgeries, and in 52.9 to 65.8% of posterior cortex surgeries. More importantly, there are clear indications that these figures are progressively improving over the last decades, reinforcing the view that epilepsy surgery is an established therapeutic option for the treatment of pharmacoresistant extratemporal epilepsies.

References

- Binder DK, Podlogar M, Clusmann H, Bien C, Urbach H, Schramm J, Kral T. Surgical treatment of parietal lobe epilepsy. *J Neurosurg* 2009; 110 (6): 1170-8.
- Binder DK, von Lehe M, Kral T, Bien CG, Urbach H, Schramm J, Clussmann H. Surgical treatment of occipital lobe epilepsy. *J Neurosurg* 2008; 109: 57-69.

- Dalmagro CL, Bianchin MM, Velasco TR, Alexandre Jr. V, Walz R, Terra-Bustamante VC, *et al*. Clinical features of patients with posterior cortex epilepsies and predictors of seizure outcome. *Epilepsia* 2005; 46: 1442-9.
- Devaux B, Chassoux F, Guenot M, Haegelen C, Bartolomei F, Rougier A, *et al*. La chirurgie de l'épilepsie en France. Évaluation de l'activité. *Neurochirurgie* 2008; 54: 453-65.
- Elsharkawy AE, Alabbasi AH, Pannek H, Schulz R, Hoppe M, Pahs G, *et al*. Outcome of frontal lobe epilepsy surgery in adults. *Epilepsy Res* 2008a; 81: 97-106.
- Elsharkawy AE, El-Ghandour NMF, Oppel F, Pannek H, Schulz R, Hoppe M, *et al*. Long-term outcome of lesional posterior cortical epilepsy surgery. *J Neurol Neurosurg Psychiatry* 2009; 80: 773-80.
- Elsharkawy AE, Pannek H, Schulz R, Hoppe M, Pahs G, Gyimesi C, *et al*. Outcome of extra-temporal epilepsy surgery experience of a single center. *Neurosurgery* 2008b; 63: 516-25.
- Jeha LE, Najm I, Bingaman W, Dinner D, Widdess-Walsh P, Lüders H. Surgical outcome and prognostic factors of frontal lobe epilepsy surgery. *Brain* 2007; 130: 574-84.
- Kim CH, Chung CK, Lee SK, Lee YK, Chi JG. Parietal lobe epilepsy: surgical treatment and outcome. *Stereotact Func Neurosurg* 2004; 82: 175-85.
- Kim DK, Lee SK, Chang-Ho Y, Kwang-Li K, Lee DS, Chun-Kee C, Kee-Hyun C. Parietal lobe epilepsy: the semiology, yield of diagnostic workup, and surgical outcome. *Epilepsia* 2004; 45: 641-9.
- Kral T, Kuczaty S, Blümcke I, Urbach H, Clusmann H, Wiestler OD, *et al*. Postsurgical outcome of children and adolescents with medically refractory frontal lobe epilepsies. *Childs Nerv Syst* 2001; 17: 595-601.
- Lee JJ, Lee SK, Lee SY, Park KI, Kim DW, Lee DS, *et al*. Frontal lobe epilepsy: clinical charac-teristics, surgical outcomes and diagnostic modalities. *Seizure* 2008; 17: 514-23.
- Mosewich RK, So EL, OʹBrien TJ, Cascino GD, Sharbrough FW, Marsh WR, *et al*. Factors predictive of the outcome of frontal lobe epilepsy surgery. *Epilepsia* 2000; 41: 843-9.
- Rasmussen T. Surgery of frontal lobe epilepsy. *Adv Neurol* 1975; 8: 197-205.
- Salanova V, Andermann F, Olivier A, Rasmussen T, Quesney LF. Occipital lobe epilepsy: elec-troclinical manifestations, electrocorticography, cortical stimulation and outcome in 42 patients treated between 1930 and 1991. Surgery of occipital lobe epilepsy. *Brain* 1992; 115: 1655-80.
- Salanova V, Andermann F, Rasmussen T, Olivier A, Quesney LF. Parietal lobe epilepsy. Clinical manifestations and outcome in 82 patients treated surgically between 1929 and 1988. *Brain* 1995; 118 (Pt 3): 607-27.
- Schramm J, Kral T, Kurthen M, Blümcke I. Surgery to treat focal frontal lobe epilepsy in adults. *Neurosurgery* 2002; 51: 644-54.
- Tailarach J, Bancaud J, Szikla G, Bonis A, Geier S, Trottier S, *et al*. Surgical therapy for frontal epilepsies. *Adv Neurol* 1992; 57: 707-32.
- Tanriverdi T, Ajlan A, Poulin N, Olivier A. Morbidity in epilepsy surgery: an experience based on 2449 epilepsy surgery procedures from a single institution. *J Neurosurg* 2009; 110: 1111-23.
- Trottier S, Landré E, Biraben A, Chassoux F, Pasnicu A, Scarabin J-M, Turak B, Devaux B. Quelles strategies pour quels résultats dans la chirurgie des épilepsies partielles frontales? *Neuro-chirurgie* 2008; 54: 388-98.
- Yu T, Wang Y, Zhang G, Cai L, Du W, Li Y. Posterior cortex epilepsy: diagnostic considerations and surgical outcome. *Seizure* 2009; 18: 288-92.

Neuropsychological outcome
of extratemporal lobe epilepsy surgery

Philip S. Fastenau

*Department of Neurology, Case Western Reserve University School of
Medicine, University Hospitals Case Medical Center, Cleveland, USA*

■ Introduction

Neuropsychology has played an integral role in epilepsy surgery since the 1950s (see Dodrill
& Matthews, 1992; Helmstaedter, 2004; Loring, 2010a). Presurgical evaluations have assis-
ted with localization of the focus (especially in the era predating current technologies),
quantification of functional disruption, exploration of patient expectations and capacity
to consent or complete complex procedures, assessment of psychosocial comorbidities that
could complicate other procedures and outcomes, and identification of risk factors for
adverse outcomes following surgery. Postsurgical evaluation has been especially beneficial
for identifying post-surgical changes that warrant rehabilitation and treatment and to
coordinate services for return to school or transition to employment. Beyond the individual patient level, neuropsychological assessment also plays a critical role in outcomes
research, quantifying cognitive changes associated with different procedures and epileptogenic sites and identifying retrospectively risk factors to guide future interventions and
to better inform patients of the risks during presurgical counseling. Neuropsychological
outcomes following temporal lobe epilepsy surgery have received a great deal of attention
in the literature. Surgical therapies for extratemporal lobe epilepsies (ETLE) have received
considerably less attention, especially with regard to neuropsychological outcomes. The
surgical techniques and seizure outcomes have been described in detail throughout this
volume. This chapter will selectively review the neuropsychological outcomes research on
various surgical therapies for ETLE and conclude with a critical analysis of the state of
our outcomes research with these therapies.

■ Callosotomy

In what appears to be the largest published series from a single site, Tanriverdi and colleagues (2009) recently conducted a retrospective review of 95 patients undergoing corpus
callosotomy to evaluate postsurgical cognitive outcomes. The sample consisted of 95 individuals with age of onset between 6 months and 31 years (M = 4.6 years) and surgery

between age 3 and 60 years (M = 24 years). Most of the patients were developmentally delayed (12 profound, 35 moderate-severe, 28 mild-borderline, 20 IQ in the normal range). The patients were followed annually for 5 to 25 years (M = 17.2 years). As depicted in *Figure 1*, IQs were stable following surgery at the group level.

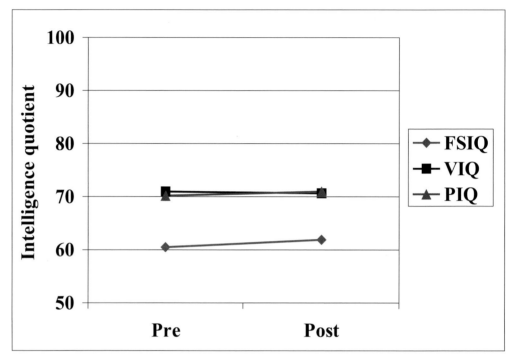

Figure 1. Change in Full Scale IQ (FSIQ), verbal IQ (VIQ), and Performance IQ (PIQ) Scores before and after surgery in 95 patients undergoing corpus callosotomy at Montreal Neurological Institute (based on data reported by Tanri-verdi *et al.*, 2009).

Mamelak and colleagues (1993) slightly expanded the typical IQ outcomes by including two additional neuropsychological measures, confrontational naming (Boston Naming Test) and verbal fluency (Controlled Oral Word Association Test). They evaluated 15 young adults, all of whom had both generalized tonic-clonic and atonic seizures (12 of those also had partial seizures with secondary generalization). Age of seizure onset averaged 6.9 years (SD = 6.6), and the average age at surgery was 22.3 years (SD = 7.1). Of the 15 patients, 5 were left-handed; these 5 and 5 right-handers were shown to have bilateral or right-hemisphere language representation on Wada exam. One patient had a complete callosotomy in a single procedure, 5 had a complete callosotomy after two procedures, and 10 had a single anterior one-half to two-thirds callosotomy. Presurgically, IQs ranged from 45 to 88 for both verbal IQ and performance IQ (M = 64, Mn = 65). At 12 months after surgery, there was minimal change in IQ (M VIQΔ = +0.4, M PIQΔ = +1.2, and all ≤ 7 points). Similarly, confrontational naming and verbal fluency were also stable following surgery. There was no relationship between IQ change and extent of resection, seizure outcome, or mixed/crossed cerebral dominance (*i.e.*, language representation contralateral to manual dominance). Informally, patients with better seizure control post-surgically were reported to have meaningful improvements in attention and behavior.

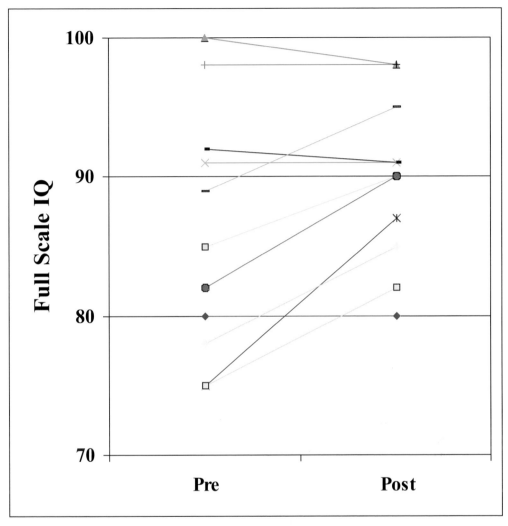

Figure 2. Change in IQ scores pre- to post-callosotomy in adults with normal intellectual development. Each line represents an individual patient (based on Cukiert, Burattini *et al.*, 2009).

In another variant of outcome in these populations, Turanli and colleagues (2006) assessed not only IQ but also other indicators of general cognitive and behavioral improvement a group of 16 children following callosotomy. Age at onset ranged from 2 to 54 months (M = 13.1 months); surgery was conducted between the ages of 2.5 and 15 years of age (M = 7.4 years), with a duration of seizures ranging from 1.5 to 15 years (M = 6.6 years). Most were developmentally delayed (7 severe, 7 mild); one was in the borderline range of intelligence, and one was in the normal range. IQ was described as stable. It should be noted that these children were tested five times within one year (pre-surgically and again 1, 4, 6, and 12 months post-surgically), which could introduce error associated with practice effects masking possible declines; however, given the stability in other samples, these

IQ results are typical. Beyond IQ scores, the investigators reported increased quality of life (as rated by their parents) and increased interest in surroundings; in addition, activities of daily living (self-care, family life, school attendance) improved in 50% of the children.

A series of patients reported by Cukiert, Burattini and colleagues (2009) was unique in that they had higher intellectual functioning. Their series consisted of 11 adults with idiopathic generalized epilepsy (11 generalized tonic-clonic & 10 generalized absence epilepsy). Age at onset ranged from 4 to 8 years old, age at surgery ranged from 21 to 53 years old, with follow-up 2 to 8 years (M = 4) after surgery. Presurgically, IQ ranged from 75 to 100 (M = 85), placing the sample in the lower half of the normal range. Results are depicted in *Figure 2*; 6 improved (not necessarily a reliable change), and 5 remained stable.

Although gross indicators of global cognitive function tend to be stable following callosotomy, neurobehavioral syndromes can emerge. Jea and colleagues (2008) recently summarized these techniques and described in some detail the various disconnection syndromes that can develop postsurgically. *Figure 3* subdivides the commissures into anatomically and behaviorally meaningful segments; *figure 4* lists the syndromes that can emerge and their anatomical correlates. In a separate review, Spencer and Huh (2008) reported that in adults these syndromes are often transient (resolving within 1 month). Persistent syndromes (in up to 17% of patients) are typically mild and unnoticeable; even the "classic disconnection syndrome" develops typically after complete callosotomy and resolves over time. Severe/disabling syndromes (*e.g.*, alien hand) are rare. By their summary, language syndromes are observed most often in individuals with crossed cerebral dominance; informal reports of improvement in attention appear to accompany better seizure control following surgery (Spencer & Huh, 2008).

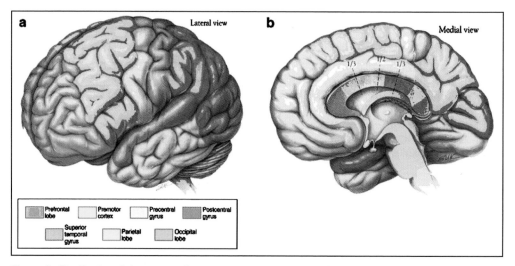

Figure 3. Classification of the corpus callosum into segments corresponding with cortical regions and neurobehavioral syndromes (from Jea et al., 2008).

In summary, individuals undergoing callosotomy typically have severe generalized syndromes with developmental delays, often with early age of onset. IQ is typically stable after surgery (no improvement but no decline), with improved subjective reports of alertness and ratings of adaptive behavior. Adults with normal IQ also show stable global cognitive outcomes. Although global cognitive indices remain stable, disconnection syndromes can result with extensive resection, postpubescent age of resection, and higher intellectual functioning; language syndromes appear to be more likely with cross-dominance.

Timing	Disconnection syndrome	Site of hemispheric disconnection	Site of callosal lesion
Acute	SMA syndrome	Premotor cortex	Unknown
Chronic	Alien hand syndrome	Precentral gyrus	Posterior 1/2
	Dichotic listening suppression	Superior temporal gyrus	Isthmus
	Tactile dysnomia	Postcentral gyrus	Unknown
	Hemispatial neglect	Postcentral gyrus	Unknown
	Nondominant hand agraphia	Parieto-occipital lobe	Splenium
	Alexia without agraphia	Parieto-occipital lobe	Splenium
	Tachistoscopic visual suppression	Occipital lobe	Splenium

Figure 4. Summary of disconnection syndromes and their corresponding anatomical sites (From Jea *et al.*, 2008).

■ Hemispherectomy/hemispherotomy

As is common in callosotomy, measures of cognitive change following hemispherectomy have been limited largely to IQ tests and developmental scales (*e.g.*, see review by Samargia & Kimberley, 2009). This is necessitated in part by the high comorbidity of mental and developmental delays in these populations, as well as the early age of surgery which precludes use of many formal neuropsychological measures that are predicated on skill sets that develop later and for which normative reference values are often unavailable below age 6.

In a recent review, Battaglia and colleagues (2006) noted that developmental delays are common in these populations and concluded that cognitive outcome following hemispherectomy depends on several variables. First, widespread cortical dysplasia (CD) – hemimegalencephaly and hemicortical dysplasia – are associated with persistent severe developmental delays postsurgically, whereas other etiologies such as Sturge-Weber syndrome, Rasmussen encephalitis, and vascular pathology carry a better prognosis. In addition, earlier age of surgery and complete seizure control after hemispherectomy are associated with improvement in cognitive ability. Verbal skills seem to improve more than visual-spatial skills, irrespective of the side of resection; although more complex linguistic deficits can be detected on laboratory measures, the right hemisphere possesses considerable capacity to support most aspects of language required for everyday communication following left hemispherectomy. Few studies have examined memory, attention, and nonlinguistic functions systematically before and after hemispherectomy. Psychosocial functioning and quality of life improve with the degree of seizure control following hemispherectomy.

Battaglia *et al.* (2006) reported on their own series of 19 children who underwent hemispherectomy on average at 2.25 years of age. All children had significant developmental delays and very low IQ presurgically. After surgery, 79% were seizure-free. Most children (*n* = 16) showed stable IQ or developmental quotient (DQ) from pre- to post-surgical testing. One patient with right hemimegalencephaly declined in IQ from 89 to 64 in spite of being seizure-free, whereas two others improved (one with hemispheric CD, IQ 38 to 50; one with Sturge-Weber, IQ 69 to 85), also being seizure-free; all three had onset before 3 months of age.

Two much larger surgical series help to further illustrate the general principles above. In a cohort of 71 patients (Pulsifer *et al.*, 2004), 53 completed both pre- and post-surgical testing. A total of 31 were diagnosed with Rasmussen's (age at onset M = 6.0 years, age at surgery at M = 9.2 years), 7 with vascular etiology (onset M = 2.4 years; surgery M = 6.8 years), and 15 with dysplasia (presumed hemimegalencephaly; onset M = 0.7 years, surgery M = 4.6 years). The dysplasia group had a significantly younger age of onset compared to the other groups, but the three groups did not differ on duration (M = 3.6 years) or on age of follow-up (M = 5.4 years). The dysplasia group had significantly lower IQ presurgically compared to the other two groups; however all groups were stable following hemispherectomy *(Figure 5)*.

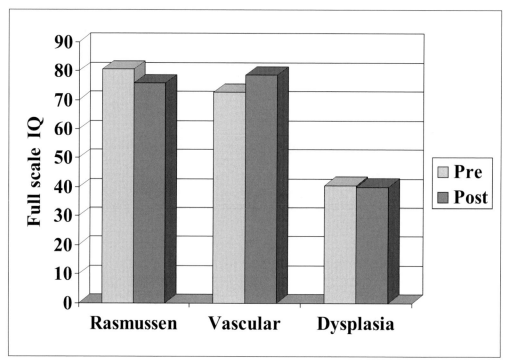

Figure 5. Change in IQ from pre- to post-hemispherectomy, by pathology (based on data presented in Pulsifer et al., 2004).

In a second large surgical series (Jonas *et al.*, 2004), 115 children completed both pre- and post-surgical testing. A total of 21 were diagnosed with Rasmussen's (age at onset M = 4.9 years, age at surgery M = 7.8 years), 27 with vascular etiology (onset M = 1.9 years; surgery M = 8.3 years), 39 with hemispheric CD (onset M = 0.5 years, surgery M = 2.7 years), and 16 with hemimegalencephaly (onset M = 0.1 years, surgery M = 1.5 years). The hemispheric CD and hemimegalencephaly groups both had very early age of onset and shorter duration before going to surgery compared to the other groups. The vascular group had longer duration before going to surgery (M = 6.4 years) compared to the other three groups (Ms ranging 1.4 to 2.9 years). On adaptive behavior, 84% across groups improved after hemispherectomy; the hemispheric CD group improved the most. On expressive language (MacArthur Communicative Development Inventories Spoken Language Rank, "SLR"), which was assessed pre- and post-surgically in only 51% of the patients, the hemispheric CD group improved dramatically; among the hemimegalencephaly patients, the mean SLR score improved, but 66% still had little or no language skills and their motor functioning worsened postsurgically *(Figure 6)*. In the sample as a whole, better adaptive behavior was associated with shorter duration of seizures before surgery and better seizure control after surgery *(Figures 7 and 8)*.

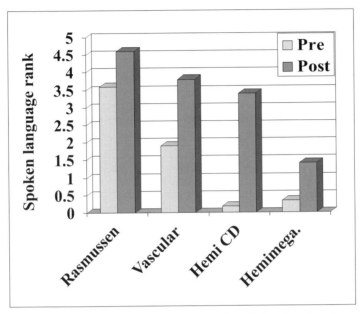

Figure 6. Change in language before and after hemispherectomy, by pathology (based on data presented in Jonas *et al.*, 2004).

Many studies of hemispherectomy outcomes have looked at sensory and/or motor functioning. In a sophisticated study examining sensorimotor outcomes in conjunction with diffuse tensor imaging, the sensorimotor outcomes were shown to improve with earlier age of surgery for the small Rasmussen's subgroup (*n* = 5), which was the only subgroup who had a sufficient range in age of surgery for measuring this relationship (Choi *et al.*, 2010).

Although hemispherectomy has been used almost exclusively in children, one center has examined outcomes in adults. Cukiert, Cukiert and colleagues (2009) recently reported on a series of 14 adults with early middle cerebral artery infarcts and hemiplegia. Age of onset ranged from 2 to 18 months, but none of these individuals underwent surgery until adulthood (ages 19-39 years old). Cognitive assessment followed surgery by 2 to 10 years (M = 5 years). Presurgically, IQ ranged from 60 to 110 (M = 82); post-surgically, all 14 improved or remained stable *(Figure 9)*.

In summary, hemispherectomy has been associated with stable cognitive development in most children. Factors associated with better cognitive outcome include better seizure control, earlier age of surgery, shorter duration of seizures, and lesser extent of the pathological substrate. In addition, certain etiologies carry a better prognosis (Rasmussen's, vascular, hemispheric CD, Sturge-Weber), whereas others carry a worse prognosis (*e.g.*, hemimegalencephaly). Limited data in adults show good cognitive outcomes.

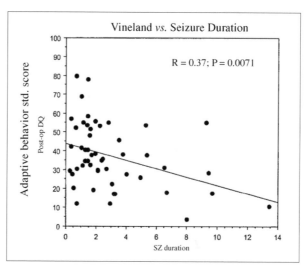

Figure 7. Relationship between duration of seizure disorder and adaptive behavior following hemispherectomy (from Jonas et al., 2004).

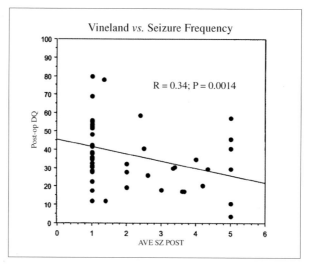

Figure 8. Relationship between seizure frequency and adaptive behavior following hemispherectomy (from Jonas et al., 2004).

■ Focal cortical resection

Mixed samples

Lee and colleagues (2010) reported on a relatively large series of 27 children and adolescents with Lennox-Gastaut syndrome (LGS), of whom 10 had focal unilobar frontal resection; the remainder of children had focal temporal resection ($n = 1$), multilobar resection that included temporal cortex ($n = 6$ frontotemporal, $n = 4$ temporo-occipital), or hemispherectomies ($n = 6$). For the 10 undergoing focal unilobar frontal resection, age of onset ranged from 0 to 12 years (M = 2.26); age at surgery ranged from 1 to 17 years (M = 8.12);

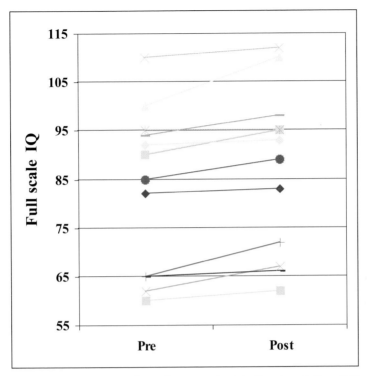

Figure 9. Change in IQ scores pre- to post- hemispherectomy in adults (based on Cukiert, Cukiert *et al.*, 2009).

duration ranged from 1.7 to 11.8 years (M = 5.87). For the total sample, follow-up ranged from 1 to 4 years post-surgery (M = 2.8), but this was not reported individually for each patient or for the frontal subgroup. Of the 10 frontal resection patients, post-surgically 4 achieved Engel Class I status, 2 were Class II and Class III, and 4 were Engel Class IV. Cognitive outcomes were reported only by seizure outcome subgroups for the entire sample (no data for frontal unilobar resections only). Developmental quotient improved for children with Engel Class I outcome only (DQ improving from 42.71 presurgically to 51.93 postsurgically); caregiver ratings also improved, especially for those children with Class I or II outcomes. The severe nature of cognitive delays in this population precluded more detailed neuropsychological assessment.

Van Oijen and colleagues (2006) reported on a series of children treated through the Dutch Collaborative Epilepsy Surgery Program over a 10-year period. Of the 69 children reported, 17 had focal resections (10 frontal, 3 parietal, 2 occipital, 1 hypothalamic, 1 multilobar). Pre- and postoperative IQs were reported for 13 of the children from 6 months to 2 years following surgery. IQ was stable for 9 children and improved for 4 children (for all 13, M IQ was approximately 85 presurgically and 90 postsurgically, based on their graph). This study from a large epilepsy surgery consortium highlights a significant challenge for outcomes research with focal ETLE resection: The number of individuals undergoing focal ETLE resection is very small by comparison to temporal lobe resections, leading investigators to combine the ETLE patients into a single – albeit, heterogeneous – group. Even after combining patients, the sample sizes are typically very small. Associated with this, these studies often use a gross nonspecific measure (IQ) for comparing these small disparate groups such that any specific effects associated with a discrete neural substrate is not reflected on the broad index score. Also common in ETLE focal resection studies, the follow-up period varied considerably across patients, and there was no control group to help correct for changes associated with progression of chronic epilepsy, medication effects, and practice effects.

Another study is commendable for the breadth of assessment across many specific neuropsychological domains. Buschmann and colleagues (2009) assessed attention, processing speed, verbal and nonverbal memory, visual-spatial skills, and executive functioning in a sample of 21 adults (M age 32.3 ± 10.6 years; 17 males, 4 females) undergoing focal ETLE resection (14 frontal, 4 occipital, 3 parietal) with a mean duration of 11.8 years (SD = 11.0). This was a higher functioning group (IQ M = 107.6 ± 16.3). The most frequent etiologies were cavernoma, benign tumors, and CD. The investigators detected no change in neuropsychological functioning after surgery, but this study shared many limitations illustrated by the previous study (e.g., small N, combining patients with heterogeneous foci and etiologies, lack of control group). In addition, there was considerable variability across procedures (18 lesionectomy, 1 complete lesionectomy and multiple subpial transection [MST], 1 incomplete resection, and 1 lobectomy).

In a much more elegant sampling design, Smith and her colleagues (2004) compared 30 surgical patients to 21 medically-refractory non-surgical controls. The two groups were equal to one another with regard to sex (48%-50% female), handedness (86-90% right-handed), IQ (M = 84, range 46-137), and age at testing (range 6-18 years; M = 13.2), with a one-year retest interval for both groups. The surgical group had an older age of onset (M = 6.7, SD = 3.7 years) compared to the control group (M = 5.4 years, SD = 4.7). The investigators assessed IQ, memory, attention, and academic skills, with no differences between groups. Unfortunately, the sample was predominantly temporal lobe epilepsy patients, and the ETLE patients were combined into single group for analysis of neuropsychological outcomes. Also, the nonsurgical control group was more likely to have multilobar or generalized epilepsy (33% vs. 13% in surgical group), and the surgical group was predominantly temporal (60% vs. 24% in control group), which further confounds comparisons between groups, especially on specific cognitive functions.

Posterior resections

In an attempt to focus on a more homogeneous sample, Luerding and colleagues (2004) limited their sample to 28 patients undergoing posterior resections (14 temporo-occipital, 5 occipital, 5 parietal, 2 parieto-occipital, and 2 temporo-parieto-occipital), with 18 in the right hemisphere and 9 on the left. Age ranged 13 to 53 years (M = 27.8). Three had right hemisphere language, and one had bilateral language by Wada exam. Full IQ ranged from 38 to 132 presurgically (M = 85.3). There was no significant change in either Verbal IQ or Performance IQ after right or left resection (Figure 10). Visual field defects were experienced by 50% of the patients after surgery, but this was unrelated to performance on IQ tests. There were no differences detected in either VIQ or PIQ by pre- vs. post-surgery, by side of resection, by seizure control following surgery, or by visual field defects. Other neuropsychological measures that depend on visual-spatial functioning were examined informally (just describing changes in age-corrected scores from pre- to post-surgery); changes were relatively small (difference in z score ranging + 0.2 for the WAIS-R PIQ subtests, Trail Making Part A, and Rey Complex Figure Copy Trial; Trail Making Part B showed a 0.6 increase, which was not meaningful by the author's informal cutoff score of 1.0 SD).

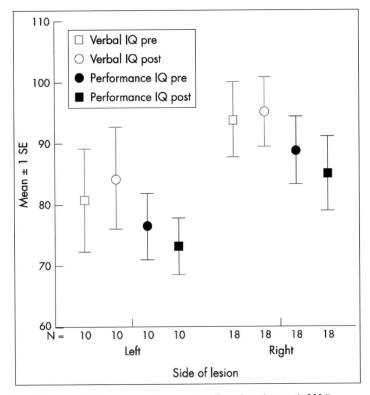

Figure 10. Stabilty of IQ scores following posterior resection (from Luerding *et al.*, 2004)

Lippé and colleagues (2010) published a very small case series (n = 5) but consisting of a homogeneous group of patients undergoing focal parieto-occipital resection (4 left hemisphere, 1 right) for Taylor-type focal CD. Age of onset ranged from birth to 20 months; age at surgery ranged from 0.7 to 7.0 years. The interval to post-surgical testing ranged from 3 to 7 years postsurgery. Four children were seizure-free after surgery (3 off medications, 1 on oxcarbazepine), and one child had "subtle seizures" (on carbamazepine). Only IQ was assessed both pre- and post-surgically for evaluation of actual change and only for 4 of the 5 children, but for those 4 children Performance IQ was very low presurgically and remained low after surgery, whereas Verbal IQ improved 15-20 points following left resection and improved 36 points following right resection *(Figure 11)*. Elaborate visual-spatial testing was conducted with all five patients, but only postsurgically so no baseline was available for comparison. Most of the children showed significant deficits on measures of visual cancellation (four of the five demonstrating hemianopsia or quadranopsia, with a corresponding hemi-inattention pattern on cancellation), visual-spatial perception/construction, and word reading skills *(Figure 12)*; however, it is unclear whether the spatial cognitive deficits were new or worsened following surgery without a baseline, especially given the stable spatial intelligence score (PIQ) from pre- to post-surgery in 4 of the 5 children.

Gleissner and colleagues (2008) reported on a large homogeneous series of patients undergoing unilobar parietal resection (6 left-hemisphere, 9 right-hemisphere) using a neuropsychological battery sampling a variety of specific domains. Age of onset ranged from

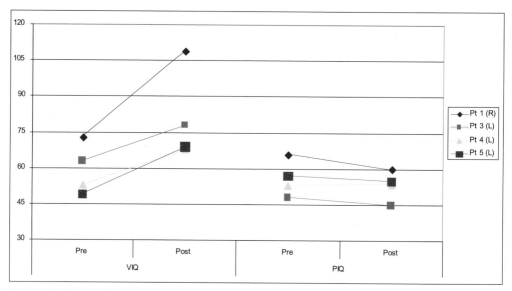

Figure 11. Change in IQ from pre- to post-surgery for focal parieto-occipital resection for Taylor-type focal cortical dysplasia, by patient number (side of resection in parentheses) (based on Lippé et al., 2010).

1 to 12 years (M = 6.1), and age at testing ranged from 6 to 15 years (M = 11.0). IQ ranged from 44 to 112 (M= 80.8; Mn = 82.5); two were left-handed, and two were ambi-dextrous. Etiologies were varied. Children were tested presurgically and one year following surgery. The authors noted that there was not a clear correspondence between left PLE and language and right PLE and spatial memory, but such relationships would not be expected with focal PLE. Postoperatively, one-half of the sample improved on attention measures, and visuospatial-dependent measures were not significantly different after surgery. The authors reported no other change that was statistically or qualitatively significant.

Frontal resections

Lendt and colleagues (2002) compared a small group of children undergoing focal resection for frontal lobe epilepsy (FLE, n = 12) associated with a variety of pathologies to a closely matched control group undergoing resection for temporal lobe epilepsy (TLE, n = 12). In the FLE group, age at surgery ranged from 7 to 15 years (M = 11.0, SD = 3.0), with age of onset between 1 and 12 years (M = 6.3, SD = 3.8); in the TLE group, age at surgery ranged from 8 to 15 years (M = 11.8, SD = 2.5), with age of onset between 1 and 11 years (M = 5.0, SD = 3.8). All children were required to have IQ > 70 (FLE IQ M = 96.8, SD = 9.9; TLE IQ M = 88.3, SD = 7.2); handedness was not reported. Groups were matched on side of surgery (6 L, 6 R), but the nature of surgery varied within and between groups. In the FLE group, 6 had lesionectomy alone, 2 had MST alone, and 4 had a combination; 10 involved the premotor area, and 9 involved the prefrontal area; in addition, 2 involved the precentral gyrus, 2 involved Brodmann area 44, and 1 involved the operculum and insula. In the TLE group, 8 children had selective amygdalohippocampectomy, 3 had two-thirds anterior temporal lobe resection, and only 1 had a pure lesionectomy. Both groups were tested presurgically and at approximately one year following surgery on a broad neuropsychological battery assessing fine motor coordination, attention,

N = 5	Deficits ≤ −1.5 SD	Average ≥ −1 SD
Visual attention		
Visual attention task (NEPSY, Bell test)	1, 2, 4, 5	3
Symptoms of neglect (BEN)		
Extinction	2, 5	1, 3, 4
Line bisection (BEN)	1	2, 3, 4, 5
Visual recognition		
Object recognition	1, 2, 3, 4, 5	
(Jambaqué et Dellatolas)		
Embedded figures (Ghent)	1, 2, 3, 4	5
Gestalt closure (K-ABC)	1, 2, 3, 4	5
Face recognition (Benton)	1, 3, 4, 5	2
Spatial perception and praxies		
Visuospatial orientation	1, 3, 4	2, 5
(Arrows and Benton JLOT)		
Visuoconstructive	1, 3, 4, 5	2
(copy of the Rey complex figure)		
Visuomotor precision (NEPSY)	1, 2, 4, 5	3
Imitation of hand movements (NEPSY)	1, 2, 3, 4, 5	
Reading skills		
Text reading (Lefavrais)[a]	1, 4, 5	2, 3
Word and pseudo-word reading	5	1, 2, 3, 4
(ODEDYS) regular word		
(errors)		
Irregular word (errors)	4, 5	1, 2, 3
Regular word (time)	1, 2, 3, 4, 5	
Irregular word (time)	2, 3, 4, 5	1
Pseudo-word (errors)	4	1, 2, 3, 5
Pseudo-word (time)	1, 2, 4, 5	3
Calculation (Zareki-R)	3	1, 2, 4, 5
number reading		
Counting	3	1, 2, 4, 5
Number writing	3	1, 2, 4, 5
Visual estimation	4	1, 2, 3, 5
Verbal estimation		1, 2, 3, 4, 5

[a]Delay of 2 years.

Figure 12. Spatial functions following focal parieto-occipital resection for Taylor-type focal cortical dysplasia (no presurgical baseline) (from Lippé et al., 2010). Numerals represent individual patients (e.g., Patient 1, Patient 2, etc.).

working memory (*e.g.*, digit span), secondary/long-term memory (word-list learning), language (token test, word fluency, verbal reasoning, object naming), and executive functions (inhibition, fluency, planning). Both groups improved on several measures, including attention, working memory (Corsi Blocks), and verbal learning (auditory-verbal learning test). There was no interaction to suggest differential effects of surgery between groups. Within the FLE group, those who were seizure-free after surgery improved on working memory; even those whose seizures continued after surgery improved on attention and long-term memory measures. With regard to language, two FLE children had resection of

Brodmann area 44 on the left, and both were determined to have bilateral language by Wada; one declined slightly on fluency and receptive language, whereas the other improved on fluency and naming. There were no changes in motor coordination.

Suchy and colleagues (2003) compared patients with FLE (8 L, 14 R) to a group with TLE (81 L, 71 R) before and after surgery on verbal and figural fluency. The four groups did not differ on age (ranging 16 – 55; Ms = 28.9 to 33.1 years; SDs = 8.1 to 10.8), education (minimum 7 years; Ms = 12.1 to 13.1 years; SDs = 2.1 to 2.7), ethnicity (> 86% Caucasian), IQ (minimum 70 required for inclusion; Ms = 87.1 to 95.1; SDs = 9.9 to 13.4), age of onset (Ms = 12.4 to 18.5 years; SDs = 9.9 to 10.5), duration (Ms = 11.1 to 20.5 years; SDs = 5.6 to 11.4), or retest interval (Ms = 14.1 to 17.0 months; SDs = 6.1 to 10.0). All patients were required to be left-hemisphere dominant for speech and language by Wada or presumed left-dominant based on right-handedness and history. After surgery, there was a higher rate of persistent seizures in the FLE groups compared to the TLE groups. FLE patients scored lower than TLE patients both at presurgical evaluation and again postsurgically, with no significant change and with no significant laterality effect for either verbal or figural fluency *(Figure 13)*.

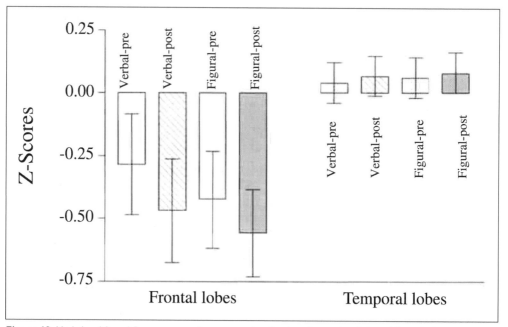

Figure 13. Verbal and figural fluency pre- and post-resection, by site of resection (adapted from Suchy et al., 2003).

These same investigators (Suchy & Chelune, 2001) examined changes in estimated IQ in a very similar but smaller sample, comparing patients undergoing surgery for FLE (15 L, 15 R) to those undergoing surgery for TLE (15 L, 15 R). Groups were matched on age (ages 16-47 years), sex (73%-80% male), and duration (Ms = 11.5 to 16.3 years; SDs = 6.1 to 9.2), as well as presurgical estimated IQ (group Ms ranging 87 – 89 across the 4 groups on a screening comprised of vocabulary and matrix reasoning subtests from the K-BIT). The FLE patients showed no significant change in fluency after surgery, whereas the TLE patients (both L and R) generally improved after surgery.

In a brief review summarizing cognitive correlates of frontal lobe epilepsy, Risse (2006) described two studies that had been reported only as abstracts from conference presentations. Very limited details are presented about these samples, the testing, or the specific analyses and results. The first series consisted of 8 children who had resection of language-dominant frontal cortex; "the most significant cognitive declines were noted on measures of verbal fluency, particularly in children with large resections of prefrontal and orbitofrontal cortex, extending to the midline;" declines in Verbal IQ, visual confrontation naming, and conceptual reasoning also were observed in some children (Risse, 2006, p. 88).

Risse (2006) summarized a second unpublished study comparing 27 children with L FLE to 14 with R FLE. Preoperatively, the two groups did not differ on IQ, phonemic fluency, design fluency, or cognitive flexibility. Postoperatively, the L FLE children scored lower than the R FLE group on phonemic fluency, and there was a trend for the R FLE group to score lower on design fluency. Further analysis by side, site and size of resection reportedly showed patterns that were specific for different cognitive functions. R FLE was associated with broader intellectual deficits (pre- and post-surgery), whereas L FLE tended to be limited to verbal intellectual deficits. Phonemic fluency was associated with lateral and dorsolateral resections but tended to be spared in prefrontal resections. Finally, perseverative responding increased after surgery for children undergoing large R frontal pole and prefrontal resections. From these studies, Risse concluded, "While these numbers are limited, they do suggest that previous failed attempts to define subtle deficits in frontal lobe functioning among patients with epilepsy may, in part, be explained by a lack of appropriately sensitive measures and limited efforts to subdivide frontal patient populations based on lateralization, localization, and size of pathological region. Whether the presence of epileptogenic cortex alone, independent of focal structural lesions from other causes, contributes any unique features to these focal cognitive deficits remains to be determined" (Risse, 2006, p. 89).

In summary, the few outcomes studies of focal resection for ETLE suffer from many different methodological limitations that greatly constrain the conclusions that can be drawn. Small sample sizes raise suspicions of insufficient power when no change is detected. Combined individuals with heterogeneous surgical sites is especially problematic in this realm because different brain regions are associated with widely varying cognitive functions, and gross nonspecific measures (IQ, developmental scales, ratings) are too gross to capture specific changes that could occur with resection of different regions. Even when using specific neuropsychological measures of discrete functions, combining patients with foci in different locations obscures cognitive changes that might be unique to specific neural substrates. Though not specific to focal resection studies, other limitations include wide-ranging follow-up periods (both within studies and across studies), lack of control groups, and lack of alternate forms of testing measures (which is especially critical with shorter follow-ups when there is no control group to correct for practice effects).

■ Multiple subpial transection

Multiple subpial transection (MST) has been evaluated with regard to neuropsychological outcomes in quite a few studies. In a "meta-analysis," Spencer and colleagues (2002) combined data from eight studies that had been conducted across six epilepsy surgery centers prior to 2001. Of 211 children and adults, 26% had MST only, and 74% had MST combined with resection; roughly two-thirds were extratemporal, and half of those were frontal. The collective sample is characterized in *figures 14 and 15*. The authors stated that "data were sparse on specific neuropsychological profile results ... before and after surgery" (Spencer *et al.*, 2002, p. 143). Persistent neurologic or cognitive deficits were reported in 19% of patients undergoing MST alone and in 23% of patients undergoing a combination of MST and resection. Most common were deficits in memory, hemiparesis, or visual field defects; rarely did any patient have multiple deficits, and no persistent aphasia or sensory changes were observed. Although this effort to combine data from multiple published studies was innovative (raw data were requested directly from the study sites using a standardized template rather than relying on published summary data only), it is not without notable limitations. First, the sample was very heterogeneous (*e.g.*, ranging in age from 1 to 75 years). Second, there was considerable variability in the amount of data available on each individual patient, but patients were not excluded for incomplete data; consequently, clinical characteristics and outcomes reported do not always represent the same group of patients. This can lead to misleading summary data; for example, one table shows that of 209 patients, only 8 undergoing MST + resection and 4 undergoing resection alone developed memory deficits (suggesting 5.7% rate of memory decline); however, elsewhere the authors stated that memory outcomes were documented for only 31 patients, 16 of whom experienced decline postsurgically (*i.e.*, 51.6% rate of memory decline). Finally, there is no information on the length of follow-up; a common clinical protocol (< 1 year) is presumed.

Several more-recent studies have expanded our understanding of outcomes from MST. In a study with longer follow-up, Blount and colleagues (2004) reported neurobehavioral outcomes an average of 3.5 years following surgery in 30 children (age M = 11.7 years, *SD* = 4.4). The majority (87%) had MST with cortical resection; only 4 children (13%) had MST without resection. MST of motor cortex (*n* = 20) resulted in transient hemiparesis in 60%; MST of language cortex (*n* = 10) resulted in transient aphasia in 60%. Detailed neuropsychological testing was not reported.

Factor	Available number	Mean	Range
Age at onset (yr)	162	10.5	0–72
Age at surgery (yr)	165	26.4	1–75
Duration (yr)	162	15.9	1–43
Pre-op sp sz freq (mo)	199	72.2	0–900
Pre-op cp sz freq (mo)	199	26.1	0–600
Pre-op gen sz freq (mo)	199	7.6	0–300
MST depth (mm)	158	5.1	4–20
MST number	120	57.7	4–180
MST spacing (mm)	160	4.9	3–10
Post-op sp sz freq (mo)	148	15.9	0–500
Post-op cp sz freq (mo)	148	4.0	0–100
Post-op gen sz freq (mo)	148	0.6	0–30

Figure 14. Sample characteristics for meta-analysis of multiple subpial transaction (part I) (from Spencer *et al.*, 2002). Freq: frequency; sp: simple partial; cp: complex partial; gen: generalized; sz: seizures

Factor	Response available, number of patients	Most common responses (number)
Etiology	55	Infection (15)
		Trauma (9)
Febrile seizures	72	No (65)
SPECT	34	Frontal (14)
		Temporal (9)
PET	41	Temporal (19)
		Frontal (9)
MRI	47	Frontal (13)
		Temporal (12)
EEG	199	Frontal (77)
		Temporal (40)
Pre-op neurol exam	166	Normal (87)
		Hemiparesis (51)
Post-op neurol exam	147	No change (111)
		Hemiparesis (12)
Memory function	31	Worse (16)
Resection	208	Yes (154)
Resection area	144	Frontal (56)
		Temporal (47)
MST orientation	161	Perpendicular (108)
		Star (48)
MST functional area	146	Sensorimotor (39)
		Motor (35)
MST depth	158	5 mm (86)
		4 mm (38)
MST spacing	160	5 mm (128)
		4 mm (29)
MST anatomic area	166	Frontal (57)
		Frontoparietal (48)
Pathology	114	Gliosis (59)
		Developmental (31)

Figure 15. Sample characteristics for meta-analysis of multiple subpial transaction (part II) (from Spencer et al., 2002).

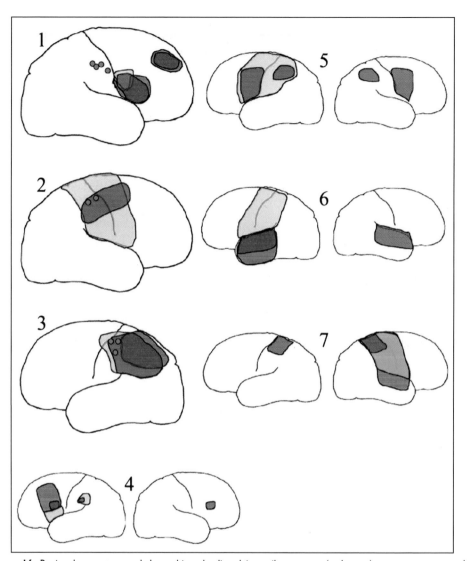

Figure 16. Regional magnetoencephalographic rolandic-sylvian spike sources (red areas), somatosensory-evoked fields (green dots), cortical excision site (grey areas), and multiple subpial transection (blue areas). Patients 4 to 7 had mirror foci (From Otsubo et al., 2001).

Two studies reported on MST in extratemporal regions for specific childhood syndromes. Otsubo and colleagues (2001) described 7 children with intractable sensorimotor seizures, centrotemporal spikes on EEG, and variable cognitive impairment, diagnosed as atypical benign rolandic epilepsy (BRE) and Landau-Kleffner Syndrome (LKS) variant and collectively labeled by the authors as "malignant rolandic-sylvian epilepsy" (MRSE). Age of onset ranged 0.6 to 6 years (M = 3.1, Mn = 3.0), and age at presentation for surgery ranged from 6 to 16 years (M = 12.1, Mn = 14.0). All had extratemporal foci; 2 children also had some temporal involvement. Epileptogenic tissue was resected to the extent that was not believed would affect functional cortex, and MST was used in eloquent cortex; 5 children had MST with resection, and 2 children had MST without resection. The areas of resection and MST are depicted in *Figure 16*. At 10 to 44 months post-surgery (M = 30 months), 3 children were seizure-free, and 4 had only very infrequent seizures. After cortical excision and MST, patients 1, 2, and 4 were seizure-free (Engel Class I), and patients 3, 5, 6, and 7 were Engel Class II. All children had presurgical neuropsychological testing, and 6 of the 7 had post-surgical testing. Of those 6 children, 3 (50%) declined (> 1 standard deviation change in age-adjusted scores), 1 experienced a mixture of decline and improvement, 1 was stable, and 1 improved. Within this narrow range of positive seizure control, there was no relationship between seizure control (Engel Class I vs. Class II) and cognitive outcome.

Irwin and colleagues (2001) reported on a small series of 5 children with LKS (3 left-hemisphere, 2 right-hemisphere foci) treated with MST without resection. Age of onset ranged 1.5 to 5.0 years (M = 3.7, Mn = 4.5), and age at initial presentation for surgery ranged from 5.5 to 10 years (M = 7.9, Mn = 8.5); one child with onset at age 4.5 who presented to surgery initially at age 5.5 repeated the procedure at age 7.5; MST was on the right side on both occasions. Postsurgical follow-up was conducted an average of 4.1 years (Mn = 3.5) after MST; age at follow-up ranged from 10 to 17 years (M = 12.4, Mn = 12.0). All children were seizure-free within 3 months after MST. On EEG, ESES was eliminated and background activity on EEG normalized in all five children; occasional spikes were detected following MST but persisted at 1 year postsurgery in only one child. Behavior improved dramatically with ongoing improvement through the last follow-up: "In each child following the procedure, attention span increased, hyperactivity resolved, and the defiant aggressive behaviour disappeared. Each child again became interested in communicating and was able to be included in normal domestic routines." Language decline was arrested, and cognitive functioning stabilized. All children showed some improvement in language during the first year following MST, and stabilized thereafter; however, they remained below age levels (even as long as 6 years after MST). IQ testing using language-reduced measures (WISC-R Performance IQ) was reported to have been stable; one table value indicates that one child improved by 24 points, but there is no reference to this in the text so it might be a clerical error.

In summary, the conclusions that can be drawn with regard to neuropsychological outcomes following MST are constrained by methodological limitations. Samples were typically very small, and larger samples were heterogeneous. MST is often used in conjunction with resection; therefore, it is difficult to discern the changes that are due to MST specifically. In addition, outcomes were often characterized in gross terms (neurobehavioral syndromes or adverse events); formal neuropsychological test data were sparse. Results vary by brain region, with deficits corresponding with the functions served in the region of MST (memory deficits, hemiparesis, aphasia or visual field loss); some deficits are transient, but others persist. Results can vary by syndrome; in LKS, language development is often stable or improved following MST, whereas in MRSE permanent deficits appear to be the rule rather than the exception.

■ Electrical stimulation

Vagus nerve stimulation

Boon and colleagues (2006) summarized six studies that examined neuropsychological functioning in patients implanted with vagus nerve stimulation (VNS). No adverse cognitive changes were detectable using pre-implantation versus post-implantation designs ranging in follow-up from 3- to 28-months. Acute changes have been detected in sham vs. stimulation designs: At subtherapeutic thresholds, favorable change was observed following stimulation; at therapeutic levels, adverse effects were noted on visual memory measures but were reversible. Thus, any changes were believed to have limited impact in daily activity.

Subsequent studies have echoed these conclusions with both children and adults. Rychlicki and colleagues (2006) examined cognitive changes in 34 children treated with VNS who ranged in age from 1.5‰ to 18 years (M = 11.5 years). Diagnoses included LGS (n = 9), multifocal with drop attacks (n = 9), and CPS without drop attacks (n = 16); all had mental retardation. Of the original 34 patients, 21 were compared to 21 "homogeneous control subjects" (no description) at 18 months. The authors reported, "No clear cognitive improvement, but also no major disruption, was evident on the clinical sample," but no data were reported. There was a "positive trend" in adaptive behavior (Vineland Adaptive Behavior Scales Motor Skills & Sociability subscales); controls reportedly declined on VABS, but no data were reported.

Rossignol and colleagues (2009) examined neuropsychological change before and after VNS implantation in 25 children with heterogeneous syndromes (5 Lennox-Gastaut syndrome, 2 severe infantile myoclonic epilepsy of Dravet, 1 myoclonic epilepsy of Doose, 5 cryptogenic generalized epilepsies, 7 cryptogenic bilateral partial epilepsies, 5 bilateral partial symptomatic epilepsies). Three additional children with absence seizures were included in the study but were not tested by the neuropsychologist. Of the 25 non-absence, 6 had severe MR, 11 moderate MR, and 8 mild MR; only 16 of these (64%) had follow-up testing and only 6 months after implantation (with no explanation for attrition and potential bias). There was no measurable change in neuropsychological functioning from pre- to post-implantation. Subjective improvement in attention/alertness was reported in 11 of the 16.

In a smaller study of children (n = 15, ages 5-17; IQs 30-74), Hallböök and colleagues (2005) noted similar findings. Two children improved in IQ (12-15 points), one declined (20 points), and the remainder were considered to be stable; at the group level of analysis, there was no statistically significant change in IQ at 3 or 9 months after implantation. Quality of life improved for 12, but this was not correlated with change in seizure control.

In one last study of children, Danielsson and colleagues (2008) followed 8 children (ages 5-18) who had medically refractory epilepsy and comorbid autism. All had moderate to profound mental retardation (IQ/DQ = 7-58) except one (IQ = 99). Over the 2-year follow-up period after VNS implantation, there was no change in seizure frequency, and IQ/DQ declined 2-22 points with minor behavior changes. This was the only study reporting decline in IQ; lack of improvement in seizure control, very low IQ, autism, or a combination of those factors might carry risk for adverse outcomes following VNS in this very impaired population.

In adults, also, there have been several noteworthy studies recently. McGlone and colleagues (2008) conducted a prospective, case control design comparing a group of medically-refractory epilepsy patients undergoing VNS (n = 16) *versus* resective surgery (n = 10) *versus* continued pharmacological management (medical control; n = 9). Compared to pre-implantation scores, objective memory scores were stable for the VNS group (no decline, no improvement).

Ghacibeh and colleagues (2006) conducted an elegant carefully controlled study using a double-blind, within-subject design comparing stimulation vs. sham (counter-balanced and using alternate forms for testing) with 5 women and 5 men (ages 26-58 years; M = 46.7). At a minimum of 3 months post-implantation, there was acute deterioration in cognitive flexibility and creativity (acute effects only) and no effect on memory.

Deep brain stimulation

Deep brain stimulation (DBS) for epilepsy has utilized multiple targets, as summarized by Jobst and colleagues (2010) and illustrated in *Figure 17*. However, very few studies have examined or reported neuropsychological outcomes.

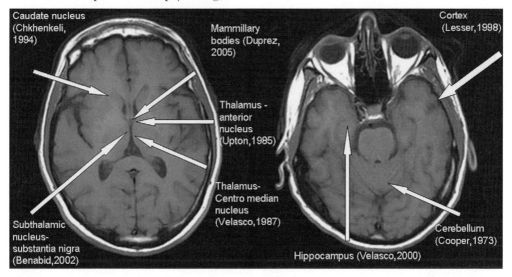

Figure 17. Targets of deep brain stimulation (DBS) for treatment of medically refractory epilepsy (from Jobst, 2010).

Fisher and colleagues (1992) stimulated the centromedian thalamus bilaterally in 7 people with medically-refractory epilepsy using a double-blind, cross-over placebo-controlled design. Patients were tested with stimulation on or off in 3-month blocks with a 3-month washout period between phases. There was no improvement in seizure frequency, and patients reported more subjective memory complaints during stimulation periods; however, there were no group differences on objective neuropsychological testing.

Raftopoulos and colleagues (Duprez *et al.*, 2005; Raftopoulos *et al.*, 2004) stimulated the mammillary body and mammillothalamic tract in 3 men with medically refractory epilepsy (ages 41 to 43 years) in a randomized double-blind, cross-over placebo-controlled design. One patient had hypothalamic hamartoma, another became refractory after prolonged convulsive status but with a normal MRI, and the third had "cryptogenic frontal lobe seizures associated with unspecific parietal lesion." All three had prior VNS implantation with poor results; VNS was turned off 6 weeks before obtaining baseline for the DBS trial. All were implanted in the mammillary body and mammillothalamic tract bilaterally (*Figure 18*). They were randomized to stimulation versus no-stimulation in 3-month blocks, with a 1-month wash-out period between treatment phases. According to the authors, "None of the three patients experienced any memory deficit, neither immediately after surgical implantation, nor during global or elective stimulations ... under close neuropsychological monitoring. Additional comprehensive cognitive tests were repeatedly performed, all of which failed to reveal any early or delayed mental decline after implantation" (Duprez *et al.*, 2005, p. 196). No neuropsychological data were reported.

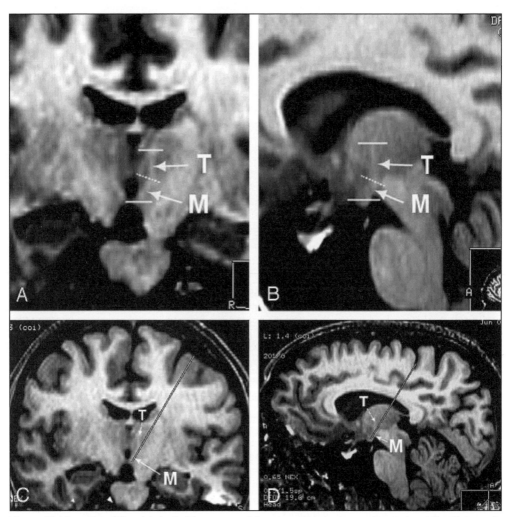

Figure 18. Mammillary (M) and thalamic (T) segments of the mammillothalamic tract (Panels A and B) and electrode trajectory simulation (Panels C and D) for DBS (from Duprez *et al.*, 2005).

Another target receiving attention is the anterior nucleus of the thalamus. A large multicenter trial is underway (Stimulation of the Anterior Nuclei of Thalamus for Epilepsy, or "SANTE"; Fisher *et al.*, 2010) examining outcomes associated with bilateral stimulation of this site. It utilizes a prospective, randomized, double-blind, parallel group design. A total of 110 patients have been enrolled (ages 18-65 years; M = 36.1, *SD* = 11.2) who have partial seizures including secondary generalized seizures (≥ 6/month, < 10/day, per 3-month daily diary) and who have been unresponsive to at least 3 antiepileptic drugs. Exclusion criteria include IQ < 70, inability to take neuropsychological tests or complete seizure diaries, progressive neurologic or medical diseases, nonepileptic seizures, or pregnancy. With regard to location of seizure onset, 60% had TLE, 27% FLE, 5% PLE, and 4% OLE; 18% were classified as diffuse, multifocal or other. Just over one-half of the sample had had previous surgery for epilepsy (29% VNS, 9% resection, and 16% both); VNS hardware was removed at the time of DBS electrode implantations. Patients were randomly assigned to treatment groups (stimulation versus control) for 3 months. The stimulation group and control group did not differ on demographic or clinical variables. The authors reported that "cognition and mood did not differ between control and stimulated groups at the end of the blinded phase," but no neuropsychological data have been reported to date. Based on adverse events reporting, there were more complaints of memory impairment in the stimulated group (13%) than in the control group (2%); according to the authors, self-reported memory adverse events resolved in 12-476 days.

Another innovative stimulation treatment is the responsive neurostimulation system (RNS). There is a randomized, double-blind, sham-stimulation controlled study in progress at 28 sites (Cascino et al., 2008), but no neuropsychological data were available at the time of this chapter.

In summary, among the stimulation treatments, VNS has more neuropsychological data than other modalities. There has been no discernable adverse cognitive impact in most VNS studies but very low IQ in this population produces a floor effect that can make it difficult to detect decline. Very low functioning children might be at risk for further cognitive decline or developmental delay, but this is based on a single study with a very small sample and warrants further investigation. DBS has been applied to a number of targets with the goal of controlling refractory epilepsy (ANT, CM thalamus, MB/MTT, cerebellum, STN, and caudate), but very few studies systematically evaluated neuropsychological functioning. RNS is a newer modality of stimulation for epilepsy, but neuropsychological results are pending.

■ Critical analysis

From this review of the scant research measuring neuropsychological outcomes following surgical management of the ETLEs, several factors have been associated with better outcomes as a general rule. Earlier age of surgery, shorter duration of epilepsy prior to surgery, better seizure control after surgery, less extensive lesions, and total lesion resection have all been associated with better outcomes.

However, this review highlights many significant methodological issues that limit our interpretation and conclusions with regard to neuropsychological outcomes in ETLE. Many themes cut across treatment approaches and studies. First, retest effects are largely uncontrolled in many studies of ETLE; even in studies where investigators tested patients numerous times, alternate forms were rarely used. Consequently, lack of improvement (especially when patients were tested multiple times within a relatively short period of time) could potentially reflect decline. Related to this, reliable change indices (RCIs) correct for retest effects when determining whether change is due to chance or extraneous factors. RCIs have been used increasingly in TLE surgery outcome studies but not for ETLE research. Regression to the mean in low-IQ populations might also obscure change such that stability in scores might actually reflect decline.

Many studies lack appropriate control groups. Refractory seizures have been associated with cognitive decline; therefore, lack of decline could reflect improvement when compared to nonsurgical medically refractory controls. Surgical candidates with epileptic foci in the same location who were re-evaluated one year apart before going to surgery could make a good control group, but imposing a 1-year delay on a "wait-list control group" might not be ethically defensible.

Studies of ETLE surgical outcomes are few in number, and sample sizes are small. This is most likely due to the relative infrequency of refractory epilepsy in ETLE compared to TLE. In an effort to combat this, investigators have combined TLE and ETLE in many studies; even within ETLE investigators have combined heterogeneous patients with foci in different lobes. Because certain regions (*e.g.*, frontal) can be neuropsychologically heterogeneous, even defining samples by lobe can be insufficient without further analysis by discrete sites.

Duration of follow-up is another methodological issue that can be improved in future studies. The vast majority of studies measure neuropsychological functioning less than one year postsurgery; longer outcome follow-up periods would be beneficial. Finally, many studies examine seizure outcome alone, without formally testing neuropsychological functions. When cognitive functioning is measured as an outcome, IQ is the most common variable assessed (which is gross and nonspecific). Greater breadth of cognitive domains needs to be assessed in ETLE outcome studies.

■ Conclusions

Improving the research methodologies for measuring outcomes associated with extratemporal epilepsies will be critical to advancing our understanding of the true outcomes following these interventions and of the protective and risk factors associated with various procedures. In particular, it will be essential to use empirically-informed assessment tools that are appropriate to the substrates and networks that are affected by the seizure focus and by the surgical intervention. Pooling data across multiple centers to examine outcomes in homogeneously defined and well characterized samples would help to increase sample sizes. Recent initiatives, such as attempts to define a common set of measures to use across studies (see Loring, 2010b) and an ILAE-commissioned task force consensus meeting held in Toronto in November, 2010 (Lassonde *et al.*, 2011) have the potential to move us forward in this regard, as long as we learn from the limitations revealed in our past research efforts.

References

- Battaglia D, Chieffo D, Lettori D, Perrino F, Di Rocco C, Guzzetta F. Cognitive assessment in epilepsy surgery of children. *Childs Nerv Syst* 2006; 22: 744-59.
- Blount JP, Langburt W, Otsubo H, Chitoku S, Ochi A, Weiss S, et al. MSTs in the treatment of pediatric epilepsy. *J Neurosurg* 2004; 100 (2 Suppl Pediatrics): 118-24.
- Buschmann F, Wagner K, Metternich B, Biethahn S, Zentner J, Schulze-Bonhage A. The impact of extratemporal epilepsy surgery on quality of life. *Epilepsy Behav* 2009; 15: 166-9.
- Boon P, Moors I, de Herdt V, Vonck K. Vagus nerve stimulation and cognition. *Seizure* 2006; 15: 259-63.

- Cascino GD. When drugs and surgery don't work. *Epilepsia* 2008; 49 (Suppl. 9): 79-84.
- Choi JT, Vining EPG, Mori S, Bastian AJ. Sensorimotor function and sensorimotor tracts after hemispherectomy. *Neuropsychologia* 2010; 48: 1192-9.
- Cukiert A, Burattini JA, Mariani PP, Cukiert CM, Argentoni-Baldochi M, Baise-Zung C, *et al.* Outcome after extended callosal section in patients with primary idiopathic generalized epilepsy. *Epilepsia* 2009; 50: 1377-80.
- Cukiert A, Cukiert CM, Argentoni M, Baise-Zung C, Forster CR, Mello VA, *et al.* Outcome after hemispherectomy in hemiplegic adult patients with refractory epilepsy associated with early middle cerebral artery infarcts. *Epilepsia* 2009; 50: 1381-4.
- Danielsson S, Viggedal G, Gillberg C, Olsson I. Lack of effects of vagus nerve stimulation on drug-resistant epilepsy in eight pediatric patients with autism spectrum disorders: a prospective 2-year follow-up study. *Epilepsy Behav* 2008; 12: 298-304.
- Dodrill CB, Matthews CG. The role of neuropsychology in the assessment and treatment of persons with epilepsy. *Am Psychol* 1992; 47: 1139-42.
- Duprez TP, Serieha BA, Raftopoulos C. Absence of memory dysfunction after bilateral mammillary body and mammillothalamic tract electrode implantation: preliminary experience in three patients. *American Journal of Neuroradiology* 2005; 26: 195-7.
- Fisher R, Salanova V, Witt T, Worth R, Henry T, Gross R, et al. and the SANTE Study Group. Electrical stimulation of the anterior nucleus of thalamus for treatment of refractory epilepsy. *Epilepsia* 2010; 51: 899-908.
- Fisher RS, Uematsu S, Krauss GL, Cysyk BJ, McPherson R, Lesser RP, *et al.* Placebo-controlled pilot study of centromedian thalamic stimulation in treatment of intractable seizures. *Epilepsia* 1992; 33: 841-51.
- Ghacibeh GA, Shenker JI, Shenal B, Uthman BM, Heilman KM. Effect of vagus nerve stimulation on creativity and cognitive flexibility. *Epilepsy Behav* 2006; 8: 720-5.
- Gleissner U, Kuczaty S, Clusmann H, Elger CE, Helmstaedter C. Neuropsychological results in pediatric patients with epilepsy surgery in the parietal cortex. *Epilepsia* 2008; 49: 700-4.
- Hallböök T, Lundgren J, Stjernqvist K, Blennow G, Strömblad LG, Rosén I. Vagus nerve stimulation in 15 children with therapy resistant epilepsy; its impact on cognition, quality of life, behaviour and mood. *Seizure* 2005; 14: 504-13.
- Helmstaedter C. Neuropsychological aspects of epilepsy surgery. *Epilepsy Behav* 2004; 5: S45– S55.
- Irwin K, Birch V, Lees J, Polkey C, Alarcon G, Binnie C, *et al.* Multiple subpial transection in Landau-Kleffner syndrome. *Dev Med & Child Neurology* 2001; 43: 248-52.
- Jea A, Vachhrajani S, Widjaja E, Nilsson D, Raybaud C, Shroff M, Rutka JT. Corpus callosotomy in children and the disconnection syndromes: a review. *Childs Nerv Syst* 2008; 24: 685-92.
- Jobst B. Brain stimulation for surgical epilepsy. *Epilepsy Research* 2010; 89: 154-61.
- Jonas R, Nguyen S, Hu B, Asarnow RF, LoPresti C, Curtiss S, *et al.* Cerebral hemispherectomy: hospital course, seizure, developmental, language, and motor outcomes. *Neurology* 2004; 62: 1712-21.
- Lassonde M, Helmstaedter C, Arzimanoglou A, Hermann B, Kahane P, eds. *Neuropsychology in the Care of People with Epilepsy.* Montrouge: John Libbey Eurotext, 2011.
- Lee YJ, Kang HC, Lee JS, Kim SH, Kim DS, Shim KW, *et al.* Resective pediatric epilepsy surgery in Lennox-Gastaut syndrome. *Pediatrics* 2010; 125; e58-e66.
- Lendt M, Gleissner U, Helmstaedter C, Sassen R, Clusmann H, Elger CE. Neuropsychological outcome in children after frontal lobe epilepsy surgery. *Epilepsy Behav* 2002; 3: 51-9.
- Lippé S, Bulteau C, Dorfmuller G, Audren F, Delalande O, Jambaqué I. Cognitive outcome of parietooccipital resection in children with epilepsy. *Epilepsia* 2010; 51: 2047-57.

• Loring DW. History of neuropsychology through epilepsy eyes. *Arch Clin Neuropsychol* 2010a; 25: 259-73.

• Loring DW. Material, modality, or method? Manageable modernization of measurement. *Epilepsia* 2010b; 51: 2357-67.

• Luerding R, Boesebeck F, Ebner A. Cognitive changes after epilepsy surgery in the posterior cortex. *J Neurol Neurosurg Psychiatry* 2004; 75: 583-7.

• Mamelak AN, Barbaro NM, Walker JA, Laxer KD. Corpus callosotomy: a quantitative study of the extent of resection, seizure control, and neuropsychological outcome. *J Neurosurg* 1993; 79: 688-95.

• McGlone J, Valdivia I, Penner M, Williams J, Sadler RM, Clarke DB. Quality of life and memory after vagus nerve stimulator implantation for epilepsy. *Can J Neurol Sci* 2008; 35: 287-96.

• Novelly RA. The debt of neuropsychology to the epilepsies. *Am Psychol* 1992; 47: 1126-9.

• Van Oijen M, De Waal H, Van Rijen PC, Jennekens-Schinkel A, van Huffelen AC, Van Nieuwenhuizen O; Dutch Collaborative Epilepsy Surgery Program. Resective epilepsy surgery in childhood: the Dutch experience 1992-2002. *Eur J Paed Neuro* 2006; 10: 114-23.

• Otsubo H, Chitoku S, Ochi A, Jay V, Rutka JT, Smith ML, *et al.* Malignant rolandic-sylvian epilepsy in children: diagnosis, treatment, and outcomes. *Neurology* 2001; 57: 590-6.

• Pulsifer MB, Brandt J, Salorio CF, Vining EP, Carson BS, Freeman JM. The cognitive outcome of hemispherectomy in 71 children. *Epilepsia* 2004; 45: 243-54.

• Raftopoulos C, van Rijckevorsel K, Abu Serieh B, de Tourtchaninoff M, Ivanoiu A, Mary G, *et al.* Chronic electrical stimulation of the mammillary bodies and mammillothalamic tracts in chronic refractory epilepsy [Abstract]. *Neuromodulation* 2004; 7: 148.

• Risse GL. Cognitive outcomes in patients with frontal lobe epilepsy. *Epilepsia* 2006; 47 (Suppl. 2): 87-9.

• Rossignol E, Lortie A, Thomas T, Bouthiller A, Scavarda D, Mercier C, Carmant L. Vagus nerve stimulation in pediatric epileptic syndromes. *Seizure* 2009; 18: 34-7.

• Rychlicki F, Zamponi N, Trignani R, Ricciuti RA, Iacoangeli M, Scerrati M. Vagus nerve stimulation: clinical experience in drug-resistant pediatric epileptic patients. *Seizure* 2006; 15: 483-90.

• Samargia SA, Kimberley TJ. Motor and cognitive outcomes in children after functional hemispherectomy. *Pediatr Phys Ther* 2009; 21: 356-61.

• Smith ML, Elliott IM, Lach L. Cognitive, psychosocial, and family function one year after pediatric epilepsy surgery. *Epilepsia* 2004; 45: 650-60.

• Spencer SS, Schramm J, Wyler A, O'Connor M, Orbach D, Krauss G, *et al.* Multiple subpial transection for intractable partial epilepsy: an international meta-analysis. *Epilepsia* 2002; 43: 141-5.

• Suchy Y, Sands K, & Chelune GJ. Verbal and nonverbal fluency performance before and after seizure surgery. *J Clin Exper Neuropsychol* 2003; 25: 190-200.

• Suchy Y, Chelune GJ. Postsurgical changes in self-reported mood and Composite IQ in a matched sample of patients with frontal and temporal lobe epilepsy. *J Clin Exper Neuropsychol* 2001; 23: 413-23.

• Tanriverdi T, Olivier A, Poulin N, Andermann F, Dubeau F. Long-term seizure outcome after corpus callosotomy: a retrospective analysis of 95 patients. *J Neurosurg* 2009; 110: 332-42.

• Turanli G, Yalnizoğlu D, Genç-Açikgöz D, Akalan N, Topçu M. Outcome and long term follow-up after corpus callosotomy in childhood onset intractable epilepsy. *Childs Nerv Syst* 2006; 22: 1322-7.

IMPRIM'VERT®

Achevé d'imprimer par   Corlet, Imprimeur, S.A.
14110 Condé-sur-Noireau
N° d'Imprimeur : 139134 - Dépôt légal : août 2011
Imprimé en France